MEXICAN AMERICAN HEALTH

MEXICAN AMERICAN HEALTH

Historical, Social, and Cultural Perspectives

Antonio L. Estrada

University of Arizona

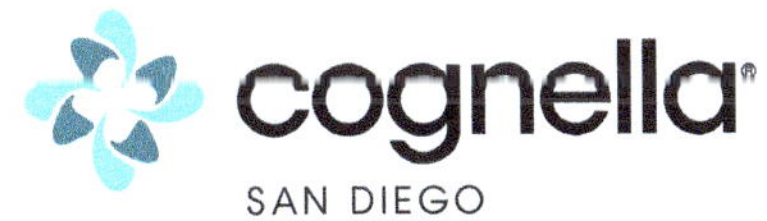

Bassim Hamadeh, CEO and Publisher
Amanda Martin, Executive Publisher
Amy Smith, Associate Editorial Manager
Rachel Kahn, Production Editor
Emely Villavicencio, Senior Graphic Designer
Kara Tatum, Licensing Coordinator
Natalie Piccotti, Director of Marketing
Kassie Graves, Senior Vice President, Editorial
Alia Bales, Director, Project Editorial and Production

Copyright © 2025 by Cognella, Inc. All rights reserved. No part of this publication may be reprinted, reproduced, transmitted, or utilized in any form or by any electronic, mechanical, or other means, now known or hereafter invented, including photocopying, microfilming, and recording, or in any information retrieval system without the written permission of Cognella, Inc. For inquiries regarding permissions, translations, foreign rights, audio rights, and any other forms of reproduction, please contact the Cognella Licensing Department at rights@cognella.com.

Trademark Notice: Product or corporate names may be trademarks or registered trademarks and are used only for identification and explanation without intent to infringe.

Cover image copyright © 2022 iStockphoto LP/Yulia Novik.
Interior image copyright © 2022 iStockphoto LP/Yulia Novik.

Printed in the United States of America.

This book is designed to provide educational information and motivation to our readers. It is sold with the understanding that the publisher is not engaged to render any type of psychological, legal, diet, health, exercise or any other kind of professional advice. The content of each chapter or reading is the sole expression and opinion of its author, and not necessarily that of the publisher. No warranties or guarantees are expressed or implied by the publisher's choice to include any of the content in this volume. Neither the publisher nor the individual author(s) shall be liable for any physical, psychological, emotional, financial, or commercial damages, including, but not limited to, special, incidental, consequential or other damages. Our views and rights are the same: You are responsible for your own choices, actions, and results and for seeking relevant topical advice from trained professionals.

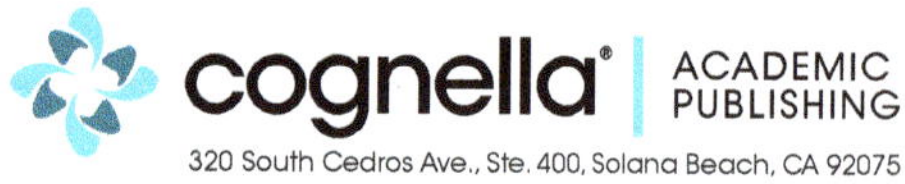

Brief Contents

Detailed Contents

Reviewers

Dr. Nashat Zuraikat, PhD, RN
Indiana University of Pennsylvania
Indiana, PA

Brandon Censon
Tacoma Community College

Audrey McCrary-Quarles, PhD, MSA, CHES, CCHW
Professor, Health Education
South Carolina State University

Renée M. Huth, PT, DPT, PhD
Radford University

Dr. Ladonna Michelle McClave, EdD, MSN, RN
Morehead State University

Introduction

Latinos are the largest ethnic minority group residing in the United States. Comprising close to 20% of the U.S. population, Latinos are heterogenous, differing with respect to place of birth, country of origin, socioeconomic status, political affiliation, and cultural beliefs and attitudes.

The Office of Management and Budget (OMB) defines *Latino/Hispanic* "as a person of Cuban, Mexican, Puerto Rican, South or Central American, or other Spanish culture or origin regardless of race" (U.S. Census Bureau, 2022b, para. 1). Hispanics/Latinos, then, can racially identify as "White," "Black," "American Indian," "Asian/Pacific Islander," or "mixed race." The Latino population represents many countries, historical origins, colonial impacts, socioeconomic status variations, and cultural practices. Currently, the Latino population represents almost 1 in 5 persons in the U.S. population. Moreover, that percentage is projected to increase to 26% of the population by 2050, representing almost 100 million people (U.S. Census Bureau, 2017a, 2017b).

Due to changes made by the U.S. Census Bureau to gain a more accurate enumeration of the Latino population in the United States, there was a notable increase in those identifying as Hispanic or Latino. Between 2010 and 2020, the number of people of Latino origin reporting two or more races increased 628.8%, from approximately 3 million (5.4%) to 18.6 million (34.1%). The number of people of Latino origin who identified as "White" alone decreased by 57.5%, down from 22.5 million to 9.5 million since 2010, and there was a 140% increase in the number of Latinos who self-identified as "American Indian/Alaska Native" (Jones et al., 2021; Krogstad et al., 2023).

According to the Office of Minority Health (n.d.), Latinos of Mexican descent account for 61.6% of the total Latino population, far more than Puerto Ricans (9.6%), Central Americans (9.3%), South Americans (6.4%), Other Hispanic/Latino (including Spanish; 5.8%), and Cubans (3.9%). In 2020, states with the largest Latino populations were Arizona, California, Colorado, Florida, Illinois, Nevada, New Jersey, New Mexico, New York, and Texas. In 2020, Latinos aged 18 and under comprised 25.7% of the population, compared to 53% of non-Latino Whites.

Overall, Latinos accounted for over 50% of the U.S. population growth between 2010 and 2020, a larger share of the U.S. population than any other racial/ethnic group (Krogstad et al., 2023). Much of this growth is not due to immigration but rather to an increase in Latino births in the United States (Osterman et al., 2023). According to Pew Research Center data (2022), between 1980 and 1990 immigration drove Latino population growth, as more Latino immigrants arrived than Latino babies were born. However, in 2020 and 2021, virtually all Latino population growth is a result of U.S. births. The challenges presented by this increased population include providing access and quality education to Mexican American youth and adolescents, providing health care services that are linguistically and culturally responsive to elderly Mexican Americans, and identifying the needs of Latinas, the majority of whom are of childbearing ages (15–44 years of age). Noted in Figure 0.1 below, Mexican Americans have a higher fertility rate than Black women and non-Mexican American White women.

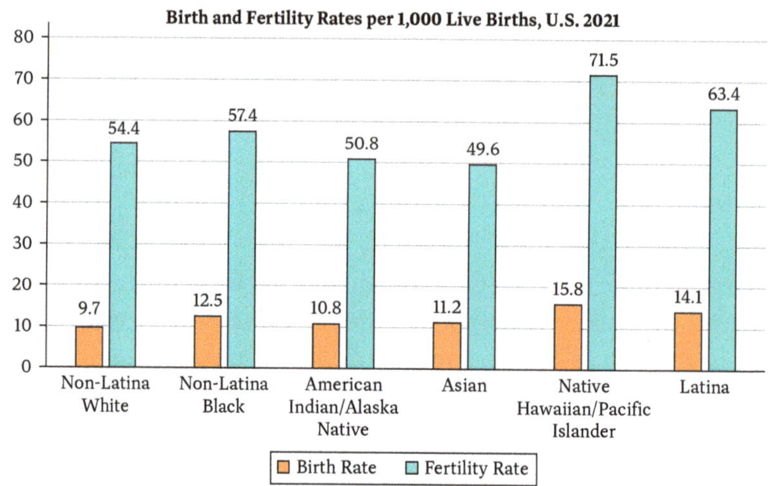

FIGURE 0.1 Birth and Fertility Rates per 1,000 Live Births by Race of Mother

Generation, Nativity, and Citizenship Status

There are additional variations in the Mexican American population in generational and nativity status that contribute to the diverse sociocultural context of Mexican Americans. Among all Mexican American subgroups, there is an even distribution of generational status, with about 34% first generation (immigrant), 31% second generation (one U.S.-born parent), and 35% third generation or higher (both parents U.S. born) (see Table 0.1). Other than Puerto Ricans and "Other" Latinos, Mexicans have the third highest percentage of third generation or higher (35.1%). Only Puerto Ricans have a higher percentage, but they are classified as U.S. citizens since Puerto Rico has been a territory of the United States since 1899 when the Treaty of Paris ceded the island to the United States, ending the Spanish American War (Nofi, 1997).

Combined with second generation (one U.S.-born parent), Mexicans represent the largest percentage of Latinos with a multigenerational presence in the United States (see Table 0.2). Moreover, 70% of Mexicans are U.S.-born, 10% are naturalized U.S. citizens, and about 20% are noncitizens, which is a counternarrative to the "all Mexicans are illegal immigrants" rhetoric inflamed by anti-immigration and anti-Mexican sentiment in the United States. The fact is Mexicans and Mexican Americans have resided in the southwestern United States for multiple generations, long before the Mexican American War (1846–1848).

TABLE 0.1 **Generation Status of Latino Populations (Percent)**

Generation status	Total Latino[1]	Mexican	Puerto Rican	Cuban	Central American	South American	Other Latino[3]
First generation[2]	33.7	29.8	0.8	59.1	58.7	60.0	34.7
Second generation[2]	31.0	35.1	6.2	23.7	31.8	30.3	29.3

Generation status	Total Latino[1]	Mexican	Puerto Rican	Cuban	Central American	South American	Other Latino[3]
Third generation[2] and higher	35.4	35.1	93.1	17.2	9.4	9.7	36.0

[1]Latino refers to people whose origin is Mexican, Puerto Rican, Cuban, Spanish-speaking Central or South American countries, or other Hispanic/Latino, regardless of race. Central American totals exclude Mexican. [2]"First generation" refers to those who are foreign born; "second generation" refers to those with at least one foreign-born parent; "third-and-higher generation" includes those with two U.S. native parents. [3]This category includes Dominicans and people who responded "Hispanic," "Latino," or provided other general terms. Source: U.S. Census Bureau (2021)

TABLE 0.2 Nativity and Citizenship Status of Latinos, 2021 (Percent)

Nativity and citizenship status[4]	Total Latino[1]	Mexican	Puerto Rican	Cuban	Central America[2]	South American	Other Latino[3]
U.S.-born	66.3	70.2	99.2	40.9	41.3	40.0	65.3
Foreign-born	33.7	29.8	0.8	59.1	58.7	60.0	34.7
Naturalized citizen	13.0	9.9	0.4	36.2	17.7	30.5	18.6
Not a citizen	20.6	19.8	0.4	22.9	41.0	29.5	16.1

[1]Latino refers to people whose origin is Mexican, Puerto Rican, Cuban, Spanish-speaking Central or South American countries, or other Hispanic/Latino, regardless of race. [2] Central American totals exclude Mexican. The foreign-born are considered first generation. [3] This category includes Dominicans and people who responded "Hispanic," "Latino," or provided other general terms. Source: U.S. Census Bureau (2021)

According to the U.S. Census Bureau (2021), among the Latino subgroups, South Americans have the lowest percentage of U.S.-born (40%) and the highest percentage of foreign-born (60%). More than one third of Cubans are naturalized U.S. citizens (36%), the highest percentage among the Latino subgroups. Central Americans have the highest percentage of non-U.S. citizens at 41%.

Also, according to the U.S. Census Bureau (Jensen et al., 2021) Latinos are most prevalent in the former territory belonging to Mexico (California, New Mexico, Texas, and Arizona) and Puerto Rico. When viewed as the second most prevalent racial/ethnic group, Latinos are widely dispersed throughout the United States. There are major geographical distinctions, with Latinos of Mexican descent primarily residing in the former territory of Mexico, Cubans in Florida, and Puerto Ricans and Central and South Americans dispersed throughout the northeastern states (see Figures 0.2 and 0.3).

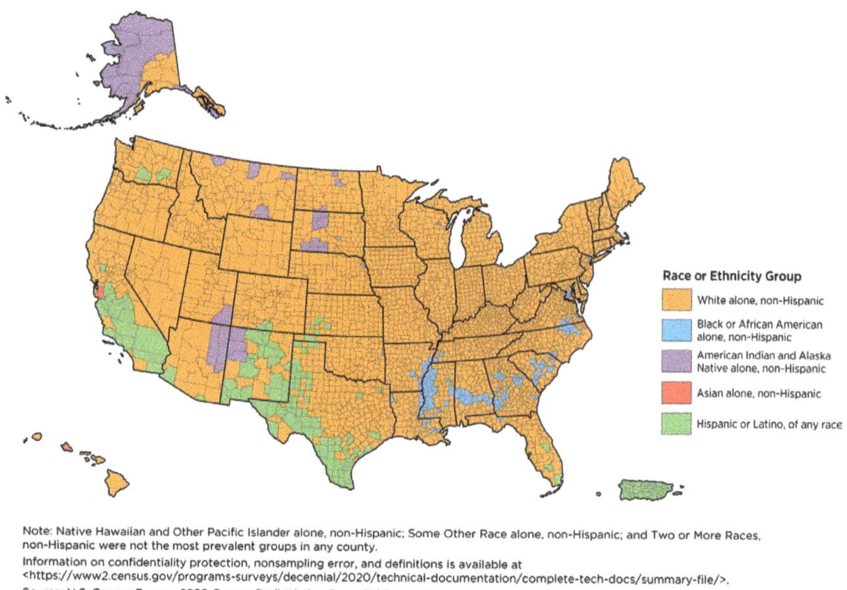

FIGURE 0.2 Most Prevalent Race or Ethnic Group by County

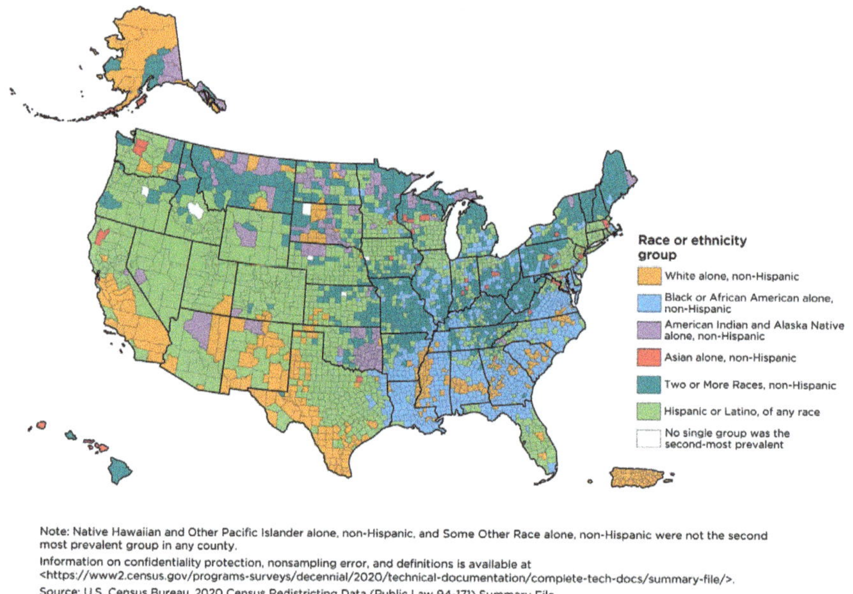

FIGURE 0.3 Second Most Prevalent Race or Ethnic Group by County

Age Structure, Marital Status, and Household Size

Age is a biological characteristic with many social and cultural ramifications. In many studies, marital status is used as a proxy measure for social support, albeit an inaccurate one. Household size determines how many persons live in a particular house or "family" and in many ways determines how much any household must spend on goods, services, and the necessities of life. Female-headed households are important given their higher poverty rates and gender wage-gap differentials.

Data from the U.S. Census Bureau (2021) show that Latinos are generally younger than other racial/ethnic groups in the United States. In 2021, the percentage of Latinos under 21 years of age was 35.3% compared to 22% for non-Latino White people and 29.6% of Black people (see Table 0.3). Latinos of Mexican descent had the highest percentage of their population under 21 years of age (37.2%) compared to the other Latino subgroups. Conversely, almost 80% of Latinos of Cuban descent were 21 years of age or older (U.S. Census Bureau, 2021).

TABLE 0.3 Age Structure of the Latino, Non-Latino, and Black Population, 2021

Age group	Non-Latino[1] White (alone)	Non-Latino Black (alone)	Total Latino	Mexican	Puerto Rican	Cuban	Central American[2]	South American	Other Latino[3]
Under 21 years	22.0	29.6	35.3	37.6	33.7	20.7	34.1	27.9	34.2
21 years and over	78.0	70.4	64.7	62.4	66.3	79.3	65.9	72.1	65.8

[1]Latino refers to people whose origin is Mexican, Puerto Rican, Cuban, Spanish-speaking Central or South American countries, or other Hispanic/Latino, regardless of race. [2] Central American totals exclude Mexican.[3] This category includes Dominicans and people who responded "Hispanic," "Latino," or provided other general terms. Source: U.S. Census Bureau (2021)

The Metropolitan Policy Program at the Brookings Institute documents the U.S. racial/ethnic profiles by generation that are generally accepted (Frey, 2018). Their generations and definitions include post-Gen Z (2016–present), Gen Z (1996–2015); millennials (1980–1994); Gen X (1965–1980); baby boomers (1946–1964); and pre-boomers (1945 and before). The Brookings Institute analyses (see Figure 0.4) reveals that in each succeeding generation (from pre-boomers to post-Gen Z), Latinos represent an increasing percentage of the population, tripling over this period (8.1% to 25.9%). The growth seen in Gen Z and post-Gen Z portends a significant presence of Latinos into the 21st century and beyond.

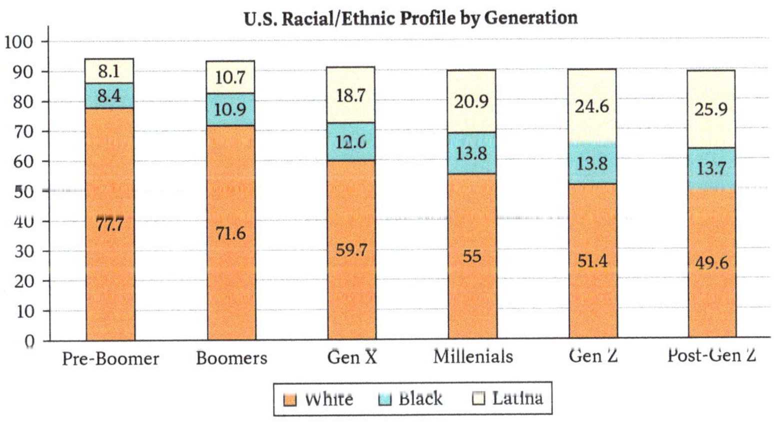

FIGURE 0.4 Generation Status by Race and Ethnicity, 2020

In terms of marital status, there is a lower percentage of married persons among Latinos of Mexican descent compared to non-Latino White people (44.2% compared to 55.2%, respectively). Among other Latino subgroups, South Americans have the highest percentage of married persons (50.8%), followed by Cubans (46.5%), and Central Americans (44.2%). Central Americans also have the highest percentage of "never married" or "single" persons (44.8%), with non-Latino White people having the lowest percentage of "never married" persons at 26.5%. In general, divorce rates are lower among Latinos than non-Latino White people and highest among Puerto Ricans and Cubans. Central Americans have the lowest divorced rate of 5.6% (see Table 0.4).

TABLE 0.4 Marital Status (Persons 15 and Older) of the Latino Population, 2022 (Percent)

Marital status	Non-Latino[1] White (alone)	Total Latino	Mexican	Puerto Rican	Cuban	Central American[2]	South American	Other Latino[3]
Married	55.2	44.0	44.2	39.0	46.5	44.3	50.8	40.6
Widowed	6.5	3.3	2.9	3.5	7.5	1.9	4.0	4.5
Divorced	10.5	7.3	6.3	10.8	10.2	5.6	8.6	9.8
Separated	1.3	2.9	2.8	2.7	2.2	3.4	1.7	4.8
Never married	26.5	42.5	43.7	44.0	33.6	44.8	35.0	40.3

[1]Latino refers to people whose origin is Mexican, Puerto Rican, Cuban, Spanish-speaking Central or South American countries, or other Hispanic/Latino, regardless of race. [2] Central American totals exclude Mexican.[3] This category includes Dominicans and people who responded "Hispanic," "Latino," or provided other general terms. Source: U.S. Census Bureau (2021)

The U.S. Census Bureau (2020a) reports that the average number of people per household is significantly larger in Latino families than non-Latino families (3.24 vs. 2.42, respectively). Also, the average number of people over 18 years of age in households is significantly larger for Latinos than non-Latinos (U.S. Census Bureau, 2020b) (see Figure 0.5).

Cohn et al. (2022) defined *multigenerational households* as including two or more adult generations (with adults mainly ages 25 or older) or a "skipped generation," which consists of grandparents and their grandchildren younger than 25. Most multigenerational households consist of at least two adult generations, such as young adults living with their parents, parents residing in their adult children's homes, or a grandparent, adult child, and adult grandchild within a single household. About 5% of multigenerational households consist of grandparents and grandchildren younger than 25 (Cohn et al., 2022). Latino and Black people are 2 times more likely than non-Latino White people to live in multigenerational households (26% for both compared to 13% for non-Latino White people; Cohn et al., 2022).

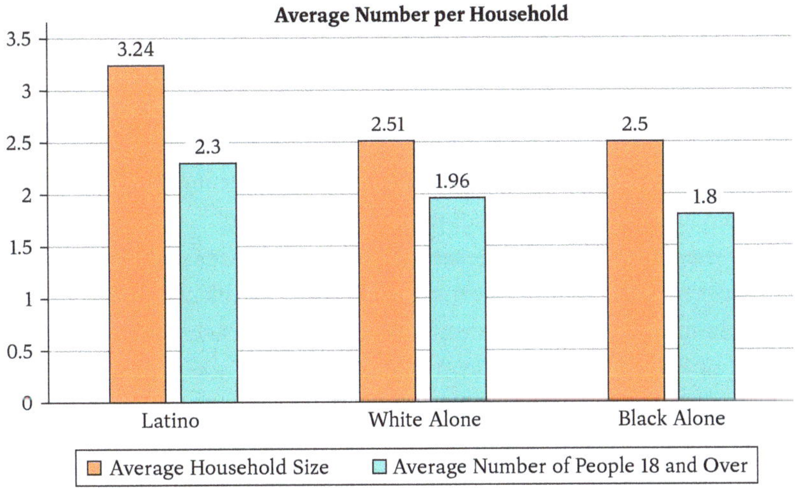

FIGURE 0.5 Average Number of Persons per Household by Race and Ethnicity, 2020

Racial Identification Among Latinos

Most social and behavioral scientists agree that "race" and "ethnicity" are social constructs reflecting the social, political, and scientific climate in any given period. The U.S. Census Bureau (2022b) notes that racial categories that are commonly used reflect "social definitions in the U.S. and are not an attempt to define race biologically, anthropologically, or genetically" (What Is Race? section). Prior to the 1930 U.S. Census, Mexicans were classified as White (U.S. Census Bureau, n.d.). There was a one-time inclusion of Mexican as a race category in the 1930 census and continued through 1939 (U.S. Census Bureau, n.d.).

The first attempt to assess the number of Latinos nationally was the 1970 U.S. Census (U.S. Census Bureau, n.d.). At the request of the White House a Hispanic self-identification question was included in the 1970 U.S. Census. The question asked, "is this person's origin or descent—"Mexican," "Puerto Rican," "Cuban," "Central or South American," "Other Spanish," and No, none of these" (U.S. Census Bureau, n.d.).

According to a Pew Research Center study (Krogstad et al., 2023), more than 2 million Latinos changed their racial identification from "Some other race" to "White." Overall, 53% of Latinos classified themselves as "White" in 2010. In 2015, the percentage had increased to 66% who identified as "White" and about 26% identified as "Some other race" (Parker et al., 2015). Clearly, even among Latinos there is confusion over racial identification. Parker et al. (2015) also found that a majority of Latinos (67%) view their Latino background as part of their racial background. Among those Latinos who identify as having a multiracial background (based on reporting two or more census races), 30% say most people would think they are White if they passed them on the street, 24% say most people would see them as Latino, 17% as mixed race, 10% as Black only and 4% as American Indian only (Parker et al., 2015, p. 103).

Are Latinos "White"? According to a Pew Research Center Report (Krogstad et al., 2023), 22.1% of Latinos identify as "Some other race," 10.2% identify as "White," 1.4% identify as "American Indian/Alaska Native," 0.9% as Black, and 0.3% as "Asian." 27.6 million Latinos identified as "more than one race" in 2021, a substantial increase from 3 million in 2010 (Krogstad et al., 2023). The Report also notes how self-identify as Latino shifts with increased generational status. For example, among those Americans with Latino ancestry who do not identify as Latino, 50% are fourth generation or higher, 23% are third generation, 8% are second generation, and only 3% are foreign-born. It appears that self-identification as "White" has little or no bearing on the experience of racial discrimination and exclusion of Latinos. Again, the Pew Research Center Report study (Krogstad et al., 2023) found that about a quarter of U.S.-born Latinos who identify as "White" indicated that discrimination was a major problem for Latinos in the United States, compared to a third of those who say they are "Some other race."

Latino subgroups in the United States represent genetic admixtures of European, African, and Native American ancestral genomes in different proportions with considerable variation depending primarily on their country of origin (Hanis et al., 1991). However, Native American ancestry predominates in all regions, whereas the proportion of European and African ancestry varies by region (Lisker et al., 1986; Bonilla et al., 2005). Furthermore, Basu et al. (2008) identified genetic variation in a Mexican American sample from Texas. They found that the sample had 39% Native American ancestry, 57% European ancestry, and 4% African ancestry. Alternatively, Bryc et al. (2015), using genome-wide ancestry estimates to examine genetic ancestry in the United States, found Latinos had 6.2% African ancestry, 18% Native American ancestry, and 65.1% European ancestry.

Found in their sample of Mexican Americans that on average, they had 50.2% Native American ancestry, 42.7% European ancestry, and 7.1% African ancestry. Other genetic studies of Mexicans living in the Federal District of Mexico, Oaxaca City, and rural Oaxaca confirm that racial admixture estimations are 69%–73% Native American, 17%–26% European, and 5%–10% African (Hernández-Hernández et al., 2020; Juárez-Cedillo et al., 2008).

Many genetic studies to date hypothesize that due to extensive migrations within Mexico and the Southwest, most Mexican populations have some level of Native American, European, and African ancestry. African ancestry in the Mexican and Mexican American population is most likely the result of the importation of enslaved people brought to Mexico by the Spanish over 500 years ago. This admixture can confer darker skin and Native American phenotypic characteristics that distinguish them from White Europeans and elicit prejudice, racism, and discrimination.

SUMMARY

This brief overview of the Latino population indicates that they have been and will continue to be an important demographic presence in U.S. society. Soon, 1 out of every 5 U.S. residents will be of Latino descent, with the majority being Mexican or Mexican American (U.S. Census Bureau, 2021). Latinos are younger than non-Latino White people and Black people, have higher fertility rates, and have a larger proportion who are single (U.S. Census Bureau, 2021). Because of this demographic transition, the United States can expect a larger percentage of Latinos, with the Mexican American population continuing to grow well into the 21st century even without immigration from Mexico. Moreover, access to quality health care will be imperative for Mexican American children, youth, adults, older adults, and women of childbearing age. Social determinants of health will become even more important for this growing population, especially educational programs, improving economic well-being, and enhancing the environments in which they live, work, recreate, worship, and learn.

ORGANIZATION OF THE BOOK

Each of the chapters in the book is organized around important issues and topics relevant to Latino health inequalities.

Chapter 1 provides a critical overview of important public health theories and concepts useful in the examination of contributing factors to the health status of Latinos of Mexican descent.

In Chapter 2, a detailed examination of the historical, political, social, and cultural influences on Latino health inequalities is presented. Latinos of Mexican descent are a historically disenfranchised and marginalized population. Beginning first with the Spanish conquest of Mexico and the establishment of the colonial model and then with the United States and the establishment of the neocolonial model, these historical, social, and political events created inequalities echoing into the present. Students will understand and appreciate how these important contexts have helped to shape health and health care of this population.

Chapter 3 examines several sociodemographic characteristics in-depth that have influenced the health of Latinos of Mexican descent. The social determinants of health (SDOH) is viewed as paradigm shift in public health in understanding the importance of "place" and its effects on population health. In this chapter, we will examine the influences of economic stability, education, the social and community context, the neighborhood and the physical environment, and access to health care from a Latino health perspective.

In Chapter 4, cultural dimensions of health among Latinos of Mexican descent are discussed. It is widely known that an individual's or group's culture influences health care attitudes, health beliefs, and health behaviors. Latino health is no exception. In this chapter, we explore several Latino cultural determinants that play an important role in the initiation and maintenance of health among Latinos. Readers will gain an appreciation of the unique Latino cultural determinants, beyond level of acculturation, that have an important influence on health.

In Chapter 5, we critically examine theories of health inequalities. A fundamental understanding of health inequality theories or hypotheses is essential if one is to understand potential mechanisms that lead to the etiology and development of disease in disenfranchised populations. This chapter highlights several health inequality theories and hypotheses pertinent to Latino health. Students will gain an understanding on their utility in developing theory-driven risk-reduction interventions commonly used in implementation science.

Chapter 6 examines the "causes of the causes"—that is, "upstream" causes of health inequalities among Latinos of Mexican descent. The field of epigenetics and social epigenomics provides a potential area of investigation that examines prenatal and maternal stress, adult origins of chronic diseases, adverse childhood experiences, and the concept of historical or intergenerational trauma as potential mechanisms for disease etiology and lack of health care access among Latinos of Mexican descent.

Chapter 7 provides an overview of important communicable diseases among Latinos. The H1N1 virus, for example, significantly impacted Latinos and foreshadowed the effects of the COVID-19 pandemic. We explore several issues surrounding vaccine hesitancy and the social and cultural determinants of HIV disease among Latinos.

In Chapter 8, we examine several important Latino chronic health disparities in reference to their incidence, prevalence, and mortality characteristics in comparison to non-Latino White people. Readers will gain insight on the underlying social and cultural dimensions of these chronic diseases.

Lastly, in Chapter 9, we discuss how to develop culturally innovative interventions for Latinos, utilizing what we have learned in the preceding chapters. Readers will learn why risk-reduction interventions with Latinos should be theoretically driven and how Latino health research needs to move beyond acculturation level and utilize other Latino cultural concepts to examine risk behaviors, risk perceptions, and culturally congruent ways of working with Latino communities to produce tangible changes.

REFERENCES

Basu, A., Tang, H., Zhu, X., Gu, C. C., Hanis, C., Boerwinkle, E., & Risch, N. (2008). Genome-wide distribution of ancestry in Mexican Americans. *Human Genetics, 124*, 207–214.

Bonilla, C., Gutiérrez, G., Parra, E. J., Kline, C., & Shriver, M. D. (2005). Admixture analysis of a rural population of the state of Guerrero, Mexico. *American Journal of Physical Anthropology: The Official Publication of the American Association of Physical Anthropologists, 128*(4), 861–869.

Bryc, K., Durand, E. Y., Macpherson, J. M., Reich, D., & Mountain, J. L. (2015). The genetic ancestry of african americans, latinos, and european Americans across the United States. *The American Journal of Human Genetics, 96*(1), 37–53.

Cohn, D., Horowitz, J. M., Minkin, R., Fry, R., & Hurst, K. 2022, March 24). *The demographics of multigenerational households.* Pew Research Center. https://www.pewresearch.org/social-trends/2022/03/24/the-demographics-of-multigenerational-households/

Frey, W. H. (2018). *The millennial generation: A demographic bridge to America's diverse future.* Metropolitan Policy Program at Brookings.

Hanis, C. L., Hewett-Emmett, D., Bertin, T. K., & Schull, W. J. (1991). Origins of U.S. Hispanics. Implications for diabetes. *Diabetes Care, 14*, 618–627.

Hernández-Hernández, O., Hernández-Zaragoza, D. I., Barquera, R., Warinner, C., López-Gil, C., Arrieta-Bolaños, E., ... & Granados, J. (2020). Genetic diversity of HLA system in two populations from Oaxaca, Mexico: Oaxaca city and rural Oaxaca. *Human Immunology, 81*(9), 553–556.

Jensen, E., Jones, N., Rabe, M., Pratt, B., Medina, L., Orozco, K., & Spell, L. (2021, August 12). The chance that two people chosen at random are of different race or ethnicity groups has increased since 2010. 2020 U.S. population more racially diverse than in 2010. Retrieved August 24, 2023, https://www.census.gov/library/stories/2021/08/2020-united-states-population-more-racially-ethnically-diverse-than-2010.html

Jones, N., Marks, R. Ramirez, R., & Rios-Vargas, M. (2021, August 12). *2020 Census illuminates racial and ethnic composition of the country.* U.S. Census Bureau. https://www.census.gov/library/stories/2021/08/improved-race-ethnicity-measures-reveal-united-states-population-much-more-multiracial.html

Juárez-Cedillo, T., Zuñiga, J., Acuña-Alonzo, V., Pérez-Hernández, N., Rodríguez-Pérez, J. M., Barquera, R., ... & Vargas-Alarcón, G. (2008). Genetic admixture and diversity estimations in the Mexican Mestizo population from Mexico City using 15 STR polymorphic markers. *Forensic Science International: Genetics, 2*(3), e37–e39.

Krogstad, J. M., Passel, J. S., Moslimani, M., & Noe-Bustamante, L. (2023, September 22). *Key facts about U.S. Latinos for National Hispanic Heritage Month.* Pew Research Center. https://www.pewresearch.org/short-reads/2023/09/22/key-facts-about-us-latinos-for-national-hispanic-heritage-month/

Lisker, R., Perez-Briceño, R., Granados, J., Babinsky, V., de Rubens, J., Armendares, S., & Buentello, L. (1986). Gene frequencies and admixture estimates in a Mexico City population. *American Journal of Physical Anthropology, 71*(2), 203–207.

Nofi, A. A. (1997). *Spanish American War, 1898.* Da Capo Press.

Office of Minority Health (n.d.). *Hispanic/Latino health—Overview (demographics).* Retrieved April 20, 2023, from https://www.minorityhealth.hhs.gov/hispaniclatino-health.

Osterman, M. J. K., Hamilton, B. E., Martin, J. A., Driscoll, A. K., & Valenzuela, C. P. (2023). Births: Final data for 2021. *National Vital Statistics Reports, 72*(1). https://doi.org/10.15620/cdc:122047

Parker, K., Menasce Horowitz, J., Morin, R. & Lopez, M.H. (2015, June 11). Multiracial in America. Pew Research Center. Retrieved April 22, 2023, from https://www.pewresearch.org/social-trends/2015/06/11/multiracial-in-america/

Pew Research Center. (2022, February 3). *Hispanic population growth and dispersion across U.S. counties, 1980–2020.* https://www.pewresearch.org/hispanic/interactives/hispanic-population-by-county.

U.S. Census Bureau. (n.d.). *Measuring race and ethnicity across the decades: 1790–2010.* https://www.census.gov/data-tools/demo/race/MREAD_1790_2010.html

U.S. Census Bureau. (2017a). *2017 national population projections*. https://www.census.gov/programs-surveys/popproj/data/tables.2017.List_1416517092.html#list-tab-List_1416517092

U.S. Census Bureau. (2017b). *Vintage 2017 population estimates*. https://www.census.gov/data/tables/2017/demo/popproj/2017-summary-tables.html.

U.S. Census Bureau. (2020a). *America's families and living arrangements: 2020. Table AVG1*. Retrieved on April 21, 2023, from https://www.census.gov/data/tables/2020/demo/families/cps-2020.html

U.S. Census Bureau. (2020b). *America's families and living arrangements: 2020. Table AVG2*. Retrieved on April 21, 2023, from https://www.census.gov/data/tables/2020/demo/families/cps-2020.html

U.S. Census Bureau. (2021). *The Hispanic population in the United States: 2021*. www.census.gov/data/tables/2021/demo/hispanic-origin/2021-cps.html

U.S. Census Bureau. (2022a, April 15). *About the Hispanic population and its origin*. https://www.census.gov/topics/population/hispanic-origin/about.html

U.S. Census Bureau. (2022b, March 1). *About the topic of race*. https://www.census.gov/topics/population/race/about.html

Figure Credits

Fig. 0.2: United States Census Bureau, "Most Prevalent Race or Ethnic Group by County: 2020," https://www.census.gov/library/stories/2021/08/2020-united-states-population-more-racially-ethnically-diverse-than-2010.html, 2021.

Fig. 0.3: United States Census Bureau, "Second-Most Prevalent Race or Ethnic Group by County: 2020," https://www.census.gov/library/stories/2021/08/2020-united-states-population-more-racially-ethnically-diverse-than-2010.html, 2021.

CHAPTER 1

Theoretical and Conceptual Foundations for Understanding Mexican American Health

LEARNING OBJECTIVES

- Evaluate the importance and contributions of modern, social, and cultural epidemiology in the investigation and identification of health inequalities and their distribution among historically marginalized groups in the United States.
- Explain the framework of critical race theory and intersectionality theory as a lens for examining the structural and institutional origins of social and health inequalities among historically marginalized groups in the United States.
- Appraise the internal colonial model as a suitable sociohistorical and political framework to examine social and health inequalities among Mexican Americans in the southwestern United States.
- Describe the five domains of the social determinants of health (SDOH) paradigm and their contribution to understanding health inequalities.
- Provide examples of how each of these theories, frameworks, and paradigms are necessary to provide a comprehensive understanding of social and health inequalities among Mexican Americans.

USEFUL EPIDEMIOLOGICAL TERMS

- Incidence: the number of new cases of a disease or injury; expressed as rates per 1,000 or 100,000 persons.
- Prevalence: the number of existing cases of a disease or injury; expressed as rates per 1,000 or 100,000 persons or as a percentage of the population.
- Age-adjusted rates: incidence, prevalence, or mortality rates that are statistically adjusted for the age distribution in the United States for a given census period (e.g., 2024).

- Crude rates: incidence, prevalence, or mortality rates that are not statistically adjusted for the age distribution in the United States for a given census period.
- Relative risk (RR): the association between a risk factor and a specific disease comparing those "exposed" to those "not exposed." It provides information on the magnitude of risk in exposed versus unexposed groups.
- Population attributable risk (PAR): the proportional reduction in disease or mortality in the population that would occur if exposure to a risk factor were reduced to an alternative ideal exposure scenario (e.g., no tobacco use).

Mexican Americans account for 62% of all Latinos, and Latinos are the largest ethnic minority group in the United States, representing approximately 19% of the nation's population (U.S. Census Bureau, 2021). It is important to understand factors that contribute to their health status since Mexican Americans are major contributors to our labor force, economy, and society. In this chapter, I briefly outline several epidemiological foundations, scientific theories, and sociopolitical paradigms and their importance in understanding the health status of Mexican Americans in the United States.

Public Health Foundations and Concepts

Modern epidemiology, social epidemiology, and cultural epidemiology are important public health disciplines that provide the basic scientific understanding of disease causation and prevention. In addition, the examination of U.S. race relations using critical race theory, intersectionality theory, and an internal colonial model provides a sociohistorical and sociopolitical context for understanding the unequal distribution of goods and services among historically marginalized groups like African Americans, Native Americans, and Mexican Americans.

Furthermore, a recent paradigm shift in public health to delineate the contributions of the social environment through the articulation of the social determinants of health (SDOH) provides a holistic approach to investigate social environmental contributions to population health. The specific addition of cultural determinants to the multilayered and integrative theories and paradigms described provides a cultural context that may be unique to each racial, ethnic, or cultural group. Also, recent research in the field of social epigenetics focuses on the "cause of the causes" in examining "upstream" factors that contribute to increased disease susceptibility across the lifespan that contributes to understanding how past social and biological environments influence present and future disease trajectories.

Modern or Classical Epidemiology

Modern or classical epidemiology has roots in the ancient past when town officials would exclude and limit the freedom of those people afflicted with leprosy or other diseases. *Quarantine,* restricting the movement of presumed infected people, was also initiated in the mid-14th century to curtail the spread of bubonic plague that ravaged Asia and Europe (Conti, 2008). The word "quarantine" is derived from the Italian *quaranta giorni*, which refers to when people were required to stay on their ships for 40 days before they could disembark at the port of Venice in order not to infect others (Gensini et al., 2004).

Infectious diseases were much more prevalent prior to the discovery of penicillin in 1929 by Sir Alexander Fleming. Cholera outbreaks, caused by bacterial infection spread by contaminated water and food, were severe during the 19th century. During the London cholera epidemic of 1854, Dr. John Snow, a physician, and the father of modern epidemiology, identified the likely source of cholera contamination and was able to have the Broad Street water pump shut down, which stopped the epidemic from spreading. Snow was the first to use epidemiological principles to investigate the spread of cholera, comparing those who received contaminated water to those who did not and determining who got ill (Frerichs, 2023).

Epidemiology is one of five traditional cornerstones in the field of public health (the others are biostatistics, health promotion/disease prevention, public health policy, and health services). *Epidemiology* is the study of the distribution and causes of disease, injuries, and other adverse conditions in human populations (Schneider & Lilienfeld, 2015).

Epidemiology has several subfields that investigate a variety of diseases, adverse events, and risk behaviors. For example, *psychiatric epidemiology* examines the incidence, prevalence, and treatment of psychological disorders. *Chronic disease epidemiology* examines the incidence, prevalence, and patterns of chronic diseases like cancer, diabetes mellitus, and heart disease. *Infectious disease epidemiology* investigates the causes and distribution of infectious diseases like COVID-19, influenza, and the Zika virus. *Behavioral epidemiology* examines behavioral risk factors for disease, like smoking behaviors, drug use behaviors, and other behaviors that place individuals at increased risk for disease.

Epidemiology uses scientific methods to examine the causes, determinants, and consequences of diseases as well as injuries, accidents, and many other adverse events that negatively influence population and individual health and access to care (Schneider & Lilienfeld, 2015). Epidemiology is data-driven, meaning that it relies on large-scale community or national studies using representative samples to examine the etiology, incidence, prevalence, and consequences of diseases or other adverse conditions. Epidemiology primarily uses quantitative rather than qualitative data analytic approaches and relies heavily on biostatistics to examine disease patterns, causes, and effects.

Important considerations in epidemiology are "person," "place," and "time"—that is, *who* is affected, *where* the event occurs, and *when* or over *what* span of time the event happens. In terms of disease causation, epidemiology acknowledges "a web of causation" indicating that in most cases, there is more than one cause of disease (Krieger, 1994). Several models have been developed to show the relationships between person, place, and time. For example, the "epidemiologic triangle" model is one of the most frequently used to show these relationships (see Figure 1.1).

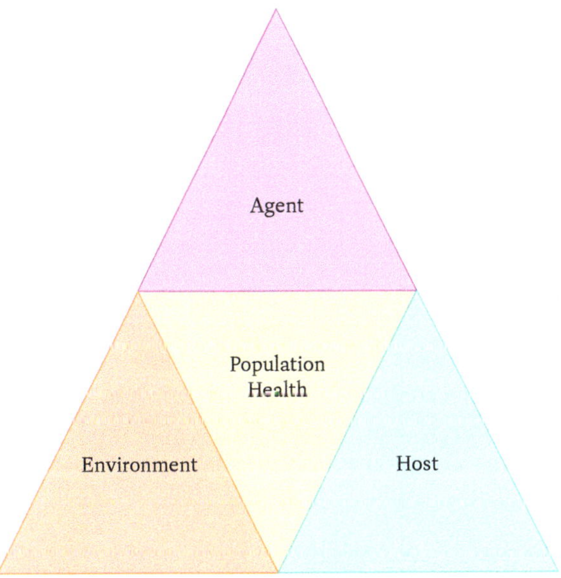

FIGURE 1.1 Epidemiologic Triangle Showing Relationships Between Agent, Host, and Environment to Population Health

In the model, "agent" is the causative factor in disease. It could be a microorganism such as a virus, bacteria, or fungus, or it could be a chemical toxin. The agent alone, however, is not considered sufficient in and of itself to cause disease. The agent also needs a "host" to affect, such as an animal, insect, or human being. Even so, the host possesses intrinsic factors such as hereditary, immune function, and other internal factors that may mitigate or enhance disease progression. Environmental conditions must be optimal for the agent to affect the host. There are four environments external to the host that are especially important to take into consideration: the biological, physical, social, and cultural environments.

The *biological environment* includes infectious agents, reservoirs of infection, and biological or mechanical vectors that transmit disease. For example, an infectious agent could be the human immunodeficiency virus (HIV); the reservoir of infection would then be those persons infected with HIV who can transmit it to others. With HIV for example, a mechanical vector, such as an infected syringe, would transmit the virus to others. In the case of dengue fever or the Zika virus, a biological vector would be a mosquito.

The *physical environment* includes sunlight exposure and exposure to heat, air pollution, contaminated water, and chemical agents that can adversely affect humans. For example, air pollution is associated with lung disease and heart disease. It is widely known that chemical carcinogens can contaminate ground water that can lead to cancer clusters observed in contaminated communities (Pratt et al., 2015). Extensive sun exposure over long periods can lead to melanoma and other skin cancers (Goodman et al., 2012).

The social environment has gained increasing attention in disease causation over the past several decades, especially in accordance with the social determinants of health paradigm advanced by the American Public Health Association (Office of Disease Prevention and Health Promotion n.d.). The *social environment* includes discrimination and racism, social support networks, social and political institutions, and socioeconomic status. For example, poverty is widely acknowledged as a major underlying cause for increased susceptibility to infectious and chronic diseases worldwide. Poverty is intrinsically associated with poor housing and living conditions, poor quality of food and water, lack of education, and lack of access to health care.

Other than documenting patterns of disease and risk, there are four basic prevention goals of epidemiology: reduce incidence and prevalence of disease, delay the onset of physical disability, ameliorate the severity of disease, and prolong the person's life. There are also several key concepts in epidemiology: incidence rate, prevalence rate, relative risk, and population attributable risk (see Useful Epidemiological Terms box). Briefly, *incidence rate* is the number of new cases of a disease, and *prevalence rate* is the number of existing cases of a disease, both measured over time. Prevalence varies with incidence and duration of disease. Usually, as incidence increases, so does prevalence. However, if a disease has a high cure rate or a high fatality rate, the prevalence rate will be low.

Using type 2 diabetes mellitus (DM) as an example, about 1.4 million new cases (*incidence*) of DM were diagnosed in 2018–2019 among U.S. adults 18 years and older, or approximately 6.9 per 1,000 persons, compared to a prevalence of 37 million people, or 11.3% of the population (Centers for Disease Control and Prevention [CDC], 2022). Prevalence estimates are higher than incidence estimates because DM is a chronic disease. The incidence varies by race/ethnicity, however. According to the CDC (2022), in 2019 the incidence rate for Mexican Americans was 7.9 per 1,000, for non-Mexican American Black people it was 6.6 per 1,000, and non-Mexican American White people had the lowest rate of 5.5 per 1,000. Prevalence also varies by race/ethnicity. The percentage of non-Mexican American White people with DM was 7.4% in 2019, compared to 12.1% for African Americans and 11.8% for Mexican Americans.

Relative risk (*RR*) is an important concept in epidemiology that conveys the risk of exposure to disease in one group compared to the risk of the unexposed group. It demonstrates the strength or magnitude of the association between a risk factor and a specific disease and is a ratio of two probabilities. For example, Mexican Americans have a relative risk of diabetes that is twice that of non-Latino White Americans. Haffner et al. (1997), using data from the San Antonio Heart Study, found that Mexican Americans 35–44 years of age had a relative risk of 5.4 for an 8-year incidence of DM compared to non-Latino White Americans, or a factor of 5 (5 times the risk for developing DM).

Population attributable risk or fraction (*PAR/PAF*) is the proportion of disease in a population that is associated with (i.e., attributable to) a certain risk factor. The formula to calculate PAR is Pe (RR-1)/1+Pe (RR-1), where Pe is the population exposed to the risk factor, and RR is the relative risk of exposure. These measures can be obtained from the Centers for Disease Control and Prevention (CDC) and the National Center for Health Statistics (NCHS) for specific diseases.

Understanding PAR is important because many of the risk factors associated with chronic diseases like cancer, heart disease, and diabetes mellitus are modifiable through public health prevention and intervention strategies. We will see this application of PAR in Chapter 6 in the discussion of adverse childhood experiences and their association with negative health consequences in later life.

Social Epidemiology

The field of social epidemiology is relatively new as public health pedagogies go but has a deep historical background. The early observation that individuals living in poverty had higher rates of disease than individuals from the upper class did foreshadow the examination of conditions in the social environment as integrally associated with both infectious and chronic diseases.

Social epidemiology is defined as the examination of "the social distribution and social determinants of states of health" (Berkman et al., 2014, p. 5). Thus, the examination of income, poverty, education, gender, occupation, age, race, and ethnicity in relation to disease incidence and prevalence established a form of "social causation." Additionally, the examination of neighborhood measures of psychosocial stress, neighborhood disorganization, school climate, community affluence, crime rates, and air pollution are crucial in the field of social epidemiology because they link the social environment to the health status of individuals and populations.

Fundamentally, causal inference is at the core of epidemiological inquiry. It is especially critical in social epidemiology because of the focus on "social" and the meaning of "causation." For example, social causation and social drift hypotheses are alternative explanations for how the social environment influences disease and socioeconomic status (Link & Phelan, 1995). The *social causation hypothesis* asserts that social conditions like social economic status (SES) cause both physical and psychological illnesses. The *social drift/selection hypothesis* asserts that a person's health influences their ability to attain or maintain optimum socioeconomic standards and resources. A study by Mulatu and Schooler (2002) found that "both social causation and health selection contribute to social inequities in health" (p. 22). Overall, the empirical evidence regarding the relative value of the social causation and health selection/drift hypotheses are mixed. It varies by how SES and health are measured and by the research design utilized (cross-sectional at one point in time or longitudinal with multiple points over time; Braveman et al., 2005).

"Burden of disease" is an important concept in the field of social epidemiology. The question of which population groups or segments of society have higher disease incidence, prevalence, and mortality or "burden" is important to direct public health disease prevention and intervention efforts for those who have a higher burden of disease, such as those who live in poverty, African Americans, Native Americans, or women.

Stress, Stressors, and Stressful Life Events (SLEs)

There currently is no single model that fully explains the relationship between social causation and the health of individuals and/or populations. A multilayered approach may prove more useful by examining which social determinants have more of an effect than others or in combination with others that place one at risk for disease, and, taken together, how they can integrate the social, physiological, and psychological characteristics of person, place, and time. The stress process model comes the closest to describing the pathways from macro-level to micro-level stressors (Aneshensel & Avison, 2015; Pearlin, 1989; Pearlin et al., 2005; Pearlin & Bierman, 2013). One of the important contributions of social epidemiology is the examination of how stress, stressors, and stressful life events are associated with chronic diseases like cancer, heart disease, and depression.

However, what is stress? We can recognize it when we feel it, but stress and stressors vary by age, gender, race, ethnicity, and other social and cultural factors. The intensity and ramifications of stress are also variable, again depending on its context and the social factors and psychological factors of the individual experiencing it. Measures of stress are both objective and subjective. Objective measures include blood pressure rates, galvanic skin response, cortisol, and adrenocorticotropic hormone (ACTH) hormonal secretions, among others. Subjective measures of stress include the experience and internalization of stressful events like racism, discrimination, the death of a loved one, the birth of a child, and other positive or negative events that require some form of personal adaptation (Cohen et al., 2019). A *stressor* is a chemical or biological agent, environmental condition, external stimulus, or an event seen as causing stress to an individual. Hans Selye, an endocrinologist, observed that many patients with tuberculosis and chronic diseases like cancer had experienced significant stressors in their lives. Selye demonstrated that stressors could interrupt the human endocrine system and lead to chronic diseases like heart disease and high blood pressure, what he termed "diseases of adaptation" (*Encyclopaedia Britannica Online*, 2023; Selye, 1936, 1950).

The fact that stress and stressors, however measured, produce strong associations and inferred causal pathways to the physical and psychological health of individuals and populations demonstrates the utility of the concept in explaining negative health outcomes among historically marginalized groups like African Americans, Native Americans, and Mexican Americans (O'Connor et al., 2021).

Thoits's research on social support, coping, and differential exposure to stressors and their relationship to health is instrumental in conceptualizing and empirically demonstrating that exposure to stressors across the lifespan can be cumulative and differentially expose women and racial/ethnic minorities to stressors that negatively impact physical and mental health (Thoits, 1995, 2010, 2011). Pearlin's and Aneshensel's major contributions to the understanding of the stress process model and how social structures within society influence and sustain the stress process over time has provided important insights on how individuals and groups experience and respond to stressors in their social environments (Aneshensel, 1992, 2009; Aneshensel & Avison, 2015; Aneshensel & Uchechi, 2014; Aneshesel et al., 1991; Pearlin, 1989; Pearlin & Bierman, 2013) (see Figure 1.2).

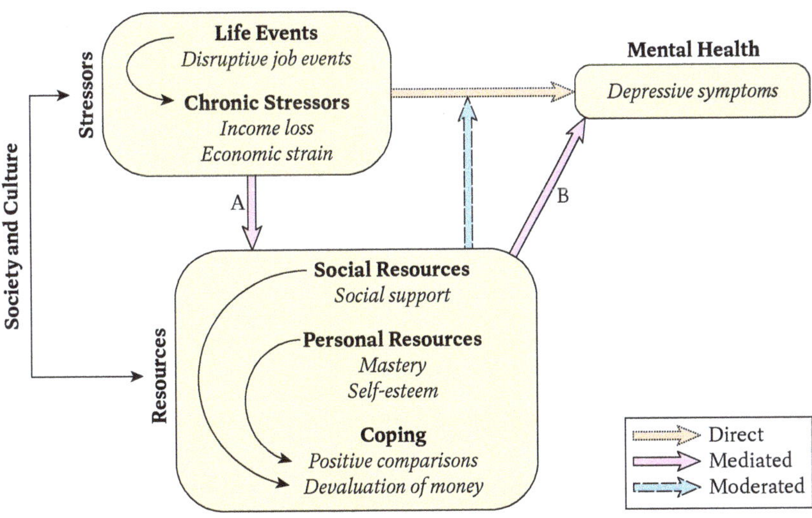

FIGURE 1.2 The Social Stress Process Model

Source: Aneshensel and Avison (2015)

Several types of psychosocial stressors are known to negatively affect health: socioenvironmental stressors such as oppression and subordination; racism, discrimination, and prejudice; microaggressions; historical or intergenerational trauma; institutional racism; acculturative stress; living in disorganized neighborhoods; and stressful life events (SLEs). Socioeconomic stressors include poverty; underemployment or unemployment; low educational attainment; and undocumented immigration status. Sociocultural stressors include alcohol and tobacco marketing in Latino communities; high prevalence of drug trafficking and use in neighborhoods; customs amenable to convivial alcohol use; positive attitudes toward drug use; and acculturative stress.

Psychosocial Stress and Social Support

The effect of psychosocial stressors on bio-physiology occurs through two major biological systems: the sympathetic-adrenal-medullary (SAM) axis and the hypothalamic-pituitary-adrenal (HPA) axis. Stressors, whether physical, psychological, or emotional, signal the brain to release hormones like ACTH and cortisol for an immediate "fight or flight" response or a delayed response once the acute stressor has passed (see Figure 1.3). These systems influence many physiological processes relevant to the maintenance of health, including metabolic regulation, cardiovascular activity, blood pressure, and immune and inflammatory functioning. In addition, these systems provide potential pathways by which socioenvironmental stressors can influence bio-physiological processes and produce disease outcomes (Elenkov & Chrousos, 2006; Ulrich Lai & Herman, 2009).

A large body of research exists on the direct, indirect, and mediating/moderating effects of social support networks on both physical and psychological health (see works by Thoits, Pearlin, and Aneshensel). The *direct effects hypothesis* holds that social support reduces the negative effects of stress on physiological and psychological health of the individual. The *indirect effect hypothesis* suggests that social support acts indirectly on stress through other mechanisms, such as through the addition of increased internal or external coping resources available to the individual. The *mediating/moderating effects hypothesis* holds that

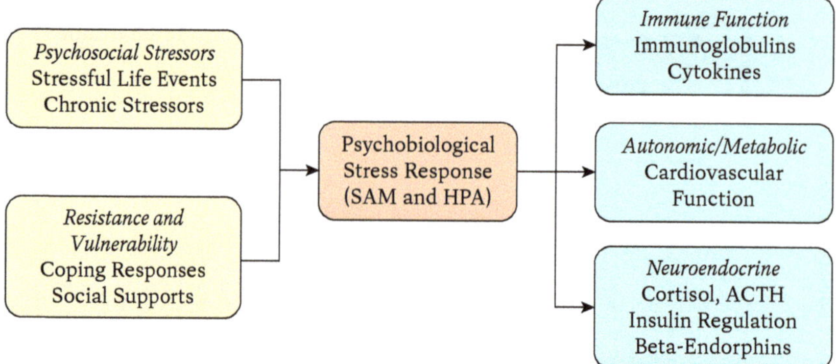

FIGURE 1.3 Major Physiological Pathways in the Psychobiological Stress Response

the individual having a social support network mediates the perception and therefore the psychological effects of stress.

Methodological approaches in social epidemiology are like those of modern epidemiology. Social epidemiologists typically conduct large-scale community or national studies using representative samples examining the social determinants of health and their consequences.

Cultural Epidemiology

At first glance, culture and epidemiology appear incongruous. Elements of culture are identified, defined, and measured using different analytical techniques and research methodologies than modern or social epidemiology. However, they are not mutually exclusive. One scientific approach can inform the other, especially when mixed methods approaches are used for data collection, as described below.

Classic epidemiologists do not usually examine the cultural environment. Cultural influences on health are generally the purview of anthropologists, who have uncovered many important cultural aspects on the etiology of disease, treatment, and its consequences. The cultural environment influences attitudes, beliefs, and practices regarding disease causation and cure. For example, the common Mexican American folk illness *susto* has a specific understanding of causation and cure, with witnessing a traumatic event as the cause and a *barrida* (sweeping) for the cure (Tafur et al., 2009).

Anthropologists and medical anthropologists have investigated cultural dimensions of health for several decades. Concerns regarding the context and content of localized "folk" illnesses were and continue to be the focus of these investigations. In the early 21st century, theoretical and conceptual arguments called for a synthesis of anthropological and epidemiological approaches to examine disease etiology, symptom manifestation, and non-Western medical treatment. The articulation and intersection of the two investigative approaches has led to the field of cultural epidemiology.

Cultural epidemiology developed in response to the perceived limitations of the quantitative and statistical approaches used in the examination of patterns of disease in classic and social epidemiology (Trostle, 2005). A synthesis of research approaches, using what is termed *mixed methods approaches*, using both qualitative and quantitative research methods to investigate disease patterns in the community and the individual, has led to an in-depth and richer understanding of how culture shapes health attitudes, beliefs, and how the manifestation of symptoms associated with specific folk illnesses are presented and treated.

Weiss (2001) has defined *cultural epidemiology* as the study of "locally valid representations of illness and their distributions in cultural context" (p. 5). I would augment this definition to include the examination of the incidence, prevalence, and cultural understanding of the etiology and treatment of "folk" diseases. Additionally, cultural risk factors for disease are important to assess within the framework of cultural epidemiology (Quintero & Estrada, 1998).

Another perspective on the definition of cultural epidemiology is that it differs from classic epidemiology by having a focus on "illness" instead of disease. According to Weiss (2017), cultural epidemiology "is concerned with the illness-related experience, meaning and behavior from the vantage point of the people directly concerned ... or otherwise involved." (p. 247). I would argue that there is room for both perspectives: disease as a manifestation of symptoms (biological and cultural) and illness (social and cultural) as a manifestation of sociocultural patterns of behavior related to disease and its symptoms.

Within the scope of cultural epidemiology are traditional and Indigenous "ways of knowing" about disease causation and potential treatments or cures. It includes an examination of cultural attitudes, beliefs, and practices based on traditional cultural worldviews of "illness" and "disease." Cultural epidemiology explores how diverse cultural worlds intersect, reflect, include, and rebuff modern Western perspectives of disease etiology and treatment. It examines the cultural influences and dimensions of health that are separate from poverty, class, or socioeconomic status influences. Cultural factors, however, overlap or combine with social influences, contributing to "risk subcultures" and creating a more complex paradigm of social and cultural influences on the health of individuals and populations (Quintero & Estrada, 1998).

Culture, Health, and Health Belief Systems

Explanatory models of disease and illness assist in disentangling social influences from cultural influences on health and wellness among cultural groups like Mexican Americans and Native Americans. Kleinman et al. (1978) introduced the *explanatory model* and defined it as a complex, culturally determined process of ascribing meanings to symptoms, causal attributions to disease, and using acceptable treatments. This explanatory model occurs within a cultural and social milieu congruent with the individual's expectations for cure and rehabilitation. Parsons's (1951) conceptualization of the "sick role" governed by social expectations has its cultural counterparts in defining the "illness" or "disease" as undesirable, a movement towards getting better, and seeking assistance from competent caregivers to get well.

Cultural health beliefs influence the meaning of the illness, the definition of the illness, the congruency of the illness with a Western medical diagnosis, the willingness or lack thereof to adhere to a plan for care, and combinations of traditional and Western biomedicine. It also influences how one communicates one's health problems, how one presents one's symptoms, when and to whom one goes for care, how long one remains in care, and how one evaluates the care received (de la Torre & Estrada, 2015).

Health belief systems, like explanatory models of disease, help define and categorize health and illness. They are based upon theories of the relationship between the cause (etiology) and the nature of illness and treatments (i.e., physical, magical, or supernatural), and they define the specific "scope" of practice for traditional healers. An important health belief system in Mexican American culture is *curanderismo*, which is discussed in more detail in Chapter 4

Epidemiology of Mexican American Folk Illnesses

The incidence and prevalence of Mexican American folk illnesses is difficult to assess. Within Mexican American culture, the topic of folk illnesses can be met with negative perceptions relating to superstitious beliefs or the works of *brujas* (witches). As a result, it can be difficult to grasp the extent of belief in folk illnesses and their treatments among Mexican Americans. During the mid-20th century, a focus on the Mexican American health subculture typically developed stereotypes and generalizations that were limited by the nonrepresentative samples studied. Findings suggested that belief in folk illnesses was widespread. However, research conducted in the 1980s suggested that only a fraction of the Mexican Americans sampled believed in folk illnesses (Estrada et al., 1990). The problem in ascertaining folk beliefs and folk illnesses lies in the research design used and who is asking the questions. Nevertheless, documented Mexican American folk illnesses and their traditional folk treatments are available in the literature (de la Torre & Estrada, 2015) (see Table 1.1).

TABLE 1.1 Select Mexican American Folk Illnesses and Their Meaning

Some Mexican American folk illnesses	Definition
Empacho	Swollen belly; upset stomach; indigestion
Mal de ojo	"Evil eye" caused by intense staring
Susto	Fright due to experiencing/witnessing a traumatic event
Ataque de nervios	Anxiety; panic attacks
Caida de mollera	Fallen fontanel
Bilis	Suppressed anger
Muina	Outward rage

(Adapted from de la Torre & Estrada, 2015)

Does culture influence health risk behaviors for disease? This is a different question than asking whether there are culturally constituted health risk factors for disease (i.e., whether certain cultural patterns of behavior increase or decrease risks associated with chronic or infectious diseases; Singer, 2005). Rather, the examination of cultural influences on risk behaviors can shed light on whether cultural values and beliefs influence behaviors that increase or decrease risk for disease beyond socioeconomic conditions and access to care.

We have used mixed method approaches in our research. For example, qualitative research methods were used to identify and define subcultural values of Mexican Americans who inject drugs (Quintero & Estrada, 1998; Estrada et al., 1999). Several Mexican American cultural values (familism, traditionalism, and religiosity) and subcultural values *(machismo)* were identified through in-depth interviews. These cultural concepts were quantified using Likert scale items to develop measures of *machismo*, familism, traditionalism, and religiosity, which proved useful in examining behavioral intentions and self-efficacy to perform HIV risk-reduction strategies (i.e., bleaching syringes, using new syringes, and condom use). We found that *machismo* values were negatively correlated with measures of self-efficacy and that familism, traditionalism, and religiosity were positively correlated with behavioral intentions and self-efficacy to perform risk reduction.

Acculturation level among Mexican Americans is the most examined cultural concept. There are numerous published articles on its definition, measures, and influences on health and risk behaviors among Mexican Americans. Research on acculturation level among Mexican Americans demonstrates that as acculturation level increases, so do alcohol and drug use risk behaviors (Ebin et al., 2001; Mainous et al., 2008). Additionally, research shows that acculturation to mainstream U.S. customs erodes traditional cultural values and beliefs (Abraido-Lanza et al., 2005; Schwartz & Unger, 2017). We will examine acculturation and acculturative stress in Chapters 4 and 5.

Theories of Racial Inequality Applicable to Mexican Americans

Several racial inequality theories applicable to Mexican Americans have been advanced to help underscore the unique social, historical, and political contexts that have influenced their health status and psychological well-being. These theories include the Internal Colonial Model (ICM), Critical Race Theory (CRT) and Latino Critical Race Theory (LatCrit), and Intersectionality Theory (IT).

The Internal Colonial Model (ICM)

Among all the Latino groups residing in the United States, Mexicans and Mexican Americans have had the longest history of interactions with non-Latino White people. Since the early 1800s, there have been tensions between the United States and Mexico, especially during the era of American "Manifest Destiny" and westward expansion.

When Tejas, a northern state of Mexico, declared its independence in 1836, it was widely viewed in Mexico as direct aggression by the United States to fulfill its Manifest Destiny, especially when the United States annexed the Republic of Texas (Acuna, 2014). The Mexican American War, known in Mexico as the "War of North American Invasion" or the "U.S. Invasion" (Velasco-Márquez, 2006), resulted with the United States acquiring an area of approximately 970,000 square miles—over half of Mexico's territory (see Figure 1.4).

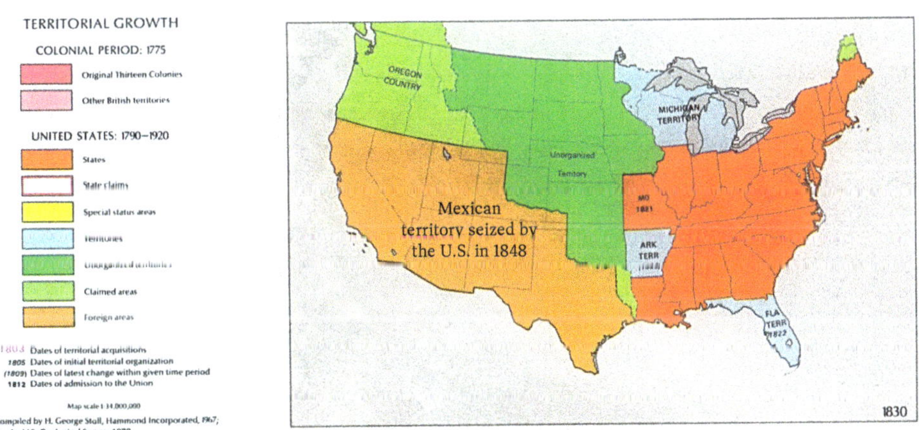

FIGURE 1.4 Territory Acquired by the United States in 1848

Originally proposed by Mario Barrera (1979), the internal colonial model is a relevant paradigm to examine racial inequality among Mexican Americans (see Figure 1.5). The internal colonial model established in the Southwest and the sociopolitical and historical context articulated by Barrera (1979) are the consequences of Manifest Destiny and the Mexican American War. The Treaty of Guadalupe Hidalgo ended the Mexican American War (1846–1848) but not the territorial expansion by the United States, which gained parts of southern Arizona and New Mexico as part of the Gadsden Purchase (1853). For almost 200 years, Mexicans and Mexican Americans residing in the United States, especially in the U.S.–Mexico borderlands (Arizona, New Mexico, Texas, and California) have experienced political disenfranchisement, discrimination, racism, cultural destruction, forced detention and removal, and many other social and cultural stressors (Barrera, 1979; Estrada, 2009; Cerdena et al., 2021).

The internal colonial model benefited the economic and political interests of non-Latino White people. It represented a structured relationship of domination and subordination, where the dominant and subordinate groups are defined by race, ethnicity, place of birth, or nationality. The interests of the dominant majority group, subordinating the interests of "colonized" populations, maintain the internal colonial system.

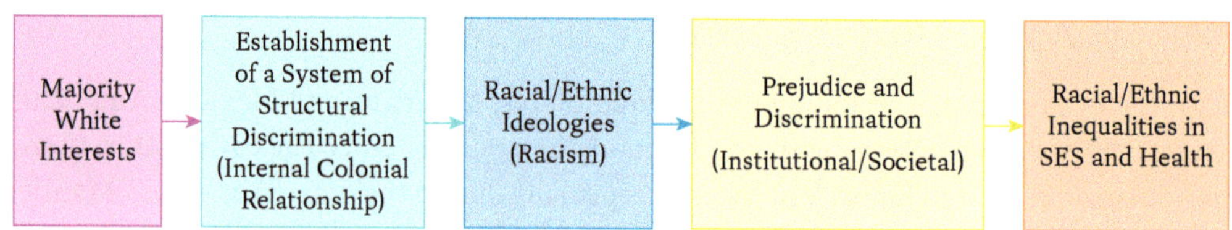

FIGURE 1.5 The Internal Colonial System (Adapted from Barrera, 1979)

Based on the 170-year sociopolitical and historical context of U.S.–Mexico relations, Mexican Americans have withstood the worst of anti-Mexican sentiment, prejudice, discrimination, and outright racism from non-Latino White Americans to the present day (Estrada, 2009; Cerdena et al., 2021). One would theorize that experiencing these stressors would lead to increased morbidity and mortality among Mexican Americans, but this is not necessarily the case. The Latino "epidemiologic paradox" references the fact that certain Latino subgroups have better health outcomes than African Americans and non-Latino White Americans (Abraido-Lanza et al., 1999; Gonzalez Burchard et al., 2005; Markides & Coreil, 1986). However, there are also specific health inequalities that Mexican Americans experience at higher rates than non-Latino White Americans (Vega et al., 2009; Zsembik & Fennell, 2005). Why would this be so? A closer examination of sociocultural influences may provide some answers as well as paradoxes associated with the health status of Mexican Americans (Scribner, 1996).

Critical Race Theory (CRT) and Latino Critical Race Theory (LatCrit)

Any discussion of critical race theory (CRT) must acknowledge the polemics the term engenders. CRT has come under increasing attack by the lay public and scholars alike who perceive the theory as underdeveloped, without testable hypotheses, and "White blaming" more than attempting to explore the complex interracial society in which we live. Critical race theory is an "aspirational theory" (Cabrera, 2018) of oppression based on racial power dynamics that non-Latino White Americans exert over minority groups in the United States. As Crenshaw (2002) states, "We would signify the political and intellectual location of the project through 'critical,' the substantive focus through 'race,' and the desire to develop a coherent account of race and law through the term 'theory'" (p. 1361). Therefore, some scholars may not see CRT as a fully developed theory in the sense of postulating testable hypotheses or axioms. Rather, it provides a useful framework for understanding the consequences of European hegemonic control on the health and social inequalities observed among minority and disenfranchised groups in the United States.

Crenshaw (1988, 1989) is widely viewed as the originator of CRT and intersectionality theory (IT). CRT developed as a response to the perceived "colorblind" criminal justice system in the United States (Crenshaw, 1991, 2011). Crenshaw's (1988) critique of U.S. discriminatory legal practices has transformed perceptions of "equal justice" under the law. In addition, Crenshaw's (1991) introduction of the term "intersectionality" describes how multiple identities of oppression can serve to reinforce one another, thus creating an "inescapable" entanglement of prejudice, discrimination, sexism, and racism. These insights demonstrate how the social environment reinforces these social stressors to produce chronic diseases in socially and historically marginalized groups (Kessler et al., 1999; Flores et al., 2008).

Similarly, Solórzano and others have adapted CRT to Latinas/os using the methodology of counter-storytelling to bring historically marginalized voices to the "center" of investigation to understand the effects of discrimination and oppression on personal and community development and to empower communities and individuals to make positive changes to overcome their negative effects. The emphasis on marginalized voices is essential to what has evolved to be Latina/o critical race theory (LatCrit; Delgado, 1990, 1993; Delgado & Stefancic, 2001; Solórzano, 1998; Solórzano & Yosso, 2001; Yosso, 2005).

Advanced in the literature are seven "central tenets" of CRT (Cabrera, 2018; Capper, 2015; Delgado & Stefancic, 2001; Solórzano, 1998) (Table 1.2).

TABLE 1.2 Central Tenets of Critical Race Theory

Tenet	Description
The centrality or permanence of race and racism in U.S. society	Asserts that race/racism is a permanent social norm in the United States and by extension is the foundation of society in the United States.
The challenge to dominant ideology/"Whiteness as property"	Challenges the claims of neutrality, objectivity, colorblindness, and meritocracy in the United States and by doing so demonstrates these concepts to be ephemeral to historically marginalized groups in U.S. society.
The centrality of experiential knowledge/counter storytelling	Claims that the experiential knowledge of socially and historically marginalized groups is appropriate, legitimate, and integral to understanding racial inequality; it empowers people of color to view their culture as a strength rather than a deficit. This tenet is at the core of most LatCrit methodologies.
Optimal interest convergence	Asserts that the White majority advances the interests of historically marginalized groups only when there is a shared interest to do so (i.e., when it benefits the dominant White population).

(continued)

TABLE 1.2 (*continued*)

Tenet	Description
Critique of neoliberalism and multiculturalism	A criticism of neoliberal ideology like colorblindness, meritocracy, and legal neutrality as serving the dominant status quo while keeping historically marginalized groups at bay. Multiculturalism is considered a neoliberal construct.
Interdisciplinary perspective to examine inequalities	Demands that race, gender, and class be viewed in both a contemporary, historical, and political context and should be examined using an interdisciplinary perspective to examine the relationships among them.
Commitment to social justice	Establishes CRT as a framework committed to eliminating all forms of subordination and oppression of historically marginalized groups in the United States.

Extended to the educational system in the United States during the 1990s, CRT and IT have gained growing acceptance in the field of public health since the 2000s. The interesting and perhaps most controversial aspect of CRT is that it situates race and race relations at the center of understanding the perpetuation of "White privilege" in the United States. CRT has a history of challenging "colorblind" approaches to social, educational, and economic justice reform in the United States. Central to CRT is viewing "hegemonic" or dominant non-Mexican American White influences on power dynamics, control, and exploitation over racial/ethnic groups in the United States that serves to influence many of the social and health inequalities observed. It also challenges the postmodern ideals of colorblindness, equal opportunity, and social justice as ephemeral and serving the goals of the dominant non-Mexican American White majority and their institutions.

Examples of negative cultural evaluations provided in the literature focus on denying cultural validity to marginalized groups like African Americans, Mexican Americans, and Native Americans (Brown, 2003). Examples include cultural destructiveness, cultural incapacity, cultural blindness, cultural insensitivity, and cultural appropriation. *Cultural destructiveness* is the forced assimilation and subjugation of racial/ethnic groups and serves to justify the rights and privileges of the dominant group. *Cultural incapacity* includes racism, the creation and maintenance of demeaning stereotypes, and discrimination practices. *Cultural blindness* ignores differences, and practitioners tend to treat everyone the same. It is a deliberate and conscious effort to minimize cultural differences and maximize the values of the dominant group. *Cultural insensitivity* blatantly ignores cultural strengths and traditions of marginalized groups and instead perpetuates dominant cultural practices and beliefs. *Cultural appropriation* is seen in the ways in which non-Western methods of healing are adopted and used by the dominant culture. For example, the New Age movement culturally appropriated many Native American practices and spiritual beliefs without undergoing an apprenticeship or learning the appropriate techniques (e.g., sweat lodges).

Taken together, these approaches of commodifying others' culture led to professional and institutional bias in educating or caring for historically marginalized groups that are non-White. As well, these conditions reinforce the status quo by limiting access to goods and services that are culturally congruent to these groups.

The major criticism of CRT leveled by its detractors is that CRT "blames" non-Meixcan American White people for past and current social problems experienced by historically marginalized population groups. Some believe that the indoctrination of their children will occur with this alternate race-conscious paradigm, and they will feel ashamed of their race. Non-White groups view CRT as a means to empower themselves and their children through resilience and proactive affirmation. It may be more useful to view CRT as a lens "of the other" to examine racial dynamics and interrogate how race relations in the United States have undermined social and health inequalities among historically marginalized groups.

Intersectionality Theory (IT)

Because individuals operate within various social, political, and cultural domains, it is important to examine how these domains complement one another to influence health and health behaviors. The socio-ecological model proposed by Bronfenbrenner (1979, 1989) and Stokols (1992, 1996) articulates micro-level interactions with macro-level structures to produce health outcomes (see Figure 1.6). The individual, embedded within the interpersonal, organizational, community, and public policy structures, interacts with and are, in turn, influenced by these various macro-level structures. Absent from this model are the interactions of historically marginalized individuals and groups with these predominantly White macro-level structures that perpetuate social and health inequalities at the individual and population level through institutionalized racism and discrimination. More attention to the public policy, community, and organizational structures within the context of CRT may provide insights on how positive health outcomes can be achieved for historically marginalized groups within a race-conscious society.

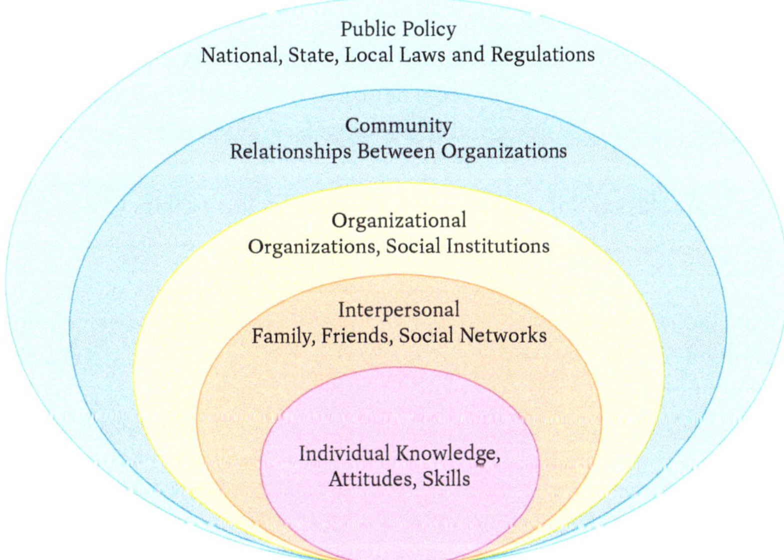

FIGURE 1.6 Bronfenbrenner's Ecologic Model

Intersectionality is the examination of the interconnected features of social constructions such as race/ethnicity, class, and gender as they apply to continued oppression of a given individual or group based on power dynamics within U.S. society (Bauer, 2014; Bowleg, 2012; Brown, 2003; Crenshaw, 1989). People have multiple intersecting identities (e.g., mother, spouse, administrator, Latina), and the power dynamics between groups and/or individuals influence the economic well-being and health of historically excluded and marginalized persons and populations (Bowleg, 2012).

According to Bowleg (2012):

> Intersectionality is a theoretical framework for understanding how multiple social identities (e.g., race, gender, sexual orientation, SES, and disability) intersect at the micro-level of the individual to reflect interlocking systems of privilege and oppression (e.g., racism, heterosexism, sexism, classism, colonialism) at the macro social-structural level. (p. 1267)

An intersectionality perspective focuses on studying the interactions and synergies of race, ethnicity, sociodemographic characteristics, and personal identities with "place." The value of employing this perspective is in uncovering how multiple identities increase or decrease morbidity and mortality. Place, then, is influenced by these micro- and macro-level intersecting characteristics that profoundly affect the lived experiences of Mexican Americans, African Americans, Native Americans, those living in poverty, and other disenfranchised groups. An example of intersectionality theory is the work of Geronimus (1992) and the proposed "weathering hypotheses" among African American women. Essentially, the *weathering hypothesis* suggests that social (racism) and environmental factors (discrimination) negatively influence the health of young African American women, making them more vulnerable (increasing risk) to physiological adversity because of increased psychological coping. The "intersectionality paradox" is one explanation for observed racial differences in health status proposing that high-status African American women have worse health outcomes than low-status White women. For example, high-SES African American women have higher rates of low-birthweight (LBW) infants than low-SES White women (Forde et al., 2019).

Both critical race theory and intersectionality theory attempt to empower individuals and communities through a focus on social justice—that is, deliberate action to enhance the social, economic, psychological, and physical well-being of historically marginalized groups (see Table 1.3).

TABLE 1.3 Comparison of Intersectionality Theory and Critical Race Theory

Intersectionality theory	Critical race theory
Social identities are not independent and unidimensional but multiple and intersecting.	Centrality of race and racism; embedded within U.S. social structures, practices, and discourses
People from historically oppressed and marginalized groups are the focal point of investigation.	Challenges dominant ideologies: traditional institutional claims of color blindness, meritocracy, equal opportunity, multiculturalism. Voices of marginalized are central.
Multiple social identities at the micro level (i.e., race, gender, SES, etc.) intersect with macro-level structural factors (i.e., poverty, racism, sexism, etc.) to produce health inequalities among historically oppressed and marginalized groups.	Multiple social identities at micro level intersect with macro-level structural factors to produce social and health inequalities based on race/ethnicity, gender, and so on.
Focuses on social justice to alleviate oppression.	Focuses on social justice to alleviate oppression.

The Social Determinants of Health (SDOH) Paradigm

The Office of Disease Prevention and Health Promotion recently announced a renewed focus on "place." Healthy People 2030 (https://health.gov/healthypeople) developed an organizing framework to examine health inequalities using a "place-based" approach. The framework reflects five key areas that are important in understanding the impact of "place" on an individual's or population's health.

People live within the constraints of their social environment that affect their health, social welfare, quality of life, and differential exposure to health risks within their communities. The social, economic, and physical environment and the institutions embedded within these environments are referred to as "place" in the SDOH paradigm (see Figure 1.7). Accordingly, "Understanding the relationship between how population groups experience 'place' and the impact of 'place' on health is fundamental to the social determinants of health—including both social and physical determinants" (Office of Disease Prevention and Health Promotion, n.d.).

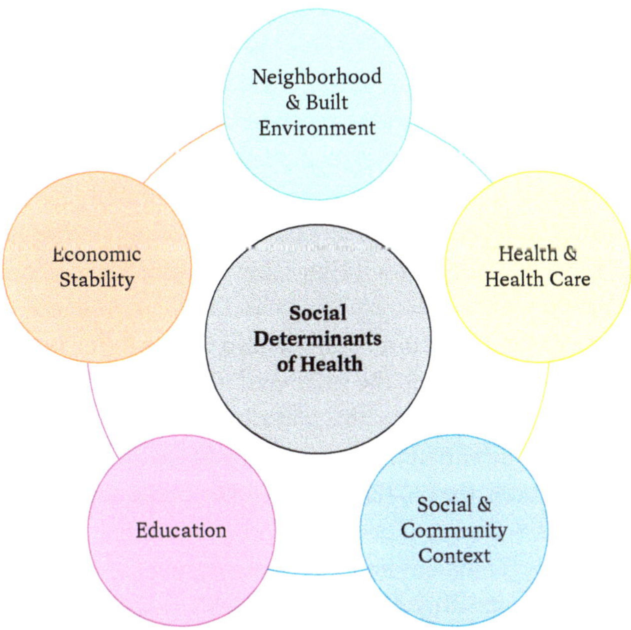

FIGURE 1.7 Social Determinants of Health

Within the SDOH framework, it is determined that 10% of negative health outcomes are attributable to the physical environment (environmental quality and the built environment). Another 20% is attributable to health care (access to care and quality of care). Another 30% is attributable to health behaviors (tobacco consumption, alcohol and drug use, diet and exercise, risky sexual behaviors). However, the majority, 40%, are attributable to SES factors (education, employment, and income), family and social support, and community safety (Magnan, 2017). There are many examples of social determinants that influence our day-to-day well-being, including (a) transportation options, (b) social support networks, (c) exposure to crime, violence, and social disorder, (d) socioeconomic conditions like concentrated poverty, (e) societal norms and attitudes like discrimination, racism, and distrust of government, (f) access to goods and services, (g) English proficiency, and (h) health literacy.

The five SDOH outlined as "place-based" are economic stability, education, social and community context, health and health care, and the neighborhood and built (human-made) environment.

Economic Stability

This social determinant includes poverty, employment and underemployment status, food security, and housing stability.

The majority of community health research indicates that poverty is the single most important determinant of an individual's or population's health status. In 2023, the federal poverty level for the 48 contiguous states was $14,580 for an individual and $30,000 for a family of four (ASPE, 2023). Data from the U.S. Census shows that 11.5%, or about 38 million people, lived in poverty in 2023 (Shrider & Creamer, 2023).

Of course, poverty rates vary by age, gender, geographic region, and race/ethnicity. For example, poverty rates increased for those 65 years and older but decreased for those aged 18 years or less. Moreover, in 2022 non-Latino White Americans 25 and older had a poverty rate of 8.6%, compared to African Americans at 17.1% and Mexican Americans at 16.9% (Shrider & Creamer, 2023).

Research findings convincingly demonstrate that poverty is a predictor of poorer health status, lower educational attainment, higher levels of unemployment, higher levels of food insecurity, higher prevalence of both communicable and chronic diseases, and overall higher morbidity and mortality rates.

Food security and housing stability are closely connected. Based on the 1996 World Food Summit, *food security* is defined as "when all people, at all times, have physical and economic access to sufficient safe and nutritious food that meets their dietary needs and food preferences for an active and healthy life" (Food and Agriculture Organization, 2008, p. 1; see also Coleman-Jensen & Nord, 2013; Nord, 2009; Nord et al., 2002, 2007). Housing stability is the increased likelihood of remaining in one's home under increasing economic difficulty and lack of accessible and affordable housing. Frederick et al. (2014) defines *housing stability* as "the extent to which an individual's customary access to housing of reasonable quality is secure" (p. 964). Chang and Chatterjee (2022) examined housing instability and food insecurity using the Food Acquisition and Purchase Survey (FoodAPS). They found that after controlling for sociodemographic characteristics and the local food environment, housing instability was a strong predictor of food insecurity, very low food security, unhealthy diet, and perceiving cost as a barrier to healthy eating among low-income households.

Education

This social determinant includes high school graduation or GED rates, enrollment in higher education, language and literacy rates, and early childhood development. These social determinants, too, vary by income and race/ethnicity. For example, in 2021, 36.7% of the U.S. population had a high school education or less. However, non-Latino White Americans had a rate of 36.5%, African Americans had a rate of 43%, and Mexican Americans had the highest rate of 57.3%. Again, research shows that those with a more than a high school education earns higher wages than those with a high school education or less (U.S. Census Bureau, 2021).

Social and Community Context

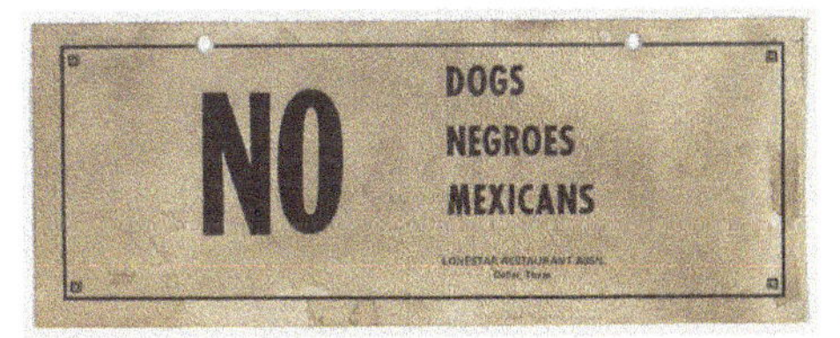

This social determinant includes social cohesion, civic participation, and incarceration and recidivism rates. It also includes racism, discrimination, and racial and ethnic segregation. *Segregation* refers to the physical separation of racial/ethnic groups by residence, housing, employment, and education. The infamous "Jim Crow Era" of the 19th and 20th centuries created and enforced legal policies that restricted the access of racial/ethnic groups to many social and public services accessible and available to White people.

There are two types of segregation. "De jure" segregation is the separation of people based on race/ethnicity and was required by law. "De facto" segregation is the separation of people based on race/ethnicity with no official law. Even though de jure segregation officially ended with the passage of the Civil Rights Act of 1964, its legacy continues to influence opportunities and upward mobility.

Within the framework of SDOH, where a person lives (i.e., place) determines the type and quality of education they receive, access and availability of quality health care, the social support networks they have access to, the types of employment they can engage in, and whether their voices will be heard regarding social justice. Racial segregation is a consistent predictor of increased morbidity and mortality among African Americans. Numerous population-based studies have demonstrated the influence of racial/ethnic segregation in higher infant mortality rates, higher adult mortality, higher rates of infectious diseases, and increased hospitalizations. There is also a correlation between racial/ethnic segregation and access to healthy foods, liquor store locations, availability of pharmacies, and availability of health care (Yang & Matthews, 2010).

Although the neighborhood and the built environment is one of the five social determinants, neighborhood disorder fits more appropriately within the social and community context. Neighborhoods are small areas within larger communities and are not necessarily defined along geographic or political boundaries. Rather, neighborhoods are social clusters that have common characteristics in terms of income, race, ethnicity, national origin, or other common characteristics.

By definition, *neighborhood disorder* is identified by visible cues of inadequate social control and an obvious lack of social order in neighborhood public places (Ross & Mirkowsy, 2001, 2009). For example, graffiti, gangs, drug transactions, violent crime, and homelessness are attributable to a lack of social control in these areas. Numerous studies have demonstrated that neighborhood disorder is related to higher levels of community mistrust and fear as well as psychological distress among community residents (Diez Roux, 2004; Plascak et al., 2018; Ross and Mirkowsy, 2009; Ross et al., 2002). In neighborhoods where community residents report high levels of disorder, they also tend to report (a) more incivility and physically threatening environments, (b) feeling intimidated by abandoned buildings, graffiti, and crime, and (c) being less likely to develop social support networks with their neighbors (Kim & Ross, 2009). Therefore, negative social, cultural, and physical perceptions of one's neighborhood characterize neighborhood disorder. The Kim and Ross (2009) study established the negative effects of neighborhood disorder with higher rates of depression, lower rates of social ties and social support, and higher rates of neighborhood disadvantage. These findings suggest that neighborhood disorder and social relationships are social mechanisms mediating the relationship between disadvantaged neighborhoods and psychological distress. Neighborhood disorder explained the negative impacts of a disadvantaged neighborhood on depression, but social relationships explained both positive and negative association between neighborhood disadvantage and depression.

Health and Health Care

This social determinant includes access to a regular source of care, health insurance coverage, and health literacy. Public health indicators of access to care include at least three areas:

- Rates of health insurance coverage
- Having a regular source of care that could include a clinic or community health center, a private physician's office or Health Maintenance Organization (HMO), or an emergency department or hospital
- "Realized" access measured using actual rates of health care utilization and barriers to health care utilization

Prior to the implementation of the Affordable Care Act, the percentage of the U.S. population with health care coverage was low. In 2014, 45% of non-Latino White Americans did not have health care coverage. Among historically marginalized groups, Mexican Americans had the highest rate of being uninsured (34%), followed by African Americans (14%; Kaiser Family Foundation, 2015). However, in 2021, the percentage of the U.S. population with health care coverage was 91.4 %, almost doubling (Branch & Conway, 2022)! Latinos still have the highest rates of being uninsured at 17.7%, but that is almost half the rate in 2014 (Table 1.4).

TABLE 1.4 Percentage of People by Health Insurance Coverage, 2021

Race and Latino origin	Private health insurance (19 and older)	Public health insurance (19 and older)	Uninsured
White, non-Latino	79.5	16.2	5.7
Black, non-Latino	62.9	29.1	9.6
Asian, non-Latino	80.7	15.0	5.8
Latino (any race)	56.8	21.8	17.7

Source: Branch & Conway, 2022

In 2022, 83.5% of persons 18 years of age and older visited a physician within the past 12 months (Schiller & Norris, 2023. When examining utilization barriers due to cost, Schiller & Norris (2023) found that only 6.1% of the population reported that they did not get needed medical care due to cost.

Neighborhood and the Built Environment

This social determinant includes many aspects of the communities in which people live. It includes access to healthy foods (food deserts and food swamps) and food insecurity, housing availability and quality, "green spaces" in the community, home ownership, traffic congestion and environmental pollution, and high rates of crime and violence.

"Food deserts" and "food swamps" are those geographic areas that do not have ready access to healthy foods (Luan et al., 2015; Richardson et al., 2014; Rose et al., 2009). *Food deserts* are defined as areas in the United States that have limited access to healthy and nutritious foods and are associated with poorer rural and urban environments. Likewise, food swamps are geographic areas where the overabundance of high-energy foods (e.g., high-caloric snacks sold at mini marts) severely limits healthy food options. A comprehensive study conducted by Kelli and associates (2017) in Atlanta found significant associations between food deserts and cardiovascular risk profile, especially hypertension and diabetes. Those residents living in food deserts also had lower incomes, lower educational levels, were predominantly African American, and had higher rates of obesity and higher rates of smoking, which suggests that risk factors for hypertension and diabetes co-occur in these communities, similar to other studies (Cooksey-Stowers et al., 2017; Ghosh-Dastidar et al., 2014; Morland et al., 2002).

These areas can be urban or rural depending on the types of food available. Studies have shown that lack of access to healthy foods is significantly associated with low income, poverty, gender, and race/ethnicity (Cook & Frank, 2008; Morland et al., 2002; Seligman et al., 2010; Walker et al., 2010; Zenk et al., 2005). *Food Security*, defined by the USDA as "access by all people at all times to enough food for an active healthy life," is an important social determinant of health for both individuals and populations (Rabbitt et al., 2023). Food insecurity, then, is the absence of access to enough food for an active healthy life. Overall, about 13% of the U.S. population is classified as having low food insecurity (Rabbitt et al., 2023).

The synergistic effects of unemployment and low income compound a household's food security status. High unemployment rates among low-income groups make it more difficult to meet basic household food needs. For example, Shrider et al. (2021) found that low-income households were twice as likely as the national average to be food insecure (28.6% versus 10.5%, respectively). Additionally, children of unemployed parents have higher rates of food insecurity compared to children with employed parents. Racial and ethnic disparities also exist related to food insecurity. Shrider et al. (2021) also reported that non-Latino Black households were over 2 times more likely to be food insecure than the national average (21.7% versus 10.5%, respectively). Among Latino households, the prevalence of food insecurity was 17.2% compared to the national average of 10.5%.

The Urban Health Penalty and the Urban Health Advantage

The number and proportion of people living in urban environments has substantially increased. More people live in urban environments. According to the World Bank, more than half of the worlds' population lived in urban areas for the first time in human history (Baeumler et al., 2021). By 2050, about 75% of the world's population will live in urban centers (Baeumler et al., 2021). The production of social and health inequalities is largely observed in urban areas where the unequal distribution of goods and services becomes manifest. For example, access and availability of health care, segregation, disadvantaged and disorganized communities, poor neighborhoods, limited green space, and food swamps are prevalent in urban areas.

According to the U.S. Census (Shrider et al., 2021), nearly one fifth of all Americans—about 52 million people—live in low-income neighborhoods (i.e., neighborhoods in which at least 30% of residents are living in poverty are classified as living in "concentrated poverty"). Between 1970 and 2000, poor families became more likely to live in neighborhoods with concentrated poverty and rich families became more likely to live in neighborhoods with concentrated wealth. Individuals from racial/ethnic groups also are more likely to live in low-income neighborhoods. Nearly half of all African Americans live in low-income neighborhoods, compared with only 1 in 10 non-Latino White Americans. Data from the U.S. Census shows that African Americans and Mexican Americans account for larger shares of those who live in low-income areas than their shares of the general population compared to non-Latino White Americans and non-Latinos (Shrider et al., 2021). The so-called "urban health penalty" proposes that high population density, food swamps, segregated housing, disorganized neighborhoods, air pollution, violence, and insufficient access to quality health care are "penalties" that people in low-income communities are exposed to that increase their risk for poor health and mental health outcomes (Freudenberg et al., 2005; McDonald et al., 2021; Miller & Vasan, 2021) (see Figure 1.8).

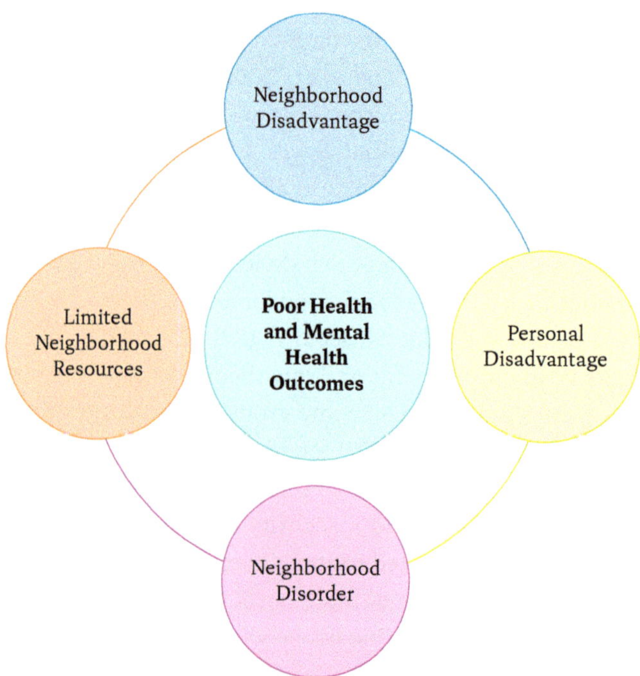

FIGURE 1.8 The Urban Health Penalty

The lack of adequate resources to enhance the quality of life for low-income urban residents leads to negative lifestyle patterns, the emergence of health-risk subcultures (e.g., prostitution, drug use, and gangs), lack of social cohesion and community capital, and low economic vitality.

Another important health problem related to urban environments is the effect of air pollution on the health of community populations (Cohen et al., 2004; Gendron-Carrier et al., 2022; Samet & White, 2004). Research has shown that the negative effects of air pollution are associated with many acute and chronic health problems (see Table 1.5).

TABLE 1.5 Adverse Effects of Air Pollution Found in the Research Literature

Adverse effects
• Premature death • Lung cancer • Exacerbation of chronic obstructive pulmonary disease (COPD) • Development of chronic lung disease • Heart attacks • Increased hospital admissions and ER visits for heart and lung disease • Decreased lung function • Increased respiratory symptoms and medication use for those who have lung disease or asthma • Preterm births • Low birth weight

Health researchers conclude that there is more than one mechanism involved in causing air pollution-related health effects (Pascal et al., 2013; National Institute of Environmental Health Sciences, 2023):

- Air pollution leads to lung irritation, which leads to increased permeability in lung tissue.
- Air pollution increases susceptibility to viral and bacterial pathogens leading to pneumonia in vulnerable persons who are unable to clear these infections (weakened immune system).
- Air pollution aggravates the severity of chronic lung diseases, causing rapid loss of airway function.
- Air pollution causes inflammation of lung tissue, resulting in the release of chemicals that impact heart function.
- Air pollution causes changes in blood chemistry that result in clots that can cause heart attacks.

Three hypothesized relationships between SES and air pollution rates are relevant (Costin & Clark, 2022):

- Exposure differentials related to SES: Traffic congestion/density, freeways, and hazardous materials located near low-income communities differentially expose them to air pollution.
- Susceptibility directly related to SES: Disadvantaged neighborhoods, reduced access to services, and co-exposure to risk factors increase susceptibility to air pollution effects.
- Susceptibility from predisposing health conditions, behaviors, or other factors: Preexisting chronic diseases, lower respiratory function, and synergism (e.g., interactions between smoking and particulate matter) increase susceptibility and risk of exposure.

Contrary to the urban health penalty, the *urban health advantage* hypothesis suggests that the urban environment has many economic and social advantages (Vlahov et al., 2005). Urban areas provide economic opportunity, upward mobility, increased access to goods and services, and social support networks, both formal and informal.

Within the concept of urban health advantage are issues of collective efficacy, informal social control, social cohesion, and community capacity (Kawachi et al., 1997; Mayer, 1996, 2003; Sampson et al.,

1997). Sampson et al. (1997) define *collective efficacy* as "the linkage of mutual trust and the willingness to intervene for the common good" (p. 919). Key components of collective efficacy are social cohesion and informal social control. Studies have shown that collective community efficacy is associated with decreases in risky sexual behaviors, decreases in asthma prevalence, decreases in obesity rates, decreases in premature mortality, and improved subjective health ratings. Similarly, *community capacity* is "the sum total of commitment, resources, and skills that a community can mobilize and deploy to address community problems and strengthen community assets" (Mayer, 1996, p. 332).

Social capital is a form of economic and cultural capital in which social networks are central and interpersonal transactions are marked by reciprocity, trust, and cooperation. Researchers note an important association between social capital and *civic participation*, which is the extent to which a person participates in or contributes to their community or country. African Americans tend to have high rates of civic participation; Mexican Americans tend to have lower rates of civic participation. Increases in social capital leads to increases in civic participation; social capital depends on external investments and the activation of internal resources. Social capital has also been shown to have both positive and negative effects on health. One study found that those with membership in voluntary groups and higher levels of social trust had a more equal income structure and had lower total and disease specific mortality rates (Kawachi et al., 1997). In another study, men with low social capital were nearly twice as likely to have a psychiatric disorder (Rose, 2000). The prevalence of poor self-rated health was higher in neighborhoods with more family ties, less integration into the wider society, and lower levels of trust. Social cohesion is in many ways like social capital. It depends on the interconnections between people; the values of trust, reciprocity, and cooperation are key components; and it depends on the mutuality of common interests for the well-being of the community and individual.

Conceptual and Theoretical Synthesis for a Holistic Understanding of Mexican American Health

The health status of any population group is fundamentally due to the interacting, reinforcing, and synergistic influences of the social, political, historical, and cultural environments. The strength of these influences will depend on the external and internal coping resources available to the population group that enable them to overcome the stressors produced by each of the environments. Likewise, the proximal and distal linkages to these various environments influence individual health.

However, among historically marginalized population groups like African Americans, Native Americans, and Mexican Americans, the historical, political, and social environments are crucial in understanding how health inequalities have persisted over time and how racism continues to be powerful stressor implicating their negative health compared to non-Latino White Americans.

Social and cultural epidemiology are the scientific foundations for understanding sociocultural influences on the incidence, prevalence, and prevention of disease and enhancing wellness among Mexican Americans. How and why social and cultural phenomena influence health are enhanced by an examination of social, political, historical, and cultural determinants that limit access to health and health care for this group.

The examination of Mexican American health inequalities includes the social environment in which a person lives, the cultural environment that influences their understanding and conceptions of health, and the political and historical context that has determined the consequences of "place," as characterized by the SDOH paradigm (e.g., were we live, work, worship, recreate, learn, etc.) (see Figure 1.9).

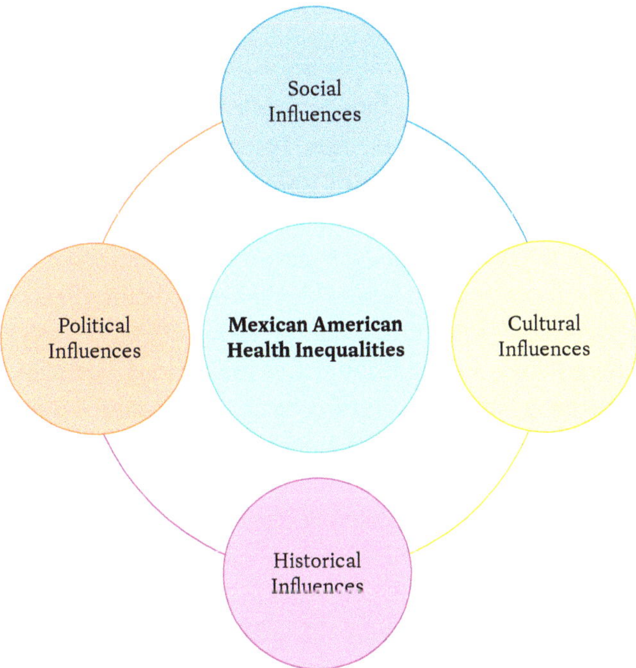

FIGURE 1.9 Influences on Mexican American Health Inequalities

Methodological approaches to understanding the influence of these domains include both quantitative and qualitative research approaches, using large data analytical techniques, along with in-depth interviewing and focus groups. Our research demonstrates that a more thorough and richer understanding of cultural phenomena can enhance the interpretation of quantitative data analyses. The two approaches are complementary and enable a thorough examination of important social, cultural, political, and historical influences on Mexican American health and health inequalities.

Intersectionality and critical race theory provide a social, political, and historical lens to examine power dynamics, past and present, between non-Latino White Americans and Mexican Americans. These theories also provide an approach for identifying solutions to health inequalities that focus on social justice in public health and equal health care access. Additionally, these theories help elucidate the complex and reinforcing influences of ethnic and cultural identities that perpetuate health inequalities among Mexican Americans. The internal colonial model is specific to the experience of racism, discrimination, and prejudice toward Mexican Americans in the southwestern United States after the Mexican American War. As such, it provides a useful sociohistorical and sociopolitical context for the examination of health inequalities experienced by Mexican Americans.

A comprehensive understanding of Mexican American health in the United States includes the interrogation of social and historical determinants and biological and cultural factors that increase morbidity and mortality and increase barriers to health care utilization. Additionally, social epigenomics provides a basis for investigating the "cause of the causes" and further the understanding of intergenerational transmission of disease, especially diabetes mellitus, cancer, cardiovascular disease, and specific psychiatric disorders known to have an epigenetic basis.

CHAPTER SUMMARY

Social epidemiology is an important field of study in public health because it locates health and disease within the social and cultural fabric of society. The "Epidemiologic Triangle" provides a schematic for understanding the relationships between the causal agents of disease, the individual, and the social, biological, physical, and cultural environments in which the individual is situated. Stress and stressful life events and personal reactions to them can produce increased allostatic load that can lead to toxic stress and negative health outcomes. Social support networks can moderate the effects of stress on the individual.

Cultural epidemiology examines the cultural interpretation of illness across various cultures. Within the scope of cultural epidemiology are traditional and Indigenous "ways of knowing" about disease causation and potential treatments or cures. Culture, health, and health belief systems can be examined through explanatory models that delves into the meanings of symptoms, casual attributions, and congruent folk treatments.

The belief in and value of Mexican American folk illnesses and their treatments depends on Latinos' generational status and acculturation level. Nevertheless, depending on the Latino community and their access to health care providers, use of folk remedies and folk healers are ubiquitous.

Several social theories of racial inequality are relevant to Latinos of Mexican descent. In particular, the Internal Colonial Model (ICM) (Barrera, 1979) appears most relevant given the socio historical and political experiences by Mexicans and Mexican Americans in the United States. Additional theories like Critical Race Theory (CRT) and Latino Critical Race Theory (LatCrit) provide a lens through which we can examine various 'oppressive' elements that underscore the predominantly non Latino White population's interactions with people of color. The increasing popularity of Intersectionality Theory in public health examines the multiple social identities of an individual in relation to the oppressive power dynamics in non-Latino White society of the United States. "Place" is influenced by micro and macro intersecting characteristics (Bowleg, 2012).

The social determinants of health (SDOH) paradigm has become fully entrenched within the field of Public Health in examining contributing factors to health inequalities among historically marginalized populations in the United States. The critical importance of identifying social inequalities in economic stability, education, the social and community context, health and health care, and the neighborhood and built environment, can assist in remediating conditions that contribute to the overall negative health and psychological well-being of people.

QUESTIONS TO CONSIDER

1. How can critical race theory and intersectionality theory assist in understanding the effects of multiple levels of oppression associated with Latino health inequalities?

2. Can colonial and/or internal colonial models assist in identifying historical, political, and social factors that underlie the social determinants of health for Latinos of Mexican descent?
3. How might the social determinants of health, singly or in combination, influence the health of Latinos of Mexican descent?
4. Evaluate the role of stressful life events, acute and chronic stressors, and their hypothesized influence on health outcomes.
5. What are the ways in which some of the urban health penalty outcomes can be interrupted?

SUGGESTED READINGS

Acuna, R. F. (2014). *Occupied America: A history of Chicanos* (8th ed.). Pearson.

Aneshensel, C. S., & Avison, W. R. (2015). The stress process: An appreciation of Leonard I. Pearlin. *Society and Mental Health, 5*(2), 67–85. https://doi.org/10.1177/2156869315585388

Barrera, M. (1979). *Race and class in the Southwest: A theory of racial inequality.* University of Notre Dame Press.

Berkman, L. F., Kawachi, I., & Glymour, M. M. (2014). *Social epidemiology* (2nd ed.). Oxford University Press.

Cerdena, J. P., Rivera, L. M., & Spak, J. M. (2021). Intergenerational trauma in Latinxs: A scoping review. *Social Science and Medicine, 270.* https://doi.org/10.1016/j.socscimed.2020.113662

Crenshaw, K. W. (1991). Mapping the margins: Intersectionality, identity politics, and violence against women of color. *Stanford Law Review, 43,* 1241–1299.

Estrada, A. L. (2009). Mexican Americans and historical trauma theory: A theoretical perspective. *Journal of Ethnicity in Substance Abuse, 8*(3), 330–340.

O'Connor, D. B., Thayer, J. F., & Vedhara, K. (2021). Stress and health: A review of psychobiological processes. *Annual Review of Psychology, 72,* 663–688. https://doi.org/10.1146/annurev-psych-062520-122331

Office of Disease Prevention and Health Promotion. (n.d.). *Healthy People 2030.* U.S. Department of Health and Human Services. Retrieved February 16, 2023, from https://health.gov/healthypeople

Pearlin, L. I., & Bierman, A. (2013). Current issues and future directions in research into the stress process. In C. S. Aneshensel, J. C. Phelan, & A. Bierman (Eds.), *Handbook of the sociology of mental health.* Springer, Dordrecht. https://doi.org/10.1007/978-94-007-4276-5_16

REFERENCES

Abraído-Lanza, A. F., Chao, M. T., & Flórez, K. R. (2005). Do healthy behaviors decline with greater acculturation?: Implications for the Latino mortality paradox. *Social Science & Medicine, 61*(6), 1243–1255.

Abraido-Lanza, A. F., Dohrenwend, B. P., Ng-Mak, D. S., & Turner, J. B. (1999). The Latino mortality paradox: A test of the "salmon bias" and healthy migrant hypotheses. *American Journal of Public Health, 89*(10), 1543–1548.

Acuna, R. F. (2014). *Occupied America: A history of Chicanos* (8th ed.). Pearson.

Aneshensel, C. S. (1992). Social stress: Theory and research. *Annual Review of Sociology, 18,* 15–38.

Aneshensel, C. S. (2009). Toward explaining mental health disparities. *Journal of Health and Social Behavior, 50*(4), 377–394.

Aneshensel, C. S., & Avison, W. R. (2015). The stress process: An appreciation of Leonard I. Pearlin. *Society and Mental Health, 5*(2), 67–85. https://doi.org/10.1177/2156869315585388

Aneshensel C. S., Rutter, C. M., & Lachenbruch, P. A. (1991). Social structure, stress, and mental health: competing conceptual and analytic models. *American Sociological Review, 56*(2), 166–178

Aneshensel C. S., & Uchechi, M. A. (2014). The stress process: Its origins, evolution, and future. In R. J. Johnson, R. J. Turner, & B. G. Link (Eds.), *Sociology of mental health: Selected topics from forty years, 1970s–2010s* (pp. 53–74). Springer.

Assistant Secretary for Planning and Evaluation. (2023). *2023 poverty guidelines: 48 contiguous states (all states execept Alaska and Hawaii).* U.S. Department of Health and Human Services. https://aspe.hhs.gov/sites/default/files/documents/1c92a9207f3ed5915ca020d58fe77696/detailed-guidelines-2023.pdf

Baeumler, A., D'Aoust, O., Das, M.D., Gapihan, A., Goga, S, Lakovits, C., Restrepo Cavadid, P., Singh, G., Terraza, H. (2021). *Demographic trends and urbanization.* World Bank. https://doi.org/10.1596/978-1-4648-1112-9

Barrera, M. (1979). *Race and class in the Southwest: A theory of racial inequality.* University of Notre Dame Press.

Bauer, G. R. (2014). Incorporating intersectionality theory into population health research methodology: Challenges and the potential to advance health equity. *Social Science and Medicine, 110,* 10–17. http://doi.org/10.1016/j.socscimed.2014.03.022

Berkman, L. F., Kawachi, I., & Glymour, M. M. (2014). *Social epidemiology* (2nd ed.). Oxford University Press.

Blauner, R. (1972). *Racial oppression in America.* Harper and Row.

Bowleg, L. (2012). The problem with the phrase women and minorities: Intertsectionality—an important theoretical framework for public health. *American Journal of Public Health, 102,* 1267–1773. http://refhub.elsevier.com/S0277-9536(14)00191-9/sref7

Branch, B. & Conway, D. (2022). *Health insurance coverage by race and Hispanic origin: 2021.* American community survey briefs. U.S. Census Bureau.

Braveman, P. A., Cubbin, C., Egerter, S., Chideya, S., Marchi, K. S., Metzler, M., & Posner, S. (2005). Socioeconomic status in health research: One size does not fit all. *JAMA, 294*(22), 2879–2888.

Bronfenbrenner, U. (1979). *The ecology of human development: Experiments by nature and design.* Harvard University Press.

Bronfenbrenner, U. (1989). Ecological systems theory. In R. Vasta (Ed.), *Annals of child development* (Vol. 6, pp. 187–249). Jessica Kingsley.

Brown T. N. (2003). Critical race theory speaks to the sociology of mental health: Mental health problems produced by racial stratification. *Journal of Health and Social Behavior, 44*(3), 292–301.

Cabrera, N. L. (2018). Where is the racial theory in critical race theory?: A constructive criticism of the crits. *The Review of Higher Education, 42*(1), 209–233.

Capper, C. A. (2015). The 20th-year anniversary of critical race theory in education: Implications for leading to eliminate racism. *Educational Administration Quarterly, 51*(5), 791–833. https://doi.org/10.1177/0013161X 15607616

Centers for Disease Control and Prevention. (2022). *National Diabetes Statistics Report: Estimates of diabetes and its burden in the United States.* https://www.cdc.gov/diabetes/data/statistics-report/index.html

Cerdena, J. P., Rivera, L. M., & Spak, J. M. (2021). Intergenerational trauma in Latinxs: A scoping review. *Social Science and Medicine, 270,* Article 113662. https://doi.org/10.1016/j.socscimed.2020.113662

Chang, Y., & Chatterjee, S. (2022). Housing instability, food insecurity, and barriers to healthy eating. *Family and Consumer Sciences Research Journal, 51*(1), 51–64. https://doi.org/10.1111/fcsr.12454

Cohen, A. J., Anderson, H. R., Ostro, B., Pandey, K. D., Krzyzanowski, M., Künzli, N., ... Smith, K. R. (2004). Urban air pollution. In M. Ezzati, A. D. Lopez, A. Rodgers, & C. J. L. Murray (Eds.), *Comparative quantification of health risks: Global and regional burden of disease attributable to selected major risk factors,* 2, 1353 1433. https://www.jstor.org/stable/resrep27829.22

Cohen, S., Murphy, M. L. M., & Prather, A. A. (2019). Ten surprising facts about stressful life events and disease risk. *Annual Review of Psychology, 70*(1), 577–597.

Coleman-Jensen, A., & Nord, M. (2013). *Food insecurity among households with working-age adults with disabilities.* U.S. Department of Agriculture, Economic Research Service.

Conti, A. A. (2008). Quarantine through history. In S. R. Quah & K. Heggenhougen (Eds.), *International encyclopedia of public health* (pp. 454–456). Academic Press.

Cook, J. T., & Frank, D. A. (2008). Food security, poverty, and human development in the United States. *Annals of the New York Academy of Sciences, 1136*(1), 193–209.

Cooksey-Stowers, J., Schwartz, M. B. & Brownell, K. D. (2017). Food swamps predict obesity rates better than food deserts in the United States. *International Journal of Environmental Research and Public Health, 14,* 1366. https://doi.org/10.3390/ijerph14111366

Costin, A., & Clark, A. (2022). *Air pollution and social determinants of health throughout U.S. counties.* Research Square. https://assets.researchsquare.com/files/rs-2351598/v1/0bd1b397-a11c-41d6-b83d-5c4ef48afcb8.pdf?c=1678807798

Crenshaw, K. W. (1988). Race, reform, retrenchment: Transformation and legitimation in anti-discrimination law. *Harvard Law Review, 101,* 1331–1387.

Crenshaw, K. W. (1989). Demarginalizing the intersection of race and sex: A Black feminist critique of antidiscrimination doctrine, feminist theory and antiracist politics. *The University of Chicago Legal Forum, 1,* 139–167.

Crenshaw, K. W. (1991). Mapping the margins: Intersectionality, identity politics, and violence against women of color. *Stanford Law Review, 43,* 1241–1299.

Crenshaw, K. W. (2002). The first decade: Critical reflections, or "A Foot in the Closing Door." *UCLA Law Review, 49,* 1343–1373.

Crenshaw, K. W. (2011). Twenty years of critical race theory: Looking back to move forward. *Connecticut Law Review, 43*, 1253–1352.

de la Torre, A., & Estrada, A. L. (2015). *Sana! Sana! Mexican Americans and health* (2nd ed.). The University of Arizona Press.

Delgado, R. (1990). When a story is just a story: Does voice really matter? *Virginia Law Review, 76*, 95–111.

Delgado, R. (1993). Rodrigo's sixth chronicle: Intersections, essences, and the dilemma of social reform. *New York University Law Review, 68*, 639–674.

Delgado, R., & Stefancic, J. (2001). *Critical race theory: An introduction*. NYU Press.

Diez Roux, A. V. (2004). Estimating neighborhood health effects: the challenges of causal inference in a complex world. *Social Science & Medicine, 58*, 1953–1960.

Ebin, V. J., Sneed, C. D., Morisky, D. E., Rotheram-Borus, M. J., Magnusson, A. M., & Malotte, C. K. (2001). Acculturation and interrelationships between problem and health-promoting behaviors among Latino adolescents. *Journal of Adolescent Health, 28*(1), 62–72.

Elenkov, I. J., & Chrousos, G. P. (2006). Stress system—organization, physiology and immunoregulation. *Neuroimmunomodulation, 13*(5–6), 257–267.

Encyclopaedia Britannia Online. (2023, January 22). Hans Selye. https://www.britannica.com/biography/Hans-Selye

Estrada, A. L. (2009). Mexican Americans and historical trauma theory: A theoretical perspective. *Journal of Ethnicity in Substance Abuse, 8*(3), 330–340.

Estrada, A. L., Estrada, B. D., & Quintero, G. (1999). The influence of cultural values on self-efficacy in reducing HIV risk behaviors [Working Paper Series No. 28]. Mexican American Studies & Research Center.

Estrada, A. L., & Quintero, G. A. (1999). Redefining categories of risk and identity: The appropriation of AIDS prevention information and constructions of risk. In W. Elwood (Ed.), *Power in the blood: AIDS, politics, and communication* (pp. 133–147). Routledge.

Estrada, A. L., Treviño, F., & Ray, L. (1990). Barriers to health care among Mexican Americans: Evidence from the Hispanic Health and Nutrition Examination Survey. *American Journal of Public Health, 80* (Suppl.), 27–31.

Flores, E., Tschann, J. M., Dimas, J. D., Bachen, E. A., & de Groat, C. L. (2008). Perceived discrimination, perceived stress, and mental and physical health among Mexican-origin adults. *Hispanic Journal of Behavioral Sciences, 30*(4), 401–424.

Food and Agriculture Organization. (2008). An introduction to the basic concepts of food security. In *Food security information for action: Practical guides*. EC-FAO Food Security Programme.

Forde, A. T., Crookes, D. M., Suglia, S. F., & Demmer, R. T. (2019). The weathering hypothesis as an explanation for racial disparities in health: A systematic review. *Annals of Epidemiology, 33*, 1047–2797. https://doi.org/10.1016/j.annepidem.2019.02.011

Frederick, T. J., Chwalek, C., Hughes, J., Karabanow, J., & Kidd, S. (2014). How stable is stable? Defining and measuring housing stability. *Journal of Community Psychology, 42*(8), 964–979.

Frerichs, R. (2023, March 11). John Snow. In *Encyclopedia Britannica Online*. https://www.britannica.com/biography/John-Snow-British-physician

Freudenberg, N., Galea, S., & Vlahov, D. (2005). Beyond urban penalty and urban sprawl: Back to living conditions as the focus of urban health. *Journal of Community Health, 30*(1), 1–11. https://doi.org/10.1007/s10900-004-6091-4

Gendron-Carrier, N., Gonzalez-Navarro, M., Polloni, S., & Turner, M. A. (2022). Subways and urban air pollution. *American Economic Journal: Applied Economics, 14*(1), 164–196.

Gensini, G. F., Yacoub, M. H., & Conti, A. A. (2004). The concept of quarantine in history: From plague to SARS. *Journal of Infection, 49*(4), 257–261.

Geronimus, A. T. (1992). The weathering hypothesis and the health of African-American women and infants: Evidence and speculations. *Ethnicity & Disease, 2*(3), 207–221. http://www.jstor.org/stable/45403051

Ghosh-Dastidar, B., Cohen, D., Hunter, G., Zenk, S. N., Huang, C., Beckman, R., & Dubowitz, T. (2014). Distance to store, food prices, and obesity in urban food deserts. *American Journal of Preventive Medicine, 47*, 587–595.

González Burchard, E., Borrell, L. N., Choudhry, S., Naqvi, M., Tsai, H. J., Rodriguez-Santana, J. R., ... Risch, N. (2005). Latino populations: A unique opportunity for the study of race, genetics, and social environment in epidemiological research. *American Journal of Public Health, 95*(12), 2161–2168.

Goodman, M., Naiman, J. S., Goodman, D., & LaKind, J. S. (2012). Cancer clusters in the USA: What do the last twenty years of state and federal investigations tell us? *Critical Reviews in Toxicology, 42*(6), 474–490. https://doi.org/10.3109/10408444.2012.675315

Haffner, S., Miettinen, H., & Stern, M. (1997). Are risk factors for conversion to NIDDM similar in high and low risk populations? *Diabetologia, 40*, 62–66. https://doi.org/10.1007/s001250050643

Kaiser Family Foundation. (2015). *Analysis of March 2015 Current Population Survey, Annual Social and Economic Supplement*.

Kawachi, I., Kennedy, B. P., Lochner, K., & Prothrow-Stith, D. (1997). Social capital, income inequality, and mortality. *American Journal of Public Health, 87*(9), 1491–1498.

Kelli, H. M., Hammadah, M., Ahmed, H., Ko, Y. A., Topel, M., Samman-Tahhan, A., ... Quyyumi, A. A. (2017). Association between living in food deserts and cardiovascular risk. *Circulation: Cardiovascular Quality and Outcomes, 10*(9), Article e003532.

Kessler, R. C., Mickelson, K. D., & Williams, D. R. (1999). The prevalence, distribution, and mental health correlates of perceived discrimination in the United States. *Journal of Health and Social Behavior, 40*, 208–223.

Kim, J., & Ross, C. E. (2009). Neighborhood-Specific and general social support: Which buffers the effect of neighborhood disorder on depression? *Journal of Community Psychology, 37*(6), 725–736. https://doi.org/10.1002/jcop.20327

Kleinman, A., Eisenberg, L., & Good, B. (1978). Culture, illness, and care: Clinical lessons from anthropologic and cross-cultural research. *Annals of Internal Medicine, 88*, 251–258.

Krieger, N. (1994). Epidemiology and the web of causation: Has anyone seen the spider? *Social Science and Medicine, 39*(7), 887–903. https://doi.org/10.1016/0277-9536(94)90202-x

Link, B. G., & Phelan, J. (1995). Social conditions as fundamental causes of disease. *Journal of Health and Social Behavior*, 80–94.

Luan, H., Law, J., & Quick, M. (2015). Identifying food deserts and swamps based on relative healthy food access: A spatio-temporal Bayesian approach. *International Journal of Health Geography, 14*, Article 37.

Magnan, S. (2017). *Social Determinants of Health 101 for health care: Five plus five*. National Academy of Medicine. https://doi.org/10.31478/201710c

Mainous, A. G., Diaz, V. A., & Geesey, M. E. (2008). Acculturation and healthy lifestyle among Latinos with diabetes. *The Annals of Family Medicine, 6*(2), 131–137.

Markides, K. S., & Coreil, J. (1986). The health of Hispanics in the southwestern United States: An epidemiologic paradox. *Public Health Reports, 101*(3), 253.

Mayer, M. (2003). The onward sweep of social capital: Causes and consequences for understanding cities, communities and urban movements. *International Journal of Urban and Regional Research, 27*(1), 110–132.

Mayer, S. E. (1996). Building community capacity with evaluation activities that empower. In D. M. Fetterman, S. J. Kaftarian, & A. Wandersman (Eds.), *Empowerment evaluation: Knowledge and tools for self-assessment and accountability* (pp. 332–378). SAGE.

McDonald, R., Beatley, T., McDonald, R., & Beatley, T. (2021). Cities as inhumane: The urban health penalty. In R. Mcdonald & T. Beatley (Eds.), *Biophilic cities for an urban century: Why nature is essential for the success of cities* (pp. 23–39). Springer.

Miller, C. E., & Vasan, R. S. (2021). The southern rural health and mortality penalty: A review of regional health inequities in the United States. *Social Science & Medicine, 268*, Article 113443.

Morland, K., Wing, S., & Roux, A. D. (2002). The contextual effect of the local food environment on residents' diets: The atherosclerosis risk in communities study. *American Journal of Public Health, 92*, 1761–1768

Mulatu, M. S., & Schooler, C. (2002). Causal connections between socio-economic status and health: Reciprocal effects and mediating mechanisms. *Journal of Health and Social Behavior, 43*(1), 22–41.

National Institute of Environmental Health Sciences. (2023). *Air pollution and your health*. https://www.niehs.nih.gov/health/topics/agents/air-pollution/index.cfm

Nord, M. (2007). *Characteristics of low-income households with very low food security: An analysis of the USDA GPRA food security indicator.* U.S. Department of Agriculture, Economic Research Service.

Nord, M. (2009). *Food insecurity in households with children: Prevalence, severity, and household characteristics*. U.S. Department of Agriculture, Economic Research Service.

Nord, M., Andrews, M., & Carlson, S. (2007). *Measuring food security in the United States: Household food security in the United States, 2001*. U.S. Department of Agriculture, Economic Research Service.

Nord, M., Andrews, M., & Winicki, J. (2002). Frequency and duration of food insecurity and hunger in U.S. households. *Journal of Nutrition Education and Behavior, 34*(4), 194–201.

O'Connor, D. B., Thayer, J. F., & Vedhara, K. (2021). Stress and health: A review of psychobiological processes. *Annual Review of Psychology, 72*, 663–688. https://doi.org/10.1146/annurev-psych-062520-122331

Office of Disease Prevention and Health Promotion. (n.d.). *Healthy People 2030*. U.S. Department of Health and Human Services. Retrieved February 16, 2023, from https://health.gov/healthypeople.

Parsons, T. (1951). *The social system*. The Free Press.

Pascal, M., Corso, M., Chanel, O., Declercq, C., Badaloni, C., Cesaroni, G., Henschel, H., Meister, K., Haluza, D., Martin-Olmedo, P., Medina, S., & Aphekom Group. (2013). Assessing the public health impacts of urban air pollution in 25 European cities: Results of the Aphekom project. *Science of the Total Environment, 449*, 390–400.

Pearlin, L. I. (1989). The sociology of stress. *Journal of Health and Social Behavior, 30*(3), 241–256.

Pearlin, L. I., & Bierman, A. (2013). Current issues and future directions in research into the stress process. In C. S. Aneshensel, J. C. Phelan, & A. Bierman (Eds.), *Handbook of the sociology of mental health* (pp. 325–340). Springer, Dordrecht. https://doi.org/10.1007/978-94-007-4276-5_16

Pearlin, L. I., Schieman, S., Fazio, E. M., & Meersman, S. C. (2005). Stress, health, and the life course: Some conceptual perspectives. *Journal of Health and Social Behavior, 46*, 205–219.

Plascak, J. J. Hohl, B., Barrington, W. E., & Beresford, S. A. A. (2018). Perceived neighborhood disorder, racial-ethnic discrimination and leading risk factors for chronic disease among women: California Behavioral Risk Factor Surveillance System, 2013. *SSM—Population Health, 5*, 227–238. https://doi.org/10.1016/j.ssmph.2018.07.001

Pratt, G. C., Vadali, M. L., Kvale, D. L., & Ellickson, K. M. (2015). Traffic, air pollution, minority and socio-economic status: Addressing inequities in exposure and risk. *International Journal of Environmental Research and Public Health, 12*(5), 5355–5372. https://doi.org/10.3390/ijerph120505355

Quintero, G. A., & Estrada, A. L. (1998). cultural models of masculinity and drug use: "Machismo," heroin, and street survival on the U.S.-Mexico border. *Contemporary Drug Problems, 25*, 147–168.

Rabbitt, M.P., Hales, L.J., Burke, M.P., & Coleman-Jensen, A. (2023). *Household food security in the United States in 2022* (Report No. ERR-325). U.S. Department of Agriculture, Economic Research Service. https://doi.org/10.32747/2023.8134351.ers

Richardson, A. S., Meyer, K. A., Howard, A. G., Boone-Heinonen, J., Popkin, B. M., Evenson, K. R., Kiefe, C. I., Lewis, C.E., & Gordon-Larsen, P. (2014). Neighborhood socioeconomic status and food environment: A 20-year longitudinal latent class analysis among cardia participants. *Health Place, 30*, 145–153.

Rose, D., Bodor, N., Swalm, C., Rice, J., Farley, T., & Hutchinson, P. (2009). *Deserts in New Orleans? Illustrations of urban food access and implications for policy*. University of Michigan National Poverty Center, USDA E conomic Research Service Research.

Rose, R. (2000). How much does social capital add to individual health? *Social Science & Medicine, 51*(9), 1421–1435.

Ross, C., & Mirowsky, J. (2009). Neighborhood disorder, subjective alienation, and distress. *Journal of Health and Social Behavior, 50*(1), 49–64.

Ross, C., Mirowsky, J., & Pribesh, S. (2002). Disadvantage, disorder, and urban mistrust. *City & Community, 1*(1), 59–82.

Ross, C. E., & Mirowsky, J. (2001). Neighborhood disadvantage, disorder, and health. *Journal of Health and Social Behavior, 42*(3), 258–276.

Samet, J. M., & White, R. H. (2004). Urban air pollution, health, and equity. *Journal of Epidemiology & Community Health, 58*(1), 3–5.

Sampson, R. J., Raudenbush, S. W., & Earls, F. (1997). Neighborhoods and violent crime: A multilevel study of collective efficacy. *Science, 277*(5328), 918–924.

Schiller, J.S. & Norris, T. (2023). Early release of selected estimates based on data from the 2022 National Health Interview Survey. National Center for Health Statistics, National Health Survey Early Release Program.

Schneider, D., & Lilienfeld, D.E . (2015). *Lilienfeld's foundations of epidemiology*. 4th ed. Oxford University Press.

Schwartz, S. J., & Unger, J. (Eds.). (2017). *The Oxford handbook of acculturation and health*. Oxford University Press.

Scribner, R. 1996. Paradox as paradigm: The health outcomes of Mexican Americans. *American Journal of Public Health, 86*(3), 303–305. https://doi.org/10.2105/AJPH.86.3.303

Seligman, H. K., Laraia, B. A., & Kushel, M. B. (2010). Food insecurity is associated with chronic disease among low-income NHANES participants. *Journal of Nutrition, 140*(2), 304–310.

Selye H. (1936). A syndrome produced by diverse nocuous agents. *Nature, 138*(3479), 32

Selye H. (1950). Stress and the general adaptation syndrome. *BMJ, 1*,1383–1392.

Shrider, E. A., Kollar, M., Chen, F., & Semega, J. (2021, September). *Income and poverty in the United States: 2020 – Current Population Reports*. U.S. Government Publishing Office.

Shrider, E. A., & Creamer, J. (2023). Poverty in the United States: 2022. U.S. Census Bureau. https://www.census.gov/library/publications/2023/demo/p60-280.html

Singer, M. (2005). Book review" "Epidemiology and culture." https://www.academia.edu/84972265/Book_review_Epidemiology_and_Culture

Solórzano, D. G. (1998). Critical race theory, racial and gender microaggressions, and the experiences of Chicana and Chicano scholars. *International Journal of Qualitative Studies in Education, 11,* 121-136.

Solórzano, D. G., & Yosso, T. (2001). Critical race and LatCrit theory and method: Counter-storytelling Chicana and Chicano graduate school experiences. *International Journal of Qualitative Studies in Education, 14,* 471-495.

Stokols, D. (1992). Establishing and maintaining healthy environments: Toward a social ecology of health promotion. *American Psychologist, 47,* 6-22. https://doi.org/10.1037/0003-066x.47.1.6

Stokols, D. (1996). Translating social ecological theory into guidelines for community health promotion. *American Journal of Health Promotion, 10*(4), 282-w98. https://doi.org./10.4278/0890-1171-10.4.282

Tafur, M. N., Crowe, T. K., &Torres, E. (2009). A review of curanderismo and healing practices among Mexicans and Mexican Americans. *Occupation Therapy International, 16*(1), 82-88. https://doi.org/10.1002/oti.265

Thoits, P. A. (1995). Stress, coping, and social support processes: Where are we? What next? *Journal of Health and Social Behavior,* 53-79.

Thoits, P. A. (2010). Stress and health: Major findings and policy implications. *Journal of Health and Social Behavior, 51*(Suppl. 1), S41-S53. https://doi.org/10.1177/0022146510383499

Thoits, P. A. (2011). Mechanisms linking social ties and support to physical and mental health. *Journal of Health and Social Behavior, 52*(2), 145-161. https://doi.org/10.1177/0022146510395592. PMID: 21673143.

Trostle, J. A. (2005). *Epidemiology and culture.* Cambridge University Press.

Ulrich-Lai, Y. M., & Herman, J. P. (2009) Neural regulation of endocrine and autonomic stress responses. *Nature Reviews Neuroscience, 10*(6), 397-409.

U.S. Census Bureau. (2021). *The Hispanic population in the United States: 2021.* https://www.census.gov/data/tables/2021/demo/hispanic-origin/2021-cps.html

Vega, W. A., Rodriquez, M. A., & Gruskin, E. (2009). Health disparities in the Latino population. *Epidemiologic Reviews, 31*(1), 99-112. https://doi.org/10.1093/epirev/mxp008

Velasco-Márquez, J. (2006). A Mexican viewpoint on the war with the United States. *Voices of Mexico.* http://www.revistascisan.unam.mx/Voices/pdfs/4111.pdf

Vlahov, D., Galea, S., & Freudenberg, N. (2005). The urban health "advantage." *Journal of Urban Health, 82,* 1-4.

Walker, R., Keane, C., & Burke, J. (2010). Disparities and access to healthy food in the United States: A review of food deserts literature. *Health Place, 16,* 876-884

Weiss, M. G. (2001). Cultural epidemiology: An introduction and overview. *Anthropology & Medicine, 8*(1), 5-29. https://doi.org/10.1080/13648470120070980

Weiss, M. G. (2017). *The sociology of health, healing, and illness* (9th ed.). Routledge. https://doi.org/10.4324/9781315626901

The World Bank. (2007, July 11). *More than half the world is now urban, UN report says.* https://www.worldbank.org/en/news/feature/2007/07/11/more-than-half-the-world-is-now-urban-un-report-says

Yang, T. C., & Matthews, S. A. (2010). The role of social and built environments in predicting self-rated stress: A multilevel analysis in Philadelphia. *Health and Place, 16*(5), 803-810.

Yosso, T. J. (2005). Whose culture has capital? A critical race theory discussion of community cultural wealth. *Race, Ethnicity and Education, 8,* 69-91.

Zenk, S. N., Schulz, A. J., Israel, B. A., James, S. A., Bao, S., & Wilson, M. L. (2005). Neighborhood racial composition, neighborhood poverty, and the spatial accessibility of supermarkets in metropolitan Detroit. *American Journal of Public Health, 95*(4), 660-667.

Zsembik, B. A., & Fennell, D. (2005). Ethnic variation in health and the determinants of health among Latinos. *Social Science and Medicine, 61,* 53-63. https://doi.org/10.1016/j.socscimed.2004.11.040

CHAPTER 2

The Historical, Geopolitical, and Social Contexts of Mexican American Health

LEARNING OBJECTIVES

- Describe how the origin myth of Mexica has shaped the perspectives of current Americans of Mexican descent in territorial claims.
- Analyze the historical and geopolitical foundations of health inequalities among Americans of Mexican descent.
- Explain the influence of the Spanish colonial and American neocolonial models on feelings of cultural and racial inferiority among Indigenous populations.
- Examine the social foundations of health inequalities that have destabilized the social determinants of health among Americans of Mexican descent.
- Appraise the influence of Manifest Destiny and the Mexican American War on Latinos of Mexican descent.
- Discuss the consequences the Treaty of Guadalupe Hidalgo had on Mexicans who remained in the Southwest.
- Critically assess the dimensions of Jim Crow laws in the American Southwest that affected Americans of Mexican descent.
- Evaluate how *colorism* still influences social relationships among Americans of Mexican descent.
- Assess how Americanization forced Mexican Americans to assimilate.
- Describe some of the unintended consequences of border militarization on the Mexican population in the Southwest.
- How does structural and symbolic violence manifest in the U.S.–Mexico border?
- Can the concept of historical trauma be applied to Americans of Mexican descent?

In this chapter, we will examine the historical, geopolitical, and social influences underpinning the health of Mexicans and Mexican Americans in the southwestern United States. Each has contributed to a foundation of institutionalized racism, anti-Mexican prejudice, and racial/ethnic segregation in which many of the social determinants of health have been destabilized.

Mexicans and Mexican Americans are a historically disenfranchised population. Beginning first with the Spanish conquest of Mexico and the establishment of a colonial model with the encomienda system that exploited Indigenous labor, and then with the United States and the establishment of a neocolonial model. Both have left a legacy of political disenfranchisement, mob violence and mass lynching of Latinos of Mexican descent, and other societal injustices that echo into the present. Readers should understand the importance of how historical, geopolitical, and social contexts have influenced the health and health care of the Mexican and Mexican American population residing in the United States.

The Pre-Columbian Historical Context

The ancestors of Latinos of Mexican descent, especially those Indigenous tribes who settled in the Valley of Mexico, were the Aztecs, who called themselves the Mexica. The origin story of the Mexica is imbued with colorful descriptions of an idyllic place. Aztlan, meaning "land of the herons" or "land of whiteness," has been characterized in the literature as semitropical or swampy and perhaps an island, with seven caves (Chavez, 1984, p. 13). According to Nahua legend, seven Chichimec tribes, including the Mexica, once lived in the area called Chicomoztoc—the land of the seven caves, also known as Aztlan (Rodríguez, 2014; Weber, 2003) (see Figure 2.1).

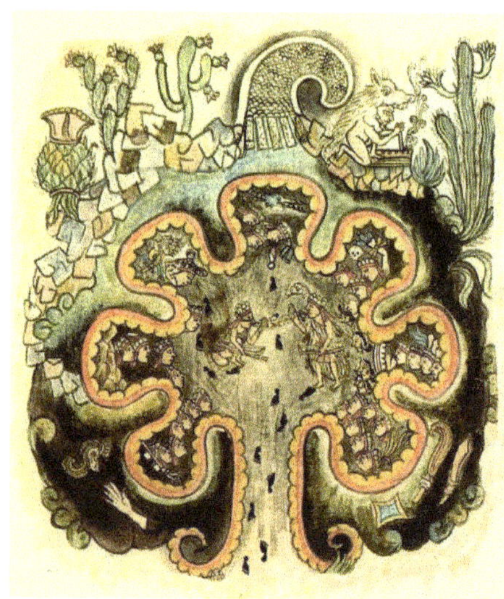

FIGURE 2.1 Chicomoztoc, Land of the Seven Caves

Some scholars have placed Aztlan in the American Southwest (Acuna, 1988; Rodríguez, 2014), while others place it in northern Mexico (Chavez, 1984; Weber, 1992). Orally preserved by the Mexica, the Aztlan origin story had been passed down through multiple generations of Mcxica by the time the Spanish arrived in 1519. Another link to the Southwest is that the Mexica spoke a Uto-Aztecan language (Nahuatl), which is found in the southwestern United States and Mexico (Shaul, 2014). Historical research shows that the Mexica were of Nahua ethnicity and originally migrated to Mexico and Central America from the "north" (Smith, 2005).

The climate in the Southwest underwent what is called the "Great Drought" from 1276–1299, which coincides with the migration of the Mexica from Aztlan (*Encyclopaedia Britannica Online*, 2012). Several Nahua-speaking tribes migrated from the "north" to the Valley of Mexico in the 1200s CE, and the Mexica were the last to arrive (Aguilar-Moreno, 2007). The Nahua currently comprise the largest Indigenous group in Mexico and the second largest in El Salvador, with about 1.5 million speakers of Nahuatl, the same language as the Mexica.

Enduring frequent attacks by the Indigenous tribes inhabiting the area around Lake Texcoco, the Mexica travelled until they came upon an island in the middle of the lake (Smith, 2005) (see Figure 2.2).

Upon the island was an eagle nesting in a nopal cactus that grew out from a rock, where legend foretold the Mexica were to build their capital city of Tenochtitlan, founded in 1325 CE, that had a population of 250,000 people at the time of Spanish contact. The number of people who inhabited the Valley of Mexico increased from 175,000 in what is called the "Early Aztec period" (1150–1350 CE) to nearly one million in the "Late Aztec period" (1350–1520 CE). Growth occurred in other parts of the Mexica Empire, with similar increases in population (Smith, 2005).

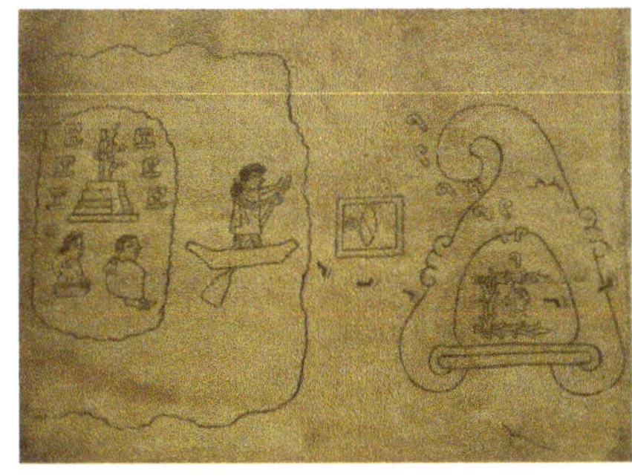

FIGURE 2.2 First Page of the Codex Boturini, Showing the Migration of the Mexica

Interestingly, the 1847 Disturnell Treaty Map of Mexico and the American West appears to show the ancient homeland of the Mexica located in modern Utah, northeast of the Great Salt Lake. A copy of the Disturnell map was used in the negotiations between Mexico and the United States that produced the Treaty of Guadalupe Hidalgo, signed on February 2, 1848, that ended the Mexican American War (1846–1848). However, the map had many errors that led to the renegotiation of the boundaries with Mexico and the Gadsden Purchase in 1853.

Real or imagined, the history and collective memory of the Mexica migration from Aztlan in the north by Latinos of Mexican descent is an important factor in the peaceful "Reconquista"—that is, the resettlement of the Mexica homeland in the Southwest. The Mexica migration story forms the basis for the ancestral claims to the Southwest by Latinos of Mexican descent (Acuna, 1988; Chavez, 1984; Meier & Rivera, 1972; Rodríquez, 2014; Weber, 1992).

Spanish Colonialism (1521–1821)

The Spanish conquest of Tenochtitlan in 1521 set the stage for the subsequent cultural destruction, oppression, and codification of a hierarchical system based on race in Mexico and New Spain (the Southwest). Conquerors write the history, and it is written that about 400 Spanish conquered Tenochtitlan and the Mexica Empire. This is not historically accurate (Smith, 2005). The conquest could not have succeeded without the assistance of a thousand Tlaxcala warriors who joined with the Spanish to overthrow the Mexica (Chavez, 1984). The "superiority myth" that the Spanish alone conquered the Mexica became well established in Mexico and their descendants for the past 500 years. Smallpox decimated the Mexica population during the final phase of the conquest in 1521, killing millions (Smith, 2003) (see Figure 2.3). Diseases for which the Mexica had no immunity against include:

- Bubonic plague
- Measles
- Smallpox
- Mumps
- Chickenpox
- Influenza
- Cholera
- Diphtheria

- Typhus
- Malaria
- Yellow fever
- Leprosy

An estimated 70%-96% of the people in the Valley of Mexico died due to these diseases, famine, and enslavement (McCaa, 1997). There were an estimated 25 million Indigenous people before the conquest and a little over a million by 1605 (McCaa, 1997). The Indigenous population did not revive until around 1650 (McCaa, 1997). The Spanish imported enslaved Africans to make up for the decrease in the Indigenous labor pool, with about 20,000 arriving in New Spain by 1553. By 1560, there were only about 20,000 Spaniards in Mexico, some of whom eventually returned to Spain.

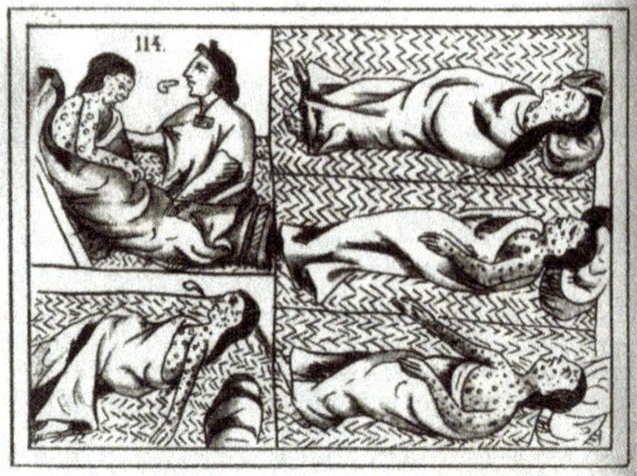

FIGURE 2.3 Introduction of Smallpox Devastated the Indigenous Populations

The Spanish Colonial Model—Subordination and Oppression

The *Spanish colonial model* was a structured relationship of domination and subordination that had at its foundation the differentiation of the social hierarchy based on nationality, race, and color that introduced social and health inequalities among the Indigenous population. A structurally designed system of exploitation and brutality that followed the initial conquest of the Mexica to control the population was introduced: the establishment of the encomienda system (Barrera, 1979; Menchaca, 1993). The relationship is established and maintained to serve the interests of all or part of the dominant group. The Spanish, then, subordinated and oppressed the Indigenous population to serve their own self-interests (see Figure 2.4).

The encomienda system was essentially slave labor, with blatant exploitation of the Indigenous population (Haring, 1947; Keith, 1971; Menchaca, 2012). The word "encomienda" is derived from the Spanish word *encomendar*, meaning "to entrust." Spanish conquistadors, civilian colonists, priests, and/or colonial officials were "entrusted" with a land grant (*repartimiento*) from the Spanish Crown from which they could exploit the land and the Indigenous people residing on it. The Indigenous people were required to provide tribute in the form of crops, foodstuffs, or animals. In many instances, Indigenous people were enslaved to work in the silver mines of Zacatecas. In return, the head of the land grant (*encomendero*) was responsible for the well-being of the Indigenous people. They were supposed to educate them in Spanish culture and convert them to Christianity. The abolishment of this brutal system occurred in 1720, some 200 years after the initial Spanish conquest of Mexico. By this time clear class distinctions

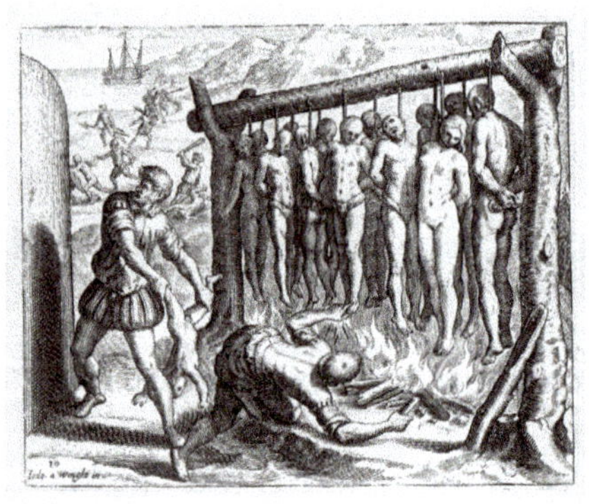

FIGURE 2.4 Spanish Hanging Indigenous Natives

had developed, as had internalized inferiority and increasing rates of alcohol abuse among the disenfranchised Indigenous population (Menchaca, 2012) (see Figure 2.5).

The Hacienda system succeeded but was not identical to the encomienda system in the northern part of New Spain—New Mexico, Arizona, California, and northern Mexico (Keith, 1971). Haciendas were less brutal in the treatment of Indigenous people but still exploited their labor. The point here is not the replacement of one system with another but rather a legacy of continued exploitation of Indigenous labor and the establishment of a hierarchical class system based on race, nationality, and color (Haring, 1947; Menchaca, 2001).

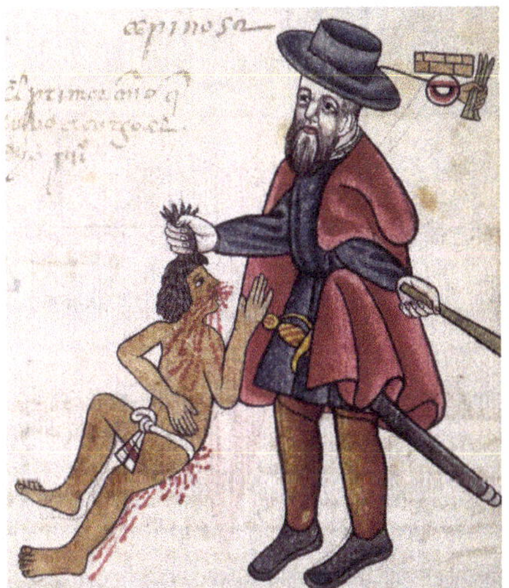

FIGURE 2.5 Mistreatment of Natives by Spanish Encomenderos

Nationality and Racial Hybrids During the Spanish Colonial Period (1521–1821)

The Spanish colonial period gave rise to social classes in the New World based on race and place of birth (Menchaca, 1993). Soon, however, the blending of Spanish and Indigenous DNA (*mestizaje*, or "racial blending") led to hybrid "racial typologies." These typologies established a hierarchical system wherein Spanish colonists and "native"-born Spaniards (those Spanish descendants of the initial conquistadores and colonists born in Mexico) were seen as superior to Indigenous peoples. The Spanish created 16 racial hybrid types (called *castas*, or "castes") based on color and "mixture percent" and enforced by law. At the top this social caste system was the White ruling class, which numbered about 1 million people by the end of the Spanish colonial period. At the top of this group were the Spanish from Spain (*peninsulares*). Below them were the Spanish born in Mexico, the Creoles (*criollos*), who by law could not hold royal office. Below them were the "hybrids" of varying skin tone with many different terms for the various, and often subjective, combinations of Europeans, Indians, and Africans (see Figure 2.6).

For example:

- *Mestizo:* persons with one peninsular parent and one Indio (Indian) parent.
- *Castizo:* persons with one mestizo parent and one Creole parent.
- *Cholos:* persons with one Indio parent and one mestizo parent.
- *Mulatos:* persons of mixed peninsular and African descent. They were sometimes enslaved.
- *Zambos:* persons who were mixed Indio and African.
- *Euromestizos:* Spanish Indian mixture with Spanish characteristics predominating.
- *Indomestizos:* Spanish Indian mixture with Indian characteristics predominating.

Español con India.
Mestizo.
Mestizo con Española
Castizo.
Castizo con Española
Español.
Español con
Mulato.

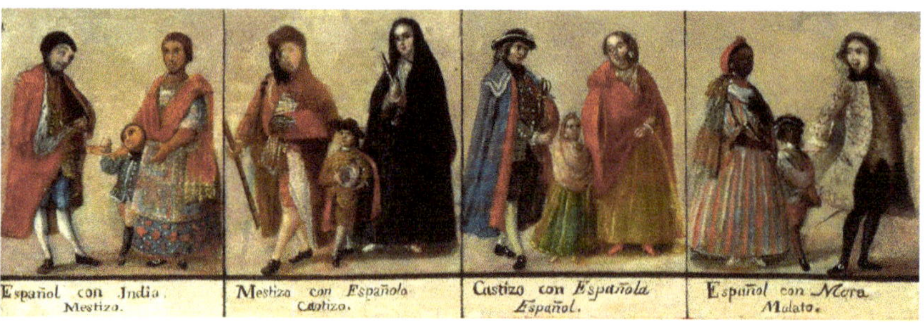

FIGURE 2.6 Spanish Colonial Racial Hybrid Types

According to Menchaca (1993), the eventual dissolution of this racialized caste system was achieved through the increase population of mestizos as well as gaining more political power among elite mestizos. Nevertheless, these Spanish colonial racial hybrids laid the foundation for continued racial and ethnic divisions based on colorism (see Figure 2.7).

Colorism is a social phenomenon that attributes privilege and power to lighter skinned individuals. It includes discriminatory practices based on skin color and is an insidious Spanish colonial legacy that continues in Mexico and among Mexican Americans to the present. For example, intraethnic preferences for lighter skinned marriage partners are ubiquitous in Mexico and Latin America (Chavez-Dueñas et al., 2014; Organista, 2009), to "cleanse the blood." The Mexican saying "*Hay que mejorar la raza o cásate con un blanco* (We need to better the race by marrying a White individual)" echoes to this prejudice based on color (Chavez-Dueñas et al., 2014, p. 17). From personal anecdotal experience, differentiation by skin tone, for example *morenos* (dark skin) and *queros* (light skin) are quite normalized, unfortunately, in everyday parlance among Mexicans and Mexican Americans in the Southwest.

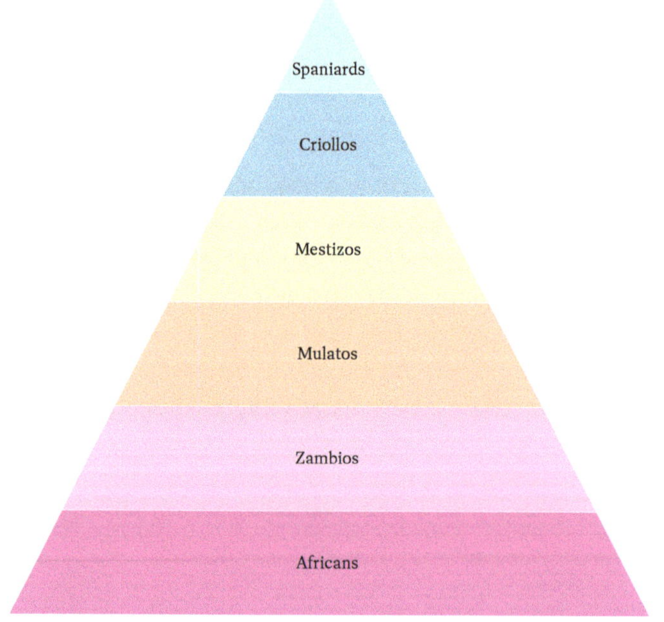

FIGURE 2.7 Abbreviated Spanish-Colonial Racial Hybrid Typology

(Adapted from Chavez-Dueñas et al., 2014, p. 7)

For almost 300 years the Spanish conquistadores and colonists viewed Mexican Indigenous populations, *mestizos*, and other racial hybrids as culturally and racially inferior to White Europeans (Menchca, 1993). As a result, the Indigenous populations of Mexico suffered from exploitation, oppression, racism, and discrimination. These social conditions led directly to cultural marginalization, destruction of Indigenous knowledge through the massive destruction of Nauahtl codices by Christian friars, with the continued perpetuation of cultural and racial inferiority, at least until Mexico declared its independence from Spain.

Mexican Independence From Spain and the Texas Revolt (1810–1836)

Mexico declared its independence from Spain in 1810, but Spain acknowledged Mexico's independence in 1821. Much of the population was now mestizo, of mixed Spanish and Mexican Indigenous heritage. Under Mexico's new constitution, racial restrictions on citizenship had been rescinded, but prejudice and discrimination toward *Indios* (Indians) remained part of Mexican society. Increased populations developed in the Mexican Southwest in areas of New Mexico (at this time Arizona was part of the New Mexico Territory), southern Texas, and the California coast, with economic sustainability derived from agriculture, mining, and ranching. Although Mexican and Spanish settlers sparsely populated the region, there was a significant Native American presence (e.g., Pueblos, Apaches, Navajos, Comanche, and Kickapoo). Like many newly emancipated former colonies of Spain, Mexico was politically and economically unstable and could not adequately protect its northern frontier.

The Mexican government invited Americans to settle in Texas, notably Stephen F. Austin and his colonists, to increase the population and help stave off attacks by Native American tribes (Brands, 2019). However, not all immigration was legal, and consequently illegal immigration by Americans into Mexican territory became a problem (Barrera, 1979).

Americans who legally migrated to the Mexican state of Texas had to become Mexican citizens, learn Spanish, become Roman Catholics, and free the people they had enslaved (Acuna, 1988). Of course, many Americans resisted. The Americans who had entered the region legally and illegally soon outnumbered the Spanish-speaking Mexicans residing there. Meier and Rivera (1972) note that an estimated ratio of six Americans to one Mexican existed in the region by 1830, thus overwhelming the Mexican population. White Americans had not encountered mestizos before. As Weber (1992) states, "From Texas to California ... Anglo Americans were shocked to meet a predominantly mestizo population. Through much of the nineteenth century, Anglo Americans generally regarded racial mixture as a violation of the laws of nature" (p. 7).

Fueled by several factors, including U.S. interest in the region (the United States had offered to purchase Texas previously), Mexico experienced a citizen uprising in 1835, and Texas declared its independence from Mexico in 1836. Weber (1992) notes that Stephen F. Austin characterized the Texas uprising against Mexico as nothing less than "a war of barbarism and of despotic principles, waged by the mongrel Spanish Indian and Negro race, against civilization and the Anglo-American race" (p. 9)

Manifest Destiny and the Mexican American War (1836–1848)

In 1845, newspaper editor John O'Sullivan coined the term "Manifest Destiny" to describe the ideology of continental expansionism (Heidler & Heidler, 2023). *Manifest Destiny* was the idea that Americans were divinely ordained to settle the entire continent of North America "from sea to shining sea." Soon, the term became a rallying cry for American expansion through Mexican territory and beyond. Since declaring its independence from Mexico, many white Texans had yearned to become annexed by the United States, and Texas did become the 28th state to enter the union in 1845. This annexation, however, led to hostilities with Mexico, coupled with a dispute over whether the Republic of Texas ended at the Nueces River (as claimed by Mexico) or the Rio Grande, which was about 150 miles further north (as claimed by Texas). It is the opinion of several scholars that President James K. Polk (1845–1849) contrived the war with Mexico and initiated the war with Mexico on May 13, 1846. Notable American leaders like Abraham Lincoln and Ulysses S. Grant were opposed to the war (Acuna, 1988; Menchaca, 2001; Weber, 2003).

Nevertheless, according to Acuna (1988) the United States waged a "brutal and violent" (p. 15) war, with indiscriminate killing of hundreds of Mexican civilians, including women and children. There were several factors that led the United States to declare war and invade Mexico. The first was the American nationalist idealism of Manifest Destiny. The second factor was greed, to gain access to the rich mineral resources, including timber, gold, and silver in the West. The third factor was the perception that Mexico and its people were culturally and racially inferior to White Americans because they were primarily Indian or of mixed-race (mestizo; Menchaca, 2012). The fourth factor was the perceived misrule by the Mexican government in the disputed territory that was under the despotic leadership of the dictator General Santa Ana (Acuna, 1988).

The Mexican American War (1846–1848) was a watershed historical and traumatic event that formed the relationship between "space" and the Mexican people inhabiting it. The United States acquired more than 500,000 square miles (1,300,000 square km) of Mexican territory through the Treaty of Guadalupe Hidalgo. Although the Mexican American War was a lopsided and short war and characterized as a stronger nation making war on a weaker one, it has had a long and lasting impact on the U.S.–Mexico border region, the people, and the ancestral claims to the land by Mexicans and Mexican Americans.

The Treaty of Guadalupe Hidalgo (1848)

The Treaty of Guadalupe Hidalgo was an imperfect treaty. Considering that Mexico lost almost 55% of its land, it benefited the United States much more than it did Mexico. With the annexation of more than 500,000 square miles, the Treaty of Guadalupe Hidalgo extended the boundaries of the United States west to the Pacific Ocean. The treaty, along with the 1853 Gadsden Purchase, created the southern border of the present-day United States with Mexico. The U.S. government paid Mexico $15 million "in consideration of the extension acquired by the boundaries of the United States" and agreed to pay American citizens debts owed to them by the Mexican government (about $3.5 million) (Treaty of Guadalupe Hidalgo, 1848) (see Figure 2.8).

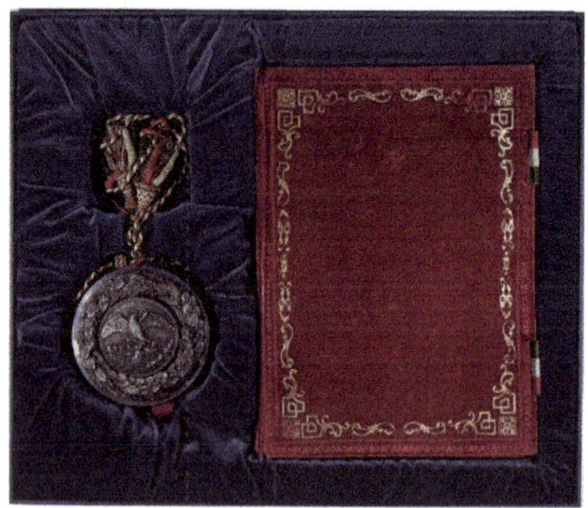

FIGURE 2.8 Treaty of Guadalupe Hidalgo, 1848

The United States ratified the treaty on March 10, 1848, and it was ratified by Mexico on May 19, 1848. On May 30, 1848, the ratifications were exchanged, and the treaty was proclaimed on July 4, 1848. Prior to ratification by the U.S. Senate, however, Article X that would have guaranteed the protection of Mexican land grants was removed without the consent of Mexico. This is an important detail given how many Mexican land grants were dissolved by legal and illegal means in what is now the American Southwest.

Other important provisions of the treaty included the protection of property and civil rights of Mexican nationals living within the new boundaries of the United States, the promise of the United States to police its boundaries because of Indian attacks, and compulsory arbitration of future disputes between the two countries. Article VIII of the treaty states:

> The said territories (the land ceded to the US), property of every kind, now belonging to Mexicans not established there, shall be inviolably respected. The present owners, the heirs of these, and all Mexicans who may hereafter acquire said property by contract shall enjoy with respect to it guarantees equally ample as if the same belonged to citizens of the United States. (Treaty of Guadalupe Hidalgo, 1848)

In addition, Article IX, states:

> The Mexicans who, in the territories aforesaid, shall not preserve the character of citizens of the Mexican Republic, conformably with what is stipulated in the preceding article, shall be incorporated into the Union of the United States, and be admitted at the proper time (to be judged of by the Congress of the United States) to the enjoyment of all the rights of citizens of the United States, according to the principles of the Constitution; and in the meantime, shall be maintained and protected in the free enjoyment of their liberty and property, and secured in the free exercise of their religion without restriction. (Treaty of Guadalupe Hidalgo, 1848)

There are no specific provisions in the treaty that preserve the Spanish language or any other "cultural rights" other than religion of Mexicans choosing to remain in the United States, as some scholars have interpreted (e.g., Acuna, 1988; Griswold del Castillo, 1992; Perrigo, 1971). On the contrary, the treaty states just the opposite, that former Mexican citizens "shall not preserve the character of citizens of the Mexican Republic, comfortably with what is stipulated in the previous article" (i.e., Article VIII) that only refers to land owned by Mexicans (Treaty of Guadalupe Hidalgo, 1848, Article IX). Many Mexicans in the now ceded territory assumed that the Spanish language would continue as a means for official transactions. However, this was not to be the case. The use of Spanish for legal and civil discourse became restricted and then eliminated altogether through legislation enacted by the conquering White Americans.

In truth, the treaty dispossessed many Mexican landowners of their homesteads, even though the treaty was supposed to protect the land rights of Mexicans remaining in the area (Acuna, 1988, p.20). Clearly, protecting Mexican land ownership was secondary to the goals of White American settlement in the region and Manifest Destiny (Griswold del Castillo, 1992).

The signing and ratification of the Treaty of Guadalupe Hidalgo in 1848 created the first Mexican Americans: those Mexicans who chose to remain in *their* native homeland and become U.S. citizens (Acuna, 1988, p. 19; Weber, 2003).

However, when the Mexican territory was annexed, the United States did not ratify the racial equality laws that had been in place in Mexico since 1821 (Menchaca, 1993). In fact, the United States enacted exclusionary Indian citizenship laws that placed the majority mestizo population in a precarious position. Mechaca (1993) states that these exclusionary laws negatively affected Mexicans with full or half-Indian ancestry, which led to political disenfranchisement of Mexicans now residing in the United States. In effect, the United States violated the Treaty of Guadalupe Hidalgo by not conferring U.S. citizenship on Mexicans who looked Indian.

In summary, although the Treaty of Guadalupe Hidalgo was supposed to protect the civil liberties of Mexicans who chose to remain in their native homeland, it did not. The United States did not enforce the recognition of Mexican or Spanish land grants, withheld full U.S. citizenship from Mexicans if they appeared Indian, and disenfranchised them politically by not outlawing poll taxes and racial segregation.

United States Neocolonialism and Creating a Neocolonial Labor Force (1848–1930)

Derived from the Spanish colonial model, the *internal colonial model* (*ICM*) instituted by the United States integrates the economic and political interests of the dominant group to maintain hegemony over subordinate minority groups. Structured to benefit White Americans, the ICM exploits Mexican labor and imposes a hierarchical segmentation of occupations of Mexican American workers. Implicit in the ICM is the creation of a "racially stratified labor force" of Mexican American workers to support the dominant White American infrastructure (Barrera, 1979, p. 35).

Ethnocentrism and racist ideologies of White superiority undergirded the relationship between White Americans and Mexican Americans. Mexican Americans were employed in the most menial and low-paying occupations (occupational stratification) and were often segregated to a particular area of the neighborhood or town "barrios." Mexicans were restricted to the most menial jobs because of their "race." One employer noted that because Mexicans were used to stooping, bending, and squatting, they were ideal for agricultural labor (Barrera, 1979).

Prejudice gave way to actual discrimination in housing, education, and employment. For example, in Arizona, mining towns had separate housing and schools that were set aside for Mexican Americans (Blakemore, 2018). These were usually of poorer quality than those for White people, with substandard education geared toward domestic and semiskilled labor. Occupationally, there was a two-wage system, with Mexicans earning less than White people for the same amount of work accomplished (Acuna, 1988; Barrera, 1979; Griswold del Castillo, 1975; Meier & Rivera, 1972).

With the advent of the railroad, silver and copper mining, increased agricultural production, and livestock, Mexicans and Mexican Americans were assigned to the more labor-intensive aspects of these occupations that were often accompanied by harsh and sometimes dangerous working conditions. Mexicans and Mexican Americans were often treated with disdain and suffered from prejudice and discrimination by White Americans (Acuna, 1988). Menial labor became synonymous with being of Mexican descent. According to Acuna (1988) Mexicans experienced "dispersal, isolation, migrancy, and poverty" (p. 163). Mexican Americans were treated as a conquered people with limited civil rights, subordination to American hegemony, and oppression (social control) by police, federal agents, and employers.

Exploitation of Mexican labor, and the hope among Mexicans for a better life in the United States conflated to increase Mexican immigration to the southwestern United States and beyond. The Mexican-origin population living in the United States increased from around 100,000 in 1900 to about 640,000 by 1930 (Barrera, 1979, p. 66). Many Mexican immigrants settled beyond the southwestern states into the Midwest, where they were employed in meat packaging and railroad yards (Acuna, 1988).

After the Great Depression, the Bracero Program officially known as the Mexican Farm Labor Program was initiated on August 4, 1942, to employ inexpensive Mexican labor to replace American labor shortages during WWII, especially in agriculture. This program increased the Mexican-origin population in the Southwest and other areas in the United States on a contractual basis, meaning that they were only temporarily allowed to work in the United States. Unionization of Mexican labor was opposed in many southwestern border states (Acuna, 1988), and in Texas unionization proved almost impossible given the disempowered status of Mexicans. As quoted in Acuna (1988), "Stuart Jamieson writes that 'Mexicans (in Texas) ... had a social and economic status similar to that of Negroes in other sections of the South. They were a large, lowly paid racial minority, and most of them were disenfranchised by the State poll tax'" (p. 164).

The historical context of Latinos of Mexican descent has placed them in a subordinate status to White Americans. Mexicans have been racialized as inferior to White people, and analogous to Black people, they have endured multiple acts of violence, discrimination, and racism beginning in the early 1800s. The prevailing idea was that if only their "inferior" culture could be changed or modified, they potentially could become more like White Americans.

Americanization Processes—Forced Assimilation (1854–Present)

Along with Native American tribes, Mexicans and Mexican Americans residing in the territory conquered by the United States became subject to Americanization processes that attempted to eradicate their traditional cultures and languages. For Mexicans and Mexican Americans, Americanization processes included forced assimilation and the enforcement of "Juan Crow" laws—that is, discrimination toward Mexicans based on their race and ethnicity.

"Mexican schools" and "Indian schools" were common in the American Southwest and lingered through the 1950s. Mexican American students continued to attend mostly segregated schools in the southwestern United States. As well, Mexican American students caught speaking Spanish in school were subject to corporal punishment, which unfortunately has continued to the present.

Unlike the South, which had explicit laws barring African American children from "White schools," laws in some southwestern states did not codify segregation. Rather, it was based on "de facto" segregation. Mexicans and Mexican Americans were excluded from restaurants, movie theaters, community swimming pools, and schools. In the states of California and Arizona, however, because of their mixed-Indian ancestry, they enacted "de jure" segregation on the basis that Mexican and Mexican American students were Indian (Donato et al., 1991). Consequently, separate Mexican schools in these states began in the 1870s and continued through the 1950s. In the beginning, these schools were set up to serve the children of Spanish-speaking laborers on rural ranches or agricultural areas. Soon, however, the concept of segregated "Mexican" schools spread to urban areas as well. In 1935, California passed legislation officially segregating Mexican students, especially those who "looked Indian" (Menchaca, 1993). Blakemore (2018) states, "Children were arbitrarily forced to attend based on factors like their complexion and last name" ("Latino Children Suffered" section).

Mexican schools were generally housed in rundown buildings. They employed less-experienced teachers than the White schools, and children of Mexican descent were given worn-out books and equipment and were taught in more crowded classrooms than non-Latino White children. The greatest difference between the schools was in their curricula. While geometry and biology were taught at the White schools, classes at the Mexican schools focused on teaching boy's industrial skills and teaching girl's vocational tasks (Arriola, 1995; Blakemore, 2018). Many White educators did not expect or encourage students of Mexican descent to advance beyond the eighth grade. For example, the school superintendent for Garden Grove, one of the schools sued, stated that Mexicans "were an alien race that should be segregated socially" (as quoted in Federal Bar Association, 2021, The Trial section). According to this individual, "Mexicans were 'less sturdy' than Whites, indifferent towards education, and needed to be taught 'social behavior,' that is, cleanliness, manners, 'cleanliness of mind,' and 'the ability to get along'" (as quoted in Federal Bar Association, 2021, The Trial section). School segregation for Mexican children was common in Arizona, Texas, and California, where 80 % of districts in 1931 were officially segregated, and the other 20% had off-the-record segregation rules (Blakemore, 2018; Gonzales, 2013).

On February 18, 1946, the sitting judge Paul McCormick issued his ruling that the school districts were in fact discriminating against Mexican Americans (*Mendez v. Westminster* 1946), which helped to end the Mexican school designation. Followed by *Brown v. Board of Education* (1954), these lawsuits effectively ended "separate but equal" schools for Mexican Americans and other historically disadvantaged minority groups in the United States.

Americanization processes continue through to the present time. English-only policies are one example. Beginning immediately after the U.S. conquest of the Mexican Southwest, the Spanish language was phased out of all legal and official documentation (Acuna, 1988). Only in 1975 were languages other than English required to be placed on certain voting materials (Al Jazeera, 2020). Interestingly, only two of the four U.S.-Mexico border states, Arizona, and California, have English-only laws, and Arizona's has been declared unconstitutional. The English-only movement has strong ties to anti-immigrant and racist ideologies (Padilla et al., 1991).

In sum, 200 years of U.S. neocolonialism has led to:

- Two thirds of Mexico being seized and occupied
- The subjugation and exploitation of Mexican landowners and laborers
- White ethnocentrism
- Denial of U.S. citizenship rights to Mexicans of Indian descent
- Discrimination and racism directed toward Latinos of Mexican descent
- Physical violence directed toward Latinos of Mexican descent
- The establishment of an internal colonial model that subjugates and oppresses Latinos of Mexican descent
- Increased U.S.-Mexico border militarization and DHS surveillance
- Internalized cultural and racial inferiority among Latinos of Mexican descent

The Geopolitical Context

"We didn't cross the line, the line crossed us" is a popular saying among Mexican Americans. Certainly, the Mexican American War (1846-1848) and the Gadsden Purchase (1853) were major geopolitical events of the middle of the 19th century. They represent a collective memory of conquest, political disenfranchisement, and land loss that resonates among Mexicans and Mexican Americans through to the present day (Chavez, 1984). Why? Because of the perpetual flow of people over millennia across a political boundary that has only existed for the past 200 years. One can argue that the growing militarization of the U.S.-Mexico border and increasing authority of U.S. Homeland Security are consequences of that war.

The U.S.-Mexico Border Patrol and U.S.-Mexico Border Militarization (1924–Present)

"Poor Mexico, so far from God, so close to the United States" is a well-known saying attributed to Mexican Dictator Porfirio Diaz (1830–1915), which captures the sentiment of Mexico's relationship with the expansionist and strong economic power of the United States (see Figure 2.9).

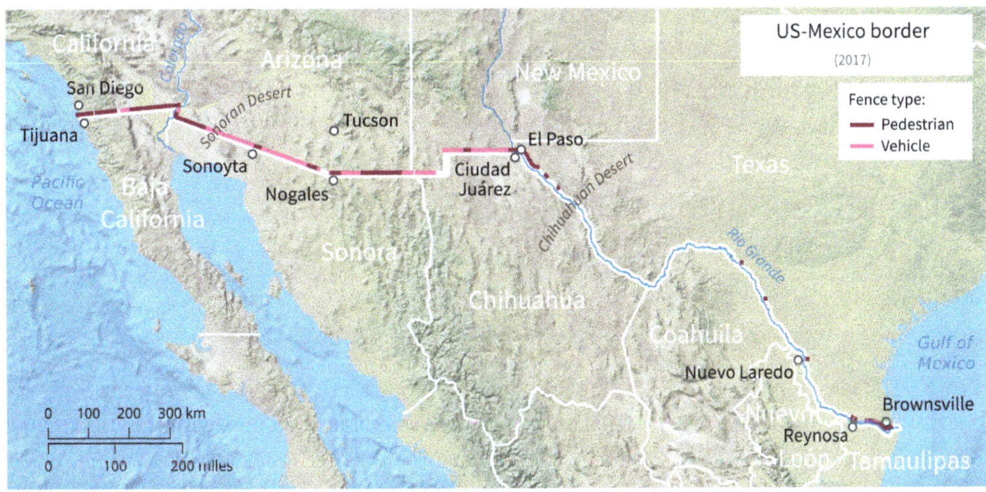

FIGURE 2.9 The U.S.-Mexico Border

Though the U.S. Border Patrol was established in 1924 and some militarization of the U.S.-Mexico border region occurred prior to recent decades, it has been in the years following the 9/11 attack that the U.S.-Mexico border has experienced unprecedented militarization. During the first 2 decades of the 21st century, militarization has steadily increased and become normalized at the U.S.-Mexico border and within U.S. border enforcement agencies. When the Department of Homeland Security (DHS) was created in 2002, the agency formerly known as Immigration and Naturalization Services (INS) was moved from the Department of Justice to DHS, and immigration enforcement programs and policy emphasized a focus on antiterrorism.

President Clinton's immigration policy— "prevention through deterrence"—had the consequences of creating "death corridors" through the Sonoran Desert and increasing migrant deaths (Binational Migration Institute, 2021).

Border militarization is the systematic intensification of the U.S.-Mexico border's security infrastructure, transforming the area from a transnational frontier to a zone of permanent vigilance, enforcement, and violence (Dunn, 1996; Kil, 2019). The term "low-intensity conflict" is used to describe these, and other actions taken up by the U.S. Department of Homeland Security, including random raids and roundups of suspected "illegals." It provides additional subordination and social control over Mexicans and Native Americans through a form of militarization where military forces take on police functions and vice versa (Dunn, 1996; Kil, 2019). In fact, some local police departments have agreed to perform these types of security checks when interacting with persons who appear to be Mexican. Scholars argue that the U.S.-Mexico border is an imagined "war zone," where the war on drugs, crime, and undocumented immigration are occurring. The consequences of the increased militarization of U.S.-Mexico border includes increased violence, civil rights violations of U.S. citizens and legal residents, unreported abuses, and death (Kil, 2019; Binational Migration Institute, 2021). Kil (2019) aptly refers to policies that directly or indirectly facilitate the deaths of migrants as *necropolitics* "that brutalizes the public and incites racial hatred toward immigrants" (Kil & Menjívar, 2006; Kil et al., 2009). Kil (2019) further contends that the border region is a "necropolitical deathscape that affects immigrants' lives well beyond the discrete border region, making them more vulnerable and exploitable" (p. xxxiv).

Mass deportations of Mexicans and Mexican Americans began during the 1930s, increased dramatically during the 1940s and 1950s, and have continued to the present. Virtually no other Latino subgroup has been singled out historically and over decades for forcible removal and detention more than Latinos of Mexican descent (see Table 2.1).

TABLE 2.1 Homeland Security Border Operations, 1954–Present

Border Patrol/ Homeland Security operation	Timeline	Description
Operation "Wet Back"	1954	Used military-style tactics to remove Mexican immigrants—some of them American citizens—from the United States.
Operation "Hold the Line"	1993	A preventative measure taken by the U.S. Border Patrol, initiated on September 19, 1993, on the U.S.-Mexico border in El Paso; 400 border agents formed a human and vehicle blockade along the border to keep illegals out.
Operation "Gate Keeper"	1994	Aimed at halting illegal immigration to the United States at the U.S.-Mexico border near San Diego, California.
Operation "Endgame"	2003–2012	A 2003–2012 plan implemented by the Office of Detention and Removal Operations (DRO) of the U.S. Department of Homeland Security Bureau of Immigration and Customs Enforcement to detain and deport all removable aliens and "suspected terrorists" currently living in the United States by 2012.
Operation "Front Line"	2004–2005	An initiative of U.S. Immigration and Customs Enforcement (ICE), a division of the Department of Homeland Security, that operated in the months leading up to the 2004 presidential election and through the 2005 presidential inauguration. It focused on immigration violators who may have imposed an enhanced public safety or national security threat.

Border Patrol/ Homeland Security operation	Timeline	Description
Operation "Streamline"	2005–Present	Created with the goal of combating drug trafficking, weapons trafficking, human smuggling, and repeat illegal immigration into the United States. Its goal is to achieve a 100% criminalization of unauthorized border crossing. Cases are not heard individually but rather in large groups, with many people caught crossing the border together generally being processed in one case.
Operation "Return to Sender"	2006–2007	A massive sweep of illegal immigrants by the ICE agency that began on May 26, 2006. According to ICE, the campaign has focused on individuals deemed to be the most dangerous, including convicted felons and gang members, as well as repeat offenders, some of whom had already been deported.
Operation "Jump Start"	2006–2008	A military operation to aid U.S. Customs and Border Protection, announced by President George W. Bush in May 2006. The mission entailed the deployment of U.S. National Guard troops along the Mexico–U.S. border for purposes of enforcement of border security and construction of a border fence. The rules of deployment were defined in a memorandum of agreement between officials in the Department of Defense and the governors of Arizona, California, New Mexico, and Texas as well as Mexico.
Operation "Phalanx"	2010–2016	Succeeded Operation Jump Start through the employment of military-style helicopters for drug and human smuggling interdiction. It was a U.S. National Guard program aimed to assist the Department of Homeland Security in the security of the Mexico–U.S. border.
Operation "Faithful Patriot"	2018–Present	A routinized domestic deployment and civil contingency operation of the U.S. Armed Forces at the Mexico–U.S. border. According to the U.S. Northern Command, the operation is being conducted to prevent potential border crossing of migrants from Central America.

The consequences of the militarized U.S.-Mexico border include increased violence, continued community disunity, unreported abuses, and death. According to a report by the Binational Migration Institute (2021), there have been several deadly "funneling" effects because of U.S. immigration law:

- *Initial Funnel Effect* (1990–1999): represented a period in southern Arizona before undocumented migration began to concentrate in the Tucson Sector. The strategy explicitly intended to prevent undocumented border crossing in urban areas such as San Diego-Tijuana and El Paso-Ciudad Juárez forcing migrants into the southwestern deserts.
- *Secondary Funnel Effect* (2000–2005): continued to divert undocumented border crossings from the San Diego-Tijuana and El Paso-Ciudad Juárez to crossing corridors into southern Arizona. This period was characterized by a relatively constant volume of apprehensions in the Tucson Sector, with at least 35% of all U.S. Border Patrol apprehensions occurring in this region.
- *Tertiary Funnel Effect* (2006–2013): was characterized by a decline in apprehensions in the Tucson Sector, while still constituting at least 20% of all southwestern border apprehensions.
- *Localized Funnel Effect* (2014–2020): represents a period in which the proportion of southwestern Border Patrol apprehensions occurring in the Tucson Sector dropped below 20%. This period was also characterized by an increase in apprehensions of Central Americans in the Tucson Sector, particularly of Guatemalans. (pp. 7–9)

Although the findings of the report are focused on immigrants from Mexico and Central America, there is a shared affinity among many Mexican Americans based on a shared hemispheric and regional area and Indigenous ancestry.

Heightened Mexican American Community Surveillance and Legal Violence

Coupled with increasing militarization and the use of local police agencies to assist in the identification of illegal immigrants, Mexican American neighborhoods have come under increasing surveillance. It is not uncommon to observe U.S. Border Patrol vehicles in these neighborhoods. As well, mass roundups of "suspected" illegal immigrants oppresses Mexican Americans who become suspects for no other reason than being brown-skinned. Critical race theory helps explain the oppressive nature of intensified surveillance by local and federal police enforcement agencies in controlling non-White populations and providing a "show of force" in Mexican American neighborhoods that places everyone with brown skin under suspicion.

The U.S. Border Patrol expanded their infrastructure, including interior checkpoints and surveillance towers, associated with its "defense in depth" strategy. This strategy sought to deploy enforcement chokepoints to force immigrants to travel greater distances and thereby increase opportunities for detection and interdiction by U.S. federal and local authorities. As mentioned previously, roundups of suspected illegal immigrants by INS were common in California and Arizona. For example, the Chandler Roundups received international attention for their obvious racialized profiling. As Romero (2006) states:

> The Chandler Roundup fits into a larger pattern of immigration law enforcement practices that produce harms of reduction and repression and place Mexican Americans at risk before the law and designate them as second-class citizens with inferior rights. Latino residents experienced

> racial affronts targeted at their "Mexicanness" indicated by skin-color, bilingual speaking abilities, or shopping in neighborhoods highly populated by Latinos. ... Individuals stopped were demeaned, humiliated and embarrassed. Stops and searches conducted without cause were intimidating and frightening, particularly when conducted with the discretionary use of power and force by law enforcement agents. In urban barrios, the costly enterprise of selected stops and searches, race-related police abuse, and harassment results in deterring political participation, identifying urban space racially, classifying immigrants as deserving and undeserving by nationalities, and serves to drive a wedge dividing Latino neighborhoods on the basis of citizenship status. (pp. 447–448)

Moreover, increased community surveillance by law enforcement officers (LEOs) increases the probability of negative encounters and encounters ending in legal homicides. Price and Khubchandani (2023) found that between 2011 and 2020, LEOs killed 1,158 Latinos. The majority of those killed were males (96.2%). with the majority being shot (89.9%). Two thirds (66.9%) of those killed were Hispanics 20–39 years of age and from the Southwest. Although California has the highest number of legal homicides, New Mexico has the highest legal homicide rate per 100,000. The rate of fatal encounters with LEOs for Latinos grew by 44.4% over the decade, with the highest rate occurring in 2020 (see Table 2.2).

TABLE 2.2 Mortality Rates of Latinos by Law Enforcement Officers in U.S.–Mexico Border States, 2011–2020

State	Number	Rate per 100,000 population
California	462	.29
Texas	144	.14
New Mexico	98	1.02
Arizona	50	.23

Source: Price and Khubchandani (2023)

Structural and Symbolic Violence in the American Southwest

Bourgois (2001) distinguished between four types of violence: political, structural, symbolic, and everyday (normalized) violence. *Political violence* refers to "targeted physical violence and terror administered by official authorities and those opposing it, such as military repression, police torture, and armed resistance" (Bourgois, 2001, Chart 1). *Structural violence* is "chronic, historically entrenched political-economic oppression and social inequality, ranging from exploitative international terms of trade to abusive local working conditions and high infant mortality rates" (Bourgois, 2001, Chart 1). Structural violence includes extreme poverty, food insecurity, homelessness, insufficient educational resources, and unemployment. Clearly, various forms of structural violence fundamentally destabilize the social determinants of health.

Symbolic violence is a term developed by Bourdieu (2001) that characterizes "the internalized humiliations and legitimations of inequality and hierarchy ranging from sexism and racism to intimate expressions of class power" (Chart 1). The insidious nature of symbolic violence is that it requires the complicity, conscious or unconsciously, of those who are being denigrated. *Everyday violence* is "expressions of interpersonal aggression that serve to normalize violence at the micro-level such as domestic, delinquent and sexual conflict, and even substance abuse" (Bourgois, 2001, para. 3). Thus, behavioral risk factors for disease, interpersonal violence against women, and gang violence are all forms of normalized societal behavior.

Structural and symbolic violence has a profound legacy in the U.S.-Mexico border region in what is described by Kil (2019) as a "necropolitical deathscape" (p. xxxiv) where immigrant deaths have little or no meaning in the larger context of U.S.-Mexico border security. Symbolic violence is enacted through covert methods and procedures that demean the human dignity of Mexicans and Mexican Americans within the U.S.-Mexico border region and beyond. Symbolic violence includes anti-Mexican sentiment, the internalization of negative stereotypes by adolescent Mexicans, feelings of inadequacy, and self-hate. Symbolic violence serves to legitimize social and health inequalities as well as the status quo of non-Latino White Americans that in turn uses racism and ethnocentrism to subordinate and oppress Latinos of Mexican descent (Sabo et al., 2014; Sabo & Lee, 2015). Fear and suspicion engendered by anti-Mexican sentiment prevents individuals and family members from accessing health care and enabling victimization because they fear deportation. The "spillover effect" of anti-Mexican sentiment, as Sabo and Lee (2015) suggest, affects Mexican Americans and legal residents of Mexican descent through the negative internalization of "illegality."

Structural violence against Latinos of Mexican descent includes:

- The indefinite separation and detention of Mexican children and families
- The continued exploitation of Mexican immigrant labor
- The continued violation of U.S. citizen civil rights of Mexican Americans by federal and local law enforcement officers
- Racial profiling and the criminalization of "Mexicanness"
- An uncertain future for Mexican minors, especially U.S.-born children deported to Mexico
- The exclusion of suspected Mexican immigrants and their children from education, health care, and social services
- The denial of other forms of socioeconomic resources necessary for upward economic mobility and assimilation into U.S. society

The Social Context

Anti-Mexican sentiment, prejudice, and discrimination in housing, voting, employment, and education serve to undermine the beneficial enhancements of the social determinants of health and provide a foundation of racial and ethnic inequality in the United States. Legal and symbolic violence toward Mexican Americans is entrenched in the Southwest due to the construction of racial and ethnic "otherness" through which non-Latino White Americans can oppress and discriminate against them.

Lynching and Mob Violence Toward Mexican Americans (1848–1928)

The dark history of mass lynching and the lynching of individuals, including Mexican women and children, is not well known outside of the southwestern United States. Lynching is a legacy shared with Black Americans, some of whom were lynched in the southern United States during the Reconstruction Era and into the mid-20th century.

Mob violence against Mexicans is not new. The earliest case of Mexican lynching occurred soon after the end of the Mexican American War in 1849 and continued into the early 20th century (Carrigan & Webb, 2017). Carrigan and Webb (2017) conducted a massive in-depth study of over 500 cases of Mexican victims of mob violence in the United States from 1848–1928 (see Figure 2.10). The majority of Mexican victims, including women, were accused of committing murder (55.4%), so perhaps "frontier justice" played a part in their demise. Additionally, a large percentage of Mexicans were hanged for property crimes such as theft or robbery (17.9%).

Carrigan and Webb (2017) state, "Allegations of property crimes were a dominant thread of history of mob violence against Mexicans and such charges provided a link across time and space for mobs executing Mexicans" (p. 67). Pejorative Mexican stereotypes, such as being conniving, unprincipled, untrustworthy, treacherous, and cowardly, grew out from these experiences with non-Latino White Americans.

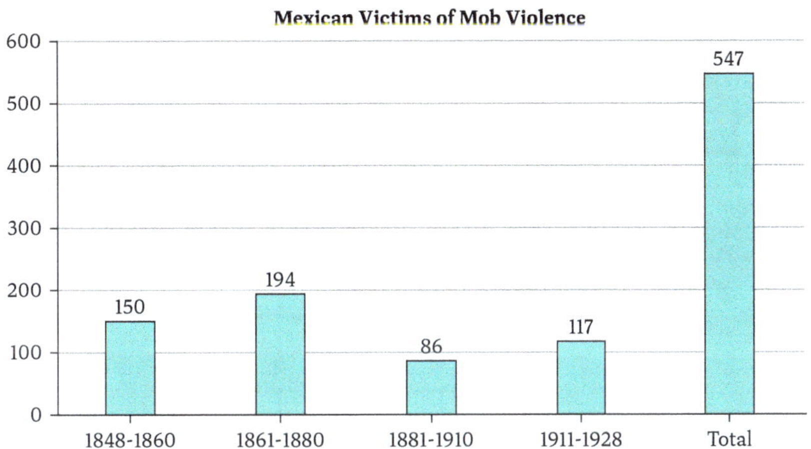

FIGURE 2.10 Confirmed Mexican Victims of Mob Violence, United States, 1848–1928

(Adapted from Carrigan & Webb, 2017, p. 30)

In July 1857, in the vicinity of Goliad, Texas, White vigilantes attacked Mexican ox cart drivers and stole their cargo, which became known as the "Ox Cart Wars" (Esquivel, 2019). It is believed that some 70 Mexican ox cart drivers were killed, and some were hanged from a tree that would come to be known as the "Cart War Oak." The tree is still there today and serves as a reminder of Mexican American social and judicial injustice.

As Carrigan and Webb (2017) note, there is overwhelming evidence that racial prejudice against Mexicans was most vehement in Texas. Their data indicates that "Texas executed more Mexicans than any other state" (Carrigan & Webb, 2017, p. 56). In fact, Texas was responsible for 92% (108 of 117) of the Mexicans

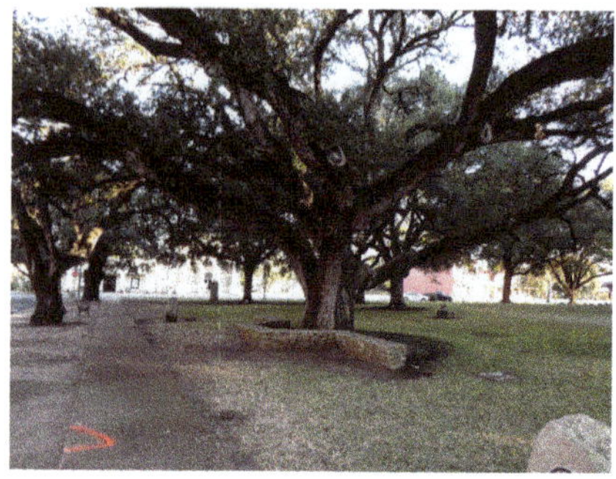

FIGURE 2.11 Cart War Hanging Tree, Goliad, Texas

executed in the early part of the 20th century. Additionally, the study documented other acts of violence, such as murder, beatings, and driving Mexicans off their lands.

The Los Angeles Times published an article in 2019 written by Paloma Esquivel that highlighted several of the atrocities committed against Mexicans by White Americans. Beginning in 1849, Mexicans were systematically excluded from gold mining operations in California, just after gold was discovered in Sutter Creek in 1848.

In 1915, *El Matanza* (The Massacre) occurred when Texas Rangers indiscriminately shot and killed dozens of Mexicans without questioning, solely based on the assumption of their allegiance to Mexican bandits in the area. In 1918, Texas Rangers, soldiers, and local White ranchers surrounded the village of Porvenir, in West Texas. Waking families from their slumber, they singled out 15 unarmed men and boys from the rest of the residents and lynched them. The mass lynching resulted in the residents of Porvenir abandoning their village and fleeing to Mexico. Again, in Texas, in 1912, 300-armed White people forced Mexican residents to leave Breckenridge, Texas. Over the years, the Texas Rangers have become notorious in the minds of Mexican Americans for their past terrorist activities and have become synonymous with hate crimes against Mexicans, Mexican Americans, and Native Americans in Texas.

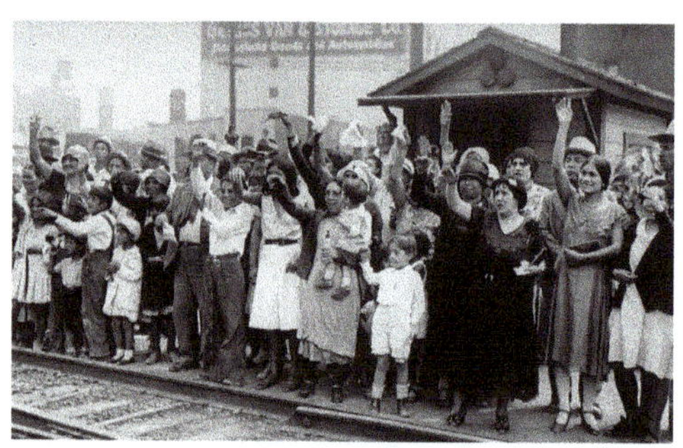

FIGURE 2.12 1930s Mexican Deportations, Los Angeles, California

During one of the mass deportations of Mexicans from 1929–1936, federal immigration agents raided Olvera Street in Los Angeles, California, a predominantly Mexican part of "old town," and began arresting Mexicans and taking them to trains to be summarily deported to Mexico (Figure 2.12). Many of these persons were Mexican Americans—that is, U.S. citizens residing legally in the United States. Some historical reports indicate that as many as 60% of Mexican children deported during this time were born in the United States but were deported because they were "culturally Mexican" nevertheless (Menchaca, 2012). Unfortunately, Mexican American children—that is, U.S. citizens—are still being deported with their Mexican parents, many of whom are suffering from depression and educational deficiencies (Lovato et al., 2018; Vargas & Ybarra, 2017).

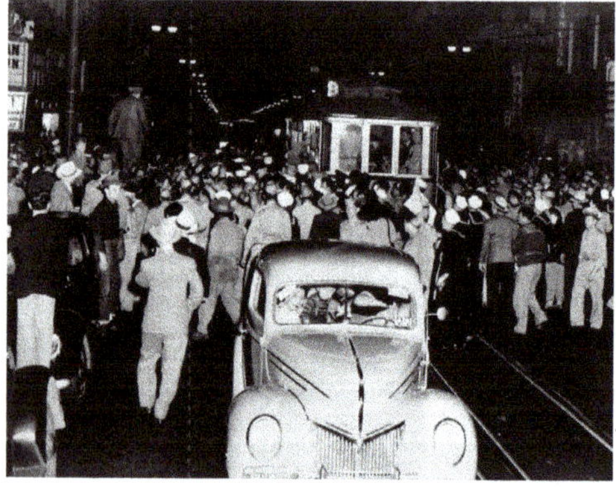

FIGURE 2.13 Zoot Suit Riots, Los Angeles, 1943

In the summer of 1943, another racially motivated incident occurred when a mob of U.S. sailors and other U.S. service men as well as White citizens roamed downtown Los Angeles searching for Mexican Americans wearing "zoot suits," a fashion at the time worn by young Black Americans and Mexican Americans. They would beat the young Mexican American men wearing the zoot suits and strip them of their clothes (see Figure 2.13).

Anti-Mexican Sentiment, Prejudice, and Discrimination

Beginning well before the Mexican American War, negative attitudes toward the Spanish and virulent anti-Mexican sentiment was prevalent among White American settlers (referred to as "Anglos" by local Mexicans). The Spanish spoke a different language, had a different religion (Roman Catholicism), and were perceived as having accomplished relatively little in developing the Southwest. After the Mexican American War, anti-Mexican sentiment became even more vicious. As Weber (1992) states:

> The bloodshed in Texas at the Alamo, Goliad, and San Jacinto, which had no parallel elsewhere in the Borderlands, hardened attitudes on both sides and left a deep reservoir of Anglo-American hatred toward Mexicans and their Hispanic forefathers. ... Hispanophobia, with its particularly vitriolic anti-Mexican variant, also served as a convenient rationale to keep Mexicans "in their place." (p. 10)

A series of incidents occurred that slowly escalated to outright brutality against Mexican Americans in the Southwest (Acuna, 1988; Carrigan & Webb, 2017; Esquivel, 2019; Weber, 1992). Similar to the experiences of Black Americans in the south, forced resettlement and violence were hallmarks of the American Southwest. Carrigan and Webb (2017) indicate that "no matter how highly regarded a Spanish speaker might be due to his or her class status or elite background ... whites reserved the prerogative to deny them basic citizenship rights" (p. 57).

Additionally, White Americans viewed Mexicans as very similar to American Indians, especially those Mexicans with darker skin and features. In fact, in Texas and California the legislatures legally identified Mexicans as Indians for political, legal, and social expediency, primarily for exclusionary policies (Menchaca, 2001). Menchaca (2001) argues that because Mexicans are partially of Indian descent, their darker skin and appearance makes them a target for discrimination by White Americans and the U.S. judicial system.

Most Americans believe that racism and discrimination are alive and well in the United States (Robert Wood Johnson Foundation, 2017). Specifically, the Robert Wood Johnson Foundation (2017) found that 92% of Black Americans and 78% of Latinos believe there is discrimination toward their group. The proportion of each group experiencing personal discrimination varied but was overall higher for Black people than Latinos. For example, when applying for jobs, 56% of Black Americans compared to 33% of Latinos felt discriminated against. In addition, 37% of Latinos reported experiencing racial or ethnic slurs, compared to 51% of Black Americans. Nevertheless, Latinos report significant personal discrimination experiences. With reference to institutional forms of discrimination, nearly a third of Latinos say they have been personally discriminated against because they are Latino when applying for jobs (33%), when being paid equally or considered for promotions (32%), and when trying to rent a room or apartment or buy a house (31%). Additionally, at least 20% of Latinos say they or a family member have been treated unfairly by the courts (20%) or unfairly stopped or treated by the police (27%) because they are Latino. The Robert Wood Johnson Foundation study also found that nonimmigrant Latinos are nearly twice as likely as immigrant Latinos to report that they or a family member have been stopped or unfairly treated by the police because they are Latino. The study concludes that Latinos continue to face personal and institutional forms discrimination, with Latinos who are younger, college educated, and nonimmigrant reporting a higher proportion of discrimination incidents than others.

In a 2021 report, the Pew Research Center reported on the discrimination experiences of Latinos (with no differentiation by Latino origin type). Overall, Latinos with darker skin report more discrimination experiences than Latinos with lighter skin. For example, 62% of Latinos indicated that darker skin color interferes with the ability to get ahead, and 57% percent indicated that "skin color shapes their daily life experiences" (Pew Research Center, 2021, p. 25). In addition, Latinos with darker skin were found to be more likely to experience discrimination incidents than those with lighter skin. There were also differences in the types of discrimination incidents experienced by Latinos based on skin color (see Table 2.3). Moreover, more than half of Latinos indicated that having lighter skin color helps to get ahead in the United States today.

TABLE 2.3 Type of Discrimination Experienced by Latinos

Type of discrimination experienced	Total (percentage)	Lighter skinned Latinos (percentage)	Darker skinned Latinos (percentage)
Experienced at least one incident	54	54	64
People acted as if you were not smart	35	34	42
Experienced discrimination by someone who is non-Hispanic	31	29	42
Experienced discrimination by someone who is Hispanic	27	25	41
Criticized for speaking Spanish*	23	22	33
Told to go back to your country	21	20	32
Feared for personal safety	21	20	27
Called offensive names	20	18	31
Been unfairly stopped by police	9	8	16

*Asked only of those who speak Spanish. Source: Pew Research Center (2021)

Key findings from the Pew Research Center (2021) report include:

- The impact of race and skin color among Latinos is a topic of conversation with relatives and friends.
- About half of Latinos say there is too little national attention on racial issues concerning Latinos.
- About half of Latinos often hear other Latinos make racially insensitive comments and jokes about Latinos and non-Latinos.

- There is an association between discrimination experiences and views about skin color among Latinos.
- Latinos experience discrimination from both Latinos and non-Latinos alike.
- Latinos with darker skin experience more discrimination than Latinos with lighter skin.
- Younger Latinos experience more discrimination than older Latinos.
- When growing up, Latinos with darker skin talked with family about likely challenges due to race or ethnicity more than those Latinos with lighter skin.
- About half of Latinos say discrimination based on race or skin color is a big problem in the United States today.

Sociohistorical influences have shaped how Mexicans and other Latinos view themselves, especially their skin color and other phenotypic features (e.g., dark hair, brown eyes, straight hair, etc.). Eurocentric values have become internalized among many lighter skinned Latinos who can "pass" as White and who self-identify as White (Hall, 2018). In turn, they discriminate against Latinos with darker skin color, and those with darker skin color experience more discrimination. The Pew Research Center (2021) study shows that colorism is deeply entrenched among Latinos, reflecting a colonial mindset inherited from the Spanish and their hybrid racial classification system and perpetuated by non-Latino White Americans in the United States (Hunter, 2007; Quiros & Dawson, 2013).

Almeida et al. (2016) found that Latinos experienced perceived discrimination at a rate similar to Black Americans (68.4%). Among Latino subgroups, Almeida et al. found the highest prevalence of perceived discrimination was among Puerto Ricans (80.7%), followed by "other" Latinos (68.7%), Mexicans (67.6%), and Cubans (45.8%). They also found that anti-immigration policies and perceived discrimination among Latinos were highly associated. Place of origin (Mexico and Cuba), generation status (third generation), and age (younger Latinos) were all positively associated with perceived discrimination, even after controlling for potential independent risk factors for discrimination (e.g., socioeconomic status).

A study by Findling et al. (2019) found significant differences between Latinos and non-Latino White Americans in personal and institutional forms of discrimination. The probability of Latinos reporting discrimination were more than 4 times that of non-Latino White Americans when trying to rent a room or buy a house, avoiding health care due to discrimination concerns, avoiding the police due to discrimination concerns, and being unfairly treated by the police. In addition, Latinos had at least 3 times the probability of non-Latino White Americans of reporting discrimination when trying to vote or participate in politics and when going to a doctor or health clinic. Latinos also had higher probabilities than non-Latino White Americans of reporting discrimination in unfair treatment by the courts, obtaining equal pay and promotions, and police interactions.

Numerous studies have shown the negative impact of discrimination on health and mental health among historically marginalized populations. The toxic effects of stress on human physiology are well known (see Chapter 1). Stress accelerates cellular aging, and chronic stressors triggered by multiple social environmental "microaggressions" can lead to wear and tear on the body that can impair multiple physiological systems and lead to premature morbidity and mortality. The term *allostatic load* represents the cumulative exposure to chronic stress and stressful life events that can overwhelm immunologic functions, causing disease (Guidi et al., 2021; McEwen & Steller, 1993).

Studies conducted with Latinos of Mexican descent clearly show an association between perceived discrimination and measures of depression (Basáñez et al., 2013; Finch et al., 2000; Flores et al., 2008; Taylor & Turner,

2002; Ward et al., 2019). For example, Ward et al. (2019) found significant associations between perceived discrimination and depression—as measured by the Center for Epidemiologic Studies-Depression Scale (CES-D)—among a sample of predominantly Mexican American adults, with those perceiving higher levels of discrimination being more likely to experience depressive symptoms than those perceiving lower levels of discrimination.

In addition to experiencing generalized stress from everyday life stressors, the overriding experiences associated with "minority stress" might create increased levels of toxic stress, leading to detrimental health and mental health outcomes among historically disenfranchised and socially marginalized populations like African Americans, Native Americans, and Latinos (Dovidio et al., 2010; Flores et al., 2008; Williams, 2018).

The Proliferation of Cultural Deficit Models

Lacayo (2017) provides an insightful theory on how non-Latino White people conjure a "perpetual inferiority" toward Latinos, and especially Mexicans. The term *cultural racism* encompasses the ideology that the culture of Mexicans and Mexican Americans is inferior to the culture of White Americans and that they "pass down their 'deficient' culture to the subsequent generation and thus are unable to change, adapt, and progress" (Lacayo, 2017, p. 566). Other scholars have used the term "cultural racism" to define the consequences of propagating negative cultural deficits of various historically excluded and marginalized populations (Griffith et al., 2010).

Ethnocentrism is the belief that one's culture is superior to others. If often consists of viewing other cultures as inferior to one's own. It also includes "blaming the victim"—that is, blaming someone for their own misfortunes. The 19th-century idea of Manifest Destiny is one example of this form of Anglo-American ethnocentrism. Thus, blaming Mexican culture for violence, crime, behaviors, beliefs, and attitudes is part of Anglo-American ethnocentrism. Cultural deficit models do not accurately portray cultural characteristics of Latinos. Rather, they oversimplify meaningful differences not related to culture but to racial/ethnic discrimination. They place the blame for any observed inequalities on the culture itself.

The promulgation of cultural deficit models to explain the "web of pathologies" hypothesized to exist among Mexican Americans began in earnest during the 1940s through the 1960s. Many of these presumed cultural deficits are nothing more than racial stereotypes (see Table 2.4). Coupled with White nativism and White nationalism in the 2000s (Huntington, 2004), negative and pejorative attitudes toward Mexicans and Mexican Americans persist—a perpetual inferiority of culture and a refusal to assimilate to American culture.

TABLE 2.4 Presumed Cultural Deficits of Mexican Americans

Social scientist and relevant work	Cultural deficit(s)	Damaging culture
Ruth D. Tuck: *Not With the First* (1946)	Passive	Change culture for Mexican Americans to become Americans
Lyle Saunders: *Cultural Difference and Medical Care: The Case of Spanish-Speaking People of the Southwest* (1954)	Irrational	Change culture to become "rational" Americans

Social scientist and relevant work	Cultural deficit(s)	Damaging culture
Munro Edmonson: *Los Manitos: A Study of Institutional Values* (1957)	Unscientific	Change culture to become scientific and modern Americans
Margaret Clark: *Health in the Mexican-American Culture: A Community Study* (1959)	Masochistic	Change culture to become "normal" Americans
Florence Kluckhohn and Fred Strodbeck: *Variations in Value Orientations* (1961)	Apathetic	Change culture to become successful Americans
William Madsen: *Mexican Americans of South Texas* (1964)	Fatalistic; lazy; lax habits; no initiative; criminally prone; present time oriented	Change culture to become healthy Americans
Peter Skerry: *Mexican Americans: The Ambivalent Minority* (1993)	Ambivalent; culturally oriented prevents assimilation	Change culture to become assimilated Americans

Source: Adapted from Romano-V (1969)

Mexican American Segregation, Social Exclusion, and Marginalization

Given the historical and geopolitical history of Latinos of Mexican descent, it is evident that this group has been politically disenfranchised, swindled out of their land, relegated to dangerous and menial occupations, provided with substandard educational resources, and saturated with a heavy dose of racial and cultural inferiority by non-Latino White people.

In Barrera's (1979) book *Race and Class in the Southwest*, he proposes what he calls "an internal colonial model" to understand the social disadvantages identified among Mexicans and Mexican Americans residing in the southwestern United States. According to Barrera, racial typologies were created in the Americas to justify the exploitation and disenfranchisement of Indians on the part of European colonists. Specifically, "racial ideologies came about in large part because they were useful in justifying classic colonialism and the neocolonial and internal colonial relationships that grew out of it" (Barrera, 1979, p. 200). The thrust of Barrera's argument is that major elements of colonialism still exist in the southwestern United States that continue to discriminate and subjugate Latinos of Mexican descent.

As previously noted, Latinos of Mexican descent have been routinely excluded and marginalized from many aspects of U.S. society by (a) "English-only" laws, (b) de facto and de jure forms of segregation, especially in education and housing, and (c) cultural racism expressed in the form of anti-Mexican prejudicial attitudes and discrimination. Over the past century, the economic and political interests of the dominant non-Latino White majority aided in the establishment of a system of structural discrimination (the colonial relationship) that perpetuated racialized occupations and division of labor. Racial ideologies developed by the dominant non-Latino White majority over the past 200 years have provided a legacy based on prejudice, discrimination, and violence toward Latinos of Mexican descent. The result established a belief in the "perpetual inferiority" of Mexican Americans and has contributed to the economic fragility and social inequality among this group vis-à-vis the non-Latino White majority.

The Concept of Historical Trauma and Latinos of Mexican Descent

Epigeneticists now know that physical and psychological trauma is transmitted across generations (see Chapter 1). The damage done to gene-signaling pathways has been shown to disrupt normal mechanisms of fetal development and human biology in general (MacDonald & Roskams, 2009; Oyama & Terry, 2016). Prior to the discovery of epigenetic modification, several scholars hypothesized about the relationship between historical events and subsequent health of populations (Fox et al., 2015) (see Figure 2.14).

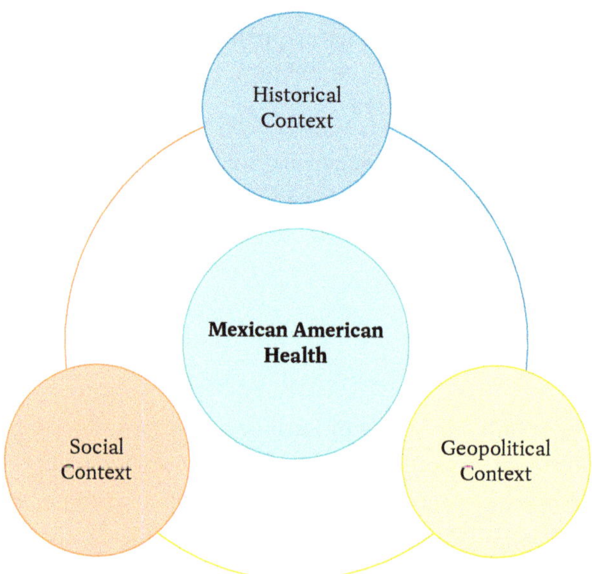

FIGURE 2.14 Influences on Mexican American Health

Brave Heart (2003), Sotero (2006), and other scholars have used the term *historical trauma* to describe the cultural destruction, genocide, and subsequent subordination and oppression of Indigenous populations (Estrada, 2009; Fox et al., 2015; Hernández-Wolfe, 2013; Kirmayer et al., 2014). A conceptual model of historical trauma developed by Sotero (2006) includes the following three sequential stages. The first stage is the exposure to a mass trauma experience where the dominant group subjugates a population, resulting in segregation and displacement, physical and psychological violence, economic destruction, and cultural dispossession. The second stage elicits a trauma response in the first or primary generation that includes physical, social, and psychological responses. In the third stage, the trauma responses are transmitted to subsequent generations through environmental factors; psychosocial factors; social, economic, and political systems; and legal and social discrimination (Estrada, 2009; Sotero, 2006).

The Spanish conquest was a mass trauma event for many of the Indigenous populations of the New World. Historical evidence confirms the increasing rates of physical and psychological violence, public intoxication, and the erosion of traditional mores among subsequent generations (Estrada, 2009; Scardaville, 1980). During the American neocolonial period, Mexicans and Mexican Americans were further subjugated with institutionalized forms of structural and symbolic violence. Mob violence toward and lynching of Latinos of Mexican descent form a shared and lasting memory of the racialized landscape that is the U.S.–Mexico border region. Historical trauma theory is aptly applied to the experiences of Latinos of Mexican descent in the Southwest. I argue that negative physical, social, and psychological responses to these historical trauma events have laid the foundation for future generations' increase in negative health and mental health through changes in epigenetic mechanisms, which we will discuss in Chapter 6.

CHAPTER SUMMARY

The Mexica origin story provides a basis for understanding the symbolic meaning of "place" for their Mexican and Mexican American descendants. Thus, the symbolic representation of the "lost land" holds real meaning—an ancestral claim to the region by this historically marginalized and disenfranchised population.

The Spanish colonial period ushered in 300 years of violence, oppression, subordination, and racialization that shadows Indigenous populations of Mexico, Central America, and South America. The establishment of a colonial model and a racial hybrid social hierarchy further subordinated Indigenous populations in the Americas. Though abolished in 1720, it laid a solid foundation for racial classifications and discrimination based on color and internalization of negative stereotypes. Once free from Spanish domination, Mexico completely abolished Spanish racial laws, but the legacy of racist ideology had been established. Mexicans who had the appearance of Indians were still discriminated against by those with lighter skin.

Americans legally immigrated to the Mexican state of Tejas (Texas) beginning in the 1820s by invitation of the Mexican government. Then a flood of illegal immigration began that quickly made White Americans the majority population in the state. Texas soon rebelled and gained independence from Mexico in 1836. This was only the beginning of American expansionism.

The White American nationalist ideal of Manifest Destiny, greed, racism, and ethnocentrism led to the subsequent invasion of Mexico and the annexation of most of today's American Southwest after the Mexican American War. Tensions between White Americans and Mexicans persisted after the war, leading to discrimination, mob violence, and the lynching of Mexicans, including women and children, especially in Texas. Texas Rangers committed acts of violence against Latinos of Mexican descent, resulting in murder. Widespread anti-Mexican sentiment was prevalent in most southwestern states, which led to mass deportations in the 1930s of both Mexican nationals and U.S. citizens. Mob violence directed toward Mexican Americans persisted into the 1950s.

The making of Mexican Americans occurred through the Treaty of Guadalupe Hidalgo. The treaty was supposed to enable Mexican Americans to become fully-fledged U.S. citizens with protected land rights. The United States violated several conditions in the Treaty of Guadalupe Hidalgo, swindling Mexicans out of their land and not providing U.S. citizenship to Indian-looking Mexicans. In fact, California and Arizona enacted legislation that prohibited Mexican Americans from U.S. citizenship and voting due to their racial status as Indians. United States neocolonialism created a working class of Mexicans who were exploited, with many assigned to work in menial and harsh conditions. Racism and discrimination continue under American occupation of the Southwest. Additionally, Americanization processes attempted to get the "Mexicanness" out of Mexicans.

U.S.-Mexico border militarization further increased suspicion of Latinos of Mexican descent. Mass deportations in the 1930s paved the way for a series of quasi-military "operations" against Latinos of Mexican descent. Heightened surveillance by Homeland Security, Border Patrol, and local police agencies further added to the idea of a population under surveillance. Increased police surveillance has led to more negative interactions with the Mexican American community that have had deadly consequences in the number of legal homicides committed against Mexicans and Mexican Americans. The conflation of Mexican immigrants with Mexican Americans meant that U.S. citizens were under suspicion. Structural and symbolic violence is enacted daily in the border states of Arizona, California, New Mexico, and Texas (formerly Mexican territory).

Anti-Mexican sentiment had fueled prejudice, discrimination, and violence directed toward Latinos of Mexican descent, leading to increased rates of depression. The proliferation of cultural deficit models to explain the "social pathology" of Mexicans has further placed this historically marginalized population into a "perpetual inferiority" and is an example of symbolic violence.

Structural violence and symbolic violence are commonplace in the U.S.-Mexico border region and elsewhere where there are large concentrations of Mexicans and Mexican Americans. The psychosocial concept of "historical trauma" aptly fits the experience of Latinos of Mexican descent from the initial Spanish conquest and the imposition of a colonial model that benefitted the conquerors and repressed the conquered to the neocolonial model and racial suppression by White Americans.

Genetic research clearly establishes an Indigenous origin of Mexicans and Mexican Americans. To suggest that this population group is not native to the Americas denies the scientific basis for migration and genetic studies. This genetic linkage also confers phenotypic characteristics, such as darker skin, that single them out for inter- and intra-ethnic discrimination.

The concept of historical trauma helps explain the negative influence of structural and symbolic violence on multiple generations of Latinos of Mexican descent. Like Black Americans and Native Americans, Mexican Americans have experienced generations of sustained prejudice, discrimination, and violence. Health inequalities among these historically marginalized groups are the result of this 500-year legacy.

QUESTIONS TO CONSIDER

1. How do historical, geopolitical, and social contexts frame the experience of Latinos of Mexican descent in the southwestern United States?
2. Discuss the health and social effects of segregation, racism, and poverty. What differences, if any, exist between White-Black and White-Latino segregation patterns, and how might these patterns impact the health of Latinos?
3. Explain how the concept of "colorism" is still pervasive among Latinos.
4. Discuss the influence of cultural deficit models on Latinos of Mexican descent.
5. How has anti-immigrant sentiment spilled over to anti-Mexican sentiment?

SUGGESTED READINGS

Acuna, R. F. (1988). *Occupied America: A history of Chicanos* (3rd ed.). Harper Collins.

Basáñez, T., Unger, J. B., Soto, D., Crano, W., & Baezconde-Garbanati, L. (2013). Perceived discrimination as a risk factor for depressive symptoms and substance use among Hispanic adolescents in Los Angeles. *Ethnicity & Health, 18*(3), 244–261.

Basu, A., Tang, H., Zhu, X., Gu, C. C., Hanis, C., Boerwinkle, E., & Risch, N. (2008). Genome-wide distribution of ancestry in Mexican Americans. *Human Genetics, 124*, 207–214. https://doi.org/10.1007/s00439-008-0541-5

Carrigan, W. D., & Webb, C. (2017). *Forgotten dead: Mob violence against Mexicans in the United States, 1848–1928*. Oxford University Press.

Chavez-Dueñas, N. Y., Adames, H. Y., & Organista, K. C. (2014). Skin-color prejudice and within-group racial discrimination: Historical and current impact on Latino/a populations. *Hispanic Journal of Behavioral Sciences, 36*(1), 3–26.

Estrada, A. L. (2009). Mexican Americans and historical trauma theory: A theoretical perspective. *Journal of Ethnicity in Substance Abuse, 8*(3), 330–340.

Kil, S. H. (2019). *Covering the border war: How the news media creates crime, race, nation, and the USA–Mexico divide*. Lexington Books. https://ebookcentral.proquest.com/lib/sjsu/detail.action?docID=5972272

Menchaca, M. (2012). Early racist discourses: The roots of deficit thinking. In R. R. Valencia (Ed.), *The evolution of deficit thinking* (pp. 13–40). Routledge.

Quiros, L., & Dawson, B. A. (2013). The color paradigm: The impact of colorism on the racial identity and identification of Latinas. *Journal of Human Behavior in the Social Environment, 23*(3), 287–297.

Sabo, S., Shaw, S., Ingram, M., Teufel-Shone, N., Carvajal, S., de Zapien, J. G., Rosales, C., Redondo, F., Garcia, G., & Rubio-Goldsmith, R. (2014). Everyday violence, structural racism and mistreatment at the US–Mexico border. *Social Science & Medicine, 109*, 66–74.

REFERENCES

Acuna, R. F. (1988). *Occupied America: A history of Chicanos* (3rd ed.). Harper Collins.

Aguilar-Moreno, M. (2007). *Handbook to life in the Aztec world.* Oxford University Press.

Al Jazeera. (2020, August 18). *Who got the right to vote when?* https://interactive.aljazeera.com/aje/2016/us-elections-2016-who-can-vote/index.html

Almeida, J., Biello, K. B., Pedraza, F., Wintner, S., & Viruell-Fuentes, E. (2016). The association between anti-immigrant policies and perceived discrimination among Latinos in the US: A multilevel analysis. *SSM-Population Health, 2*, 897–903.

Arce, J. (2021, September 29). Racial segregation of Latino students continues with English-only laws. *UnidosUS*. https://unidosus.org/blog/2021/09/29/racial-segregation-of-latino-students-continues-with-english-only-laws/

Arriola, C. (1995). Knocking on the schoolhouse door: *Mendez v. Westminster*, equal protection, public education, and Mexican Americans in the 1940s. *La Raza LJ, 8*, 166.

Barrera, M. (1979). *Race and class in the Southwest: A theory of racial inequality.* University of Notre Dame Press.

Basáñez, T., Unger, J. B., Soto, D., Crano, W., & Baezconde-Garbanati, L. (2013). Perceived discrimination as a risk factor for depressive symptoms and substance use among Hispanic adolescents in Los Angeles. *Ethnicity & Health, 18*(3), 244–261.

Basu, A., Tang, H., Zhu, X., Gu, C. C., Hanis, C., Boerwinkle, E., & Risch, N. (2008). Genome-wide distribution of ancestry in Mexican Americans. *Human Genetics, 124*, 207–214. https://doi.org/10.1007/s00439-008-0541-5

Becerra, D., Androff, D., Cimino, A., Alex Wagaman, M., & Blanchard, K. N. (2013). The impact of perceived discrimination and immigration policies upon perceptions of quality of life among Latinos in the United States. *Race and Social Problems, 5*, 65–78.

Binational Migration Institute. (2021). *Migrant deaths in Southern Arizona: Recovered undocumented border crosser remains investigated by the Pima County Office of the Medical Examiner, 1990–2020.* https://bmi.arizona.edu/sites/bmi.arizona.edu/files/BMI-Migrant-Deaths-in-Southern-Arizona-2021-English.pdf

Blakemore, E. (2018). *The long history of anti-Latino discrimination in America.* History.com. https://www.history.com/news/the-brutal-history-of-anti-latino-discrimination-in-america

Bonilla, C., Gutierrez, G., Parra, E., Kline, C., & Shriver, M. (2005). Admixture analysis of a rural population of the state of Guerrero, Mexico. *American Journal of Physical Anthropology, 128*, 861–886.

Bourdieu, P. (2001). *Male domination.* Blackwell.

Bourgois, P. (2001). The power of violence in war and peace: Post-Cold War lessons from El Salvador. http://istmo.denison.edu/n08/articulos/power.html

Brave Heart, M. Y. H. (2003). The historical trauma response among natives and its relationship with substance abuse: A Lakota illustration. *Journal of Psychoactive Drugs, 35*(1), 7–13.

Brown v. Board of Education, 347 U.S. 483 (1954). https://www.oyez.org/cases/1940-1955/347us483

Carrigan, W. D., & Webb, C. (2017). Forgotten dead: Mob violence against Mexicans in the United States, 1848–1928. Oxford University Press.

Chavez, J. R. (1984). *The Lost Land: The Chicano image of the Southwest.* University of New Mexico Press.

Chavez-Dueñas, N. Y., Adames, H. Y., & Organista, K. C. (2014). Skin-color prejudice and within-group racial discrimination: Historical and current impact on Latino/a populations. *Hispanic Journal of Behavioral Sciences, 36*(1), 3–26.

Donato, R., Menchaca, M., & Valencia, R. (1991). Segregation, desegregation, and integration of Chicano students: Problems and prospects. In R. Valencia (Ed.), *Chicano school failure and success: Research and policy agendas for the 1990s* (pp. 27–63). Falmer Press.

Dovidio, J. F., Gluszek, A., John, M. S., Ditlmann, R., & Lagunes, P. (2010). Understanding bias toward Latinos: Discrimination, dimensions of difference, and experience of exclusion. *Journal of Social Issues, 66*(1), 59–78.

Dunn, T. (1996). *The militarization of the U.S.-Mexico border, 1978–1992: Low-intensity conflict doctrine comes home.* CMAS Books.

Encyclopaedia Britannica Online. (2012, November 26). Great Drought. https://www.britannica.com/event/Great-Drought

Esquivel, P. (2019, August 16). El Paso Massacre was just the latest in long line of anti-Latino violence in the U.S. *Los Angeles Times.* https://www.latimes.com/california/story/2019-08-16/el-paso-massacre-timeline-of-anti-latino-violence-in-united-states

Estrada, A. (2009). Mexican Americans and historical trauma theory: A theoretical perspective. *Journal of Ethnicity in Substance Abuse, 8*(3), 330–340. https://doi.org/10.1080/15332640903110500

Federal Bar Association. (2021, June 16). Mendez v. Westminster: *The Mexican-American fight for school integration and social equity pre-*Brown v. Board of Education. https://www.fedbar.org/blog/mendez-v-westminster-the-mexican-american-fight-for-school-integration-and-social-equality-pre-brown-v-board-of-education/ Accessed 5/12/2023

Finch, B. K., Kolody, B., & Vega, W. A. (2000). Perceived discrimination and depression among Mexican-origin adults in California. *Journal of Health and Social Behavior, 41*(3), 295–313.

Findling, M. G., Bleich, S. N., Casey, L. S., Blendon, R. J., Benson, J. M., Sayde, J. M., & Miller, C. (2019). Discrimination in the United States: Experiences of Latinos. *Health Services Research, 54*(Suppl. 2), 1409–1418. https://doi.org/10.1111/1475-6773.13216

Flores, E., Tschann, J. M., Dimas, J. M., Bachen, E. A., Pasch, L. A., & de Groat, C. L. (2008). Perceived discrimination, perceived stress, and mental and physical health among Mexican-origin adults. *Hispanic Journal of Behavioral Sciences, 30*(4), 401–424.

Fox, M., Entringer, S., Buss, C., De Haene, J., & Wadhwa, D. (2015). Intergenerational transmission of the effects of acculturation on health in Hispanic Americans: A fetal programming perspective. *American Journal of Public Health, 105*, S409–S423. https://doi.org/10.2105/AJPH.2015.302571

Gee, G. C., & Ford, C. L. (2011). Structural racism and health inequities: Old issues, new directions. *Du Bois Review: Social Science Research on Race, 8*(1), 115–132.

Gonzalez, G. G. (2013). *Chicano education in the era of segregation* (Vol. 7). University of North Texas Press.

Griffith, D. M., Johnson, J., Ellis, K. R., & Schulz, A. J. (2010). Cultural context and a critical approach to eliminating health disparities. *Ethnicity & Disease, 20*, 71–76.

Griswold del Castillo, R. (1975). "Myth" and reality: Chicano economic mobility in Los Angeles, 1850–1880. *Aztlan, 6*(2), 151–171.

Griswold del Castillo, R. (1992). *The Treaty of Guadalupe Hidalgo: A legacy of conflict.* University of Oklahoma Press.

Guardado-Estrada, M., Juarez-Torres, E., Medina-Martinez, I., Wegier, A., Macías, A., Gomez, G., Cruz-Talonia, F., Roman-Bassaure, E., Piñero, D., Kofman-Alfaro, S., & Berumen, J. (2009). A great diversity of Amerindian mitochondrial DNA ancestry is present in the Mexican mestizo population. *Journal of Human Genetics, 54*(12), 695–705.

Guidi, J., Lucente, M., Sonino, N., & Fava, G. A. (2021). Allostatic load and its impact on health: A systematic review. *Psychotherapy and Psychosomatics, 90*(1), 11–27. https://doi.org/10.1159/000510696

Hall, R. E. (2018). Media stereotypes and "coconut" colorism: Latino denigration vis-à-vis dark skin. *American Behavioral Scientist, 62*(14), 2007–2022.

Hanis, C. L., Hewett-Emmett, D., Bertin, T. K., & Schull, W. J. (1991). Origins of U.S. Hispanics. Implications for diabetes. *Diabetes Care, 14*(7), 618–627.

Haring, C. H. (1947). *The Spanish Empire in America*. Harbinger.

Heidler, D. S., & Heidler, J. T. (2023, May 16). Manifest Destiny. *Encyclopedia Britannica Online*. https://www.britannica.com/event/Manifest-Destiny.

Hernández-Hernández, O., Hernández-Zaragoza, D. I., Barquera, R., Warinner, C., López-Gil, C., Arrieta-Bolaños, E., Clayton, S., Bravo-Acevedo, A., Del Rocío Ramos-de la Cruz, F., Méndez-Mani, P., de Los Ángeles Pavón-Vargas, M., Zúñiga, J., Yunis, E. J., Bekker-Méndez, C., & Granados, J. (2020). Genetic diversity of HLA system in two populations from Oaxaca, Mexico: Oaxaca city and rural Oaxaca. *Human Immunology, 81*(9), 553–556.

Hernández-Wolfe, P. (2013). *A borderlands view on Latinos, Latin Americans, and decolonization: Rethinking mental health*. Jason Aronson.

Hoffman, A. (2018). *Unwanted Mexican Americans in the Great Depression: Repatriation pressures, 1929–1939*. The University of Arizona Press.

Hu, H., Huff, C. D., Yamamura, Y., Wu, X., & Strom, S. S. (2015). The relationship between Native American ancestry, body mass index and diabetes risk among Mexican-Americans. *PloS One, 10*(10), Article e0141260.

Hunter, M. (2007). The persistent problem of colorism: Skin tone, status, and inequality. *Sociology Compass, 1*(1), 237–254.

Huntington, S. (2004). The Hispanic challenge. *Foreign Policy*. http://www.foreignpolicy.com/story/cms.php?story_id=2495&print=1

Jamieson, S. M. (1976). *Labor unionism in American agriculture*. Arno Press.

Juárez-Cedillo, T., Zuñiga, J., Acuña-Alonzo, V., Pérez-Hernández, N., Rodríguez-Pérez, J. M., Barquera, R., Gallardo, G. J., Sánchez-Arenas, R., García-Peña, Maria Del Carmen, Granados, J., & Vargas-Alarcón, G. (2008). Genetic admixture and diversity estimations in the Mexican Mestizo population from Mexico City using 15 STR polymorphic markers. *Forensic Science International. Genetics, 2*(3), e37–e39.

Keith, R. G. (1971). Encomienda, hacienda and corregimiento in Spanish America: A structural analysis. *Hispanic American Historical Review, 51*(3), 431–446. https://read.dukeupress.edu/hahr/article/51/3/431/152265/Encomienda-Hacienda-and-Corregimiento-in-Spanish

Kil, S. H. (2019). *Covering the border war : How the news media creates crime, race, nation, and the USA–Mexico divide*. Lexington Books. http://ebookcentral.proquest.com/lib/sjsu/detail.action?docID=5972272

Kil, S. H., & Menjívar, C. (2006). The "war on the border": The criminalization of immigrants and militarization of the USA-Mexico border. In R. Martinez, Jr. & A. Valenzuela Jr. (Eds.), *Immigration and crime: Race, ethnicity, and violence* (pp. 164–188). New York University Press.

Kil, S. H., Menjívar, C., & Doty, R. L. (2009). Securing borders: Patriotism, vigilantism and the brutalization of the U.S. American public. In W. F. McDonald (Ed.), *Immigration, crime and justice: Sociology of crime, law and deviance* (Vol. 13, pp. 297–312). Emerald/JAI Press. https://doi.org/10.1108/S1521-6136(2009)0000013019.

Kirmayer, L. J., Gone, J. P., & Moses, J. (2014). Rethinking historical trauma. *Transcultural Psychiatry, 51*(3), 299–319.

Lacayo, C. O. (2017). Perpetual inferiority: Whites' racial ideology toward Latinos. *Sociology of Race and Ethnicity, 3*(4), 566–579.

Lisker, R. (1981). *Estructura Genetica de la Poblacion Mexicana*. Salvat.

Long, J. C., Williams, R. C., McAuley, J. E., Medis, R., Partel, R., Tregellas, W. M., South, S. F., Rea, A. E., McCormick, S. B., & Iwaniec, U. (1991). Genetic variation in Arizona Mexican Americans: Estimation and interpretation of admixture proportions. *American Journal of Physical Anthropology, 84*(2), 141–157.

Lovato, K., Lopez, C., Karimli, L., & Abrams, L. S. (2018). The impact of deportation-related family separations on the well-being of Latinx children and youth: A review of the literature. *Children and Youth Services Review, 95*, 109–116.

MacDonald, J. L., & Roskams, A. J. (2009). Epigenetic regulation of nervous system development by DNA methylation and histone deacetylation. *Progress in Neurobiology, 88*, 170–183. https://doi.org/10.1016/j.pneurobio.2009.04.002

McCaa, R. (1997). The peopling of Mexico from origins to revolution. In R. Steckel & M. Haines (Eds.), *The population history of North America*. Cambridge University Press.

McEwen, B. S., & Stellar, E. (1993). Stress and the individual: Mechanisms leading to disease. *Archives of Internal Medicine, 153*(18), 2093–2101. https://doi.org/10.1001/archinte.1993.00410180039004

Meier, M., & Rivera, F. (1972). *The Chicanos*. Hill and Wang.

Menchaca, M. (1993). Chicano Indianism: A historical account of racial repression in the United States. *American Ethnologist, 20*(3), 583–603.

Menchaca, M. (2001). *Recovering history, constructing race: The Indian, Black, and White roots of Mexican Americans.* University of Texas Press. http://www.jstor.org/stable/10.7560/752535.6

Menchaca, M. (2012). Early racist discourses: The roots of deficit thinking. In R. R. Valencia (Ed.), *The evolution of deficit thinking* (pp. 13–40). Routledge.

Mendez v. Westminster, 64 F.Supp. 544 (C.D. Cal. 1946).

Organista, K. C. (2009). Latino clinical perspective on Montalvo's ethnoracial gap in clinical practice with Latinos. *Clinical Social Work Journal, 37,* 287–293. https://doi.org/10.1007/s10615-009-0231-3

Oyama, S., & Terry, S. F. (2016). Epigenetics and racial health inequities. *Genetic Testing and Molecular Biomarkers*, 20(9), 483–484. https://doi.org/10.1089/gtmb.2016.29021.sj

Padilla, A. M., Lindholm, K. J., Chen, A., Duran, R., Hakuta, K., Lambert, W., & Tucker, G. R. (1991, February 1). *The English-only movement—Myths, reality, and implications for psychology.* American Psychological Association. https://www.apa.org/pi/oema/resources/english-only

Perrigo, L. I. (1971). *The American Southwest.* Holt, Rinehart, and Winston.

Pew Research Center. (2015, June 11). *Multiracial in America.* https://www.pewresearch.org/social-trends/2015/06/11/multiracial-in-america/

Pew Research Center. (2021, November). *Majority of Latinos say skin color impacts opportunity in America and shapes daily life.* https://www.pewresearch.org/hispanic/wp-content/uploads/sites/5/2021/11/RE_2021.11.04_Latinos-Race-Identity_FINAL.pdf

Price, J. H., & Khubchandani, J. (2023). Lethal force usage by law enforcement officers against Hispanics, 2011–2020. *Journal of Community Health, 48,* 819–923 https://doi.org/10.1007/s10900-023-01222-8

Quiros, L., & Dawson, B. A. (2013). The color paradigm: The impact of colorism on the racial identity and identification of Latinas. *Journal of Human Behavior in the Social Environment, 23*(3), 287–297.

Robert Wood Johnson Foundation. (2017, October 24). *Discrimination in America: Experiences and views.* https://www.rwjf.org/en/insights/our-research/2017/10/discrimination-in-america--experiences-and-views.html. Accessed 4/24/2023

Rodríguez, R. C. (2014). *Our sacred maíz is our mother: Indigeneity and belonging in the Americas.* University of Arizona Press.

Romano-V, O. I. (1969). *The anthropology and sociology of the Mexican-Americans: The distortion of Mexican-American history.* Quinto Sol.

Romero, M. (2006). Racial profiling and immigration law enforcement: Rounding up of usual suspects in the Latino community. *Critical Sociology, 32*(2–3), 447–473. https://doi.org/10.1163/156916306777835376

Sabo, S., & Lee, A. E. (2015). The spillover of US immigration policy on citizens and permanent residents of Mexican descent: How internalizing "illegality" impacts public health in the borderlands. *Frontiers in Public Health, 3,* 155.

Sabo, S., Shaw, S., Ingram, M., Teufel-Shone, N., Carvajal, S., De Zapien, J. G., Rosales, C., Redondo, F., Garcia, G., & Rubio-Goldsmith, R. (2014). Everyday violence, structural racism and mistreatment at the US–Mexico border. *Social Science & Medicine, 109,* 66–74.

Scardaville, M. C. (1980). Alcohol abuse and tavern reform in late colonial Mexico City. *Hispanic American Historical Review, 60*(4), 643–671.

Shaul, D. L. (2014). *A prehistory of western North America: The impact of Uto-Aztecan languages.* University of New Mexico Press.

Smith, M. E. (2003). *The Aztecs* (2nd ed.). Blackwell.

Smith, M. E. (2005). Life in the provinces of the Aztec Empire. *Scientific American.* https://www.scientificamerican.com/article/life-in-the-provinces-of-the-aztec-2005-01/

Sotero, M. M. (2006). A conceptual model of historical trauma: Implications for public health practice and research. *Journal of Health Disparities Research and Practice, 1,* 93–108

Taylor, J., & Turner, R. J. (2002). Perceived discrimination, social stress, and depression in the transition to adulthood: Racial contrasts. *Social Psychology Quarterly,* 213–225.

Treaty of Guadalupe Hidalgo. (1848, February 2). National Archives. https://www.archives.gov/milestone-documents/treaty-of-guadalupe-hidalgo

U.S. Census Bureau. (2018). *Questions planned for the 2020 Census and American Community Survey: Federal legislative and program uses.* U.S. Department of Commerce, Economics and Statistics Administration. https://www2.census.gov/library/publications/decennial/2020/operations/planned-questions-2020-acs.pdf

Vargas, E. D., & Ybarra, V. D. (2017). U.S. citizen children of undocumented parents: The link between state immigration policy and the health of Latino children. *Journal of Immigrant and Minority Health, 19*, 913–920.

Wang, S., Ray, N., Rojas, W., Parra, M. V., Bedoya, G., Gallo, C., Poletti, G., Mazzotti, G., Hill, K., Hurtado, A. M., Camrena, B., Nicolini, H., Klitz, W., Barrantes, R., Molina, J. A., Freimer, N. B., Bortolini, M. C., Salzano, F. M., Petzl-Erler, J. L., ... Ruiz-Linares, A. (2008). Geographic patterns of genome admixture in Latin American mestizos. *PLoS Genetetics, 4*(3), Article e10000037. https://doi.org/10.1371/journal.pgen.1000037

Ward, J. B., Feinstein, L., Vines, A. I., Robinson, W. R., Haan, M. N., & Aiello, A. E. (2019). Perceived discrimination and depressive symptoms among US Latinos: The modifying role of educational attainment. *Ethnicity & Health, 24*(3), 271–286.

Weber, D. J. (1992). The Spanish legacy in North America and the historical imagination. *The Western Historical Quarterly, 23*(1), 5–24.

Weber, D. J. (Ed.). (2003). *Foreigners in their native land: Historical roots of the Mexican Americans*. UNM Press.

Williams, D. R. (2018). Stress and the Mental health of populations of color: Advancing our understanding of race-related stressors. *Journal of Health and Social Behavior, 59*(4), 466–485. https://doi.org/10.1177/0022146518814251

Williams, D. R., & Mohammed, S. A. (2009). Discrimination and racial disparities in health: Evidence and needed research. *Journal of Behavioral Medicine, 32*(1), 20–47. https://doi.org/10.1007/s10865-008-9185-0

Figure Credits

Fig. 2.1: "Chicomoztoc, Land of the Seven Caves," https://commons.wikimedia.org/wiki/File:ToltecaChichimeca_Chicomostoc.jpg, 1550.

Fig. 2.2: "First page of the Codex Boturini," https://commons.wikimedia.org/wiki/File:Tira-1.jpg, 1556.

Fig. 2.3: "Introduction of Smallpox," https://commons.wikimedia.org/wiki/File:Aztec_smallpox_victims.jpg, 1501.

Fig. 2.4: Johann Theodor de Bry, "Spanish Hanging Indigenous Natives," https://commons.wikimedia.org/wiki/File:De_Bry_1c.JPG, 1552.

Fig. 2.5: "Mistreatment of Natives by Spanish Encomenderos," https://commons.wikimedia.org/wiki/File:Kingsborough.jpg, 1550.

Fig. 2.6: "Spanish Colonial Racial Hybrid Types," https://commons.wikimedia.org/wiki/File:Casta_painting_all.jpg, 1750.

Fig. 2.7: Adapted from Nayeli Y. Chazev-Duenas, Hector Y. Adames, and Kurt C. Organista, "Abbreviated Spanish-Colonial Racial Hybrid Typology," Skin-Color Prejudice and Within-Group Racial Discrimination: Historical and Current Impact on Latino/a Populations. Copyright © 2013 by SAGE Publications.

Fig. 2.8: Governments of USA and Mexico, "Treaty of Guadalupe Hidalgo, 1848," https://commons.wikimedia.org/wiki/File:TreatyOfGuadalupeHidalgoCover.jpg, 1848.

Fig. 2.9: Copyright © by Földhegy (CC by 3.0) at https://commons.wikimedia.org/wiki/File:US-Mexico_barrier_map.png.

Fig. 2.10: Adapted from William D. Carrigan and Clive Webb, "Confirmed Mexican Victims of Mob Violence, US, 1848-1928," Forgotten Dead: Mob Violence Against Mexicans in the United States, 1848-1928. Copyright © 2017 by Oxford University Press.

Fig. 2.11: Copyright © by Ken Lund (CC BY-SA 2.0) at https://commons.wikimedia.org/wiki/File:Hanging_Tree,_Goliad_County_Courthouse,_Goliad,_Texas_(16075147710).jpg.

Fig. 2.12: NY Daily News Archive, "1930s Mexican Deportations, Los Angeles, CA," https://commons.wikimedia.org/wiki/File:Mexican_Repatriation,_1931.jpg, 1931.

Fig. 2.13: AP Images, "Zoot Suit Riots, Los Angeles 1943," https://commons.wikimedia.org/wiki/File:Soldier,_sailors,_and_marines_stop_a_streetcar_during_their_search_for_pachuca_%E2%80%9Czoot_suiters%E2%80%9D_in_Los_Angeles,_June_7,_1943.jpg, 1943.

CHAPTER 3

Social Determinants of Health Among Mexican Americans

LEARNING OBJECTIVES

- Describe the five domains of the social determinants of health.
- Compare and contrast several of the social determinants of health between non-Latino White Americans, non-Latino Black Americans, and Americans of Mexican descent.
- Evaluate how intersectionality contributes to increases in negative life events and health outcomes among Mexican Americans.
- Summarize the effects of the poverty cycle.
- Critically assess the gender gap in income and wealth and how Mexican Americans are negatively impacted vis-à-vis other historically marginalized groups.
- Assess the components of the behavior model for vulnerable populations and their contribution to understanding health care utilization.
- Describe Community Resilience Estimates (CRE) and the Social Vulnerability (SV) Index for the U.S.–Mexico border developed by the Centers for Disease Control and Prevention (CDC), the Agency for Toxic Substances and Disease Registry (ATSDR), and the Office of Minority Health (OMH).

A thorough understanding of the social determinants that have shaped and influenced the health status of Mexican Americans is required to appreciate their individual and combined effects. *Social determinants of health* (*SDOH*) are the conditions in the social and physical environments in which people live, learn, work, play, and age. These conditions affect a wide range of health, functioning, quality of life, and individual and population exposures to health risks (Office of Disease Prevention and Health Promotion, n.d.). According to the SDOH paradigm, the conditions in these environments (e.g., social, economic, political, and physical) and settings (e.g., social institutions, workplaces) are referred to as "place." However, historical, and cultural factors have played a major role in the real and imagined perceptions of "place" as we have seen in Chapter 2.

Krieger (2001) provides the following definition of social determinants: "social determinants of health refer to both specific features of and pathways by which societal conditions affect health and that potentially can be altered by informed, community action and health policy" (p. 697). James (2002) adds that social determinants of health are "life-enhancing resources, such as food supply, housing, economic and social relationships, transportation, education, and health care, whose distribution across populations effectively determines length and quality of life." These life-enhancing resources include:

- Safe and affordable housing, which has become problematic in emerging urban areas, with increasing cost burden and homelessness
- Access to quality education, job training, and job opportunities, which are limited in low-income, historically disadvantaged communities
- Public safety and crime free environments, without Homeland Security surveillance and racial profiling
- Availability of community-based resources in support of community living and opportunities for recreational and leisure-time activities, which are diminished by gentrification and displacement
- Availability of and access to healthy foods, depending on the prevalence of "food swamps" and "food deserts" that are more prevalent in low-income and historically disadvantaged communities
- Availability of and access to local emergency/health services, again dependent upon where a person lives
- Living environments free of life-threatening toxins, depending on the built and neighborhood physical environment. Unfortunately, a high prevalence of hazardous waste facilities are co-located with historically disadvantaged communities.

The World Health Organization (WHO, n.d.) indicates that social determinants "are the conditions in which people are born, grow, work, live, and age, and the wider set of forces and systems shaping the conditions of daily life. These forces and systems include economic policies and systems, development agendas, social norms, social policies, and political systems."

Thus, as overlapping "social policies and political systems," the use of the term "structural violence" is apt to describe health inequities resulting from "place." Gilligan (1997) defines *structural violence* as "the increased rates of death and disability suffered by those who occupy the bottom rungs of society, as contrasted with the relatively lower death rates experienced by those who are above them" (p. 200). According to Farmer et al. (2006), structural violence represents the "social arrangements that put individuals and populations in harm's way. ... The arrangements are structural because they are embedded in the political and economic organization of our social world; they are violent because they cause injury to people" (para. 4; see Chapter 2).

Structural violence, then, is a condition built into the social structure of U.S. society that serves to limit the ability of historically marginalized populations to live long and healthy lives. The probability of experiencing structural violence is disproportionately found among historically marginalized populations (Farmer, 2003).

In this chapter, several of the major social determinants of health that are embedded in the political and economic structure of U.S. society are examined relative to Latinos. These major social determinants include (a) economic stability, (b) quality education and access, (c) the social and community context, (d) health care access and quality, and (e) the neighborhood and built environment. Prior to this examination, however, it is important to view other social determinants that play a pivotal role in the need for quality and access to quality health care.

Major Social Determinants of Health

Where a person resides influences what they will experience in the physical and social environment in which they live. Moreover, where a person resides is influenced by socioeconomic status, as measured by income, poverty, and educational attainment that limit where a person resides in any given environment. A powerful social determinant is poverty, which is more prevalent in rural (nonmetro) areas in comparison to urban (metro). For example, in 2022 the USDA (n.d.-a) reported that the nonmetro poverty rate was 15.5% compared to 12.1% for metro areas. Can you think of other differences between urban and rural environments that affect access to and quality of education, health care, and social support networks?

The social determinants of health (SDOH) paradigm have gained widespread popularity as an explanation for health inequalities found among historically excluded populations, like Native Americans, Black Americans, and Latino Americans (see Figure 3.1). The SDOH paradigm theorizes that the social environments in which people interact with formal and informal institutions create circumstances that have an impact on a wide range of health outcomes, quality of life circumstances, and health risk behaviors (Office of Disease Prevention and Health Promotion, n.d.). From an intersectionality perspective, it is more useful to view these social determinants as intersecting, which mirrors the dynamic quality experienced. The SDOH areas tend to reinforce and synergize both positive and negative aspects of the social environment. They are also seen as intersecting forms of oppression (e.g., structural violence) when they come together in denying access to quality education, health care, and healthy social environments.

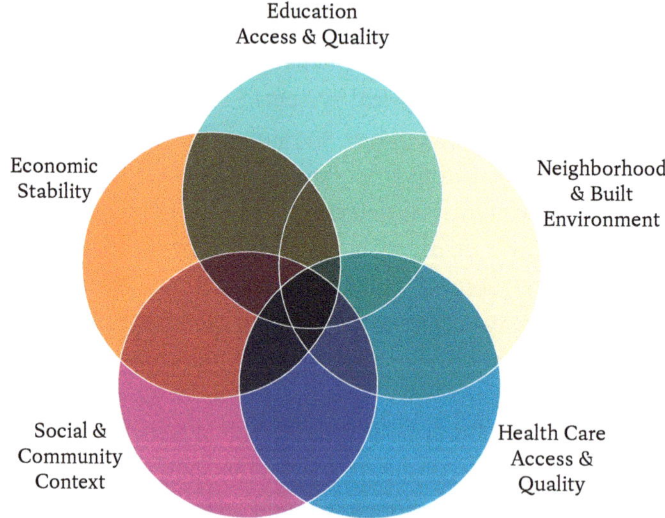

FIGURE 3.1 Intersecting Social Determinants of Health

The "place-based" approach of SDOH provides a useful framework to examine the health impact of each of the social influences as well as the potential synergy among them. For example, economic stability is associated with educational access and quality, access to health care, exposure to air pollution, and poverty. "Place" as conceived within a socioecological framework has become an increasingly important construct to understand the influence of social determinants on health. Moreover, the intersection of place, culture, and historical factors provides a much richer understanding of the complex nature of social and health inequalities that increase the social and health burden among historically marginalized populations in the United States. With respect to chronic diseases, social determinants affect access to prevention and early detection of heart disease, cancer, and type 2 diabetes, their incidence and timely diagnosis, their treatment and rehabilitation, posttreatment quality of life, and survival and mortality rates (Betancourt & Maina, 2004; Freeman, 2004). "Understanding the relationship between how population groups experience 'place' and the impact of 'place' on health is fundamental to the social determinants of health—including both social and physical determinants" (Office of Disease Prevention and Health Promotion, n.d.).

Economic Stability

Measures of economic stability include household income, income inequality or the wealth divide, poverty rates, employment status, occupation, food insecurity, and housing stability. *Economic well-being*, defined as having both present and future financial security to meet one's needs, is one of the more important social determinants of health (Office of Disease Prevention and Health Promotion, n.d.). Overall, Mexicans and Mexican Americans fare better on these measures than Black Americans but worse in comparison to than non-Latino White Americans.

Household Income

The U.S. Census Bureau (Guzman & Kollar, 2023) measures household income in several different ways. One informative measure is the amount of total earnings from full-time year-round workers 15 years and older. Non-Latino Whites have higher annual incomes than either non-Latino Blacks or Latinos. Almost 25% non-Latino White Americans earn $100,000 or more compared to almost 12% of non-Latino Black Americans and 8.5% of Americans of Mexican descent (see Table 3.1). Among the higher income groups in Table 3.1 ($75,000 or more), both non-Latino White Americans and Black Americans fare better than Americans of Mexican descent.

Among the Latino subgroups in the U.S. Census Bureau (2021) data, the highest percentage earning $100,000 or more is among South Americans (15.6%), with the lowest among Central Americans (6%). Latinos of Cuban, Central American, and Mexican descent have higher proportions of earning less than $25,000 annually than Latinos of Puerto Rican and South American descent. Non-Latino Black Americans have double the percentage, earning less than $25,000 annually compared to non-Latino White Americans (14.4% compared to 7.0%, respectively) but lower than Latinos (16.4%). Overall, among those earning more than $50,000 annually, non-Latino Black Americans (47%) have higher incomes than Latinos (40%) and 10% higher incomes than Mexican Americans (37.6%).

TABLE 3.1 Earnings of Full-Time, Year-Round Workers 15 Years and Over by Race and Latino Origin, 2020 (Percent)

Total money income in past year	Total White (alone)	Total Black (alone)	Total Latino[2]	Mexican	Puerto Rican	Cuban	Central American[3]	South American	Other Latino[4]
≤ $24,999	7.0	14.4	16.4	17.0	12.4	19.0	18.9	11.6	14.5
$25,000 to $34,999	10.3	16.1	19.9	21.1	13.2	18.6	21.8	15.5	20.3
$35,000 to $49,999	17.4	22.6	23.7	24.3	23.7	20.4	24.9	24.8	19.1
$50,000 to $74,999	27.2	25.7	22.5	21.5	28.0	20.0	22.1	23.3	25.6
$75,000 to $99,999	14.4	9.2	8.2	7.6	12.0	9.1	6.5	9.3	9.7
$100,000 and more	23.6	12.0	9.4	8.5	10.8	12.9	6.0	15.6	10.8

[2]Latino refers to people whose origin is Mexican, Puerto Rican, Cuban, Spanish-speaking Central or South American countries, or other Hispanic/Latino, regardless of race. [3] Central American totals exclude Mexican.[4] This category includes Dominicans and people who responded "Hispanic," "Latino," or provided other general terms. Source: U.S. Census Bureau (2021b)

Examining median family income with children under 18 present shows non-Latino White Americans have significantly higher income than Black Americans or Latino Americans (see Figure 3.2). The income

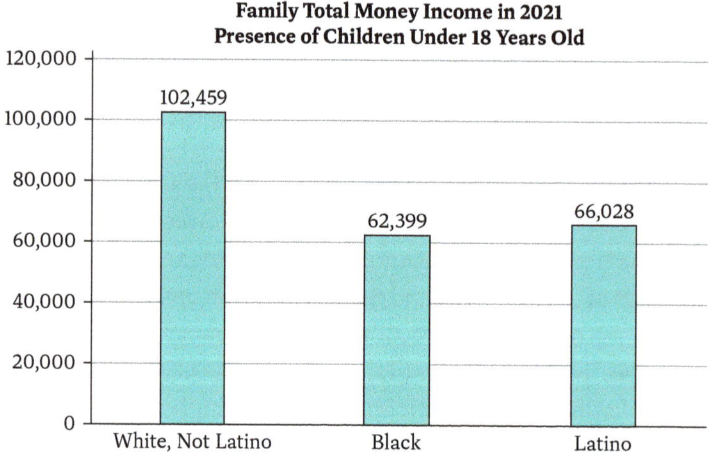

FIGURE 3.2 Family Total Income With Children Under 18 in 2021

Source: U.S. Census Bureau (2022)

gap between non-Latino White Americans and Black Americans is about $40,000/year, while the income gap between non-Latino White Americans and Latino Americans is smaller, at $36,400/year. Latino Americans earned about $2,600/year more than Black Americans in 2021, which provides a slightly different picture than the one above. Black families are slightly worse off than Latino families.

Income Inequality and the Racial Wealth Divide

In the United States, income inequality (the gap between the rich and everyone else) has been growing significantly for the last 30 years. The top 10% now average more than 9 times as much income as the bottom 90%. Moreover, the top 1% average over 40 times more income than the bottom 90% and, the top 0.1% are averaging over 198 times the income of the bottom 90% (Aladangady & Forde, 2021). This difference is even starker comparing non-Latino White Americans to Black Americans and Mexican Americans.

What is the difference between "wealth" and "income"? *Wealth* is the "net worth" of a person or household—the total value of assets minus liabilities. *Income* is the amount of money that a person or household receives in return for services, sale of goods, or profit from investments. Income generates wealth, while having wealth can enable a person or household to enjoy the benefits of their labor. Wealth takes time to acquire, while income is earned immediately. Wealth includes cash, real estate, and personal properties, such as jewelry and cars, while income is represented by a certain amount of money.

Much of the information provided below comes from the most recent Federal Reserve documentation and analyses of disparities in wealth from the 2019 Survey of Consumer Finances (Bhutta et al., 2020).

TABLE 3.2 Median Wealth by Age Group and by Race and Ethnicity in Thousands of 2019 U.S Dollars

	Non-Latino White	Non-Latino Black	Latino	Other
Under 35 years of age	25.4	0.6	11.2	13.5
35–54 years of age	185.0	40.1	46.1	154.5
Over 55 years of age	315.0	53.8	111.5	213.2

Source: Bhutta et al. (2020)

Bhutta et al. (2020) shows there are large wealth divides are apparent across racial and ethnic groups (see Table 3.2). Even among younger families (under 35 years of age) who have had relatively little time to accumulate wealth, there are sizeable gaps in wealth by race and ethnicity, most blatantly between younger Black families and younger non-Latino White families. The median younger Black family has almost no wealth ($600). In contrast, the median younger non-Latino White family has a wealth of $25,400. Younger Latinos and other families fall in between, with $11,200 and $13,500 in median wealth, respectively. Taken together, Table 3.2 shows that Latinos have more wealth at each age group than Black Americans (even doubling at the over 55 age group), but non-Latino White Americans have substantially higher wealth than both Latino and Black Americans at each successive age. Again, relative to non-Latino White Americans, Latinos are more financially disadvantaged. Moreover, even though Black Americans have higher median household earnings than Latinos, they are not accumulating wealth at the same rate.

Median net worth is another important measure of accumulated wealth. Bhutta et al. (2020) found that Black and Latino families have considerably less median net worth than non-Latino White families (see

TABLE 3.3 Median Net Worth by Race and Ethnicity in 2019 in Thousands of U.S Dollars

Race/ethnicity	Median net worth
Non-Latino White	188.2
Black	24.1
Latino	36.1
Other race	74.5

Source: Bhutta et al. (2020)

Table 3.3). Non-Latino White families have 7.8 times the median net worth of Black families and 5.2 times the median net worth for Latino families. Other families (those identifying as Asian, American Indian, Alaska Native, Native Hawaiian, Pacific Islander, and other race) have lower median net worth than non-Latino White families but higher median net worth than Black or Latino families.

More importantly, households with negative net wealth are more likely to be Latino and Black. According to analyses of Federal Reserve data from 2019, 14% of non-Latino White households had negative net wealth, compared to 28% of Black households and 26% of Mexican American households (Bhutta et al., 2020).

As seen above, racial, and ethnic wealth inequality persists among Mexican American and Black people in comparison to non-Latino White people. Additional research shows that non-Latino White Americans have *more opportunities* to acquire wealth through stocks/bonds, home ownership, inheritances, and other financial means than Mexican Americans and Black Americans (Aladangady & Forde, 2021). Many other factors contribute to the racial/ethnic wealth divide, including total earnings, the ability to save, and initial wealth. Studies have shown that generational wealth is more likely to occur among non-Latino White Americans than Mexican Americans or Black Americans (Feiveson & Sabelhaus, 2018; Thompson & Suarez, 2019). Non-Latino White families are substantially more likely to receive inheritances, gifts, and other family support than Black and Mexican American families.

Additionally, across all age groups, Black and Mexican American families are far less likely to have retirement accounts (Table 3.4). Moreover, non-Latino White families and to a lesser extent "other" families have more widespread access to employer-sponsored retirement plans than Black or Mexican American families. The disproportionate access for non-Latino White families relative to Mexican American families

TABLE 3.4 Access and Participation in Employee-Sponsored Retirement Plans

	Access	Participation
Non-Latino White	68	60
Latino	56	44
Black	44	34
Other	61	54

Source: Bhutta et al. (2020)

is the most blatant: For every three non-Latino White families that can access an employer-sponsored retirement plan, only two Mexican American families have similar access. With less opportunity to acquire wealth through, the economic well-being of Mexican Americans will continue to suffer, and they will never achieve wealth equity with non-Latino White people.

Economic Poverty

Numerous studies convincingly demonstrate the negative impact poverty has on poorer health status, higher levels of food insecurity, higher prevalence of chronic conditions, higher prevalence of infectious diseases, and overall higher morbidity rates (Abernathy et al., 2002; Chokshi, 2018; Hodgetts & Stolte, 2017; Starfield, 1992; Wagstaff, 2002).

According to Shrider et al. (2021), the poverty rate in the United States in 2020 was $30,000 for a family of four for the 48 contiguous states (i.e., not including Alaska or Hawaii). The overall poverty rate in 2020 was 15.3%. However, non-Latino White Americans have the lowest total poverty rates at 8.2%, compared to Black Americans (19.5%) and Mexican American (17%).

Among the Latino subgroups (see Figure 3.3), Central Americans have the highest poverty rate (21.1%) followed by Mexicans (17.5%) and Puerto Ricans (16.6%; U.S. Census Bureau, 2021a). However, the U.S. Census Bureau (2021a) reports that non-Latino Black Americans have higher poverty rates than Mexicans, Puerto Ricans, Cubans, South Americans, and "other" Latino subgroups. Coupled with the lack of wealth accumulation, the higher poverty rates among Black Americans are cause for concern.

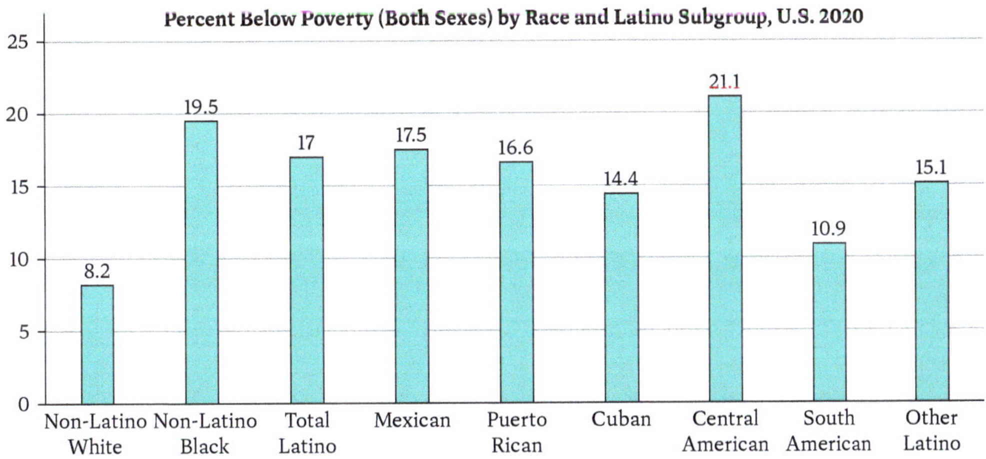

FIGURE 3.3 Percent Below Poverty by Latino Subgroup and Race, 2020

Source: U.S. Census Bureau (2021a)

Also, according to U.S. Census Bureau data (2021a) poverty rates are higher among women compared to their male counterparts (Figure 3.4). For every Latino subgroup, women have higher poverty rates, with the highest rate being among Central American women (23.7%), who have higher poverty rates than non-Latino Black women (21.5%), similar to the above documentation.

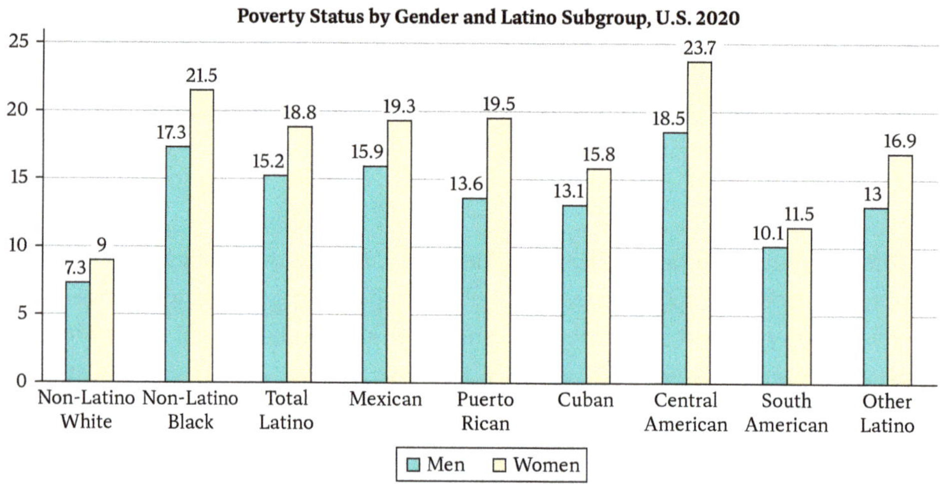

FIGURE 3.4 Poverty Status by Gender and Latino Subgroup, 2020

Source: U.S. Census Bureau (2021a)

Among single-headed female households, the poverty rates are higher (Figure 3.5). Other social factors that contribute to higher rates of poverty among women include lower educational attainment, higher unemployment rates, and the difference in pay between men and women, referred to as the *gender wage gap*.

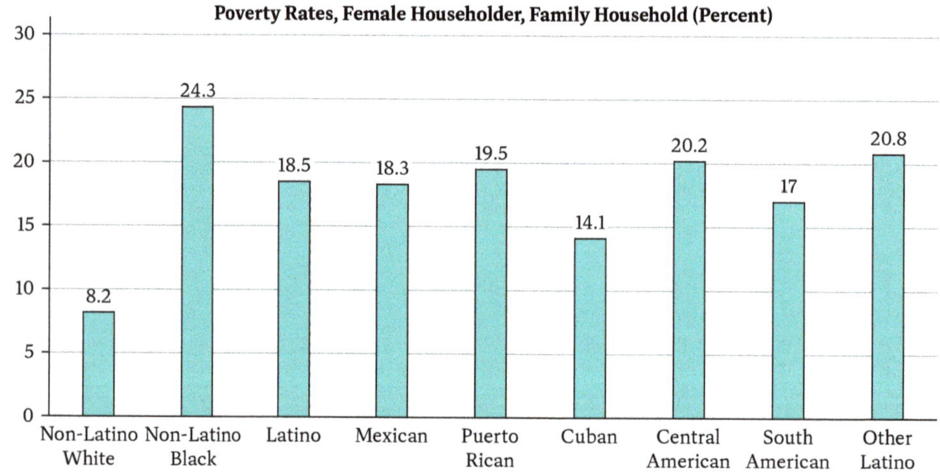

FIGURE 3.5 Female Householders Poverty by Race and Latino Subgroup, 2021

Source: U.S. Census Bureau (2021a)

Non-Latina Black women have significantly higher poverty rates, almost 3 times the rate, than non-Latina White women (24.3% vs. 8.2%, respectively). Mexican women have twice the poverty rate compared to non-Latina White women but 6% lower than non-Latina Black women. Among Latina subgroups, about 20% of Central American and "other" Latina female households live in poverty. The lowest female householder poverty rate is among Latinas of Cuban descent (14.1%), which is still almost twice the rate of non-Latina female households (U.S. Census Bureau, 2021a).

Poverty status among Latino youth 18 years of age and younger are problematic (U.S. Census Bureau, 2021a) (Figure 3.6). Overall, almost 1 in 4 Latino youth are living in poverty, usually with female-headed households, as noted above. More than a one fifth of Puerto Rican, Cuban, Central American, and Mexican youth are living below the poverty level. The lowest youth poverty rates are among South Americans and other Latinos. Non-Latino Black people have higher rates of poverty in each age group than non-Latino White people and Latinos. Central American adults 18–64 have the highest poverty rate among the Latino subgroups (18.8%), and South Americans have the lowest poverty rate in the same age group (9%). The high poverty rates among elderly Latinos and non-Latino Black people (65 and older) are of great concern because of the intersection of poverty, food insecurity, and housing stability as well as feelings of alienation, higher rates of depression, and chronic conditions.

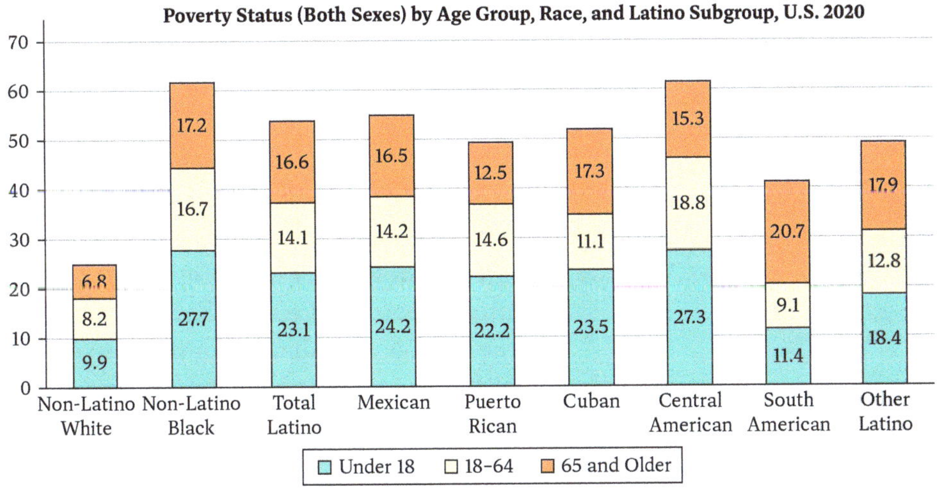

FIGURE 3.6 Poverty Status by Age Group, Race, and Latino Subgroup

Source: Semega et al. (2020)

According to Semega et al. (2020), family households maintained by women with no spouse present had the lowest median income ($48,098). For families with a female householder, the poverty rate was 22.2%, representing 3.3 million families in 2019, a decline from 24.9 percent and 3.7 million families in 2018, respectively. Non-Latino Black families have the highest percentage of households that are female headed (no spouse present), almost 3 times the rate as non-Latina White women (Figure 3.7). Among the Latina subgroups, "other" Latina and Central American women have the highest percent of households headed by women, followed by Puerto Rican women.

In 2020, almost 60% of all children in poverty lived in families headed by an unmarried mother (Javaid & Tucker, 2021). The U.S. Census Bureau (2021a) reports that among families with children under age 18, Latina mother-only families had higher poverty rates than other families: 46.3% for Latina families, compared to 45.6% for Black families, 32.0 % for non-Latino White families, and 28.9% for Asian families. Even in mother-only families with children under age 18 where the householder works full-time year-round,

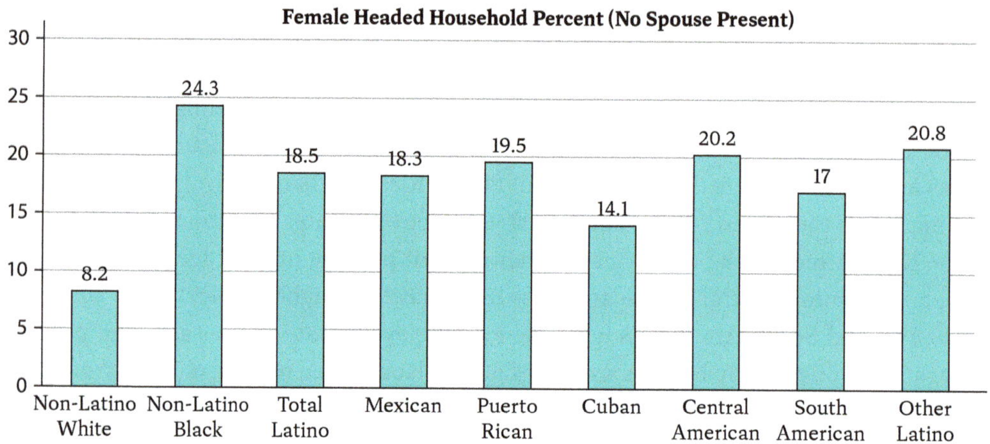

FIGURE 3.7 Female-Headed Households (Percent) by Race and Latino Subgroup, 2021

Source: U.S. Census Bureau (2021a)

Latinas experienced higher poverty rates than others: 19.8% of Latina families, compared to 17.5% of Black families, 13.0% of Asian families, and 7.5% of non-Latino White families.

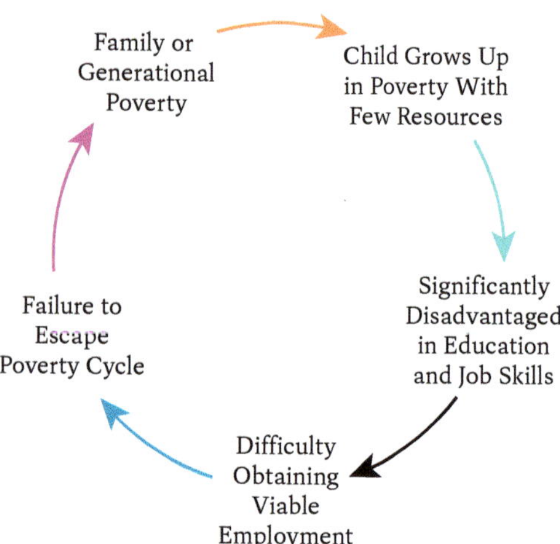

FIGURE 3.8 The Poverty Cycle

Poverty is not only about low income. Poverty influences psychological well-being, hopefulness about the future, and resiliency in coping with diminished opportunities. Decades of research shows that poverty is one of the strongest predictors for poor physical and mental health and increased mortality among populations. Among younger age groups, poverty is correlated with poor nutrition, inadequate housing, inadequate sanitation, poorer quality education, less access to health care, less access to high-paying occupations, as well as a higher incidence of infectious and chronic diseases (Abernathy et al., 2002; Chokshi, 2018). Stopping the cycle of poverty will enhance the physical and emotional well-being of historically marginalized populations in the United States (see Figure 3.8).

Employment and Unemployment Status

Latinos have been and continue to be a major driving force in the U.S. labor market, projected to account for almost 80% of net new workers between 2020 and 2030 (U.S. Bureau of Labor Statistics, 2023c). In fact, the number of Latinos in the labor force has almost tripled from 10.7 million in 1990 to 29.0 million in 2020. Latino workers are also younger on average than other racial/ethnic groups (U.S. Bureau of Labor Statistics, 2023c)

Even though Latinos are a major driver of the U.S. labor force, the types of occupations that they are employed in are often more dangerous and underpaid (e.g., farming, construction, and transportation).

As we have seen, total family income in 2021 was much lower for Latinos than it was for non-Latino White families ($66,028 and $102,459, respectively), representing a $36,000 difference in annual earnings (U.S. Census Bureau, 2022b).

According to the U.S. Department of Labor Statistics (2023a), 61.7% of the U.S. civilian population over the age of 16 were in the labor force. Unemployment rates were higher for non-Latino Blacks and Latinos than for non-Latino Whites (see Figure 3.9). Black people had double the rate of unemployed compared to non-Latino White people (10.1%, compared to 4.9%, respectively). Latinos had lower unemployment rates than Black Americans but higher than non-Latino White Americans. Among the Latino subgroups, "other" Latino had the highest unemployment rate (9.8%), followed by Puerto Ricans (9.5%).

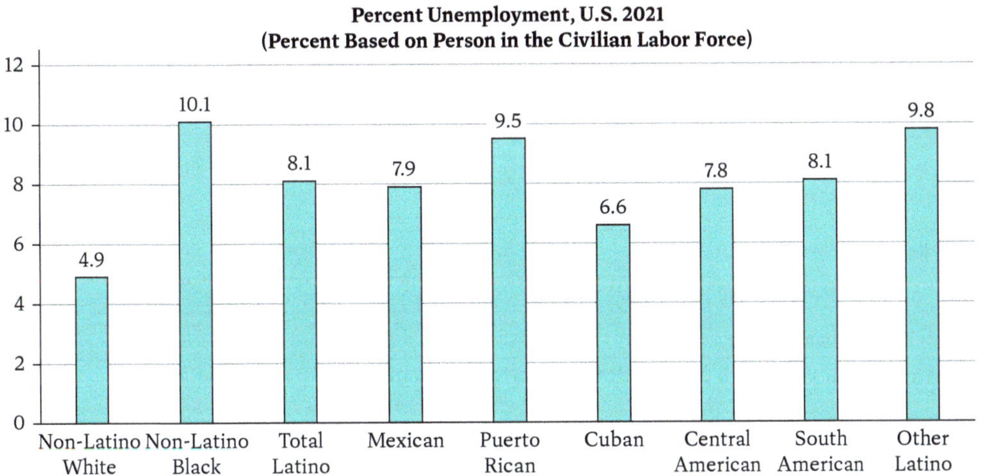

FIGURE 3.9 Percent Unemployment in the United States 2021

Source: U.S. Census Bureau (2021a)

The Gender-Wage Gap

Women remain underpaid relative to men (see Table 3.5). Women's earnings as a percentage of men's have increased from 62.3 cents per dollar in 1979 to 83.1 cents per dollar in 2021 (U.S. Bureau of Labor Statistics, 2023b). Even though there has been an increase of 21 cents/dollar, that rate varies by race, ethnicity, occupation, and educational status. For example, in 2021, among 25–34-year-olds for full-time wage and salary workers, the rate was 90.1 cents per dollar, and among workers 35–44 years, it was 79.9 cents per dollar (see Figure 3.10).

For Latinas, available data from the U.S. Bureau of Labor Statistics (2023a) shows that they earn 87.6% of what their Latino male counterparts earn weekly. Latinas' earnings as a percentage of Latino men's earnings are relatively high in comparison to non-Latina White women due to the low earnings of Latino and Black men relative to non-Latino White men. For example, Black men earned 57% as much ($825) as non-Latino White men ($1,125), and Latino men earned 56% as much ($820) as non-Latino White men (U.S. Bureau of Labor Statistics, 2023a).

TABLE 3.5 Women's Earnings as a Percentage of Men's, 2021

Race/ethnicity	Percentage of men's earnings (per $1.00)
Total women to men 16 years and older	83.1
White women to White men	82.2
Black women to Black men	94.1
Latinas to Latinos	87.6

Source: U.S. Bureau of Labor Statistics (2023b)

The Gender Wage Gap Is Much Wider for Most Women of Color
Comparing 2020 Median Earnings of Full-Time, Year-Round Workers by Race/Ethnicity and Sex

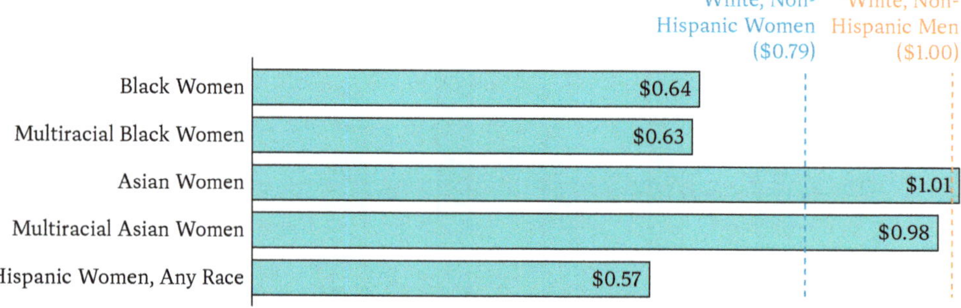

Note: The gender wage gap is calculated by finding the ratio of women's and men's median earnings for full-time, year-round workers and then taking the difference. People who have identified as Hispanic or Latino may be of any race.

Source: For all groups, authors calculated the gender wage gap using data from U.S. Census Bureau, "Current Population Survey: PINC-05. Work Experience-People 15 Years Old and Over, by Total Money Earnings, Age, Race, Hispanic Origin, Sex, and Disability Status: 2020," available at https://www.census.gov/data/tables/time-series/demo/income-poverty/cps-pinc/pinc-05.html (last accessed September 2021).

FIGURE 3.10 The Gender Wage Gap in the United States, 2021

In the United States, higher levels of education are associated with higher employment rates and higher income among persons aged 25 and older (U.S. Bureau of Labor Statistics, n.d.-b). Among persons with a bachelor's degree, Latinos earned the least ($66,300), non-Latino Whites earned the most ($88,640), and non-Latino Blacks were in between earning $72,680 (Statista, n.d.).

Intersectionality provides a method to disentangle the differential effects of gender, income, education, and their influences on health and psychological wellbeing (Hankivsky, 2012). For example, several researchers have noted that the intersection of education level, income, and gender can influence occupational status (Zimmerman & Seiler, 2019), health status (Iyer et al., 2009), and depression (Assari, 2017) among women. In 2021, the National Center for Education Statistics (2023) showed stark wage gaps between women, their level of education and median annual earnings. For example, women compared to men with a bachelor's degree earned $14,000 less ($56,000 vs. $70,000). Moreover, at the master's degree level or higher, women earned $25,000 less than their male counterparts ($64,000 vs. $89,600).

The National Center for Education Statistics (2023) also shows major differences in median earnings by gender and educational attainment. Non-Latina White, full-time, year-round workers with a bachelor's degree had higher median earnings than their peers who were Black ($50,000), Latina ($49,900), and women of two or more races ($49,300). Among those with a master's or higher degree, those who were non-Latina White ($69,700) had higher median earnings than those who were Latina ($59,200) and Black ($53,300).

Data released by the U.S. Department of Labor Women's Bureau (n.d.-a) reveals stark contrasts between women's earning as a percentage of non-Latino White men's annual earnings that are most pronounced at beyond the bachelor's degree. In comparison to non-Latino White men's earnings, non-Latino White women holding an advanced degree earned 75.8%, Latinas earned 72%, and non-Latina Black women earned 70.5%.

Additionally, in comparison to their racial/ethnic male counterparts, the earnings ratio for non-Latina White women is 80%, for non-Latina Black women it is 95.8%, and for Latinas it is 86.7%. One reason the ratios are higher for non-Latina Black women and Latinas in comparison to their respective male counterparts is due to the low earnings of non-Latino Black men and Latino men relative to non-Latino White men (U.S. Department of Labor Women's Bureau, n.d.-b). According to the World Economic Forum's (2023) *Global Gender Gap Report*, women will not achieve wage parity with their male counterparts for 131 years, or the year 2154 (p.5)

Data from the U.S. Department of Labor, Women's Bureau (n.d.-b) on median annual earnings by race, gender, and ethnicity reveal stark differences between non-Latino Whites, non-Latino Blacks, and Latinos (Figure 3.11). Latino men earn significantly less than their non-Latino White counterparts and earn less than non-Latino Black men. Latinas have the lowest median annual earnings compared to other women.

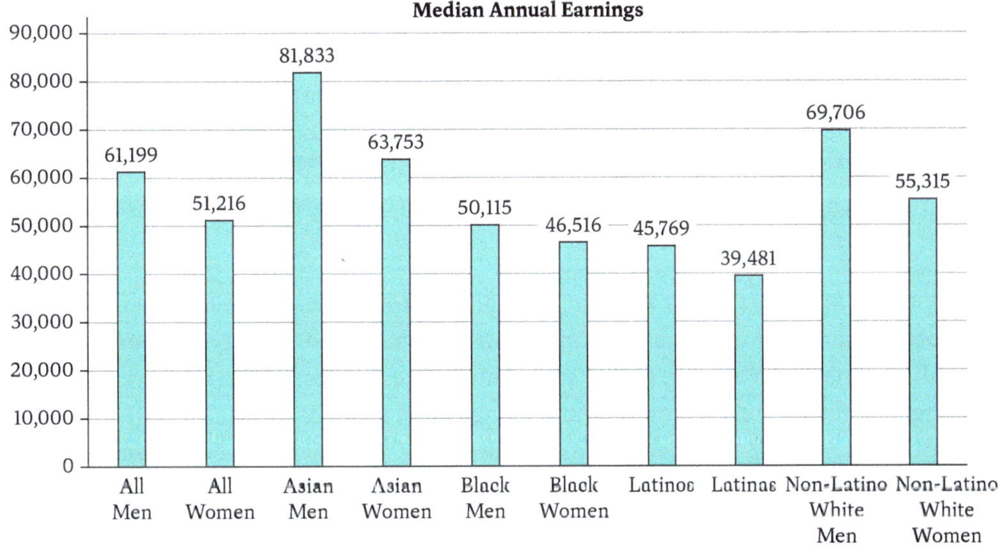

FIGURE 3.11 Median Earnings by Race, Gender, and Ethnicity, 2022

Source: U.S. Department of Labor, Women's Bureau (n.d.-b)

Occupation

Occupation influences one's income, employment, and health insurance coverage. For example, in 2021 over 54% of persons received employment-based health insurance (U.S. Census Bureau, 2021a). Some occupations are seasonal only, typically in the farming and construction areas, while the majority are year-round (see Figure 3.12). Occupations like farming and construction are also more hazardous, resulting in many more injuries, functional limitations, and contributing to chronic conditions like osteoarthritis and other musculoskeletal conditions (Kirkhorn et al., 2003; Thelin et al., 2004; Xiao et al., 2013).

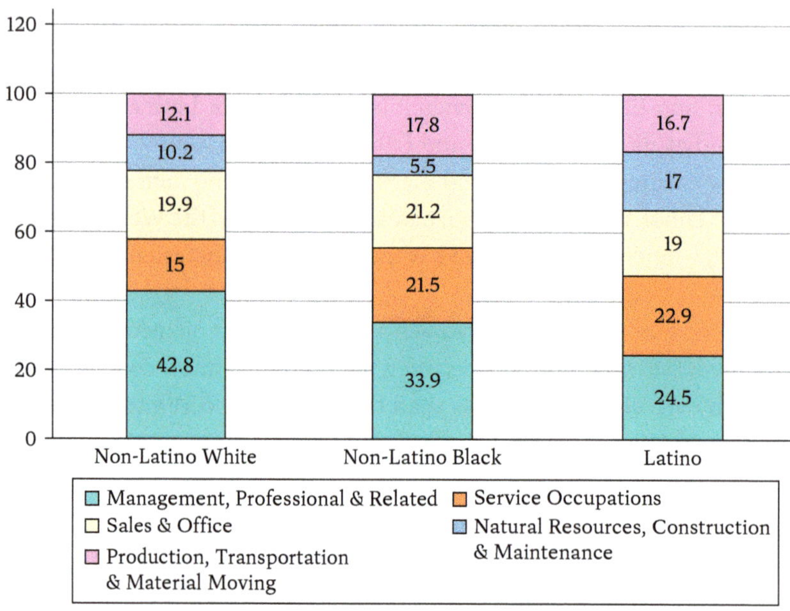

FIGURE 3.12 Occupation of the Civilian Employed Population 16 Years and Over by Sex, Race, and Latino Subgroup, United States, 2021, Percent Distribution

Source: U.S. Bureau of Labor Statistics (2021)

Some Latinos are at increased risk for occupational injuries and death due to their overrepresentation in hazardous occupations, low educational attainment, discrimination, immigration status, and language barriers, including signage. Among the Latino subgroups, more Mexicans than others are employed in the farming, fishing, and forestry occupations, and a higher percentage of Central Americans are employed in the construction, extraction, and maintenance occupations. There is a higher percentage of non-Latino White people in the management and professional occupations and sales and office occupations than Latinos (U.S. Department of Labor, 2022).

Agricultural workers are at very high risk for morbidity and mortality. It is one of the most hazardous occupations with associated health issues including accidents, pesticide-exposure related illnesses, heat-related illnesses, communicable diseases, and musculoskeletal problems, like low back pain, hip arthritis, degenerative arthritis of the knee, and upper extremity neck and shoulder problems. Communicable diseases are common among migrant farmworkers, including COVID-19, hepatitis A, B, and C, HPV, and several types of sexually transmitted diseases, like syphilis, gonorrhea, chlamydia, and HIV/AIDS (Hansen & Donohoe, 2003; Lewnard et al., 2021; Rhodes et al., 2010; Scott, 2009).

Pesticide exposure is one of the more insidious dangers because it can be absorbed through the skin, lungs, and mouth. Pesticides are directly sprayed through aerial or ground application to vegetables and fruits that can drift to where workers are. Also, reentering freshly sprayed fields increases the likelihood of pesticide contamination. Contact with dry pesticide residue can cause illness as well as eating or smoking with contaminated hands. Agricultural workers are also exposed to pesticides by eating newly harvested vegetables or fruit without washing them first, drinking from common containers in the field or bathing in canals, and using steel/aluminum containers for water storage that had previously been used to store pesticides.

The health effects of pesticide poisoning are both short and long term. Neurological effects such as slurred speech and inability to walk are known to occur. Dermatitis is also common. Long-term effects can include cancers like leukemia, Hodgkin's disease, multiple myeloma, and cancers of the lip, skin, brain, and prostate (Arcury et al., 2014; Calvert et al., 2008; Quandt et al., 2016). Moreover, indirect exposure occurs through contaminated clothing. Women who are pregnant can have spontaneous abortions and miscarriages, mutagenic and teratogenic effects on the developing fetus, and contaminated breast milk (Eskenazi et al., 1999; Hernández-Valero et al., 2003; Perfecto, 2019).

Health insurance coverage is associated with occupational status, with 54.5% of people having employee-based health coverage (Keisler-Starkey et al., 2023). Among those occupations that routinely provide health insurance coverage to their employees, the majority are "white collar" (i.e., management, professional and related occupations). Boal and Sussel (2018), using 2014 BRFSS survey data, found that the highest rates of uninsured were among construction and extraction (18.6%), farming, fishing, and forestry (19.4%), food preparation and serving related (19.3%), and building and grounds cleaning and maintenance (16.7%), all occupations with high percentages of Latino workers). The three occupations with the highest work-related mortality are in the transportation area (tractor-trailer drivers), farmers and ranchers, and construction laborers. In 2021, there were 2.6 million nonfatal injuries and illnesses in the private sector and 5,190 work-related fatalities in all sectors (U.S. Bureau of Labor Statistics, 2023b).

Food Insecurity

Food insecurity—that is, the inability to acquire and consume adequate and appropriate amounts of foodstuffs—is directly associated with poverty. The U.S. Department of Agriculture (USDA, 2023) defines *food insecurity* as "a household-level economic and social condition of limited or uncertain access to adequate food" ("CNSTAT Review" section). Food insecurity is inextricably linked to poverty, affordable housing, social isolation, health problems, and unemployment.

Food insecurity undermines the health of Latinos who live in poverty and must make a difficult choice between putting food on the table and paying the bills. Even when food is available, it may not be nutritious. Food insecurity is also associated with lack of affordable housing, health problems, social isolation, and unemployment. The southwestern states of Arizona, New Mexico, and Texas have food insecurity rates higher than the U.S. national average (Coleman-Jensen et al., 2022).

The overabundance of high caloric and high saturated fat foods in a community is referred to as a *food swamp*. Alternatively, those communities that do not have access to more nutritious foods are referred to as *food deserts*. Food deserts are defined by the USDA as "areas where people have limited access to a variety of healthy and affordable food" (Dutko et al., 2012, p. iii).

Food insecurity in the United States varies by race and ethnicity (Hales & Coleman-Jensen (2024). For example, in 2021 19.8% of non-Latino Black households were food insecure, compared to 16.2% of Latino households and 7% of non-Latino White households. Hales & Coleman-Jensen (2024) also found that food insecurity varied by Latino subgroup. For example, 11.4% of Cuban households compared to 21% of Dominican households were food insecure. Additionally, Central American (19.1%), Dominican (21%), and Puerto Rican (19%) households had significantly higher food insecurity than all Latino households (16.9%). Alternatively, Cuban (11.4%) and South American (12.1%) households had significantly lower food insecurity than all Latino households. 17.2% of Latinos of Mexican descent had a prevalence of low food security, slightly above the overall Latino household prevalence. Several chronic conditions are found to be more prevalent in food deserts, such as obesity, cardiovascular disease, and diabetes mellitus (type 2 diabetes) (Kelli et al., 2017; Cooksey-Stowers et al., 2017).

Housing Stability and Affordability

Homeownership has not changed dramatically in the United States over the past decade. According to USA-Facts (2023), in 2012, the rate of homeownership was 65.4% and in 2022 it was 65.8%, a difference of only 0.4 percentage points. Homeownership in the United States varies significantly by race and ethnicity. In 2019, the homeownership rate among non-Latino White Americans was 73.3%, compared to 47.5 percent for Latinos and 42.1% among non-Latino Black Americans. This represents a 25.8% difference between Latinos and non-Latino White people. Additionally, homeownership is lower for Latinos and non-Latino Black Americans in comparison to non-Latino White Americans across all age groups (see Figure 3.13). However, homeownership rates increased by over 6 percentage points among Latinos.

Housing instability is created when the affordability and demand for housing increases. In 2019, prior to the COVID-19 pandemic, homeownership and rentals among Latinos varied, with 10.2% of Latinos being

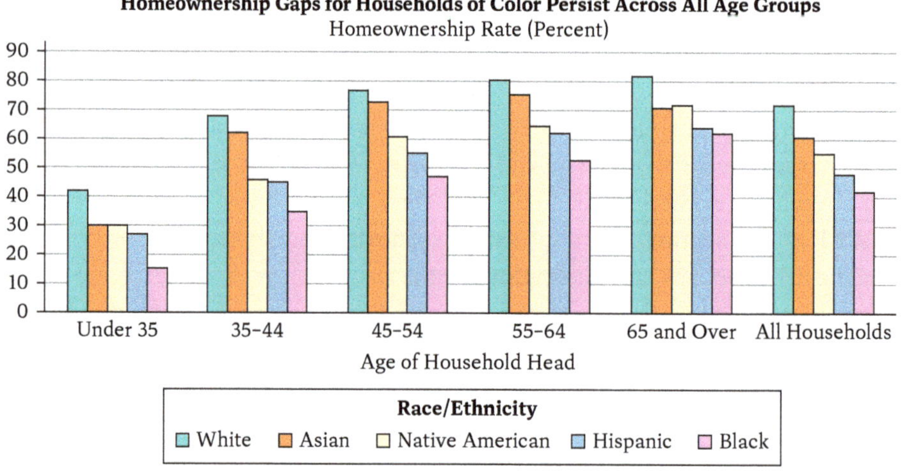

FIGURE 3.13 Homeownership, Age, and Race/Ethnicity, 2019

homeowners and 19.7% renters (DeSilver, 2021). According to DeSilver (2021) renters are more likely to be lower incomes and less wealth than homeowners.

A financial rule of thumb is that housing costs should not exceed 30% of a household's income. A report by the Joint Center for Housing Studies of Harvard University (JCHS, 2021) indicated that 37.1 million households were "housing cost burdened," spending 30% or more of their income on housing, which represented 30.2% of all households nationally. They also found that 1 in 7 households—17.6 million in total—were "severely cost burdened," spending 50% or more of their income on housing. Renters were more cost burdened than homeowners, with 46% of renters "cost burdened," compared to 21% of homeowners. In addition, 24% of renters and 9% of homeowners were "severely cost burdened" (JCHS, 2021).

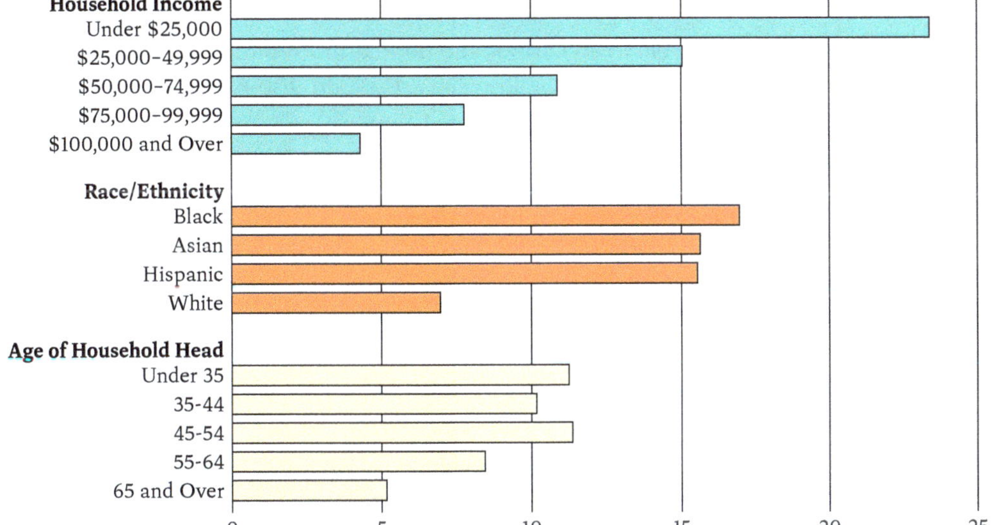

FIGURE 3.14 Percentage Behind on Mortgage, Early 2021

According to the JCHS (2021) report, Black renters had the highest share of cost burden (53.7%), followed closely by Latino renters (51.9%) and households identifying as multiracial or another race (46.6%). By comparison, 41.9% of non-Latino White renters were cost burdened, along with 42.2% of Asian renters. Furthermore, as of early 2021, the JCHS (2021) report shows that 17% of Black, 16% of Latino, and 16% of Asian homeowners were behind on their mortgage payments, which was more than twice the 7% share of non-Latino White homeowners (see Figure 3.14). Homeowners of color earning between $25,000 and $50,000 were also disproportionately behind on mortgage payments. Similarly, 23% of Black, 20% of Latino, and 19% of Asian renters were late on their rents, compared to 10% of non-Latino White renters.

The Latino Policy Forum (n.d.) indicates that Mexican Americans are overburdened with housing costs, and their housing instability places them at increased risk of losing their homes. As the number of evictions increase post-pandemic, so will the number of Mexican Americans who experience homelessness. The interconnectedness among unemployment, poverty, and lack of housing will undoubtedly lead to increased homelessness, lack of proper nutrition, and increased risk for chronic and infectious diseases among Mexican Americans.

In the area of economic stability, Mexican Americans appear to fare better than Black Americans: Their median income is higher (though household income is lower), their poverty rates are lower, their employment rates are higher, homeownership is higher, and overall net worth is higher. When data was available by Latino subgroup, Mexican Americans tend to fare better than Black Americans in most measures of economic stability but fare worse than non-Latino White Americans in all measures of economic stability considered.

Education Access and Quality

There is a substantial educational gap between Latinos and non-Latino White Americans and Black Americans that continues to persist (Murphey et al., 2014; Reardon & Galindo, 2009). The causes are multifaceted, including poverty, English learning ability, lack of parental support, and failing school (Gándara & Mordechay, 2017; Good et al., 2010; Madrid, 2011). Increasing attention to the developmental needs of Latino children has resulted in more preschool enrichment activities that enhance their chances for success in elementary, middle, and high school (Cabrera, 2013). For example, a study conducted by Bustamante and Hindman (2020) found that Mexican Americans preschoolers do well in social emotional and executive functioning skills that positively predict academic school readiness, and leveraging these strengths may decrease the educational gap. A report by the National Research Center on Hispanic Children & Families (2018) shows that Mexican American parents are as likely as other parents to engage their children in Early Care and Education (ECE) programs. They showed that about half of low-income Mexican American children 0–5 years of age were in ECE arrangements. Research also shows that Mexican American children benefit in academic achievement and social skills when interacting with their non-Latino peers (Riegle-Crumb & Callahan, 2009; Fuller & García Coll, 2010).

Educational Attainment

Unfortunately, Latinos have had higher high school dropout rates than non-Latino White students. *Dropout rates* are the percentage of 16- to 24-year-olds who are not enrolled in high school and who lack a high school credential (either a diploma or an alternative credential such as a GED certificate; National Center for Educational Statistics [NCES], 2024). In 2010, the Latino dropout rate was 15.1%, compared to 5.1% for non-Latino White students and 8.0% for Black students. In 2020, however, the dropout rate decreased to 7.4% among Latino students but was still higher than non-Latino White students (4.8%) and Black students (4.2%). According to the National Center for Education Statistics (2023), "the overall status dropout rate for 16–24-year-old decreased from 8.3% in 2010 to 5.2% in 2021."

Irwin et al. (2022) found that status dropout rates vary significantly by generational status among Latinos (see Figure 3.15). Latinos born outside the United States have more than twice the dropout rate as first generation Latinos and 3 times the dropout rate as second generation Latinos. Interestingly, first generation Latinos have almost 3 times the dropout rate as non-Latino Whites, but Latino and non-Latino second generation groups have similar dropout rates. Dropout rates also varied by gender, with Latinas 16–24 years of age having lower dropout rates than Latinos of the same age (5.9% compared to 8.9%, respectively).

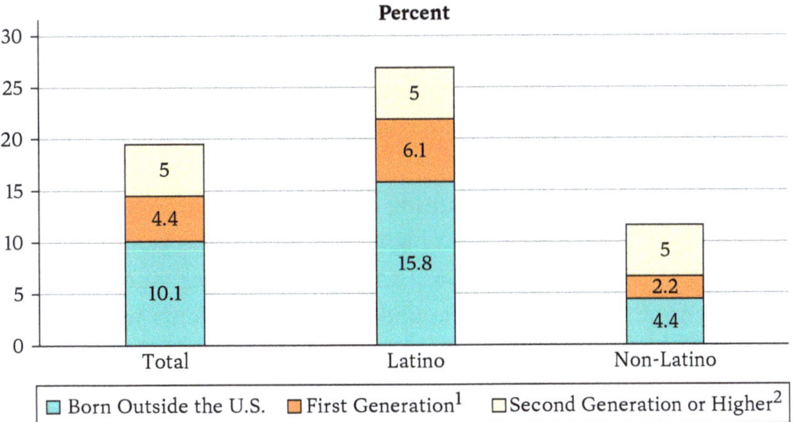

[1]Individuals defined as "first generation" were born in the United States, but one or both of their parents were born outside the United States.

[2]Individuals defined as "second generation or higher" were born in the United States, as were both of their parents.

FIGURE 3.15 Dropout Rates of Latino and Non-Latino 16- to 24-Year-Olds, by Generation, 2020

Nationally, Latino high school dropout rates have fallen substantially since 1996, from 34% to 10% in 2016 (Gramlich, 2017). Nevertheless, U.S. Census Bureau data (2021a) shows that 25.8% of Latinos have less than a high school diploma, compared to only 4.9% of non-Latino Whites. Moreover, 20.6% of Latinos have a bachelor's degree or more, compared to 41.9% of non-Latino Whites. Clearly, Latino students still lag non-Latinos in high school graduation rates.

According to the National Center for Educational Statistics (NCES, 2022), the overall college enrollment rate was 40% in 2020 and was not appreciably different from 2010. However, the college enrollment rates for 2-year and 4-year institutions changed in opposite directions over this 10-year period. The rate for 2-year institutions *decreased* from 13% to 9% between 2010 and 2020, while the rate for 4-year institutions *increased* from 28% to 31% during this period. The college enrollment rate for Latinos 18- to 24-year-olds was higher in 2020 (36%) than in 2010 (32%) but still lower than non-Latino White Americans (41% in 2020) and similar to Black Americans (36%). The college enrollment rate for those who were non-Latino White was higher than the rate for those who were Black in every year from 2010 to 2018, as well as in 2020; the two rates were not appreciably different in 2019. The college enrollment rate for those who were non-Latino White was also higher than the rate for those who were Latino in every year from 2010 to 2020, except for 2016, when the rates were not appreciably different.

The NCES (2022) also found that in every year since 2010, the college enrollment rate for 18- to 24-year-olds overall was higher for women than for men. This pattern was also observed for both non-Latino White and Latino 18- to 24-year-olds. Among those who were Black, the college enrollment rate was higher for women than for men in 7 of the last 11 years for which data were available. The rates were not appreciably different in 2012, 2015, 2016, and 2019. The college enrollment rate was higher in 2020 than in 2010 for Latinas (42% vs. 36%).

College enrollment does not always translate to college completion rates. The NCES provides information on the 6-year completion rate (150% of normal time to completion) of first-time undergraduate students at 4-year institutions by race and ethnicity using the 2010 cohort (NCES, 2019).

NCES (2019) information (Figure 3.16) clearly shows Latino students lagging non-Latino White students in in 4-year completion rates (45% vs. 32%, respectively), with Black students faring far worse (21% completion at 4 years and 14% at 5 years). Among college students of different racial/ethnic groups who began seeking a bachelor's degree at a 4-year-degree-granting institution in fall 2010, the 6-year graduation rate for first-time, full-time undergraduate students was highest for non-Latino White students (64%), students of two or more races (60%), and Latino students (54%) and lowest for Black students (40%). In comparison, the 4-year graduation rates for first-time, full-time undergraduate students were 50% or less for Latino, Black, and two or more race's students.

Additionally, NCES (2019) show that at 2-year degree-granting institutions, 30% of first-time, full-time undergraduate students who began seeking a certificate or associate degree in fall 2013 attained it within 150% of the normal time required for completion of these programs (e.g., completing a 2-year degree within 3 years). The 150% graduation rate was highest for non-Latino White students (32%) and Latino students (30%) but lower for students of two or more races (25%) and Black students (23%).

As expected, there are dynamic variations in level of educational attainment among Latinos depending on their subgroup (e.g., Mexican, Puerto Rican, Cuban, etc.). According to the U.S. Census Bureau (2021b) Central Americans and Mexicans have the lowest percentages of college graduates among Latinos 25 years and older, compared to Cubans and South Americans, who have the highest percentages of college graduates (Figure 3.16).

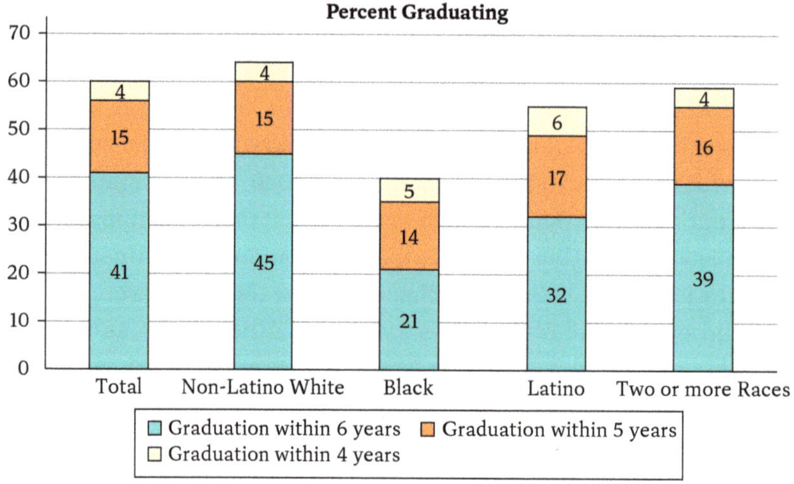

FIGURE 3.16 Percent Graduating From College in 6, 5, and 4 years, 2019

Educational attainment is associated with income level, occupation, and poverty status, all of which are important influences on the health of individuals and populations. Together, they act synergistically to increase or decrease individual and population health risks.

In comparing Latino subgroups in Figure 3.17, South Americans have the highest educational attainment (43.4% have a bachelor's degree or higher), with Mexicans having the second lowest rate (15.9% have a bachelor's degree or higher). Overall, about 79% of Latinos do not have a bachelor's degree compared to 72.5% of non-Latino Blacks and 58.1% of non-Latino Whites. Rates of not having a bachelor's degree are highest for Central Americans (85.3%) and Latinos of Mexican descent (84.1%).

Several educational barriers among Latinos are documented in the research literature (Becerra, 2012; Giraldo-García et al., 2019; Marrero, 2016; Martinez et al., 2004). These include socioeconomic barriers like parental poverty, unemployment, and work responsibilities of the student to contribute to the family. Other barriers cited include what researchers call *cultural barriers*, like limited English skills, low educational aspirations, and not as hard working as non-Latino students. Additional factors include lack of Latino parental involvement and important institutional factors, like segregation and institutionalized racism, attacks on Latino cultural studies, and lack of teacher education and preparation in cultural humility (Ellerbrock et al., 2016; Gay, 2002; Villegas & Lucas, 2002).

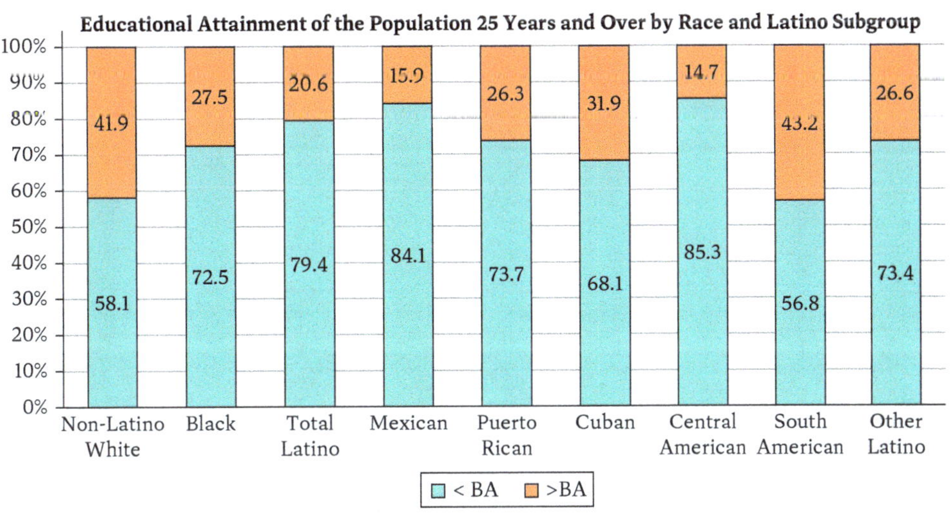

FIGURE 3.17 Educational Attainment by Race and Latino Subgroup, 2020

Source: U.S. Census Bureau (2021b)

English Language Proficiency and Literacy Rates

In 2021, almost one-third (31.8%) of Latinos residing in the United States speak only English (Statista, n.d.). Additionally, 40.1% speak English "very well," with only a combined 15.5% of Latinos speaking English "not well or not at all," indicating that most Latinos speak English, another popular myth buster. Latino youth are the main drivers of this trend toward English only. Among foreign-born Latinos, data shows that English language proficiency improves with length of residence in the United States and is generally increasing among subsequent generations born in the United States (Krogstad et al., 2022).

According to data released by Statista (Korhonen, 2023) the percentage of Latinos in the United States who speak English proficiently is increasing (see Figure 3.18). In 2021, almost three quarters of Latinos ages 5 and older spoke English proficiently, up from 59% in 2000. Driving this growth are U.S.-born Latinos, as their percentage has grown from 81% to 91% during the same time span (Krogstad et al., 2023). By comparison, 37% of Latino immigrants spoke English proficiently in 2021, a percentage that has increased only somewhat since 2000. Taken together, 41.7 million Latinos in the United States spoke English proficiently in 2021. At the same time, the proportion of Latinos who speak Spanish at home declined by 10% (78% in 2000 to 68% in 2021). Among U.S.-born Latinos, slightly more than half (55%) speak Spanish at home. Nearly all Latino immigrants (93% in 2021) indicate they speak Spanish at home.

Even though English language proficiency among Latinos is increasing, most Latinos are bilingual English-Spanish speakers. Pew Research Center (2013) data indicates that among those who speak English, 59% are bilingual. Additionally, 50% of second-generation and 23% of third-generation or higher Latinos were bilingual. One can conclude that Spanish language is still important among all Latino subgroups, which provides a common linguistic foundation and a shared cultural element.

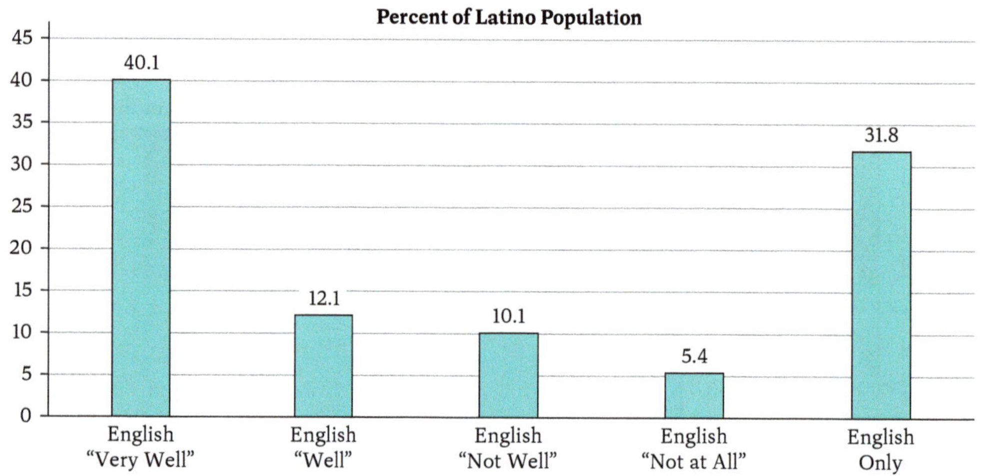

FIGURE 3.18 Distribution of English Language Proficiency Among Latinos, United States, 2022

According to the NCES (2014), about 4 out of 5 U.S. adults (79%) have medium-to-high English literacy skills. Medium-to-high English literacy levels are sufficient to compare information, paraphrase, and make low-level inferences. About 1 in 5 U.S. adults (21%) have low literacy skills. Of those who have low English literacy skills, 35% are White, 23% are Black, 34% are Latino, and 8% are of other races/ethnicities. Non-U.S.-born adults comprise 34% of the U.S. population with low literacy skills. States with the largest Latino populations also have low literacy rates—Arizona (87%), California (77%), Florida (80%), Nevada (84%), New Mexico (84%), New Jersey (83%), New York (78%), and Texas (81%)—that fall below the national literacy rate average of 88 % (World Population Review, n.d.-a).

As noted above, Latinos have high rates of English language proficiency. There are many Latinos, however, who have limited English language skills, known as limited English proficient (LEP) individuals. Research has shown that Latino LEP patients receive less information about therapeutic treatment options, understand less of the instructions related to prescription medication use, are less likely to keep follow-up appointments, and are more likely to overutilize emergency departments for health care (Pares-Avila & Sobralske, 2011; Saha et al., 2007). Additionally, LEP patients are less likely to receive preventive services; more likely to be misdiagnosed due to lack of communication, may receive poorer medical care, or be prescribed inappropriate medications, and may perceive less quality in the medical care received (Fernández et al., 2017; Jih et al., 2015).

The NCES (2014) defines *literacy* as "the ability to understand, evaluate, use and engage with written texts to participate in society, to achieve one's goals, and to develop one's knowledge and potential." According to this definition, the adult literacy rate in the United States is 79%, and the illiteracy rate is 21% (NCES, 2014). In addition, among low-English-literacy adults, 66% were born in the United States, and 34% were born outside of the United States. Non-Hispanic White and Latino adults make up the largest percentage of U.S. adults with low levels of English literacy, 35% and 34%, respectively.

Research by Rampey et al. (2016) show that by race/ethnicity and nativity status, the largest percentage of those with low English literacy skills are non-Latino White U.S.-born adults, who represented one third of the low-English-skilled population (33 %). Latino adults born outside the United States comprised about a quarter (24%) of the low-English-literacy adults in the United States, while Black adults comprised 20%, the majority of whom are born in the United States.

Health Literacy

Health literacy intersects with income, poverty, educational attainment, occupation, gender, language, and race/ethnicity. Data from the National Center for Education Statistics (NCES, 2019) indicates that "four in five U.S. adults (79%) have English literacy skills sufficient to complete tasks that require comparing and contrasting information, paraphrasing, or making low-level inferences—literacy skills at level 2 or above." According NCES (2019), of those adults born in the United States with low English literacy skills, 33% were White, 20% were Black, and 24% were Latino.

An important part of literacy is the ability to read and comprehend medical information, especially for prescription medications. The National Institutes of Health (NIH, 2021) defines *health literacy* as the "degree to which individuals have the ability to find, understand, and use information and services to inform health-related decisions and actions" (para. 1). Parker et al. (1999) state, "Poor health literacy is a stronger predictor of a person's health than age, income, employment status, education level, and race."

Health literacy assists individuals in making informed decisions about symptoms they may be experiencing, when to seek care, what questions to ask the health provider, understanding the providers' questions and prescription directions, and following care instructions and follow-up care.

A national study on health literacy published in 2006 derived from the 2003 National Assessment of Adult Literacy measured health literacy in the following manner (Kutner et al., 2006):

- *Below basic* indicates no more than the most simple and concrete literacy skills.
- *Basic* indicates skills necessary to perform simple and everyday literacy activities.
- *Intermediate* indicates skills necessary to perform moderately challenging literacy activities.
- *Proficient* indicates skills necessary to perform more complex and challenging literacy activities.

The findings from the study (Kutner et al., 2006) revealed that 53% of adults had intermediate health literacy; 22% had basic health literacy; 14% had below basic health literacy; and only 12% of adults had proficient health literacy. Latino adults had lower average health literacy than adults in any other racial/ethnic group examined, at 41% compared to 24% for Black adults and 9% of non-Hispanic White adults. Only 4% of Latinos have the proficient health literacy necessary to make appropriate health decisions.

Non-native English speakers, or limited English proficiency (LEP) speakers, are more likely to have low health literacy (Sentell & Braun, 2012), Latino immigrants are more likely to have difficulty navigating the U.S. health care system (Galvan et al., 2021), and linguistic and cultural barriers further compound the challenges related to health literacy among this population (Timmins, 2002). In a more recent study, Calvo (2016) found that about 60% of LEP Latinos reported adequate health literacy.

Increasing health literacy among Latinos is imperative for them to make informed and appropriate health care decisions that potentially could reduce the costs associated with health care, increase quality of care, and improve health outcomes. In the Latino community, the *promotora de salud* (lay community health worker) model is a widely successful culturally and linguistically appropriate educational approach that delivers simple bilingual content with pictures through interactive learning, community presentations, and other events in English-limited, low-literacy Latino communities. *Promotores* (community health workers) help bridge the Latino community and the health care system through their knowledge and understanding of the language, culture, and health behaviors common in Latinos. Promotora-based programs are ideal avenues for improving health literacy in underserved Latino communities. Not only do they actively engage "hard-to-reach" populations, the flexibility of the promotora model allows promotores to meet the needs of the community while also disseminating information more rapidly than through traditional health education methods (Calderón et al., 2014; Calvo, 2016; Pagán et al., 2012).

Social and Community Context

In 2020, approximately 87% of the U.S. population lived in metro/urban areas according to the U.S. Census Bureau (n.d.-a). Figueroa et al. (2021) found upward of 30% of Latinos living in rural parts of California and Texas, with about 25% living in rural parts of Arizona in 2017, with most Latinos being of Mexican descent (90% or more) in these three states.

Important economic and health inequalities exist between urban and nonurban residents. I use the term "metro" as equivalent to "urban" and "nonmetro" as equivalent to "rural," which is common. Acknowledging there are numerous distinctions within these umbrella terms, with additional classifications by economic and policy types (USDA, ERS, n.d.-b). Most U.S. Census data is collected at the county level, but counties can have both metro and nonmetro populations. According to the USDA, ERS (n.d.-b), "nonmetro counties include some combination of (a) open countryside, (b) rural towns (places with fewer than 2,500 people), and (c) urban areas with populations ranging from 2,500 to 49,999 people that are not part of larger labor market areas (metropolitan areas)."

According to data extracted from the Rural Health Information Hub, Rural Data Explorer (n.d.), there are six states where the Latino population accounts for 15% of the rural population or more (see Table 3.6). What is interesting is that five of the largest Latino rural population states were the ones acquired by the United States through the Mexican-America War. The primary Latino subgroup represented in these rural areas is Mexican Americans.

TABLE 3.6 States With the Largest Percentage of Latino Rural Residents, 2022

State	Metro (percent)	Nonmetro (percent)
New Mexico	50.5	48.3
Texas	40.6	33.3
Arizona	32.3	26.4
California	40.1	19.1
Nevada	30.5	18.7
Florida	26.8	16.7

Source: Rural Health Information Hub, Rural Data Explorer (n.d.)

Latino communities traditionally have had both social and cultural capital. Latinos have always been engaged in community action and advocacy for equal rights and social justice. Social cohesion has always depended on the interactions between individuals, which is prevalent in Latino communities. Shared common interests in improving community living conditions and electing officials whose interests are in common with Latino constituents are a driving force in those Latino communities that have achieved a sense of community or collective efficacy. *Compadrazgo*, usually intended to define godmother/godfather relationships in Latino culture has taken on a new meaning of caring and assisting the Latino community in achieving collective efficacy. *Communidad* means more than just community. Rather, the term conveys a sense of belonging, a shared history and culture, a togetherness, a social and cultural bond. Social capital in the form of community social support networks, informal institutions, and formalized AID societies are all marked by reciprocity, cooperation, and trust.

As defined by Sampson et al. (1997, abstract), *collective efficacy* is *"social cohesion among neighbors combined with their willingness to intervene on behalf of the common good."* Studies have shown that collective efficacy is associated with *decreases* in risky sexual behaviors, asthma prevalence, obesity rates, and premature mortality as well as improved subjective health ratings (Butel & Braun, 2019; Cohen et al., 2008).

Gentrification and Displacement

Gentrification is an aspect of urban renewal that increases housing values in low-income communities and eventually leads historically marginalized populations to move because of increased rent or housing costs. Gentrification affects a community's sense of history, culture, and belonging (i.e., "place"). The intersection of oppression regarding class, gender, race, and ethnicity occurs through gentrification processes. Although several theories on the causes of gentrification are advanced (e.g., Palen & London, 1984), there are few positive effects and many more negative effects of gentrification. Stabilization of declining neighborhoods, increased property values, and enhanced viability for additional development are positive aspects of gentrification. Negative aspects include displacement, secondary psychological costs of displacement, community resentment and conflict, cultural destructiveness, and loss of affordable housing that contributes to housing instability and homelessness (Lees et al., 2008; Massey & Denton, 1993). Some in the Latino community view gentrification as the "new colonialism."

There are both direct and indirect costs of gentrification on the health of communities. Direct costs include loss of community services and institutions and overcrowded and substandard housing conditions. Displaced residents experience relocation costs, longer commutes to work, disruption of health care access, and negative impacts on mental and psychological well-being. Some scholars view gentrification as a form of structural violence that harms communities as a whole by exacerbating segregation, increasing social and health inequalities, and contributing to increased rates of chronic and infectious diseases. Gentrification also contributes to less neighborhood cohesion and increased feelings of separation and loss.

The terms "homelessness" and "unsheltered" are frequently used interchangeably, but their meanings are distinct. According to the The Content Authority website (n.d.), "unsheltered persons are individuals who live on the streets, parks, or other public places without any form of shelter. Homeless ... is a broader term that includes individuals who are living in emergency shelters, transitional housing, or other temporary accommodations."

Homelessness rates in the United States have increased since 2010 and were increasing before the COVID-19 pandemic. According to a 2020 report from the U.S. Department of Housing and Urban Development, Latinos have significantly lower rates of homelessness. Among all homeless people, the report found that 48.3% were White, 39.4% were Black, and 22.5% were Latino. For the unsheltered, the rates of homelessness were 57% White, 27.2% Black and 23.5% Latino. Between 2019 and 2020, the number of Latinos experiencing homelessness increased by 5%. This reflects a considerable increase in the number of Latino unsheltered people, which increased by 10% between 2019 and 2020. With increasing home and rental costs, many Latinos are either overburdened financially or living on the streets without shelter.

Concentrated Poverty

The U.S. Department of Agriculture (2022b) measures poverty at different levels:

- *High poverty:* areas with a poverty rate of 20% or more in a single time period.
- *Extreme poverty:* areas with a poverty rate of 40% or more in a single time period.
- *Persistent poverty:* areas with a poverty rate of 20% or more for four consecutive time periods, about 10 years apart, spanning approximately 30 years (baseline time period plus three evaluation time periods).
- *Enduring poverty:* areas with a poverty rate of 20% or more for at least five consecutive time periods, about 10 years apart, spanning approximately 40 years or more (baseline time period plus four or more evaluation time periods).

According to information released by the ERS, USDA (n.d.-c) persistent poverty counties and tracts are predominantly in the Latino Southwest, White Appalachia in the mid-Atlantic states, and the Black Sunbelt in the southeastern states (Figure 3.19). Similarly, enduring poverty counties and tracts are in the same geographic regions (Figure 3.20) and coincide with high and extreme poverty counties and tracks (Figure 3.21).

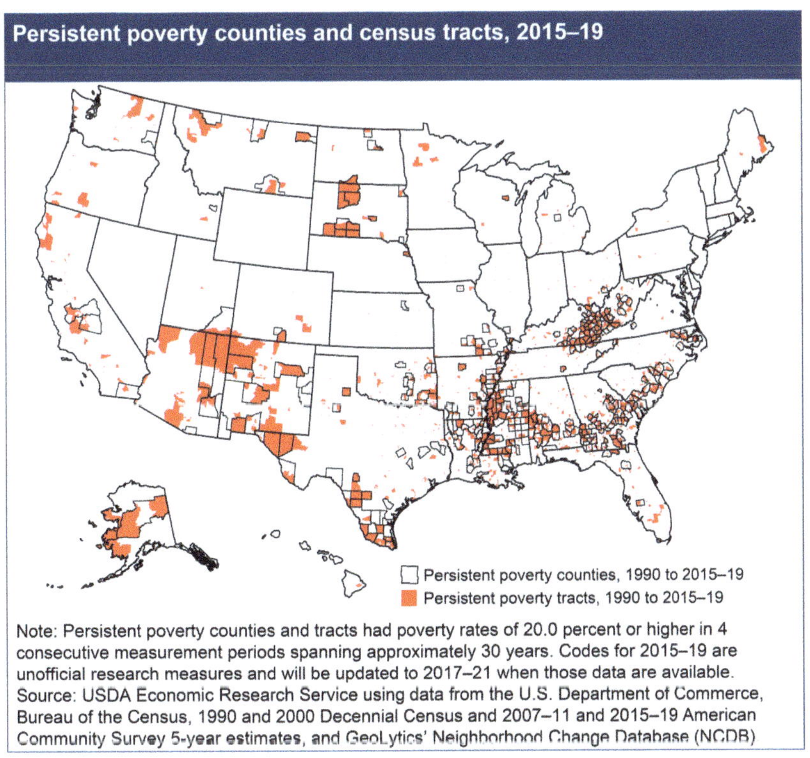

FIGURE 3.19 Persistent Poverty Counties and Census Tracts, 2015–2019

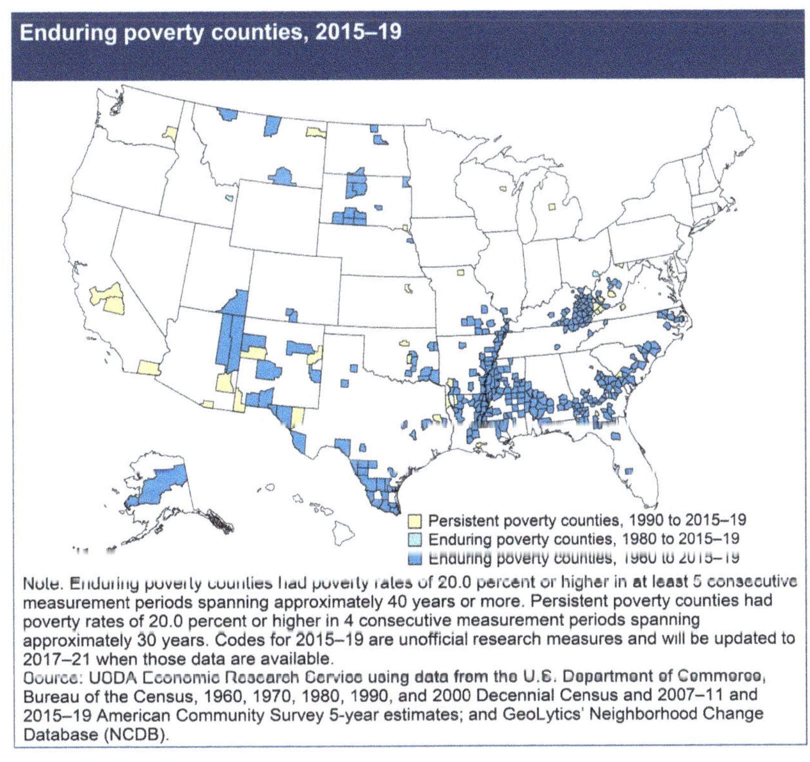

FIGURE 3.20 Enduring Poverty, United States, 2015–2019

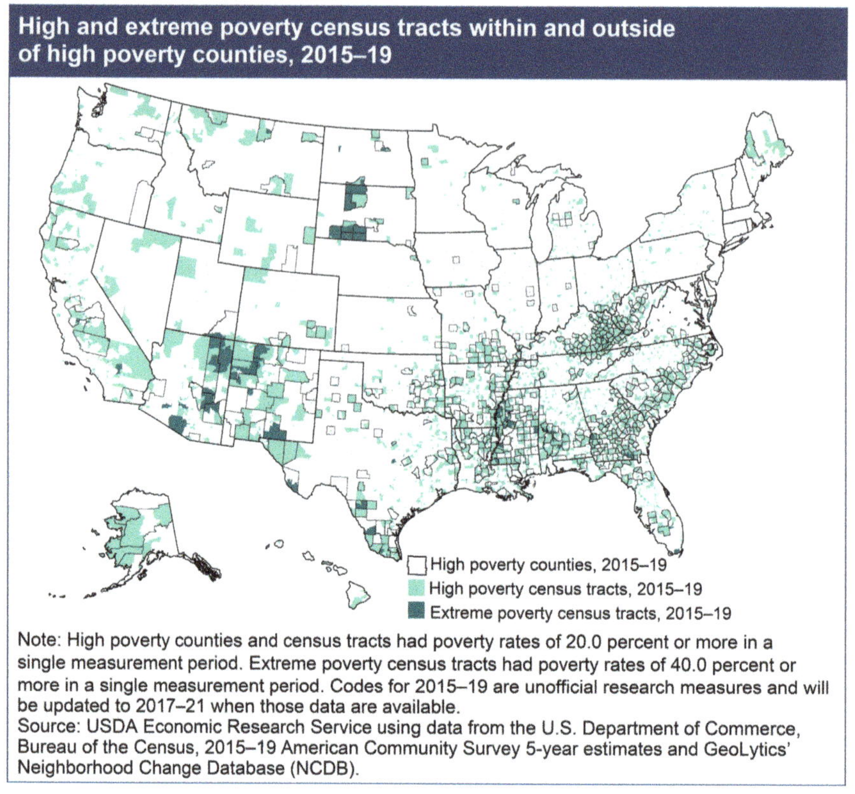

FIGURE 3.21 High and Extreme Poverty Census Tracts

Ethnic Enclaves and Increasing Segregation of Latino Neighborhoods

Research has also shown that many Latinos live in *ethnic enclaves*, or areas where there is a higher concentration of Latinos or *Latinidad* (Latino identity) and economic cultural activity such as specialty restaurants, bodegas, and auto repair shops (Moore & Vigil, 2000). Historically, in large part due to de facto segregation initiated by non-Latino White people, Latinos have concentrated in *barrios,* or neighborhoods with a distinct Latino cultural ambiance. According to the U.S. Census Bureau (n.d.-b), the "Dissimilarity Index" is the most used measure of segregation between two groups, reflecting their relative distributions across neighborhoods within the same city or metropolitan area. It ranges from 0 to 100, with 100 being the most integrated and 0 being the most segregated. In a recent report, Logan and Stults (2021) found that Latino segregation has remained unchanged since 1980 due to several complex dynamics. Higher fertility rates and movement from more segregated to less segregated metropolitan areas are part of this dynamic. According to the report, over one half of the Latino population (55.3%) in 1980 lived in metro areas with Hispanic-White segregation of 50 and above. Only 37.4% of Latinos lived in these same areas in 2010, which is a substantial decrease. At the same time, the share of Latinos living in the least segregated metro areas in 1980 was 20.2%; these same metropolitan areas accounted for 35.1% of Hispanics in 2010. There was a substantial movement away from regions of high segregation. Nevertheless, the movement of the Latino population toward areas of low segregation but with increasing segregation in those destinations contributed to the persistence of unchanged segregation among Latinos (Figure 3.22).

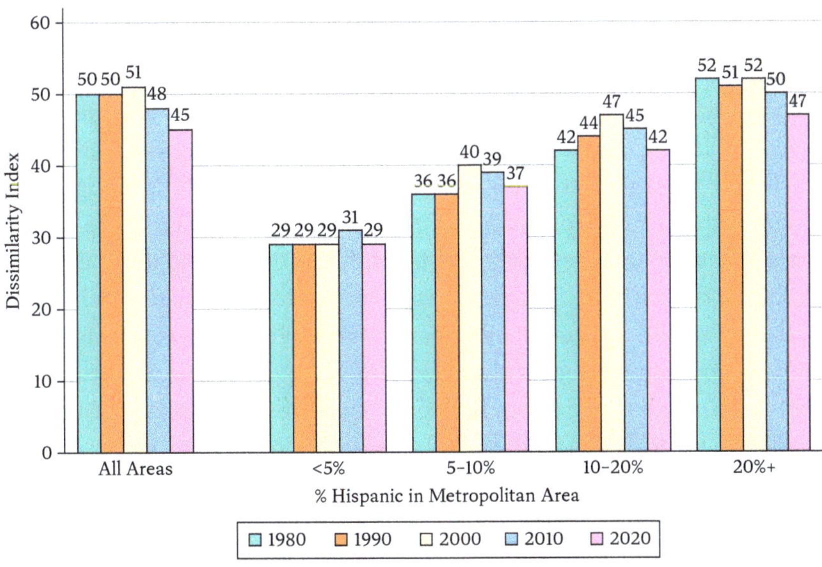

FIGURE 3.22 Percent Latino Population: Segregation Persists

The negative health and mental health impact of segregation include higher incidence and prevalence of infectious diseases, a lack of healthy food stores/alternatives, increased location of liquor stores, a lack in the availability of pharmaceuticals and health care, and an increase in predatory loan venues. Segregation is a consistent predictor of negative health outcomes and increased morbidity and mortality and serves as a partial explanation for disparities in the health of Latinos (Frank et al., 2007; Gallo et al., 2022).

Neighborhood and the Built Environment

Neighborhoods are small clusters of dwellings, from single to several blocks, which have certain characteristics in common, such as similar racial or ethnic composition, housing conditions, and recreational activities. Neighborhood disorder is identified by visible cues of poor social control and lack of social order in neighborhood public places (e.g., streets, parks, etc.; Ross & Mirowsky, 1999). Studies have shown that neighborhood disorder is associated with higher levels of mistrust and fear, both of which are associated with higher levels of psychological distress experienced by residents (Hong et al., 2014). Additionally, neighborhood disorder is negatively associated with social support, social cohesion, and social capital. Research conducted with Latinos has documented the positive association between increased social support and decreased depression (Alegría et al., 2014). Social cohesion was found to fully mediate the association between neighborhood poverty and mental health among Latinos. In neighborhoods where Latino community residents report high levels of social disorder, they also report (Alegría et al., 2014):

- Higher rates of incivility and physically threatening environments
- Feelings of intimidation by unkempt and noisy surroundings, abandoned and derelict buildings, graffiti, crime, violence, and public loitering.
- A lesser likelihood of developing social ties with their neighbors, especially if undocumented
- Less social interactions and limited social support with neighbors

Do perceptions of neighborhood disorder differ among racial/ethnic groups? A study conducted by Sampson and Raudenbush (2004) found that Black participants in the study were not significantly more or less likely than non-Latino White participants to perceive predominately Black neighborhoods as high in disorder. A notable exception was the interaction between Latino ethnicity and block-group percent Black. Perceptions of disorder increased as a function of percent Black for members of each ethnic group, but this tendency was significantly pronounced for Latinos. For example, in neighborhoods that were less than 25% Black, White participants and Latino participants essentially did not differ in their perceptions of disorder. However, at roughly 25% Black, Latino participants began to depart sharply from non-Latino White participants. When neighborhoods reached 75% Black or more, Latino participants perceived substantially more disorder than did non-Latino White participants. A recent study found that neighborhood deprivation and disorder were related to worse metabolic health in San Diego Latino adults of mostly Mexican heritage (Gallo et al., 2022).

Increased surveillance in Mexican American communities by local police, county sheriffs, and Homeland Security is not new (Morales, 1970). Two contexts are involved in police surveillance of these communities: social and historical. Within the social context are the perceptions of "disordered" populations, "crime-infested" neighborhoods, "low morals" of residents, and different "value systems" of racial/ethnic minorities. The historical context includes racism, discrimination, segregation, racial profiling, lack of understanding (i.e., language, culture), and miscommunication.

Racial and ethnic disparities also exist in the U.S. criminal justice system. According to a report by The Sentencing Project (Nellis, 2021), at the national level Black people are incarcerated at a rate of 1,240 per 100,000, while White people are incarcerated at a rate of 261 per 100,000. Black Americans are incarcerated at 4.8 times the rate of White Americans. Nationally, Latino Americans are incarcerated at a rate of 349 per 100,000 residents, producing a disparity ratio of 1.3 to 1 when compared with non-Latino White Americans (see Figure 3.23). The states with the highest Latino imprisonment rates are New Mexico (60%), California (44%), Arizona (39%), and Texas (32%).

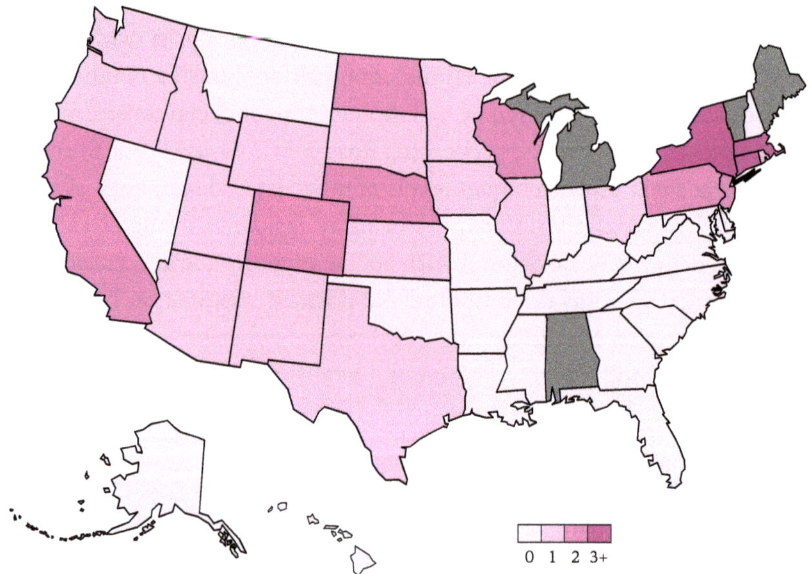

Data Source: Carson, E. A. (2021). Prisoners in 2019. Bureau of Justice Statistics; U.S. Census Bureau (n.d.). Age, sex, race, and Hispanic origin-6 race groups. (SC EST 2019-ALLDATA6).

■ = Data was not provided.

FIGURE 3.23 Latino–White Incarceration Rate Ratios

Even with increased surveillance and incarceration rates, attitudes toward police are more favorable among non-Latino White Americans compared to Black Americans and Latino Americans. Studies have shown that Black individuals tend to distrust police, do not believe police treat them equally, and about half feel that police use excessive force (MacDonald & Stokes, 2006; Liberman, 2021). In general, research has shown that Latino Americans perceive police as unfair, impolite, and unhelpful and that they tend to use excessive force, linguistic and cultural barriers exist, there is a fear of police, and the threat of deportation also shape Latino perceptions of police (Flores, 2022). Research has found that attitudes toward police among Latino Americans vary by immigration status (Salinas Thomas, 2023). Immigrants tend to view police more positively than nonimmigrant Latinos do; however, this could change with increasing detention and threat of family separation (Krogstad, 2014). Krogstad (2014) found that more than half of non-Latino Blacks feel the police do a good job in enforcing the law and that Latino attitudes toward police were intermediate between non-Latino Whites and non-Latino Blacks.

Environmental Justice in Latino Neighborhoods

The U.S. Environmental Protection Agency (n.d.) defines *environmental justice* as "the fair treatment and meaningful involvement of all people, regardless of race, color, national origin or income with respect to the development, implementation and enforcement of environmental laws, regulations, and policies" (para. 1). Nevertheless, historically marginalized populations have had little voice in policy regarding the placing of toxic waste facilities without their knowledge or input. As a result, historically excluded populations have disproportionately suffered from the placement of toxic waste facilities in their communities (Pastor et al., 2001). Data shows that tracts with 15% or more Latino Americans are exposed to 84.3% more toxic waste than an average tract from 1990–2000 (Hipp & Lakon, 2010). Even when controlling for income, race continues to be the primary predictor for placement of a toxic waste facility. De facto environmental racism is occurring in these communities, where individuals have little or no community input or knowledge on the types of potential health hazards they are exposed to.

The built environment contributes to environmental pollution through the construction of roadways and freeways. Again, research demonstrates that living near traffic-congested areas increases lung diseases like asthma and bronchitis and contributes to heavy mineral exposure (Badyda et al., 2013; Pedde et al., 2017; Zheng et al., 2022). There is generally more than one factor involved in the cause of air pollution and health effects.

The lifetime prevalence of asthma among Latino children is increasingly a cause for concern. Carter-Pokras et al. (2007) reported the highest rates are among Cubans and Puerto Ricans (23% and 22.8%, respectively), and intermediate rates are among Central and South Americans (14.4% and 17.7%, respectively). The lowest rates are among Mexican American children (13.2%). Latinos of Mexican descent present a mixed picture regarding the neighborhood and built environment. There is little doubt that they are disadvantaged relative to non-Latino White Americans but varies in relation to Black Americans.

Health Care Access and Quality

The behavioral model for vulnerable populations (Andersen, 1995; Gelberg et al., 2000) has proven to be a useful heuristic to identify factors that predict health care utilization and health outcomes among vulnerable populations, such as racial/ethnic groups, people experiencing homelessness, older adults, undocumented immigrants, and other populations that face barriers in accessing health care (see Table 3.7). The model consists of three main categories of predictors and two potential health outcomes: predisposing characteristics, including health beliefs; enabling characteristics; and need characteristics. Potential outcomes include health behaviors (e.g., preventive health behaviors) and health outcomes (e.g., negative and positive outcomes related to physical and mental health). Health beliefs would include religion/spirituality, knowledge of disease and symptoms, attitudes toward health services, values concerning health and illness, and conceptions of health and illness.

TABLE 3.7 Predisposing, Enabling and Need Characteristics

Predisposing characteristics	Enabling characteristics	Need characteristics
Age	Regular source of care	Perceived health status
Gender	Health insurance coverage and type	Perceived need
Marital status	Income	Prevalence and severity of health conditions
Veteran status	Poverty	Prevalence and severity of health inequalities
Race/Ethnicity	Social support	
Education	Personal and family resources	
Employment	Community resources	
Occupation	Residence/region	
Citizenship status	Perceived barriers	
Family size	Actual barriers	
Immigration status		

Source: Adapted from Gelberg et al. (2000)

Access to health care fundamentally changed with the passage of the Patient Protection and Affordable Care Act (ACA) of 2010. The ACA was the most significant and controversial reform of the U.S. health care system since the establishment of Medicare and Medicaid in 1965. Beginning in 2014, the ACA filled gaps in Medicaid coverage for adults by extending eligibility to 138% of the federal poverty level ($30,000 for a family of four in 2023). Undocumented immigrants face eligibility restrictions for Medicaid and continue to face eligibility restrictions for ACA health coverage options under coverage expansions.

According to the Kaiser Family Foundation (Hill et al., 2023), before full implementation of the ACA, nonelderly adult Latinos had the highest uninsured rates in the United States at 27%. In comparison, 16% of non-Latino Blacks and 11% of non-Latino Whites were uninsured. In reference to household type, only 7% of married adult Latino Americans were uninsured, compared to 35% of single Latino adults and 58% of Latino families with children.

The Commonwealth Fund (Collins et al., 2015) showed that the percentage of Latinos aged 19–64 who were uninsured fell from 36% to 23% during 2013–2016. Additionally, in states that expanded Medicaid, including California, the uninsured rate among working-age Latino adults dropped by about half, from 35% to 17%. The study found that three years after implementation of the ACA (2013–2016), among uninsured adults 19–64 years of age, 55 % of Latinos, compared to 22% of non-Latino Whites and 44% of non-Latino Blacks were still unaware of insurance marketplaces under the ACA.

A study conducted by the Commonwealth Fund (Collins et al., 2015), found that the overall uninsured rate for U.S. adults 19–64 years of age decreased from 37 million in 2013 to 24 million in 2016. According to Collins et al. (2013) uninsured Latinos comprised 29% in 2013, but 40% in 2016. A possible reason for this discrepancy is that foreign-born Latinos who are undocumented are ineligible for ACA coverage and are likely to be uninsured. Collins et al. (2013) reported that 43% of foreign-born Latinos were uninsured.

U.S. Census Bureau data (2021c) shows that the uninsured rate in 2021 was 18.8% for the Latino population (see Table 3.8). The uninsured rate varies considerably by Latino subgroup, with Puerto Ricans having the lowest rate (8.9%) of uninsured and Central Americans having the highest rate (29.4%), followed by Mexicans (20.9%).

TABLE 3.8 Health Insurance Status by Race and Latinos Subgroups (Percent)

Health insurance status	Non-Latino White	Non-Latino Black	Total Latino	Mexican	Puerto Rican	Cuban	Central American	South American	Other Latino[5]
Insured	94.1	89.0	81.2	79.1	91.1	85.2	70.6	88.0	90.2
Not insured	5.9	11.0	18.8	20.9	8.9	14.8	29.4	12.0	9.8

Source: U.S. Census Bureau (2021c)

Health care access barriers are well established for Latinos. Health insurance coverage and having a regular source of care are important factors in health care utilization rates (Alcalá et al., 2017; Chen et al., 2016; Estrada et al., 1990; Lillie-Blanton & Hoffman, 2005). Differences among Latino subgroups have been noted as well. For example, Vargas Bustamante et al. (2009) compared Latinos of Mexican ancestry with non-Mexican Latinos. The study found that Latinos of Mexican ancestry consistently demonstrated lower health care access and utilization patterns than non-Mexican Latinos. Additionally, health insurance coverage and region of residence were the most important factors that explained differences between Latinos of Mexican descent and non-Mexican Latinos. Language and citizenship status were found to be relatively unimportant. Similarly, Vargas Bustamante et al. (2010) found that Latinos of Mexican and Central/South American descent are much less likely to receive guideline-recommended preventive care services than non-Latino White people and other Latino subgroups.

Results from the Kaiser Family Foundation study (Hill et al., 2023) clearly show continuing disparities in access to health care. The study found that 34% of Latino adults and 18% of Black adults reported not having a personal health care provider, compared to 16% of non-Latino White adults. Additionally, Latino (18%) and Black (14%) adults were more likely than non-Latino White adults (9%) to report not seeing a doctor in the past 12 months because of cost. Latino adults (36%) were more likely than non-Latino White adults (30%) to say they went without a routine checkup in the past year, while Black adults (21%) were less likely to report going without a checkup. All Latino and Black adults were more likely than non-Latino White adults to report going without a visit to a dentist or dental clinic in the past year as of 2020.

Among children, the Kaiser Family Foundation study (Hill et al., 2023) found that 9% of Latino children and 7% of Black children lacked a usual source of care when sick, compared to 4% of non-Latino White children as of 2021. Latino children were more likely than non-Latino White children to report going without a health care visit in the past year (12% and 8%, respectively).

Barriers to Health Care Access and Quality

Utilization barriers consist of four general types: cost and insurance coverage barriers, access and availability barriers, patient-provider barriers, and cultural and linguistic barriers.

- *Cost of care and health insurance coverage*: This barrier includes direct costs for medical care, out of pocket payments for prescription medications, copayments for those with insurance coverage, lack of knowledge regarding what one's insurance plan covers, and lack of insurance coverage mobility (Ortega et al., 2007; Vargas Bustamante et al., 2015).
- *Access and availability of care:* These barriers include appointment delays, transportation issues, hours of service if not a 24/7 medical facility, family and childcare responsibilities, inability to take time off work, and continuity of care (Vargas Bustamante et al., 2009).
- *Patient–provider relationship:* Patient-provider barriers include perceptions of untrustworthiness, disrespectful behavior, lack of appropriate communication, and health literacy. In addition, physician bias leads to discrimination and racism and/or stereotypes about the behavior of Latino patients (Perez et al., 2009; Smedley et al., 2003). Perceptions of the quality of care received in comparison to White Americans clearly shows that many Latinos believe they are receiving lower quality care.
- *Cultural and linguistic differences:* These barriers include differences in language spoken by medical personnel or their inability to speak Spanish (Becerra et al., 2015; González et al., 2010; Rodríquez

et al., 2009). Other important utilization barriers among Latinos include mixed-status families (documented children and undocumented parents), fear of detention and deportation by Homeland Security, and lack of knowledge about the U.S. health care system.

- *Lack of Latino medical professionals*: This is a barrier that is frequently overlooked when examining utilization rates and utilization barriers among Latinos. In 2018, the percentage of full-time medical school faculty that identified as Latino was only 5.5% (Association of American Medical Colleges, 2019). Additionally, among active physicians in 2018, 5.8% identified as Latinos. In 2021, of the 4,037 Latino applicants to U.S. medical schools, 1,646, or 41%, of Latinos were accepted, with 39% matriculating (Shemmassian Academic Consulting, 2024).
- *Lack of Latino cultural competency:* Many health professionals are not linguistically or culturally competent to deal with the increasing diversity of the U.S. population. There is a lack of understanding of Latino culture, especially related to health beliefs, lack of respect for religious or spiritual beliefs, cultural scripts that may hinder health-seeking behaviors (e.g., familism, *machismo*, and *marianismo*), lack of appropriate interpreters, and lack of bilingual and/or bicultural personnel (de la Torre and Estrada, 2015).

Access to quality health care continues to be a major impediment for some Latino subgroups, primarily those of Mexican descent and those who are undocumented. Overall, Americans of Mexican descent fare worse in health care access than Black Americans and non-Latino White Americans. Even with improvements in the ACA, access is still restricted to undocumented Latinos, and rates of lack of health insurance coverage and not having a regular source of care remain higher for Latinos of Mexican descent than others.

Immigration and Documentation Status

Although the U.S. Census reveals that most of the Latinos of Mexican descent are U.S. born, it is nevertheless possible for them to be deported and/or detained by police and Homeland Security. This is exactly what occurred during the 1930s mass deportation of Mexicans where the United States deported an estimated half-million U.S. citizens of Mexican descent (Baderrama & Rodriguez, 2006). It is impossible to distinguish between documented and undocumented Mexicans by physical appearance, and concerns regarding human rights violations of American citizens have been raised (Koulish et al., 1994; Romero, 2008; Romero & Serag, 2004). "Driving while Latino," analogous to "driving while Black," has become a euphemism for official harassment and racial profiling among Latinos of Mexican descent that causes increased psychosocial stress (Anderson & Finch, 2014; Mucchetti, 2005; Romero, 2006).

According to the Department of Homeland Security (Baker, 2021), *legally authorized persons* include naturalized citizens, persons granted lawful permanent residence, persons granted asylum, persons admitted as refugees, and persons admitted as resident nonimmigrants (i.e., students and temporary workers, as opposed to tourists) who have unexpired authorized periods of admission. *Unauthorized persons* are those who are not included in these categories. Deferred Action for Childhood Arrivals (DACA) students (about 800,000 persons), or those who are residing in the United States while awaiting removal proceedings in immigration court, are included among the estimates of the unauthorized population.

The true number of unauthorized persons living in the United States is impossible to know. The Department of Homeland Security (Baker, 2021) estimates that 11.4 million unauthorized immigrants were living in the United States on January 1, 2018, roughly unchanged from 11.4 million on January 1, 2015. Slightly fewer than 50% of the unauthorized immigrants in 2018 were from Mexico, compared to nearly 55% in 2015, but still represented the largest share of unauthorized immigrants in the United States. Nevertheless, the Mexican unauthorized population continued to decline, dropping by an average of 260,000 people per year in 2015–2018. California and Texas are the primary states for unauthorized residents.

Most unauthorized immigrants live with spouses, partners, their children, or other relatives, some of whom may be U.S. citizens. An estimated 45 million immigrants lived in the United States in 2019, and that number is projected to reach 78 million by 2065 (Krogstad et al., 2022). Immigration and documentation status influence many social determinants of health, including educational attainment, economic well-being (i.e., income, poverty rates, and employment status), and place of settlement. For many Latinos, especially those who have immigrated from Mexico and Central America, immigration and residency status are important social determinants. Undocumented Latino immigrants face many social and legal barriers that limit their access to goods and services in the United States. For example, undocumented Latinos are not eligible for ACA coverage.

Citizenship status allows access to social and public services that are typically denied to noncitizens. Similarly, documentation status contributes not only to limited access to goods and services but additionally to increased crime, increased victimization, and legal detention and deportation if reported. Research shows that undocumented Latinos are less likely to utilize health care, call the police, or report crime or victimization for fear of deportation (Berk & Schur, 2001; Martinez-Donate et al., 2017; Rivers & Patino, 2006). As well, mixed-status families, where a parent is undocumented and a child is not, are also subject to negative encounters with Homeland Security, local police, or sheriffs, jeopardizing their financial and psychological well-being (Almeida et al., 2016; Morey, 2018; Salas et al., 2013; Vargas et al., 2017).

Therefore, Latinos born in the United States are not immune to the subjection of detention and deportation by legal authorities. The anti-Mexican sentiment fomented by former president Donald Trump and some media outlets has led to more scrutiny of Latinos and their communities, as well as places of employment. The legitimized harassment of Mexican Americans, legally born in the United States, leads to increased anxiety, depression, posttraumatic stress disorder (PTSD), and substance abuse disorders.

The U.S.–Mexico Border Region

No discussion of "place" and Latinos would be complete without reference to the U.S.–Mexico border, where most Latinos of Mexican and Mexican American descent reside (Moslimani et al., 2023). Acquired from Mexico through the Treaty of Guadalupe Hidalgo that ended the Mexican American War, the region is historically, demographically, and culturally unique.

The U.S.–Mexico border is approximately 2,000 miles long, stretching from San Ysidro, California, to Brownsville, Texas. It consists of 23 counties in four U.S. states (Arizona, California, New Mexico, and Texas), some of the poorest in the United States, and six Mexican states, 80 municipalities, and 14 pairs of sister cities (Healthy Border, 2020) (see Figure 3.24).

Several factors make the U.S.–Mexico border unique from other regions of the country: It has a rapid population growth from immigration and emigration, younger ages, higher poverty rates, higher rates of uninsured, higher rates of medical professional labor shortage areas, a shared commercial infrastructure with Mexico, and increased militarization and Homeland Security surveillance.

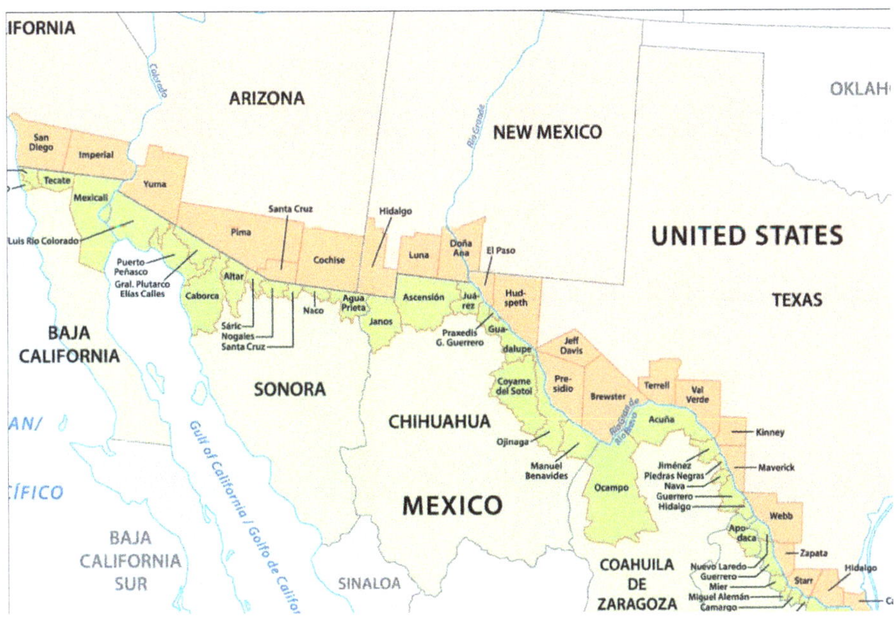

FIGURE 3.24 The U.S.–Mexico Border Region

Latinos, primarily of Mexican descent, comprise upwards of 30% of the population in the four border states (World Population Review, n.d.-b). In New Mexico, Latinos account for over 50% of the population and can trace their presence in the region for hundreds of years (Figure 3.25).

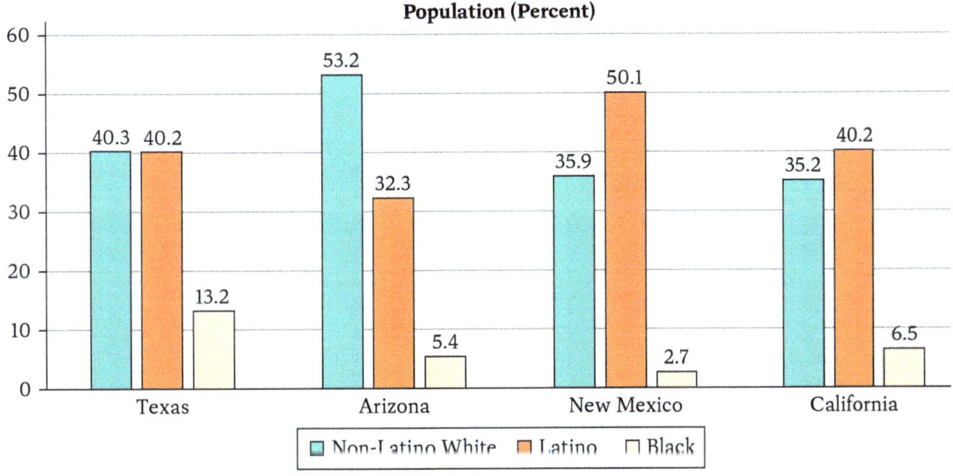

FIGURE 3.25 The Non-Latino, Latino, and Black Population of the U.S.–Mexico Border States, 2020

The U.S.-Mexico border states have higher poverty rates in comparison to the rest of the United States (U.S. Census Bureau, 2022a). In New Mexico, 1 in 5 Latinos lives in poverty (Figure 3.26), and in Texas, the Latino poverty rate is similar to the Black poverty rate (19.4%, compared to 19.5%). Poverty among Latino is lowest in California. However, the poverty rates for Black Americans are higher than the poverty rates for Latino Americans in New Mexico and California.

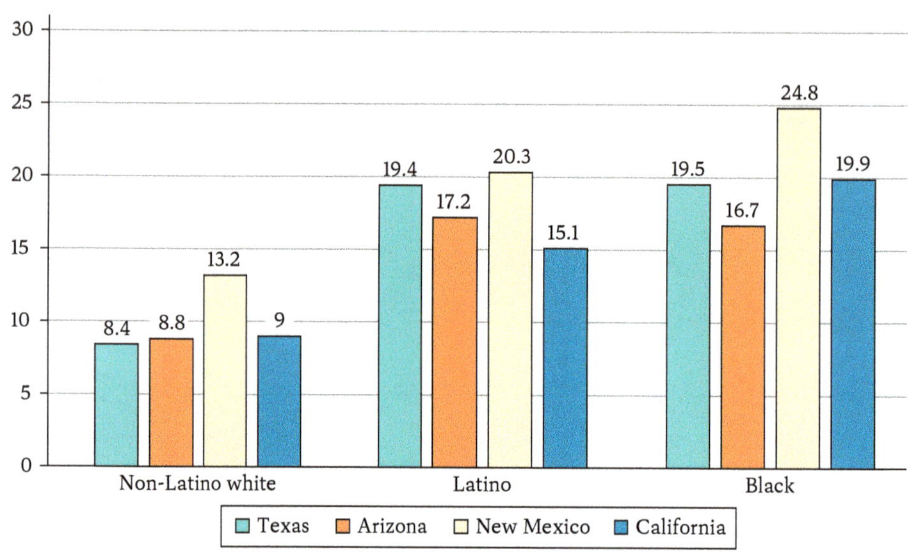

FIGURE 3.26 Poverty Rates in the U.S.–Mexico Border States, 2020

Exploring the CRE Interactive Tool (U.S. Census Bureau, 2022a), in the four U.S.–Mexico border states, Latinos have the lowest rates of health insurance coverage in comparison to non-Latino White Americans and Black Americans (Figure 3.27). Although most of the rates are above 82%, Texas has the lowest rate of 72% coverage, which is 10% lower than the Latino national average.

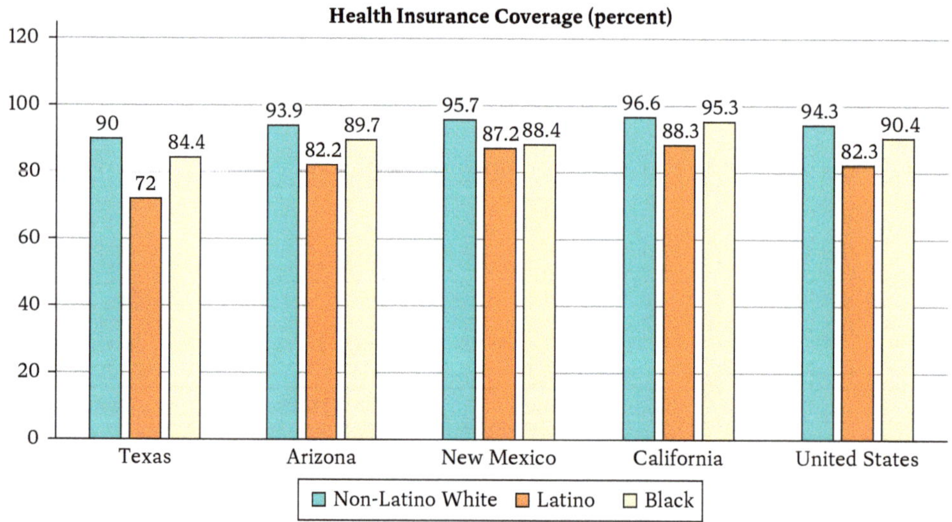

FIGURE 3.27 Health Insurance Coverage in the U.S.–Mexico Border States, 2020

Source: U.S. Census Bureau (2022)

The percent of the population with a bachelor's degree or higher varies by race/ethnicity and state (U.S. Census Bureau, 2022a) (Figure 3.28). Rates are highest for non-Latino Whites and non-Latino Blacks but very low for Latinos. The border state with the highest percentage of Latinos with a bachelor's degree or higher is New Mexico (17.3%). In contrast, Black Americans have significantly higher rates than Latino Americans of obtaining a bachelor's degree, above 25% in all border states and approaching 30% in New Mexico.

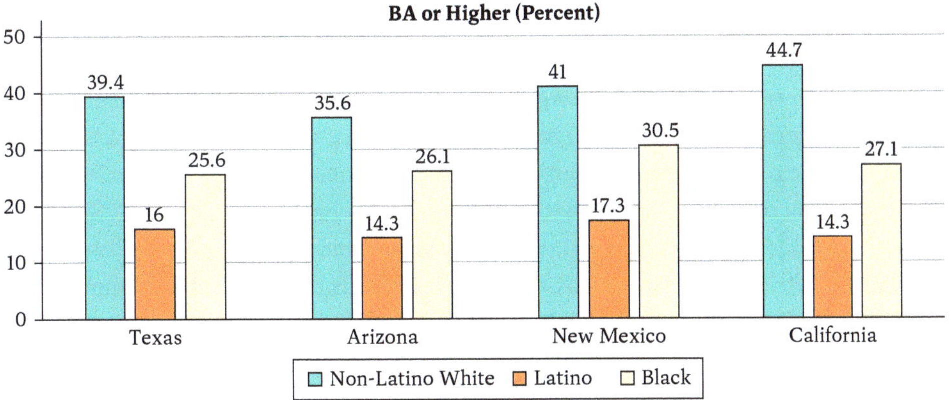

FIGURE 3.28 Percent of the Population With a Bachelor's Degree or Higher in the U.S.-Mexico Border States, 2020

Source: U.S. Census Bureau (2022a)

Equally disturbing is the low high school graduation rates for Latinos in the U.S.-Mexico border region (U.S. Census Bureau, 2022a). While non-Latino White Americans and Black Americans have high school graduation rates above 90% in every border state, Latino Americans lag far behind (Figure 3.29). The lowest Latino graduate rates are in California (66.2%), and the highest are in New Mexico (78.7%). The future earnings and economic well-being of Latinos will be significantly diminished by these low high school graduation rates.

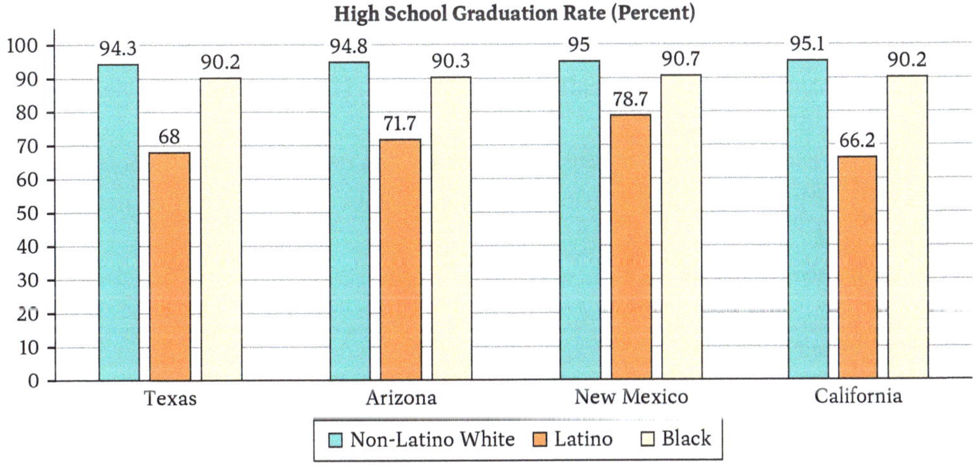

FIGURE 3.29 High School Graduation Rates in the U.S.-Mexico Border States, 2020

Source: U.S. Census Bureau (2022a)

CDC/ATSDR Community Resilience Estimates (CRE) for the U.S.-Mexico Border

The Community Resilience Estimates (CRE) and Social Vulnerability Estimates (SV) examines several different risk factors, from income to age and health insurance coverage, to measure how resilient and how at-risk communities are to the impacts of disasters. The U.S. Census Bureau launched the CRE in the summer of 2020 in response to the COVID-19 pandemic to provide a snapshot measurement of the risk and resilience of every neighborhood in the United States (Agency for Toxic Substances and Disease Registry, 2022). Similarly, the CDC and the Agency for Toxic Substances and Disease Registry (ATSDR) created the Social Vulnerability Index (SVI) to determine county risk profiles. The ATSDR (n.d.) defines *social vulnerability* as "the potential negative effects on communities caused by external stresses on human health," including natural disasters, exposure to dangerous toxins and disease (para. 1). Social vulnerability uses measures of socioeconomic status, certain household characteristics, housing type, transportation access, and racial and ethnic minority status to classify communities into a continuum from low risk to high risk. The U.S.-Mexico border was one of the regions examined.

Results of the CRE estimates show that about a quarter of the people living in the U.S.-Mexico border counties are considered high risk, with the rate higher in Texas than in the two other border states—California and Arizona. The rate between Texas and New Mexico was not statistically different (ATSDR, 2020).

The ATSDR (2020) CRE shows that there is great variation both in the selected 23 U.S.-Mexico border counties and within the four states (Arizona, California, New Mexico, and Texas) that make up the U.S. side of the region. According to Welton (2022, paragraph 8) the CRE measures "the presence of high-risk individuals within a given community using a score based on 10 preselected risk factors." These risk factors include:

- "Household income-to-poverty ratio (total family income divided by the poverty threshold of less than 130%).
- Single or zero caregiver household with one or no individuals ages 18–64.
- Unit-level crowding (less than 0.75 persons per room).
- Communications barrier (limited English-speaking household or no one in the household over 16 with a high school diploma).
- No one in the household is employed full-time, year-round. (This is not applicable if all household residents are ages 65 years or older.)
- Disability posing constraints to daily activity. (People who report any one or more of the following six disability types: hearing, vision, cognitive, ambulatory, self-care, or independent living difficulties.)
- No health insurance coverage.
- Ages 65 or older.
- Households without a vehicle.
- Households without broadband internet access."

The list includes several important social determinants of health that, taken together, cover a wide range of social inequalities present among Mexican Americans in the U.S.-Mexico border region, as previously discussed.

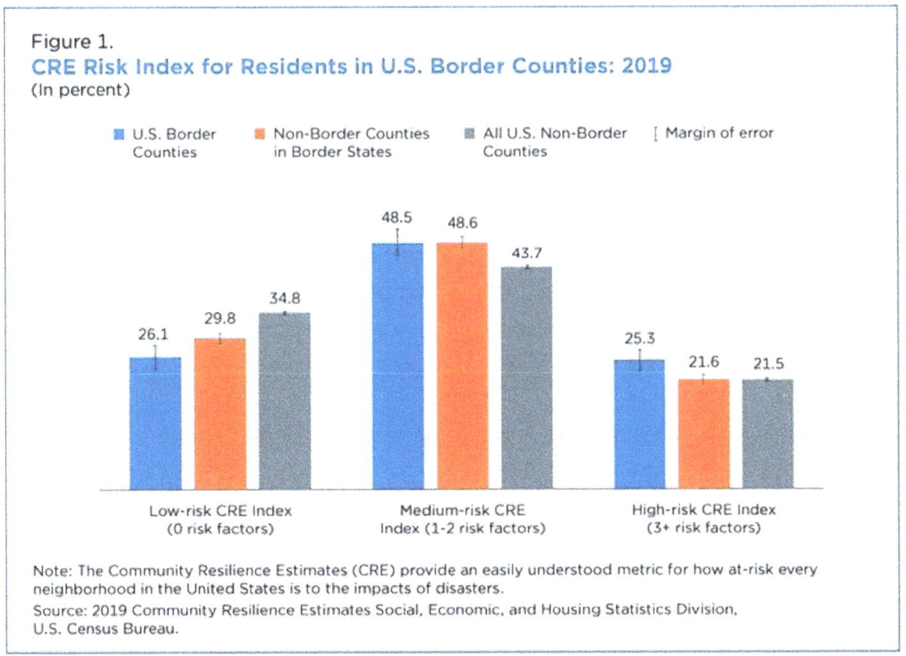

FIGURE 3.30 CRE Risk Index for Residents in U.S Border Counties: 2019 (in Percent)

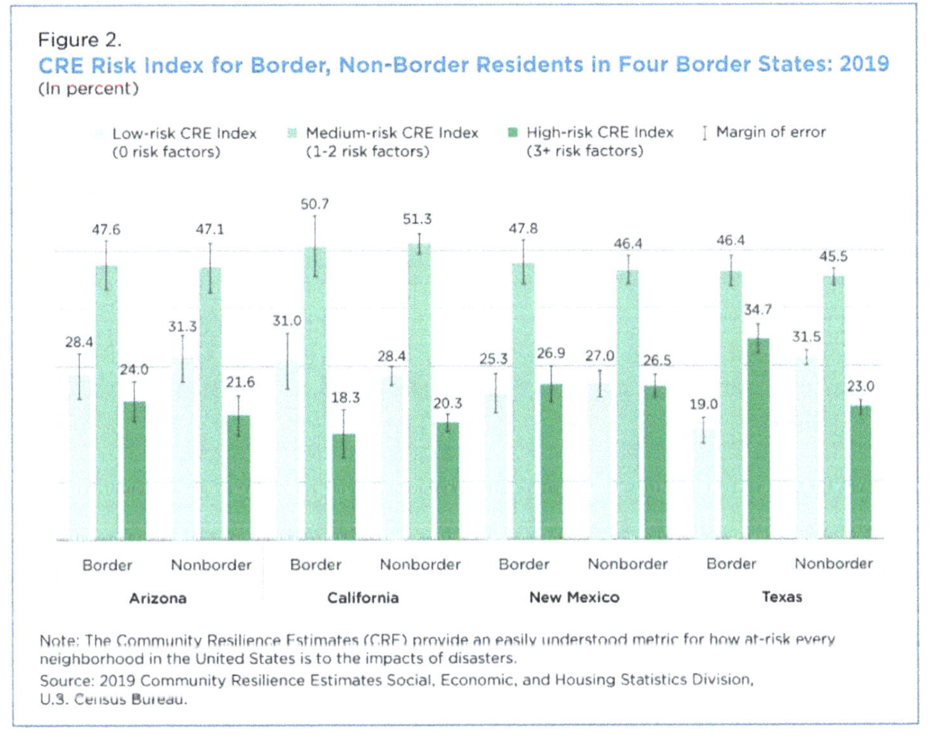

FIGURE 3.31 CRE Risk Index for Border, Non-Border Residents in Four Border States: 2019 (Percent)

The CRE groups individuals within each of the three risk categories by the number of associated risk factors: low risk (0 risk factors), medium risk (1-2 risk factors) and high risk (3+ risk factors).

According to Welton (2022), the population residing along the U.S.-Mexico border have a higher risk profile than persons residing in other parts of the United States. For example, 25.3% of U.S.-Mexico border counties compared to 21.6% of non-U.S.-Mexico in border states were classified as high-risk according to the CRE Risk Index. Additionally, Welton (2022) indicated that "the high-risk rate for people who live in border counties in Texas was 1.4 times higher than in Arizona, and 1.9 times higher than in California." In reviewing the CRE risk profiles, consideration for the large Mexican American resident population should increase health and social services in the region. Some of the poorest counties in the United States are within the U.S.-Mexico border region.

CDC/ATSDR Social Vulnerability Index (SVI) for the U.S.-Mexico Border

The CDC/ATSDR Social Vulnerability Index (SVI) is very comprehensive and includes measures of six thematic areas inclusive of many of the social determinants of health. The following measures comprise each of the four SVI thematic areas (ATSDR 2022):

- Socioeconomic status: below 150% poverty, unemployment, housing cost burden, no high school diploma, no health insurance.
- Household characteristics; aged 65 or older, aged 17 or younger, civilian with a disability, single-parent households, English language proficiency.
- Racial and ethnic minority status: Hispanic or Latino (of any race); Black, Not Hispanic or Latino; American Indian and Alaska Native, Not Hispanic or Latino; Asian, Not Hispanic or Latino; Native Hawaiian and Other Pacific Islander, Not Hispanic or Latino; Two or More Races, Not Hispanic or Latino; Other Races, Not Hispanic or Latino.
- Housing type and transportation: multi-unit structures, mobile homes, crowding, no vehicle, group quarters.

The results of the SVI analyses show that all 23 border counties in the U.S.-Mexico region meet the criteria for a high level of vulnerability (ATSDR, 2020). Several studies show that SVI scores are associated with cardiovascular disease outcomes, cardiovascular risk factors and CHD prevalence, HIV/AIDS, and COVID-19 (Bevan et al., 2023; Dailey et al., 2024; Elenwa et al., 2023; Islam et al., 2021; Oates et al., 2021; Tortolero et al., 2022).

Office of Minority Health's Social Vulnerability Index

Similarly, the Office of Minority Health (OMH; 2023) developed an extension of the original CDC/ATSDR SVI that includes several themes developed using 5-year estimates of sociodemographic data from the U.S. Census Bureau's American Community Survey (ACS). A comparison of CDC/ATSDR SVI and Minority Health SVI themes are included in Table 3.9 (adapted from OMH, 2023, p. 5-6).

TABLE 3.9 Comparison Between CDC/ATSDR SVI and Minority Health SVI

Overall vulnerability	CDC/ATSDR Social Vulnerability Index	Minority Health Social Vulnerability Index
Socioeconomic status	Below poverty	Below poverty
	Unemployed	Unemployed
	Income	Income
	No high school diplomas	No high school diplomas
Household composition & disability	Aged 65 or older	Aged 65 or older
	Aged 17 or younger	Aged 17 or younger
	Older than age 5 with a disability	Older than age 5 with a disability
	Single-parent households	Single-parent households
Minority status & language	Minority	American Indian/Alaska Native
		Asian
		African American
		Native Hawaiian/Pacific Islander
		Hispanic or Latinx
		Some other race
	Speak English less than "very well"	Spanish speakers*
		Chinese speakers*
		Vietnamese speakers*
		Korean speakers*
		Russian speakers*
Housing type & transportation	Multi-unit structures	Multi-unit structures
	Mobile homes	Mobile homes
	Crowding	Crowding
	No vehicle	No vehicle
	Group quarters	Group quarters
Health care infrastructure & access		Hospitals
		Urgent care clinics
		Pharmacies
		Primary care physicians
		Health insurance
Medical vulnerability		Cardiovascular disease
		Chronic respiratory disease
		Obesity
		Diabetes
		Internet access

*Those who speak English less than "very well"

U.S. Department of Health and Human Services, "Comparison Between CDC/ATSDR SVI and Minority Health SVI, from "Minority Health Social Vulnerability Index Overview"," p. 3, 2021.

The Minority Health SVI is an extension of the CDC/ATSDR SVI "that contribute to social vulnerability, such as health care access and chronic disease prevalence" (OMH, 2023, p. 1). Additionally, the Minority Health Social Vulnerability Index includes elements specific to health care infrastructure and access and medical vulnerability, which also includes several chronic diseases (e.g., cardiovascular disease, diabetes) and internet access.

Like findings from the CDC/ATSDR SVI (Agency for Toxic Substances and Disease Registry, n.d.), almost all the 23 contiguous border counties in the U.S.-Mexico border states are high risk (Table 3.10). The percentage of Latinos, primarily of Mexican descent, varies widely from a low of 33.5% in San Diego County, California, to 99.1% in Starr County, Texas. Overall, Latinos comprise the majority minority population residing along the U.S.-Mexico border. Few Black Americans are represented in the U.S.-Mexico border states, varying from no presence (0%) to a high of 5% of the population in San Diego County, California.

TABLE 3.10 Minority Health Sociodemographic Characteristics of the Four Border States and 23 Border Counties, 2020

Border states and counties	% below poverty	% Latino	% Black	% 17 years or younger	% Spanish speaking
Arizona (4)					
• Yuma	20.1	63.4	2.2	25.6	22.7
• Pima	17.8	37.0	3.5	21.4	6.8
• Santa Cruz	24.0	83.5	0.5	27.6	26.5
• Cochise	17.2	35.3	3.7	22.0	8.6
California (2)					
• San Diego	12.5	33.5	5.0	22.0	10.1
• Imperial	24.2	83.8	2.5	28.7	32.1
New Mexico (3)					
• Hidalgo	28.1	58.0	0.6	22.9	9.8
• Luna	30.2	66.6	1.4	26.3	18.3
• Dona Ana	27.7	68.0	1.9	25.1	14.6
Texas (14)					
• El Paso	21.3	82.4	3.4	27.8	30.0
• Hudspeth	28.2	78.4	1.6	23.9	38.2
• Presidio	33.4	83.6	0.0	27.2	36.2
• Brewster	12.4	44.5	0.2	19.3	5.8
• Terrell	15.0	63.6	2.7	13.1	4.9
• Zapata	39.5	94.2	0.0	33.6	47.6

Border states and counties	% below poverty	% Latino	% Black	% 17 years or younger	% Spanish speaking
• Val Verde	19.9	81.8	1.6	28.8	23.3
• Kinney	18.6	62.5	0.0	17.8	14.8
• Maverick	26.8	95.2	0.6	31.8	43.5
• Dimmit	29.8	86.7	0.0	30.0	18.0
• Webb	30.1	95.5	0.4	33.6	41.2
• Hidalgo	31.2	92.0	0.5	33.2	31.6
• Cameron	30.6	89.5	0.5	31.1	28.8
• Starr	35.3	99.1	0.0	33.1	51.4

Health care infrastructure, medical vulnerability, and overall vulnerability percentiles are ranked from 0–100, with "0" being the lowest and "100" being the highest level of vulnerability based on the individual items that comprise each.

Source: OMH (n.d.-a)

The percentage of the population living below the federal poverty level ($31,200 for a family of four in 2023 according to Health and Human Services (HHS, 2024) also varies considerably (OMH, 2023). Nevertheless, 16 of the 23 (69.6%) contiguous border counties exhibit poverty rates above 20%, with 7 of 23 (30.4%) contiguous border counties exceeding 30% of the population living below the federal poverty level. The border county population is young as well, exceeding one third of the population in several border counties. The percentage speaking Spanish varies with each of the border counties, from a low of 4.9% in Terrell County, Texas, to a high of 51.4% in Starr County, Texas. Together, this information indicates that the four U.S.–Mexico border states are primarily Mexican or Mexican American with few Black Americans, have very high rates of people living below the federal poverty line, have a significant population of persons under 17 years of age, and are bilingual Spanish speaking to a large degree.

Through the examination of the minority health thematic social vulnerability areas, we can determine the kinds of social determinants experienced by the U.S.–Mexico border county population. In Table 3.11, each border county displays the six thematic area scores and the overall level of social vulnerability as described earlier.

With this largely Latino population, the Minority Health Social Vulnerability Index Explorer data dashboard (OMH, n.d.-a) shows there are extremely high percentile rankings (greater than the 75th percentile) in social vulnerability for socioeconomic status (19/23, 82.6% of counties), housing and transportation (16/23, 69.6% of counties), and in their overall vulnerability percentiles (19/23, 82.6% of counties). The thematic areas of household composition and disability (13/23, 56.5%) and health care infrastructure (11/23, 47.8% of counties) had the lowest percentile rankings compared to the others. However, Maverick County, Texas, had the highest percentile (71) for medical vulnerability and San Diego, California, had the lowest (2).

When viewed from a regional perspective, the social determinants of health examined place Latinos of Mexican descent at high risk for disease and social vulnerability, more so than non-Latino White Americans. This picture belies the findings at the national level where Mexican Americans tend to do better than Black Americans but worse than non-Latino White Americans. Upon closer examination, the social determinants of health are negatively distributed in the U.S.–Mexico border region, conveying an

TABLE 3.11 Minority Health Social Vulnerability Areas and Overall Vulnerability (Percentiles), U.S.–Mexico Border States

Border states & counties	Socioeconomic status	Household composition & disability	Minority status & language	Housing & transportation	Health care infrastructure	Medical vulnerability	Overall vulnerability
Arizona (4)							
• **Yuma**	94	76	94	98	71	39	100
• **Pima**	67	57	99	98	38	6	93
• **Santa Cruz**	95	84	73	45	86	11	81
• **Cochise**	67	89	94	94	21	18	89
California (2)							
• **San Diego***	39	6	100	84	49	2	76
• **Imperial**	99	78	93	99	73	25	99
New Mexico (3)							
• **Hidalgo**	96	79	35	79	66	15	53
• **Luna**	100	95	72	98	82	63	99
• **Dona Ana**	93	69	88	97	52	17	94

Border states & counties	Socioeconomic status	Household composition & disability	Minority status & language	Housing & transportation	Health care infrastructure	Medical vulnerability	Overall vulnerability
Texas (14)							
• El Paso	88	71	97	86	74	17	98
• Hudspeth	98	81	42	79	100	56	91
• Presidio	99	100	59	70	90	43	94
• Brewster*	42	49	46	75	40	14	28
• Terrell*	78	17	40	2	99	44	47
• Zapata	100	95	36	70	99	20	81
• Val Verde	85	78	61	94	91	18	83
• Kinney	88	29	46	63	92	16	58
• Maverick	99	84	72	62	96	71	99
• Dimmit	100	99	38	93	65	45	82
• Webb	90	61	82	85	94	37	97
• Hidalgo	97	71	86	83	71	41	97
• Cameron	96	71	85	86	72	32	96
• Starr	100	93	46	55	96	57	89

Each thematic area percentile and the overall vulnerability percentile are ranked from 0–100, with "0" being the lowest and "100" being the highest level of social vulnerability based on the individual items that comprise each.

Source: OMH (n.d.-a)

increased risk for morbidity and mortality among Latinos of Mexican descent, especially from obesity, respiratory diseases, and cardiovascular disease (OMH, n.d.-a).

CHAPTER SUMMARY

Latinos are one of the fastest growing populations in the United States. There is remarkable differentiation among the various Latino groups with respect to each of the major social determinants of health, as well as differences between Latinos, Latino subgroups, and African Americans. Overall, one third of Latinos are third generation or higher, meaning that they have lived in the United States for multiple generations. Contrary to popular opinion, most Latinos are U.S. born (66%). As a group, Latinos are younger than non-Latino White Americans and Black Americans. Among Latino subgroups, South Americans and Cubans have a higher proportion of persons in the 21 and over age category. A much larger proportion of Latinos than non-Latino White Americans have never been married.

Economic stability among Latinos, a major social determinant of health, is more fragile among Latino Americans than non-Latino Black Americans and White Americans. This is especially the case for Central Americans, Cubans, and Latinos of Mexican descent. However, the median family income for Latino Americans was about $4,000 more than non-Latino Black Americans in 2021. Median wealth, another important indicator of economic stability, is higher among Latinos than non-Latino Black Americans but lags significantly behind non-Latino White Americans. Median net worth is also higher for Latino Americans than Black Americans but woefully behind non-Latino White Americans. Poverty rates are higher among non-Latino Black Americans than for Latino Americans of Mexican descent and non-Latino White Americans. Only Central Americans have a higher poverty rate than non-Latino Black Americans. Poverty is much more pronounced among women of color, with rates between 2 and 3 times higher than non-Latino White women. Black women heads of households have much higher poverty rates than Latinas and non-Latina White women. Children living in these households are negatively impacted by a lack of financial resources. Black Americans also have higher unemployment rates than any of the Latino subgroups and twice the rate of non-Latino White Americans. The gender-wage gap continues to place women and their dependent children at a disadvantage, especially for women of color. Persistent poverty is a major concern for all groups.

Access to quality education provides the necessary foundation for personal and interpersonal development. Economic success is predicated on educational attainment. Interestingly, Latinos have lower educational attainment rates than non-Latino Black Americans and White Americans. In fact, the majority of Mexican Americans have less than a bachelor's degree. English language proficiency and health literacy levels are relatively low for Latinos in comparison to non-Latino Black Americans and White Americans.

Community context is another major social determinant of health. Among Latinos, there is higher ethnic segregation, which also provides resources like social support, social cohesion, and social capital that help mitigate the detrimental effects of poverty, crime, and homelessness. Nevertheless, issues around urban renewal like gentrification erodes the cultural capital of Latino ethnic enclaves. The neighborhood and built environment places Latinos and other historically marginalized groups at a disadvantage, with increased neighborhood pollution, freeways, and food deserts.

Access to quality health care is extremely important for timely diagnosis and treatment of disease. The behavioral model for vulnerable populations provides a useful framework for examining the contribution of predisposing, enabling, and need characteristics in the utilization of health care services. Important utilization barriers exist for Latinos that need to be eliminated in order to gain full access to state-of-the-art technologies that can save and prolong lives.

Immigration and documentation status is a unique social determinant affecting those populations immigrating to the United States. Among Latinos of Mexican and Central American descent, immigration status determines the quality of life they will experience and the barriers they may encounter in achieving the "American Dream."

The U.S.-Mexico border region is an important "place" for Latinos of Mexican descent. Mexican Americans comprise over 50% of the population in the region, many of whom can trace their presence in the area for generations. Most of the SDOH are underdeveloped in the region, with higher poverty rates than in other parts of the country. Educational attainment is much lower for Latinos in this region than other parts of the United States.

The creation of Community Resilience Estimates (CRE) and Social Vulnerability Index (SVI) for the U.S.-Mexico border region by the CDC, ATSDR, and OMH contribute to our understanding of the problems facing the area in the aftermath of COVID-19 and other potential natural and manmade disasters. Overall, the U.S.-Mexico border is highly vulnerable to epidemics and other calamitous events.

Overall, this chapter presents a mixed and complex analysis of the social determinants of health among Latinos and Latinos of Mexican descent relative to non-Latino White Americans and Black Americans. In almost every instance, Latino Americans were found to be worse off than non-Latino White Americans but perhaps better-off than non-Latino Black Americans in some areas.

QUESTIONS TO CONSIDER

1. How are sociodemographic characteristics associated with access to health care for Latinos of Mexican descent?
2. How do non-Latino White Americans, non-Latino Black Americans, and Latinos differ on the social determinants of health?
3. Compare and contrast the wage gap between Latinas, non-Latina Black women, and non-Latina White women. Why does the gap appear smaller in among Black women and Latinas?
4. Describe the behavioral model for vulnerable populations and its potential application to Hispanic/Latino access to health care?
5. What do the Community Resilience Estimates and the Social Vulnerability Index reveal about Latinos living in the U.S.-Mexico border region?

SUGGESTED READINGS

Alcalá, H. E., Chen, J., Langellier, B. A., Roby, D. H., & Ortega, A. N. (2017). Impact of the Affordable Care Act on health care access and utilization among Latinos. *The Journal of the American Board of Family Medicine*, 30(1), 52–62.

Alegría, M., Molina, K. M., & Chen, C. N. (2014). Neighborhood characteristics and differential risk for depressive and anxiety disorders across racial/ethnic groups in the United States. *Depression and Anxiety, 31*(1), 27–37.

Becerra, D., Androff, D., Messing, J. T., Castillo, J., & Cimino, A. (2015). Linguistic acculturation and perceptions of quality, access, and discrimination in health care among Latinos in the United States. *Social Work in Health Care, 54*(2), 134–157.

Calvo, R. (2016). Health literacy and quality of care among Latino immigrants in the United States. *Health & Social Work, 41*(1), e44–e51.

Dailey, A., Gant, Z., Hu, X., Lyons, S. J., Okello, A., & Johnson, A. S. (2024). A census tract-level examination of diagnosed HIV infection and social vulnerability themes among Black/African American, Hispanic/Latino, and White Adults, 2019—USA. *Journal of Racial and Ethnic Health Disparities, 11*(1), 468–491

Enchautigui, M. E. (1997). Latino neighborhoods and latino neighborhood poverty. *Journal of Urban Affairs, 19*(4), 445–467.

Farmer, P. E., Nizeye, B., Stulac, S., & Keshavjee, S. (2006). Structural violence and clinical medicine. *PLoS Med, 3*(10), e449. https://doi.org/10.1371/journal.pmed.0030449

Gallo, L. C., Savin, K. L., Jankowska, M. M., Roesch, S. C., Sallis, J. F., Sotres-Alvarez, D., Talaera, G. A., Perreira, K. M., Isasi, C. R., Penedo, F. J., LLabr, M. M., Estrealla, M. L., Chamber, E. C., Daviglus, M. L., Brown, S. C., & Carlson, J. A. (2022). Neighborhood environment and metabolic risk in Hispanics/Latinos from the Hispanic Community Health Study/Study of Latinos. *American Journal of Preventive Medicine, 63*(2), 195–203.

Guzman,G. & Kollar, M. (2023, September). Income in the United States: 2022. U.S. Census Bureau, Current Population Reports, P60–279. U.S. Government Publishing Office, Washington, DC. Retrieved April 15, 2023 from: Income in the United States: 2022 (census.gov)

Hacker, K., Auerbach, J., Ikeda, R., Philip, C., & Houry, D. (2022). SDOH Task Force. Social determinants of health—An approach taken at CDC. *Journal of Public Health Management and Practice, 28*(6), 589–594.

Hilmers, A., Hilmers, D. C., & Dave, J. (2012). Neighborhood disparities in access to healthy foods and their effects on environmental justice. *American Journal of Public Health, 102*(9), 1644–1654.

Lewnard, J. A., Mora, A. M., Nkwocha, O., Kogut, K., Rauch, S. A., Morga, N., Hernandez, S., Wong, M. P., Huen, K., Andrejko, K., Jewell, N. P., Parra, K. L., Holland, N., Harris, E., Cuevas, M., & Eskenazi, B. (2021). Prevalence and clinical profile of severe acute respiratory syndrome Coronavirus 2 infection among farmworkers, California, USA, June–November 2020. *Emerging Infectious Diseases, 27*(5), 1330.

Marrero, F. A. (2016). Barriers to school success for Latino students. *Journal of Education and Learning, 5*(2), 180–186.

Pedroza, J. M. (2022). Housing instability in an era of mass deportations. *Population Research and Policy Review, 41*, 2645–2681. https://doi.org/10.1007/s11113-022-09719-1

Saha, S., Fernandez, A., & Perez-Stable, E. (2007). Reducing language barriers and racial/ethnic disparities in health care: An investment in our future. *Journal of General Internal Medicine, 22*, 371–372.

Xiao, H., McCurdy, S. A., Stoecklin-Marois, M. T., Li, C. S., & Schenker, M. B. (2013). Agricultural work and chronic musculoskeletal pain among Latino farm workers: The MICASA study. *American Journal of Industrial Medicine, 56*(2), 216–225.

REFERENCES

Abernathy, T. J., Webster, G., & Vermeulen, M. (2002). Relationship between poverty and health among adolescents. *Adolescence, 37*(145), 55–68.

Agency for Toxic Substances and Disease Registry. (n.d.). *CDC/ATSDR Social Vulnerability Index*. Retrieved June 22, 2023, from https://www.atsdr.cdc.gov/placeandhealth/svi/index.html#:~:text=Social%20vulnerability%20refers%20to%20the,human%20suffering%20and%20economic%20loss

Agency for Toxic Substances and Disease Registry. (2020). *CDC/ATSDR SVI Analyses 2020*. https://www.atsdr.cdc.gov/placeandhealth/svi/interactive_map.html.

Agency for Toxic Substances and Disease Registry. (2022, August 5). *CDC/ATSDR SVI Documentation 2020*. www.atsdr.cdc.gov/placeandhealth/svi/documentation/SVI_documentation_2020.html

Aladangady, A., & Forde, A. (2021, October 22). *Wealth inequality and the racial wealth gap*. Board of Governors of the Federal Reserve System. https://doi.org/10.17016/2380-7172.2861

Alcalá, H. E., Chen, J., Langellier, B. A., Roby, D. H., & Ortega, A. N. (2017). Impact of the Affordable Care Act on health care access and utilization among Latinos. *The Journal of the American Board of Family Medicine, 30*(1), 52–62.

Alegría, M., Molina, K. M., & Chen, C. N. (2014). Neighborhood characteristics and differential risk for depressive and anxiety disorders across racial/ethnic groups in the United States. *Depression and Anxiety, 31*(1), 27–37.

Almeida, J., Biello, K. B., Pedraza, F., Wintner, S., & Viruell-Fuentes, E. (2016). The association between anti-immigrant policies and perceived discrimination among Latinos in the US: A multilevel analysis. *SSM-Population Health, 2*, 897–903.

Andersen, R. M. (1995). Revisiting the behavioral model and access to medical care: Does it matter? *Journal of Health and Social Behavior, 36*(1), 1–10.

Anderson, K. F., & Finch, J. K. (2014). Racially charged legislation and Latino health disparities: The case of Arizona's SB 1070. *Sociological Spectrum, 34*(6), 526–548.

Annie E. Casey Foundation. (2019, September 24). *Children living in high-poverty, low-opportunity neighborhoods*. https://www.aecf.org/resources/children-living-in-high-poverty-low-opportunity-neighborhoods

Arcury, T. A., Nguyen, H. T., Summers, P., Talton, J. W., Holbrook, L. C., Walker, F. O., Chen, H., Howard, T. D., Galván, L., & Quandt, S. A. (2014). Lifetime and current pesticide exposure among Latino farmworkers in comparison to other Latino immigrants. *American Journal of Industrial Medicine, 57*(7), 776–787.

Assari, S. (2017). Social determinants of depression: The intersections of race, gender, and socioeconomic status. *Brain Sciences, 7*(12), 156.

Association of American Medical Colleges. (2019). *Diversity in medicine facts and figures*. https://www.aamc.org/data-reports/workforce/interactive-data/figure-18-percentage-all-active-physicians-race/ethnicity-2018

Badyda, A. J., Dabrowiecki, P., Lubinski, W., Czechowski, P. O., Majewski, G., Chcialowski, A., & Kraszewski, A. (2013). Influence of traffic-related air pollutants on lung function. *Neurobiology of Respiration*, 229–235.

Baker, B. (2021, January). *Estimates of the unauthorized immigrant population residing in the United States: January 2015–January 2018*. Department of Homeland Security. https://www.dhs.gov/immigration-statistics/population-estimates/unauthorized-resident.

Balderrama, F., & Rodriquez, R. (2006). *Decade of betrayal: Mexican repatriation in the 1930s*. University of New Mexico Press.

Becerra, D. (2012). Perceptions of educational barriers affecting the academic achievement of Latino K–12 students. *Children & Schools, 34*(3), 167–177.

Becerra, D., Androff, D., Messing, J. T., Castillo, J., & Cimino, A. (2015). Linguistic acculturation and perceptions of quality, access, and discrimination in health care among Latinos in the United States. *Social Work in Health Care, 54*(2), 134–157.

Berk, M. L., & Schur, C. L. (2001). The effect of fear on access to care among undocumented Latino immigrants. *Journal of Immigrant Health, 3*, 151–156.

Betancourt, J. R., & Maina, A. W. (2004). The Institute of Medicine report "Unequal Treatment": Implications for academic health centers. *The Mount Sinai Journal of Medicine, 71*(5), 314–321.

Bevan, G., Pandey, A., Griggs, S., Dalton, J. E., Zidar, D., Patel, S., Khan, S. U., Nasir, K., Rajagopalan, S., & Al-Kindi, S. (2023). Neighborhood-level social vulnerability and prevalence of cardiovascular risk factors and coronary heart disease. *Current Problems in Cardiology, 48*(8), Article101182. https://doi.org/10.1016/j.cpcardiol.2022.101182

Bhutta, N., Chang, A. C., Dettling, L. J., & Hsu, J. W. (2020, September 28). *Disparities in wealth by race and ethnicity in the 2019 Survey of Consumer Finances*. Board of Governors of the Federal Reserve System. https://www.federalreserve.gov/econres/notes/feds-notes/disparities-in-wealth-by-race-and-ethnicity-in-the-2019-survey-of-consumer-finances-20200928.html

Boal, W. L., Li, J., & Sussell, A. (2018). Health insurance coverage by occupation among adults aged 18–64 years—17 states, 2013–2014. *Morbidity and Mortality Weekly Report, 67*, 593–598. https://doi.org/10.15585/mmwr.mm6721

Bustamante, A. V., Chen, J., Rodriguez, H. P., Rizzo, J. A., & Ortega, A. N. (2010). Use of preventive care services among Latino subgroups. *American Journal of Preventive Medicine, 38*(6), 610–619.

Butel, J., & Braun, K. L. (2019). The role of collective efficacy in reducing health disparities: A systematic review. *Family & Community Health, 42*(1), 8.

Cabrera, N. (2013). Positive development of minority children. *Social Policy Report, 27*(2), 1–30.

Calderón, J. L., Shaheen, M., Hays, R. D., Fleming, E. S., Norris, K. C., & Baker, R. S. (2014). Improving diabetes health literacy by animation. *The Diabetes Educator, 40*(3), 361–372.

Calvert, G. M., Karnik, J., Mehler, L., Beckman, J., Morrissey, B., Sievert, J., Barrett, R., Lackovic, M., Mabee, L., Schwartz, A., Mitchell, Y., & Moraga-McHaley, S. (2008). Acute pesticide poisoning among agricultural workers in the United States, 1998–2005. *American Journal of Industrial Medicine, 51*(12), 883–898.

Calvo, R. (2016). Health literacy and quality of care among Latino immigrants in the United States. *Health & Social Work, 41*(1), e44–e51.

Carter-Pokras, O., Zambrana, R. E., Poppell, C. F., Logie, L. A., & Guerrero-Preston, R. (2007). The environmental health of Latino children. *Journal of Pediatric Health Care, 21*(5), 307–314.

Chen, J., Vargas-Bustamante, A., Mortensen, K., & Ortega, A. N. (2016). Racial and ethnic disparities in health care access and utilization under the Affordable Care Act. *Medical Care, 54*(2), 140.

Chokshi, D. A. (2018). Income, poverty, and health inequality. *JAMA, 319*(13), 1312-1313.

Cohen, D. A., Inagami, S., & Finch, B. (2008). The built environment and collective efficacy. *Health & Place, 14*(2), 198–208.

Coleman-Jensen, A., Rabbitt, M. P., Gregory, C. A., & Singh, A. (2022, September). *Household food security in the United States in 2021, ERR-309.* U.S. Department of Agriculture, Economic Research Service.

Collins, S. R., Gunja, M., Rasmussen, P. W., Doty, M. M., & Beutel, S. (2015, September). *Are marketplace plans affordable? Consumer perspectives from the Commonwealth Fund Affordable Care Act Tracking Survey, March–May 2015.* The Commonwealth Fund.

The Content Authority. (n.d.) Unsheltered vs homeless: When and how can you use each one? Accessed on April 20, 2024, from https://thecontentauthority.com/blog/unsheltered-vs-homeless

Cooksey-Stowers, J., Schwartz, M. B., & Brownell, K. D. (2017). Food swamps predict obesity rates better than food deserts in the United States. *International Journal of Environmental Research and Public Health, 14,* 1366. https://doi.org/10.3390/ijerph14111366

Dailey, A., Gant, Z., Hu, X., Lyons, S. J., Okello, A., & Johnson, A. S. (2024). A census tract-level examination of diagnosed HIV infection and social vulnerability themes among Black/African American, Hispanic/Latino, and White Adults, 2019—USA. *Journal of Racial and Ethnic Health Disparities, 11*(1), 468–491.

DeSilver, D. (2021, August 2). As national eviction ban expires, a look at who rents and who owns in the U.S. Pew Research Center Short Reads. Accessed on April 20, 2024 from https://www.pewresearch.org/short-reads/2021/08/02/as-national-eviction-ban-expires-a-look-at-who-rents-and-who-owns-in-the-u-s/

Dietrich, S., & Hernandez, E. (2022, August). *Language use in the United States: 2019.* U.S. Census Bureau. https://www.census.gov/content/dam/Census/library/publications/2022/acs/acs-50.pdf

Dutko, P., Ver Ploeg, M., & Farrigan, T. (2012, August). *Characteristics and influential factors of food deserts, EER-140.* U.S. Department of Agriculture, Economic Research Service. Accessed on April 20, 2024 from https://www.ers.usda.gov/webdocs/publications/45014/30940_err140.pdf

Elenwa, F., Gant, Z., Hu, X., & Johnson, A. S. (2023). A census tract-level examination of HIV care outcomes and social vulnerability among Black/African American, Hispanic/Latino, and White adults in the Southern United States, 2018. *Journal of Community Health, 48*(4), 616–633.

Ellerbrock, C. R., Cruz, B. C., Vásquez, A., & Howes, E. V. (2016). Preparing culturally responsive teachers: Effective practices in teacher education. *Action in Teacher Education, 38*(3), 226–239.

Enchautigui, M. E. (1997). Latino neighborhoods and Latino neighborhood poverty. *Journal of Urban Affairs, 19*(4), 445–467.

Eskenazi, B., Bradman, A., & Castorina, R. (1999). Exposures of children to organophosphate pesticides and their potential adverse health effects. *Environmental Health Perspectives, 107*(Suppl. 3), 409–419.

Estrada, A. L., Trevino, F. M., & Ray, L. A. (1990). Health care utilization barriers among Mexican Americans: Evidence from HHANES 1982–84. *American Journal of Public Health, 80*(Suppl.), 27–31.

Farmer, P. (2003). *Pathologies of power: Health, human rights, and the new war on the poor.* University of California Press.

Farmer, P.E., Nizeye, B., Stulac, S., & Keshavjee, S. (2006). Structural violence and clinical medicine. *PLoS Med, 3*(10), e449. https://doi.org/10.1371/journal.pmed.0030449

Feiveson, L., & Sabelhaus, J. (2018, June 1). *How does intergenerational wealth transmission affect wealth concentration?* Board of Governors of the Federal Reserve System. http://doi.org/10.17016/2380-7172.2209

Fernández, A., Quan, J., Moffet, H., Parker, M. M., Schillinger, D., & Karter, A. J. (2017). Adherence to newly prescribed diabetes medications among insured Latino and White patients with diabetes. *JAMA Internal Medicine, 177*(3), 371–379.

Figueroa, C. M., Medvin, A., Phrathep, B. D., Thomas, C. W., Ortiz, J., & Bushy, A. (2021). Healthcare needs of US rural Latinos: a growing, multicultural population. *Online journal of rural nursing and health care: the official journal of the Rural Nurse Organization, 21*(1), 24.

Flores, A. (2022). *Distrust of Police Officers due to the Perception of Racial Profiling Practices in Latino Communities* (Doctoral dissertation, The Chicago School of Professional Psychology).

Frank, R., Cerda, M., & Rendon, M. (2007). Barrios and burbs: Residential context and health-risk behaviors among Angeleno adolescents. *Journal of Health and Social Behavior, 48*(3), 283–300.

Freeman H. P. (2004). Poverty, culture, and social injustice: Determinants of cancer disparities. *CA: A Cancer Journal for Clinicians, 54*(2), 72–77. https://doi.org/10.3322/canjclin.54.2.72

Fuller, B., & García Coll, C. (2010). Learning from Latinos: contexts, families, and child development in motion. *Developmental Psychology, 46*(3), 559.

Gallo, L. C., Savin, K. L., Jankowska, M. M., Roesch, S. C., Sallis, J. F., Sotres-Alvarez, D., Talavera, G. A., Perreira, K. M., Isasi, C., R., Penedo, F. J., Llabre, M. M., Estrealla, M. L., Chambers, E. C., Daviglus, M. L., Brown, S. C., & & Carlson, J. A. (2022). Neighborhood environment and metabolic risk in Hispanics/Latinos from the Hispanic Community Health Study/Study of Latinos. *American Journal of Preventive Medicine, 63*(2), 195–203.

Galvan, T., Lill, S., & Garcini, L. M. (2021). Another brick in the wall: Healthcare access difficulties and their implications for undocumented Latino/a immigrants. *Journal of Immigrant and Minority Health, 23*, 885–894.

Gándara, P., & Mordechay, K. (2017, April). Demographic change and the new (and not so new) challenges for Latino education. *The Educational Forum, 81*(2), 148–159.

Garcés, I. C., Scarinci, I. C., & Harrison, L. (2006). An examination of sociocultural factors associated with health and health care seeking among Latina immigrants. *Journal of Immigrant and Minority Health, 8*, 377–385.

Gay, G. (2002). Preparing for culturally responsive teaching. *Journal of Teacher Education, 53*(2), 106–116.

Gelberg, L., Andersen, R. M., & Leake, B. D. (2000). The behavioral model for vulnerable populations: Application to medical care use and outcomes for homeless people. *Health Services Research, 34*(6), 1273–1302.

Gilligan, J. (1997). *Violence: Reflections on a national epidemic.* Vintage Books.

Giraldo-García, R. J., Galletta, A., & Bagakas, J. G. (2019). The intersection of culture and institutional support for Latino students' academic success: Remediation or empowerment? *Journal of Latinos and Education, 18*(1), 68–80.

González, H. M., Vega, W. A., & Tarraf, W. (2010). Health care quality perceptions among foreign-born Latinos and the importance of speaking the same language. *The Journal of the American Board of Family Medicine, 23*(6), 745–752.

Good, M. E., Masewicz, S., & Vogel, L. (2010). Latino English language learners: Bridging achievement and cultural gaps between schools and families. *Journal of Latinos and Education, 9*(4), 321–339.

Gramlich, J. (2017, September 29). Hispanic dropout rate hits new low, college enrollment at new high. Pew Research Center Short Reads. Accessed on April 20, 2024 from https://www.pewresearch.org/short-reads/2017/09/29/hispanic-dropout-rate-hits-new-low-college-enrollment-at-new-high/

Hacker, K. Auerbach, J., Ikeda, R., Philip, C., & Houry, D. (2022). Social determinants of health—An approach taken at CDC. *Journal of Public Health Management and Practice, 28*(6), 589–594. https://doi.org/10.1097/PHH.0000000000001626

Hacker, K., & Houry D. (2022). Social needs and social determinants: The role of the Centers for Disease Control and Prevention and Public Health. *Public Health Reports, 137*(6), 1049–1052. https://doi.org/10.1177/00333549221120244

Hales, L.J. & Coleman-Jensen, A. (2024). Household food insecurity across race and ethnicity in the United States, 2016–21, Report No. EIB-269, Table 6. U.S. Department of Agriculture, Economic Research Service. Retrieved on April 21, 2024, from: https://www.ers.usda.gov/publications/pub-details?pubid=108904

Hankivsky, O. (2012). Women's health, men's health, and gender and health: Implications of intersectionality. *Social Science & Medicine, 74*(11), 1712–1720.

Hansen, E., & Donohoe, M. (2003). Health issues of migrant and seasonal farmworkers. *Journal of Health Care for the Poor and Underserved, 14*(2), 153–164.

Health and Human Services (HHS). (2024). HHS poverty guidelines for 2024. Retrieved on April 15, 2023 from Poverty Guidelines | ASPE (hhs.gov)

Healthy Border 2020. (n.d.): A prevention & health promotion initiative. Retrieved on April 22, 2024 from https://www.hhs.gov/sites/default/files/res_2805.pdf

Hernández-Valero, M. A., Hajek, R. A., & Jones, L. A. (2003). Potential pathways of exposure for DDE and mirex and reported health problems in Mexican-American migrant and seasonal farmworker children residing in Texas. *Journal of Children's Health, 1*(2), 241–255.

Hill, L., Ndugga, N., & Artiga, S. (2023, March 15). *Key data on health and health care by race and ethnicity.* Kaiser Family Foundation. https://www.kff.org/report-section/key-data-on-health-and-health-care-by-race-ethnicity-report/#endnote_link_581600-1

Hilmers, A., Hilmers, D. C., & Dave, J. (2012). Neighborhood disparities in access to healthy foods and their effects on environmental justice. *American Journal of Public Health, 102*(9), 1644–1654.

Hipp, J. R., & Lakon, C. M. (2010). Social disparities in health: Disproportionate toxicity proximity in minority communities over a decade. *Health & Place, 16*(4), 674–683.

Hodgetts, D., & Stolte, O. (2017). *Urban poverty and health inequalities: A relational approach.* Routledge.

Hong, S., Zhang, W., & Walton, E. (2014). Neighborhoods and mental health: Exploring ethnic density, poverty, and social cohesion among Asian Americans and Latinos. *Social Science & Medicine, 111*, 117–124.

Irwin, V., De La Rosa, J., Wang, K., Hein, S., Zhang, J., Burr, R., Roberts, A., Barmer, A., Bullock Mann, F., Dilig, R., and Parker, S. (2022*). Report on the Condition of Education 2022 (NCES 2022-144).* U.S. Department of Education. Washington, DC: National Center for Education Statistics. Retrieved March 15, 2023 from https://nces.ed.gov/pubsearch/ pubsinfo.asp?pubid=2022144

Islam, S. J., Nayak, A., Hu, Y., Mehta, A., Dieppa, K., Almuwaqqat, Z., Ko, Y. A., Patel, S. A., Goyal, A., Sullivan, S., Lewis, T. T., Vaccarino, V., Morris, A. A., & Quyyumi, A. A. (2021). Temporal trends in the association of social vulnerability and race/ ethnicity with county-level COVID-19 incidence and outcomes in the USA: An ecological analysis. *BMJ Open, 11*(7), Article e048086. https://doi.org/10.1136/bmjopen-2020-048086

Iyer, A., Sen, G., & Östlin, P. (2009). Inequalities and intersections in health: a review of the evidence. *Gender Equity in Health*, 92–117.

James, S. (2002). *Social determinants of health: Implications for intervening on racial and ethnic health disparities* [Paper presentation]. 24th Annual Minority Health Conference, Chapel Hill, North Carolina, United States.

Javaid, S. & Tucker, J. (2021, September). National snapshot: poverty among women & families, 2021. National Women's Law Center, September 2021. Fact Sheet. https://nwlc.org/wp-content/uploads/2021/11/NationalSnapshotFS-1.pdf

Jih, J., Vittinghoff, E., & Fernandez, A. (2015). Patient-physician language concordance and use of preventive care services among limited english proficient Latinos and Asians. *Public Health Reports, 130*(2), 134–142.

Joint Center for Housing Studies of Harvard University. (2021). *The state of the nation's housing 2021.* https://www.jchs.harvard.edu/state-nations-housing-2021

Keisler-Starkey, K., Bunch, L.N., & Lindstrom, R.A. (2023, September). *Health insurance coverage in the United States: 2022. U.S. Census Bureau, Current Population Reports, P60-281.* U.S. Government Publishing Office, Washington, DC. Retrieved on April 19, 2024 from Health Insurance Coverage in the United States: 2022 (census.gov)

Kelli, H. M., Hammadah, M., Ahmed, H., Ko, Y. A., Topel, M., Samman-Tahhan, A., Awad, M., Patel, K., Mohammed, K., Sperling, L. S., Pemu, P., Vaccarino, V., Lewis, T., Taylor, H., Martin, G., Gibbons, G. H., & Quyyumi, A. A. (2017). Association between living in food deserts and cardiovascular risk. *Circulation: Cardiovascular Quality and Outcomes, 10*(9), Article e003532.

Kingsley, G. T., & Pettit, K. L. (2005). *Severe distress and concentrated poverty: Trends for neighborhoods in Casey cities and the nation.* The Urban Institute.

Kirkhorn, S., Greenlee, R. T., & Reeser, J. C. (2003). The epidemiology of agriculture-related osteoarthritis and its impact on occupational disability. *Wisconsin Medical Journal, 102*(7), 38–44.

Korhonen, V. (2023, June 2). *Distribution of English language proficiency among Hispanics in the United States as of 2022.* Statista, 2024. Accessed on March 10, 2023, from https://www.statista.com/statistics/639745/us-hispanic-english-proficiency/

Koulish, R. E., Escobedo, M., Rubio-Goldsmith, R., & Warren, J. R. (1994). *US immigration authorities and victims of human and civil rights abuses: The Border Interaction Project Study of South Tucson, Arizona, and South Texas.* University of Arizona.

Krieger, N. (2001). A glossary for social epidemiology. *Journal of Epidemiology and Community Health, 55*(10), 693–700.

Krotgstad, J. M. (2014). *Latino confidence in local police lower than among Whites.* Pew Research Center. https://www.pewresearch.org/short-reads/2014/08/28/latino-confidence-in-local-police-lower-than-among-whites/

Krogstad, J.M., Passel, J.S., Moslimani, M., & Noe-Bustamante, L. (2023, September 22). Key facts about U.S. latinos for national hispanic heritage month. Pew Research Center Short Reads. Accessed on March 6, 2024, from https://www.pewresearch.org/short-reads/2023/09/22/key-facts-about-us-latinos-for-national-hispanic-heritage-month/#:~:text=The%20U.S.%20Hispanic%20population%20reached,increase%20in%20the%20Asian%20population

Krogstad, J. M., Passel, J. S., & Noe-Bustamante, L. (2022, September 23). *Key facts about U.S. Latinos for National Hispanic Heritage Month.* Pew Research Center. Accessed on March 5, 2024 from https://www.pewresearch.org/short-reads/2023/09/22/key-facts-about-us-latinos-for-national-hispanic-heritage-month/#:~:text=The%20U.S.%20Hispanic%20population%20reached,increase%20in%20the%20Asian%20population.

Kutner, M., Greenberg, E., Jin, Y., & Paulsen, C. (2006). *The health literacy of America's adults: Results from the 2003 National Assessment of Adult Literacy.* U.S. Department of Education, National Center for Education Statistics.

Latino Policy Forum. (n.d.). *Affordable housing.* Retrieved March 23, 2023, from https://www.latinopolicyforum.org/issues/housing/affordable-housing

Lees, L., Slater, T., & Wyly, E. (2008). Gentrification reader. In A. Rowland & G. Bridge (Eds.), *Gentrification in a global context: The new urban colonialism* (p. 196). Routledge.

Lewnard, J. A., Mora, A. M., Nkwocha, O., Kogut, K., Rauch, S. A., Morga, N., Hernandez, S., Wong, M. P., Huen, K., Andrejko, K., Jewell, N. P., Parra, K. L., Holland, N., Harris, E., Cuevas, M., & Eskenazi, B. (2021). Prevalence and clinical profile of severe acute respiratory syndrome Coronavirus 2 infection among farmworkers, California, USA, June–November 2020. *Emerging Infectious Diseases*, *27*(5), 1330–1342.

Liberman, A. (2021). "I Feared For My Life": Police Killings, Epistemic Injustice, and Social Distrust. In *Social Trust* (pp. 151–176). Routledge.

Lillie-Blanton, M., & Hoffman, C. (2005). The role of health insurance coverage in reducing racial/ethnic disparities in health care. *Health Affairs*, *24*(2), 398–408.

Logan, J. R., & Stults, B. (2021). *The persistence of segregation in the metropolis: New findings from the 2020 Census*. Diversity and Disparities Project, Brown University. https://s4.ad.brown.edu/Projects/Diversity downloaded on 8/3/2022.

MacDonald, J., & Stokes, R. J. (2006). Race, social capital, and trust in the police. *Urban Affairs Review*, *41*(3), 358–375.

Madrid, E. M. (2011). The Latino achievement gap. *Multicultural Education*, *19*(3), 7–12.

Marrero, F. A. (2016). Barriers to school success for Latino students. *Journal of Education and Learning*, *5*(2), 180–186.

Martinez, C. R., Jr., DeGarmo, D. S., & Eddy, J. M. (2004). Promoting academic success among Latino youths. *Hispanic Journal of Behavioral Sciences*, *26*(2), 128–151.

Martinez-Donate, A. P., Ejebe, I., Zhang, X., Guendelman, S., Lê-Scherban, F., Rangel, G., Gonzalez-Fagoaga, E., Hovell, M. F., & Amuedo-Dorantes, C. (2017). Access to health care among Mexican migrants and immigrants: A comparison across migration phases. *Journal of Health Care for the Poor and Underserved*, *28*(4), 1314–1326.

Massey, D. S., & Denton, N. A. (1993). Segregation and the making of the underclass. *The Urban Sociology Reader*, *2*, 191–201.

Moore, J., & Vigil, J. D. (2000). Barrios in transition. In P. Kivisto & G. Rundblad (Eds.), *Multiculturalism in the United States: Current issues, contemporary voices* (pp. 355–369). Pine Forge Press.

Morales, A. (1970). Police deployment theories and the Mexican American community. *El Grito*, *4*(1), 52–64.

Morey, B. N. (2018). Mechanisms by which anti-immigrant stigma exacerbates racial/ethnic health disparities. *American Journal of Public Health*, *108*(4), 460–463.

Moslimani, M., Noe-Bustamante, L., & Shah, S. (2023, August). *Facts on Hispanics of Mexican origin in the United States, 2021*. Pew Research Center. https://www.pewresearch.org/race-and-ethnicity/fact-sheet/us-hispanics-facts-on-mexican-origin-latinos/

Mucchetti, A. E. (2005). Driving while brown: A proposal for ending racial profiling in emerging Latino communities. *Harvard Latino Law Review*, *8*, 1.

Murphey, D., Guzman, L., & Torres, A. (2014). *America's Hispanic children: Gaining ground, looking forward*. Child Trends. https://www.childtrends.org/publications/americas-hispanic-children-gaining-ground-looking-forward

National Center for Education Statistics. (2014). *Program for the International Assessment of Adult Competencies (PIAAC), U.S. PIAAC 2012/2014*. Accessed on March 22, 2023, from https://nces.ed.gov/surveys/piaac/national_results.asp.

National Center for Education Statistics. (2019). *Indicator 23: Postsecondary graduation rates*. U.S. Department of Education, Institute of Education Sciences. https://nces.ed.gov/programs/raceindicators

National Center for Education Statistics. (2022b). *College enrollment rates*. U.S. Department of Education, Institute of Education Sciences. https://nces.ed.gov/programs/coe/indicator/cpb.

National Center for Education Statistics. (2023). Annual Earnings by Educational Attainment. *Condition of Education*. U.S. Department of Education, Institute of Education Sciences. Retrieved April 17, 2024, from https://nces.ed.gov/programs/coe/indicator/cba.

National Center for Education Statistics. (2024). *Status dropout rates*. U.S. Department of Education, Institute of Education Sciences. Retrieved June 12, 2024, from https://nces.ed.gov/programs/coe/indicator/coj

National Institutes of Health. (2021, July 7). *Health Literacy*. www.nih.gov/institutes-nih/nih-office-director/office-communications-public-liaison/clear-communication/health-literacy

National Research Center on Hispanic Children & Families. (2018, May 23). Looking at Latino families' access to early care and education through multiple dimensions: Slides. https://www.hispanicresearchcenter.org/research-resources/looking-at-latino-families-access-to-early-care-and-education-through-multiple-dimensions-slides/

Nellis, A. (2021). *The color of justice: Racial and ethnic disparity in state prisons*. The Sentencing Project. https://www.sentencingproject.org/reports/the-color-of-justice-racial-and-ethnic-disparity-in-state-prisons-the-sentencing-project/

Oates, G. R., Juarez, L. D., Horswell, R., Chu, S., Miele, L., Fouad, M. N., Curry, W. A., Fort, D., Hillegass, W. B., & Danos, D. M. (2021). The association between neighborhood social vulnerability and COVID-19 testing, positivity, and incidence in Alabama and Louisiana. *Journal of Community Health*, *46*(6), 1115–1123. https://doi.org/10.1007/s10900-021-00998-x

Office of Disease Prevention and Health Promotion. (n.d.). *Healthy People 2030*. U.S. Department of Health and Human Services. Retrieved April 16, 2024, from https://health.gov/healthypeople

Office of Minority Health. (n.d.-a). *Minority Health Social Vulnerability Index Explorer*. Retrieved April 22, 2024, from https://onemap.cdc.gov/Portal/apps/MapSeries/index.html?appid=3384875c46d649ee9b452913fd64e3c4

Office of Minority Health. (n.d.-b). *Profile: Hispanic/Latino Americans*. Retrieved April 15, 2023, from https://www.minorityhealth.hhs.gov/omh/browse.aspx?lvl=3&lvlid=64

Office of Minority Health. (2021a, July 16). *Minority Health Social Vulnerability Index fact sheet*. https://www.minorityhealth.hhs.gov/Assets/PDF/MH%20SVI%20Fact%20Sheet_7.14.2021.pdf?utm_medium=email&utm_source=govdelivery

Office of Minority Health. (2023). Minority health social vulnerability index. Retrieved on April 16, 2024 from Minority Health Social Vulnerability Index Overview | Updated June 2023, pp 5–6.

Organization for Economic Cooperation and Development. (2013). *OECD Skills Outlook 2013: First results from the Survey of Adult Skills*. http://doi.org/10.1787/9789264204256-en

Ortega, A. N., Fang, H., Perez, V. H., Rizzo, J. A., Carter-Pokras, O., Wallace, S. P., & Gelberg, L. (2007). Health care access, use of services, and experiences among undocumented Mexicans and other Latinos. *Archives of Internal Medicine, 167*(21), 2354–2360.

Pagán, J. A., Brown, C. J., Asch, D. A., Armstrong, K., Bastida, E., & Guerra, C. (2012).. Health literacy and breast cancer screening among Mexican American women in South Texas. *Journal of Cancer Education, 27*, 132–137. https://doi.org/10.1007/s13187-011-0239-6

Palen, J. J., & London, B. (Eds.). (1984). *Gentrification, displacement, and neighborhood revitalization*. State University of New York Press.

Pares-Avila, J., & Sobralske, M. C. (2011). No comprendo: Practice considerations when caring for Latinos with limited English proficiency in the United States health care system. *Hispanic Health Care International, 9*(4), 159–167.

Parker, R., Williams, M., Weiss, B. D., Barker, D. W., Davis, T. C., Doak, C. C., Doak, L. G., Hein, K., Meade, C. D., Nurrs, J., Schwartzberg, J., Somers, S. A., Davis, R. M., Riggs, J. A., Champion, H. C., Howe, J. P. Altman, R. D., Dietchman, S., Genel, M., ... Dickinson, B. D. (1999). Health literacy: Report of the Council on Scientific Affairs. *JAMA, 281*(6), 552–557. https://doi.org/10.1001/jama.281.6.552

Pastor, M., Sadd, J., & Hipp, J. (2001). Which came first? Toxic facilities, minority move-in, and environmental justice. *Journal of Urban Affairs, 23*(1), 1–21.

Pedde, M., Szpiro, A. A., & Adar, S. D. (2017). Traffic congestion as a risk factor for mortality in near-road communities: a case-crossover study. *American journal of epidemiology, 186*(5), 564–572.

Pedroza, J. M. (2022). Housing instability in an era of mass deportations. *Population Research and Policy Review, 41*, 2645–2681. https://doi.org/10.1007/s11113-022-09719-1

Perez, D., Ang, A., & Vega, W. A. (2009). Effects of health insurance on perceived quality of care among Latinos in the United States. *Journal of General Internal Medicine, 24*, 555–560.

Perfecto, I. (2019). Pesticide exposure of farm workers and the international connection. In B. Ryant & P. Mohai Eds.), *Race and the incidence of environmental hazards* (pp. 177–203). Routledge.

Pew Research Center. (2013). *2013 National Survey of Latinos*. https://www.pewresearch.org/hispanic/dataset/2013-national-survey-of-latinos/

Quandt, S. A., Walker, F. O., Talton, J. W., Summers, P., Chen, H., McLeod, D. K., & Arcury, T. A. (2016). Olfactory function in Latino farmworkers: Subclinical neurological effects of pesticide exposure in a vulnerable population. *Journal of Occupational and Environmental Medicine/American College of Occupational and Environmental Medicine, 58*(3), 248–253.

Rampey, B. D., Finnegan, R., Goodman, M., Mohadjer, L., Krenzke, T., Hogan, J., & Provasnik, S. (2016). *Skills of U.S. unemployed, young, and older adults in sharper focus: Results from the Program for the International Assessment of Adult Competencies (PIAAC) 2012/2014: First look (NCES 2016-039)*. U.S. Department of Education, National Center for Education Statistics. Retrieved on March 24, 2023 from https://nces.ed.gov/pubs2016/2016039.pdf

Reardon, S. F., & Galindo, C. (2009). The Hispanic-White achievement gap in math and reading in the elementary grades. *American Educational Research Journal, 46*(3), 853–891.

Rhodes, S. D., Bischoff, W. E., Burnell, J. M., Whalley, L. E., Walkup, M. P., Vallejos, Q. M., Quandt, S. A., Gryzwacz, J. G., Chenm,, H., & Arcury, T. A. (2010). HIV and sexually transmitted disease risk among male Hispanic/Latino migrant farmworkers in the Southeast: Findings from a pilot CBPR study. *American Journal of Industrial Medicine, 53*(10), 976–983.

Riegle-Crumb, C., & Callahan, R. M. (2009). Exploring the academic benefits of friendship ties for Latino boys and girls. *Social Science Quarterly, 90*(3), 611–631.

Rivers, P. A., & Patino, F. G. (2006). Barriers to health care access for Latino immigrants in the USA. *International Journal of Social Economics, 33*(3), 207–220.

Rodríguez, M. A., Vargas Bustamante, A., & Ang, A. (2009). Perceived quality of care, receipt of preventive care, and usual source of health care among undocumented and other Latinos. *Journal of General Internal Medicine, 24*, 508–513.

Romero, M. (2006). Racial profiling and immigration law enforcement: Rounding up of usual suspects in the Latino community. *Critical Sociology, 32*(2–3), 447–473.

Romero, M. (2008). Crossing the immigration and race border: A critical race theory approach to immigration studies. *Contemporary Justice Review, 11*(1), 23–37.

Romero, M., & Serag, M. (2004). Violation of Latino civil rights resulting from INS and local police's use of race, culture and class profiling: The case of the Chandler Roundup in Arizona. *Cleveland State Law Review, 52*, 75.

Ross, C. E., & Mirowsky, J. (1999). Disorder and decay: The concept and measurement of perceived neighborhood disorder. *Urban Affairs Review, 34*(3), 412–432.

Rural Health Information Hub. (n.d.). *Rural Data Explorer.* Retrieved April 19, 2024, from https://www.ruralhealthinfo.org/data-explorer?id=183 for year 2022.

Saha, S., Fernandez, A., & Perez-Stable, E. (2007). Reducing language barriers and racial/ethnic disparities in health care: An investment in our future. *Journal of General Internal Medicine, 22*, 371–372.

Salas, L. M., Ayón, C., & Gurrola, M. (2013). Estamos traumados: The effect of anti-immigrant sentiment and policies on the mental health of Mexican immigrant families. *Journal of Community Psychology, 41*(8), 1005–1020.

Salinas Thomas, E. (2023). Between trust and resentment: Examining competing views toward the police in Latino neighborhoods. *Politics, Groups, and Identities*, 1–20.

Sampson, R. J., & Raudenbush, S. W. (2004). Seeing disorder: Neighborhood stigma and the social construction of "broken windows." *Social Psychology Quarterly, 67*(4), 319–342.

Sampson, R. J., Raudenbush, S. W., & Earls, F. (1997). Neighborhoods and violent crime: A multilevel study of collective efficacy. *Science, 277*(5328), 918–924.

Scott, D. (2009). Tuberculosis, sexually transmitted diseases, HIV, and other infections among farmworkers in the eastern United States. In T. A. Arcury & S. A. Quandt (Eds.), *Latino farmworkers in the eastern United States* (pp. 131–152). Springer.

Semega, J., Kollar, M., Shrider, E. A., & Creamer, J. F. (2020, September). *Income and poverty in the United States: 2019. Current Population Reports.* U.S. Census Bureau. https://www.census.gov/content/dam/Census/library/publications/2020/demo/p60-270.pdf

Sentell, T., & Braun, K. L. (2012). Low health literacy, limited English proficiency, and health status in Asians, Latinos, and other racial/ethnic groups in California. *Journal of health communication, 17*(sup3), 82–99.

Shemmassian Academic Consulting. (2024). *Medical school acceptance rates by race (2024): Does ethnicity play a role?* https://www.shemmassianconsulting.com/blog/medical-school-acceptance-rates-by-race

Shrider, E.A., Kollar, M., Chen, F. & Semega, J. (2021, September). *Income and Poverty in the United States: 2020. U.S. Census Bureau, Current Population Reports, P60-273.* U.S. Government Publishing Office, Washington, DC.

Smedley, B. D., Stith, A. Y., & Nelson, A. R. (Eds.). (2003). *Unequal treatment: Confronting racial and ethnic disparities in health care.* National Academies Press.

Starfield, B. (1992). Effects of poverty on health status. *Bulletin of the New York Academy of Medicine, 68*(1), 17.

Statista. (n.d.). Mean earnings in the United States in 2022, by highest educational degree earned and ethnicity/race. Accessed on April 20, 2024 from Earnings by educational attainment and ethnicity/race U.S. 2022 | Statista

Thelin, A., Vingård, E., & Holmberg, S. (2004). Osteoarthritis of the hip joint and farm work. *American Journal of Industrial Medicine, 45*(2), 202–209.

Thompson, J. P., & and Suarez, G. (2019). *Accounting for racial wealth disparities in the United States.* Federal Reserve Bank of Boston. https://doi.org/10.29412/res.wp.2019.13

Timmins, C. L. (2002). The impact of language barriers on the health care of Latinos in the United States: a review of the literature and guidelines for practice. *Journal of midwifery & women's health, 47*(2), 80–96.

Tortolero, G. A., Otto, M. O., Ramphul, R., Yamal, J. M., Rector, A., Brown, M., Peskin, M. F., Mofleh, D., & Boerwinkle, E. (2022). Examining social vulnerability and the association with COVID-19 incidence in Harris County, Texas. *Frontiers in Public Health, 9*, Article 798085. https://doi.org/10.3389/fpubh.2021.798085

USAFacts. (2023). *U.S. homeownership rates by race.* https://usafacts.org/articles/homeownership-rates-by-race/

U.S. Bureau of Labor Statistics. (n.d.-a). *10.Employed persons by occupation, race, Hispanic or Latino ethnicity, and sex.* Retrieved April 20, 2024, from https://www.bls.gov/cps/aa2021/cpsaat10.pdf

U.S. Bureau of Labor Statistics. (n.d.-b). *Education pays.* Accessed on April 20, 2024 from Education pays : U.S. Bureau of Labor Statistics (bls.gov)

U.S. Bureau of Labor Statistics. (2021). *Household data annual averages: Employed persons by occupation, race, Hispanic or Latino ethnicity, and sex.* https://www.bls.gov/cps/aa2021/cpsaat10.pdf

U.S. Bureau of Labor Statistics. (2023a, March). *BLS Reports: Highlights of women's earnings in 2021.* https://www.bls.gov/opub/reports/womens-earnings/2021/home.htm

U.S. Bureau of Labor Statistics. (2023b, December 19). *National Census of Fatal Occupational Injuries in 2022.* https://www.bls.gov/news.release/pdf/cfoi.pdf

U.S. Bureau of Labor Statistics. (2023c). *Civilian labor force participation rate by age, sex, race, and ethnicity.* https://www.bls.gov/emp/tables/civilian-labor-force-participation-rate.htm

U.S. Census Bureau. (n.d.-a). 2020 *Census urban areas facts.* Accessed on April 20, 2024 from 2020 Census Urban Areas Facts

U.S. Census Bureau. (n.d.-b). *Housing patterns: Appendix B: measures of residential segregation.* Accessed on April 19, 2023 from Housing Patterns: Measures of Residential Segregation (census.gov)

U.S. Census Bureau. (n.d.-c). Hispanic or latino population in the US (Current ACS). Retrieved on April 21, 2023 from Hispanic or Latino Population in the US (Current ACS) - Overview (arcgis.com)

U.S. Census Bureau. (2021a). *The Hispanic population in the United States: 2021. Table 22.* Retrieved on April 20, 2023 from: The Hispanic Population in the United States: 2021 (census.gov)

U.S. Census Bureau. (2021b). *The Hispanic population in the United States: 2021. Table 6.* Retrieved on April 20, 2023 from: The Hispanic Population in the United States: 2021 (census.gov)

U.S. Census Bureau. (2021c). *The Hispanic population in the United States: 2021. Table 28.* Retrieved on April 20, 2023 from: The Hispanic Population in the United States: 2021 (census.gov)

U.S. Census Bureau. (2022b). *Current Population Survey, Annual Social and Economic Supplement, 2022.*

U.S. Census Bureau. (2022a). Community Resilience Estimates. CRE Interactive Tool. Retrieved on April 19, 2024, from Community Resilience Estimates (census.gov)

U.S. Department of Agriculture, Economic Research Service. (n.d.-a). U.S. poverty rates in metro and nonmetro areas, 1962–2022. Retrieved 2/15/2023 from: USDA ERS - Chart Detail

U.S. Department of Agriculture, Economic Research Service. (n.d.-b). Overview. Retrieved on February 15, 2023, from ttps://primary.ers.usda.gov/topics/rural-economy-population/rural-classifications.aspx#:~:text=ERS%20researchers%20and%20others%20who%20analyze%20conditions%20in,track%20and%20explain%20regional%20population%20and%20economic%20trends.

U.S. Department of Agriculture, Economic Research Service. (n.d.-c). Persistent poverty counties and census tracts, 2015–19. Accessed on February 13, 2023 from persistentcountytracts.png (6248×5669) (usda.gov)

U.S. Department of Agriculture, Economic Research Service. (2022a). *Descriptions and maps.* https://www.ers.usda.gov/data-products/poverty-area-measures/descriptions-and-maps/ Retrieved 2/15/2023

U.S. Department of Agriculture, Economic Research Service. (2022b). *Poverty area measures.* www.ers.usda.gov/data-products/poverty-area-measures

U.S. Department of Agriculture, Economic Research Service. (2023). *Definitions of food security.* https://www.ers.usda.gov/topics/food-nutrition-assistance/food-security-in-the-u-s/definitions-of-food-security/#:~:text=Food%20insecurity—the%20condition%20assessed,may%20result%20from%20food%20insecurity.

U.S. Department of Housing and Urban Development. (2020). *The 2020 Annual Homeless Assessment (AHAR) Report to Congress.* https://www.huduser.gov/portal/sites/default/files/pdf/2020-AHAR-Part-1.pdf

U.S. Department of Labor. (2022). *Earnings and earnings ratios by sex, race and occupation group.* www.dol.gov/agencies/wb/data/earnings/wage-gap-race-occupation

U.S. Department of Labor. Women's Bureau. (n.d.-a). *Women's earnings by race, ethnicity, and educational attainment as a percentage of White men's earnings (annual).* Accessed April 23, 2024 from Women's earnings by race, ethnicity, and educational attainment as a percentage of White men's earnings (annual) | U.S. Department of Labor (dol.gov)

U.S. Department of Labor. Women's Bureau. (n.d.-b*). Gender earnings ratio and wage gap by race and Hispanic ethnicity.* Accessed April 23, 2024 from Gender earnings ratio and wage gap by race and Hispanic ethnicity | U.S. Department of Labor (dol.gov)

U.S. Department of Labor Statistics (2023a, January). Labor force characteristics by race and ethnicity, 2021. BLS Reports, Report 1100. Retrieved April 10, 2023 from Labor force characteristics by race and ethnicity, 2021 : BLS Reports: U.S. Bureau of Labor Statistics

U.S. Department of Labor Statistics (2023b, March). Highlights of women's earnings in 2021. Table13. BLS Reports, Report 1102. Retrieved April 10, 2023, from https://www.bls.gov/opub/reports/womens-earnings/2021/home.htm

U.S. Environmental Protection Agency. (n.d.). *Environmental justice*. Retrieved April 11, 2023, from https://www.epa.gov/environmentaljustice

Vargas, E. D., Sanchez, G. R., & Juárez, M. (2017). Fear by association: perceptions of anti-immigrant policy and health outcomes. *Journal of Health Politics, Policy and Law, 42*(3), 459–483.

Vargas Bustamante, A., Fang, H., Rizzo, J. A., & Ortega, A. N. (2009). Understanding observed and unobserved health care access and utilization disparities among U.S. Latino adults. *Medical Care Research and Review*, 66(5), 561–577. https://doi.org/10.1177/1077558709338487

Villegas, A. M., & Lucas, T. (2002). Preparing culturally responsive teachers: Rethinking the curriculum. *Journal of Teacher Education, 53*(1), 20–32.

Wagstaff, A. (2002). Poverty and health sector inequalities. *Bulletin of the World Health Organization, 80*, 97- 105.

Welton, T.A. (2022, October). *More than a quarter of people who live in counties along the U.S. southern border are considered high-risk.* Retrieved April 20, 2024, from https://www.census.gov/library/stories/2022/10/how-resilient-are-communities-along-border.html

World Economic Forum. (2023). *Global gender gap report.* https://www.weforum.org/publications/global-gender-gap-report-2023/

World Health Organization. (n.d.). *Social determinants of health.* Retrieved April 19, 2024 from Social determinants of health (who.int)

World Population Review. (n.d.-a). *U.S. literacy rates by state.* Retrieved August 22, 2022, from https://worldpopulationreview.com/state-rankings/us-literacy-rates-by-state?123

World Population Review. (n.d.-b). Hispanic population by state 2024. Retrieved on August 22, 2024 from Hispanic Population by State 2024 (worldpopulationreview.com)

Xiao, H., McCurdy, S. A., Stoecklin-Marois, M. T., Li, C. S., & Schenker, M. B. (2013). Agricultural work and chronic musculoskeletal pain among Latino farm workers: The MICASA study. *American Journal of Industrial Medicine, 56*(2), 216–225.

Zheng, J., Liu, S., Peng, J., Peng, H., Wang, Z., Deng, Z., ... & Ran, P. (2022). Traffic-related air pollution is a risk factor in the development of chronic obstructive pulmonary disease. *Frontiers in Public Health, 10*, 1036192.

Zimmermann, B., & Seiler, S. (2019). The relationship between educational pathways and occupational outcomes at the intersection of gender and social origin. *Social Inclusion*, 7(3), 79–94.

Figure Credits

Fig. 3.19: Economic Research Service U.S. Department of Agriculture, "Persistent Poverty Counties and Census Tracts, 2015-2019," https://www.ers.usda.gov/data-products/chart-gallery/gallery/chart-detail/?chartId=105109, 2019.

Fig. 3.20: Economic Research Service U.S. Department of Agriculture, "Enduring Poverty, 2015-2019, US," https://www.ers.usda.gov/data-products/poverty-area-measures/descriptions-and-maps/, 2019

Fig. 3.21: Economic Research Service U.S. Department of Agriculture, "High and Extreme Poverty Census Tracts," https://www.ers.usda.gov/data-products/poverty-area-measures/descriptions-and-maps/, 2019.

Fig. 3.22: John R. Logan and Brian Stults, "Percent Latino Population: Segregation Persists," The Persistence of Segregation in the Metropolis: New Findings from the 2020 Census. Copyright © 2021 by Brown University.

Fig. 3.23: Adapted from A. Nellis, "Latino-White Incarceration Rate Ratios," The Color of Justice: Racial and Ethnic Disparity in State Prisons. Copyright © 2021 by The Sentencing Project.

Fig. 3.23a: Copyright © 2016 Depositphotos/pyty.

Fig. 3.24: U.S. Census Bureau, "The US-Mexico Border Region," https://www.census.gov/library/stories/2022/10/how-resilient-are-communities-along-border.html, 2022.

Fig. 3.30: U.S. Census Bureau, "CRE Risk Index for Residents in U.S. Border Counties: 2019 (in percent)," How Resilient are Communities along the US-Mexico Border? https://www.census.gov/library/stories/2022/10/how-resilient-are-communities-along-border.html, 2022.

Fig. 3.31: U.S. Census Bureau, "CRE Risk Index for Border, Non-Border Residents in Four Border States," https://www.census.gov/library/stories/2022/10/how-resilient-are-communities-along-border.html, 2019.

CHAPTER 4

Cultural Determinants of Health Among Mexican Americans

LEARNING OBJECTIVES

- Define and operationalize cultural determinants of health among Latinos.
- Describe the historical origins of Latino cultural health beliefs and their cultural continuity to the present.
- Assess the influences of Latino cultural values in help-seeking behaviors, patient–provider interactions, and risk reduction interventions.
- Compare and contrast differences in the meaning of cultural competency and cultural humility.
- Assess the Mexican American folk healing system of *curanderismo* and its potential application in today's society.
- Describe several common Mexican American folk illnesses.
- Explain the Latino familial context and cultural transmission of traditional gender roles and cultural expectations to children.
- Synthesize the dynamic interplay between acculturation, cognitive referents of acculturation, and acculturative stress.
- Assess the concept of Latino cultural resiliency and Latino cultural wealth in mediating the effects of social and cultural stressors.

The *cultural determinants of health* are those factors that coalesce to provide meaning to and a remedy for physical and mental health symptoms. Like social determinants, cultural determinants of health are intersecting and complementary domains. Cultural values and beliefs about health are formed within the familial context, as are expected gender roles. Acculturation level, or the extent of assimilation into the dominant culture, influences the degree to which one continues to endorse traditional cultural values and beliefs (see Figure 4.1).

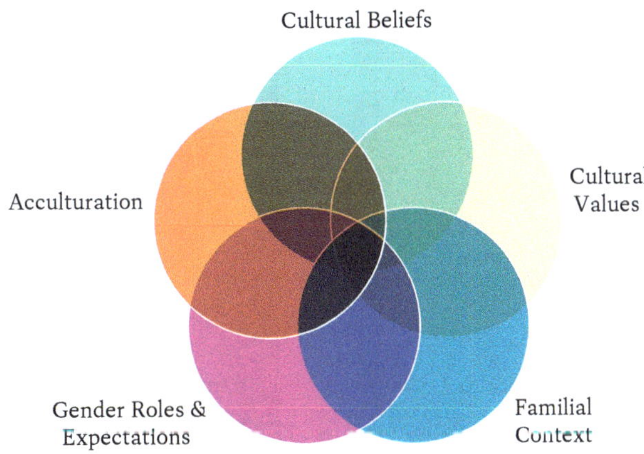

FIGURE 4.1 Cultural Determinants of Health

One's cultural upbringing shapes one's values, beliefs, perceptions, and behaviors. It also influences how one feels about, manifests, and treats health, illness, and physical and psychological challenges. Symbolically, culture is exemplified in one's language preference (i.e., English, Spanish, Spanglish), communication style, social interactions, and physical adornment. Essentially, culture shapes our worldview and perspectives of one another and our social interactions.

Culture can be thought of as lying on continuum, from more to less traditional, along which people move throughout their lives, and interpersonal and group experiences over a lifetime contribute to movement along this cultural continuum. Culture does not include socioeconomic conditions like poverty or educational attainment that cut across all cultures. Rather, culture is a synthesis of cognition, behavior, and feelings about traditional ways of living that are influenced by socioenvironmental conditions. Alternatively, culture can be conceived as a multidimensional construct including language, customs, norms, beliefs, behaviors, and personal space, among others.

Latino health beliefs are a synthesis of Mesoamerican and Spanish worldviews regarding the well-being of the individual, family, and community. Integrating the physical, mental, and spiritual aspects of personal experiences contributes to the concept of "being healthy" (Ailinger & Causey, 1995). Also, the intertwining of mind, body, and spirit provides a holistic approach to disease etiology and treatment.

Latino Cultural Health Beliefs and Values

Our personal understanding of what causes disease comes from our families, social media, educational institutions, and friends, which are also within a cultural context. In today's world, one can obtain accurate (and inaccurate) information on almost any medical condition and assorted symptoms through the internet (e.g., WebMD). However, prior to having information readily available, one relied on the oral transmission of treatments and cures for specific types of "folk" ailments. The Mesoamerican origin of traditional cultural health beliefs and values among Latinos of Mexican descent is deeply rooted in the cultural beliefs and practices of the Mexica. As with many Indigenous cultures, the Mexica believed that health was holistic and that states of health were closely related to a condition of equilibrium or disequilibrium. For good health, one had to be in balance physically, socially, and spiritually (Ortiz de Montellano, 1990).

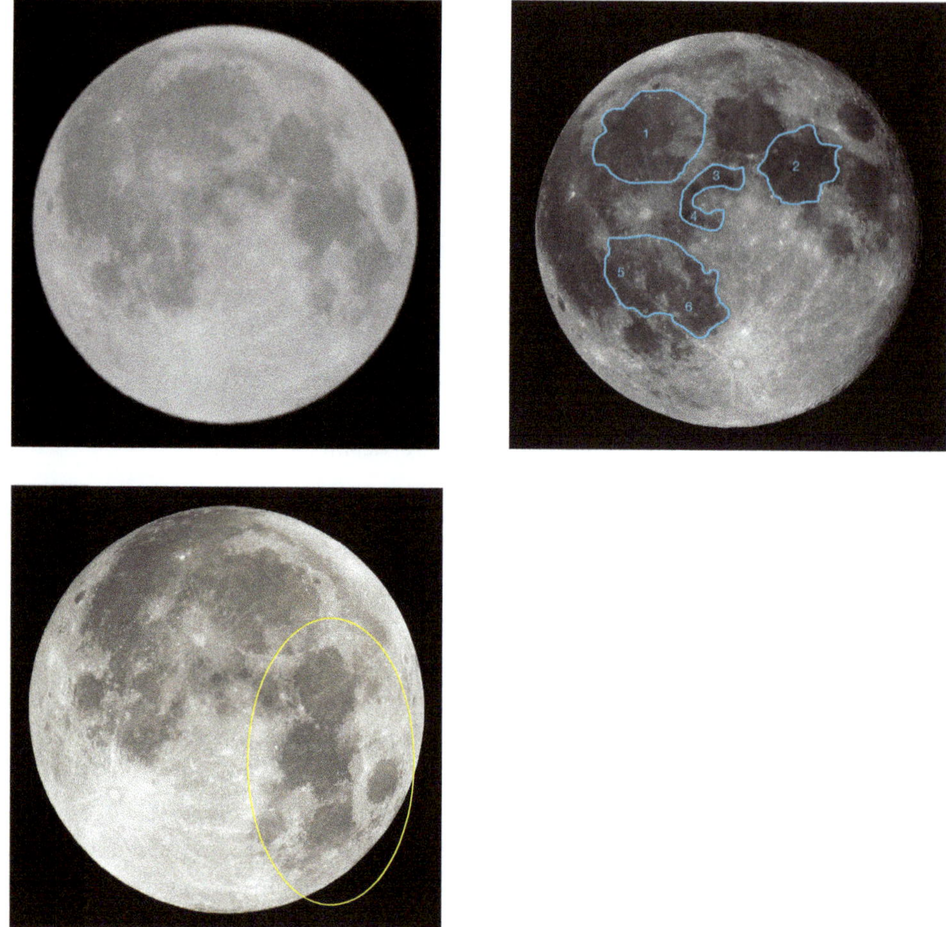

FIGURE 4.2 Rabbit (top left) and Frog (lower left) in the Moon

Culture shapes our worldview and vice versa. For example, what do you see when you look at the full moon? Some western cultures see "the man in the moon." Other cultures see a frog, and still others see a rabbit (see Figure 4.2).

I have told a story that resonates with my classes that was originally discussed by Ortiz de Montellano (1990, pp. 142–143) and associated with lunar eclipses. Pregnant Mexica women would wear an amulet or knife made of obsidian to ward off the negative influences of a lunar eclipse on the developing fetus. They believed that through magical causation, if they were exposed to a lunar eclipse without protection, their baby would be born with a cleft lip. According to Ortiz de Montellano (1990), this belief is derived from the Mexica creation myth, which tells how the face of a rabbit was imprinted on the moon. The Mexica name for a lunar eclipse conveys how the crescent moon is "bitten" via the eclipse, resulting in "bites" taken from the developing fetus's lips (*tenqualo*, "the eating of the lips") (see Figure 4.3).

Today, many pregnant Latinas wear a key or metal to ward off the negative influence of a lunar eclipse. Remarkably, this story has been passed down from generation to generation for over 500 years! This is just one of several examples of how oral transmission of folk beliefs sustains cultural continuity over time.

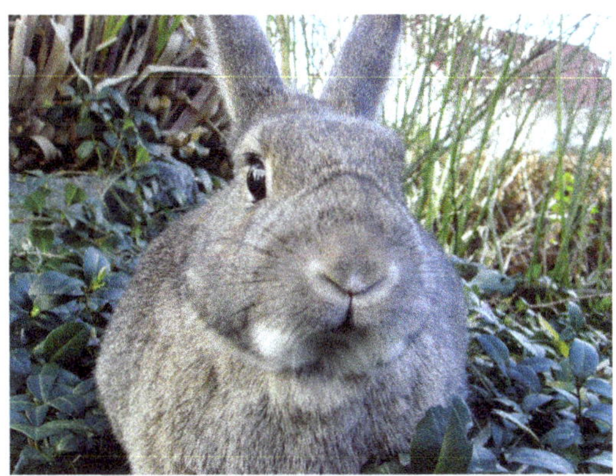

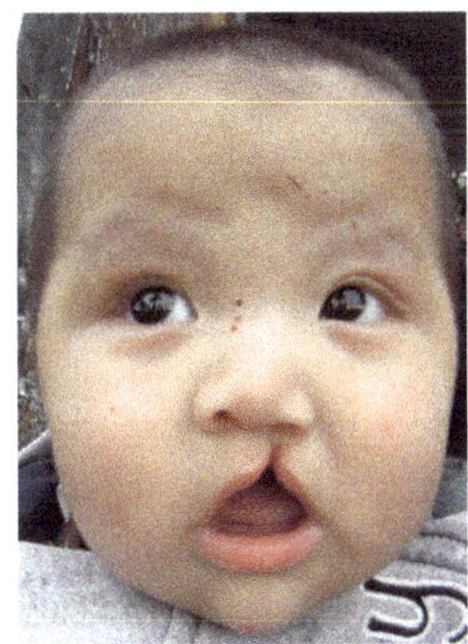

FIGURE 4.3 "Hare" Lip of Rabbit

Preconquest Mexica Health Beliefs

Two historical documents are the foundation of our knowledge regarding Mexica medicine: the Badianus Codex and the Sahagun Codices (Guerra, 1966). The Badianus Codex is sourced to Martin de la Cruz, an Indian physician who wrote about Mexica medicine just after the conquest. The Sahagun Codices, commonly known as the Florentine Codex, are a group of manuscripts on the Mexica written by the Franciscan friar Bernardino de Sahagun (1499–1590), who arrived in Mexico 8 years after the Spanish conquest (1529). According to Guerra (1966), both historical sources are believed to be definitive descriptions of Mexica health beliefs and practices at the time of Spanish contact (or soon thereafter) from the Mexica informants themselves. The codices explain that illness could be the result of natural, supernatural, or magical phenomenon (Ortiz de Montellano, 1990).

According to historical accounts, there were both male and female physicians (*ticitl*) in Mexica society who provided treatments and cures for supernatural and natural causation of disease.

As quoted in Guerra (1966):

> The physician ticitl is a curer of people, a restorer and provider of health. A good physician is a diagnostician, experienced and well versed in the virtues of herbs, stones, trees and roots. He is moderate in his acts, cures people by setting bones, providing splints, knows how to purge and to give emetics and potions, he knows how to bleed, he stitches wounds, makes incisions and revives the sick. A bad physician is a fraud, a half-hearted worker, unskilled, a killer with his medicines because of over dosage, he worsens the condition of the sick, endangers others' lives, he pretends to be a counsellor, adviser and chaste. He bewitches, is a sorcerer, a soothsayer, a caster of lots, he seduces women and bewitches them.
>
> A woman physician is knowledgeable in herbs, roots, trees and stones; she has experience in them. She can make prognoses and can be trusted because of her professional skill. The good woman physician restores and provides health, revives and relaxes, makes people feel well, covers one with ashes. She can cure people, she lances them, bleeds them in various places with the lancet. She gives potions, purges and medicines. (pp. 321–322)

According to these historical accounts, "good" Mexica physicians possessed diagnostic and treatment knowledge that could cure disease and had a positive ethical approach to their patients. Bad physicians were frauds and endangered others' lives with their quackery.

The Mexica also believed that disease was a punishment from the gods for committing a sin. Guerra (1966) states that "a close relationship existed between a god and a specific type of disease as far as cause and treatment were concerned" (p. 320). The Mexica also believed that disease could be the result of enemies, witchcraft, and natural causation—but only in certain circumstances. The process of making a diagnosis among the Mexica included the professional gift in identifying the pathological syndrome of the patient together with the supernatural influences affecting their case. The latter was the result of the religious concept of disease and therefore involved practices related to one's horoscope and religious ceremonies alongside sound medical discovery. Pre-Columbian codices portray a human figure showing the influence of certain signs upon specific parts of the body (see Figure 4.4).

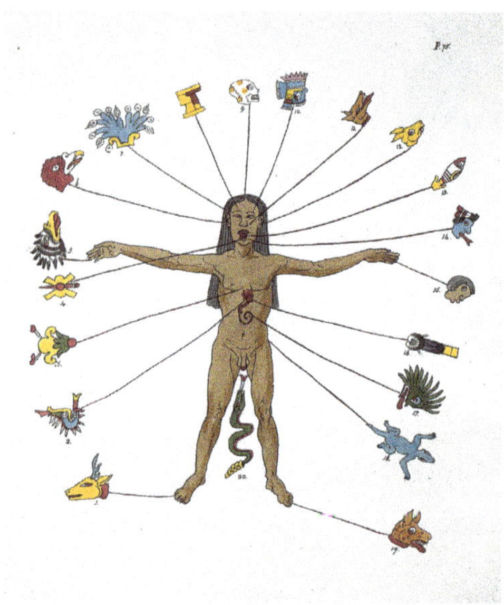

FIGURE 4.4 Horoscope Signs and Their Bodily Influences

The Mexica medical arts were called *ticiotl* and included knowledge of herbs and plants that could heal or kill the individual. Physicians either applied treatments with medicinal herbs and plants (*tepatiani*) or used religious ceremonies, horoscopes, predictions, and "secret" ingredients to achieve a cure (*nahualli*). Moreover, a steam bathhouse (*temazcalli*) was used as a frequent therapeutic procedure combining bodily cleanliness with spiritual purification. According to Guerra (1966), "The extent of anatomical and botanical nomenclature, professional ethics, some sound clinical observations, and the importance given to psychological factors in the genesis and treatment of disease were outstanding in the Aztec culture" (p. 334).

Two health belief systems continue to influence the health of Latinos of Mexican descent. The basis for healing derived from both "hot-cold" syndromes and "wet-dry" beliefs regarding illnesses and their associated treatments (Currier, 1966; Foster, 1953, 1987; Messer, 1987). Indigenous healing beliefs merged with Spanish beliefs in Greek humoral theory that was believed to regulate bodily functions—what scholars refer to as *syncretism*, or the synthesis of cultural health beliefs (Messer, 1987). In this system, "adoption and adaptation are made selectively from incoming systems; where essential indigenous elements may be reinforced and modified by the incoming elements, but where basic structures, objectives, and characteristics of the indigenous remain identifiable and a continuity is achieved" (Colson & de Armellado, 1983, p. 1229).

The bodily fluids, or four humors, and associated wet/dry/cold/hot concepts are blood (hot and wet), yellow bile (hot and dry), black bile (cold and dry) and phlegm (cold and wet). Healing involves correcting imbalances by the addition or subtraction of heat, cold, dryness, or wetness by a folk practitioner because any imbalance of these four humors could cause disease (Currier, 1966; Lopez Austin, 1980; Messer, 1987). Among the Mexica the hot-cold system included states of health and illness, types of foods, and types of medicines, as well as cosmological beliefs (Messer, 1987). A duality system of corresponding opposites was widespread among the Mexica, and they were usually conceptualized as lying on a continuum and acted as guides to the use of medicinal herbs and plants (Foster, 1987; García-Hernández et al., 2021) (see Table 4.1).

A study by García-Hernández et al. (2021) found that climate of the region appears to influence the hot-cold system of Mexican traditional medicine, with temperate areas exhibiting more cold illnesses treated with hot medicinal plants and warm-tropical areas having more hot illnesses treated with cold medicinal plants (see Figure 4.5). The historical importance of Mexica health beliefs has a cultural continuity with modern day folk systems of healing: *curanderismo.*

TABLE 4.1 Mexican Duality System of Beliefs

Father	Mother
Heavens	Earth
Shining	Dark
Fire	Water
Hot	Cold
Wet	Dry

Source: Messer (1987)

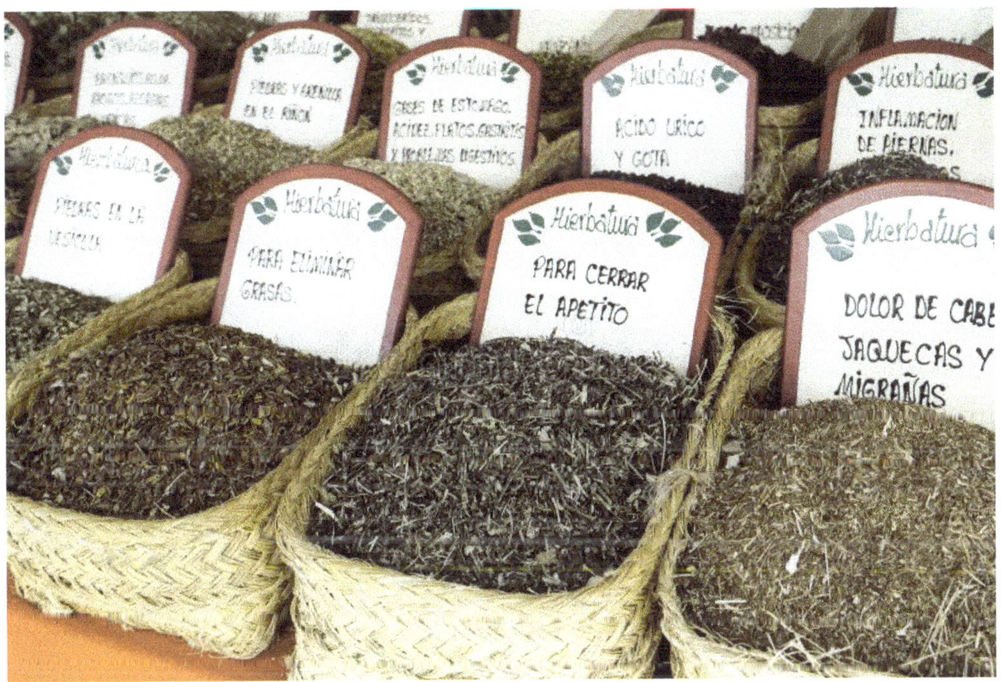

FIGURE 4.5 Mexican Medicinal Herbs

Also of importance to the Mexica was the belief in multiple souls or animistic forces (Ortiz de Montellano, 1990, pp. 55–67). The health of a person depended on the relative amounts of each soul at a given time and, on the maintenance, and balance among them. The three souls are *tonalli, teyolia,* and *ihiyotl. Tonalli* was believed to reside in the head. It provided a vital hot force. Tonalli gave a person bravery, vigor, warmth, and made growth possible. Involuntary loss of tonalli caused illness and death. *Teyolia* was believed to be in the heart. It imparted vitality, knowledge, and vocational ability. The heart was believed to be the center of thought and personality, involved in will, memory, emotion, and mental activity. *Ihiyotl* was believed to be in the liver. It gave people vigor, passion, and feelings such as desire, envy, and anger. Sins, particularly of a sexual nature, were believed to harm the liver and made it emit ihiyotl involuntarily, which could harm others.

Curanderismo—Mexican American Folk Medicine

Curanderismo is a term used to describe the entire Mexican and Mexican American folk health belief system (de la Torre & Estrada, 2015; Maduro, 1983). It involves a coherent worldview of healing that has deep historical roots. Modern curanderismo is syncretic, holistic, and eclectic. It is a synthesis of beliefs derived from Indigenous and Spanish beliefs, spiritualism, and modern biomedicine. There are eight major philosophical principles that underlie the health explanatory model of curanderismo (Arizaga, 1999; Maduro, 1983; Ortiz de Montellano, 1990):

- Strong emotional states, such as rage, fear, envy, or mourning, may cause disease (e.g., *muina,* derived from the Mexica belief in ihiyotl).
- Being out of balance and harmony with one's environment may cause disease (e.g., *empacho,* derived from both Mexica and Spanish beliefs).
- A patient is often seen as the victim of malevolent forces (e.g., *mal de ojo,* derived from both Mexica and Spanish beliefs).
- The soul may become separated from the body (e.g., *susto,* derived from the Mexica belief in tonalli).
- Cure requires the participation of the entire family (*familismo*).
- The natural world is not always distinguishable from the supernatural.
- Sickness often serves a social function through increased attention and rallying of the family around the patient and reestablishing a sense of belonging (resocialization).
- Latinos respond better to an open interaction with their healer (*personalismo*).

In *curanderismo,* the cause of the disease usually dictates its treatment. For example, if the disease is believed to be due to supernatural causes, then the required treatment would be prayer and placation. If the cause is believed to be magical, then the treatment is counter-magic. If the cause is natural, then the required treatment is physical measures (Abril, 1977; Maduro, 1983; Ortiz de Montellano, 1990).

Mexican American folk healers *(curanderos)* become so due to a "calling" or "gift" (*el don*) from God that one receives as a youth or as an adult. Apprenticeships to curanderos are also a method of learning how to diagnose and treat folk illnesses and symptoms. These apprenticeships can last for 20 years or more to become knowledgeable on how to "call the spirits" from the herbs and plants used to obtain a cure. *Curanderos* possess three levels of knowledge: the material, spiritual, and mental (Arizaga, 1999). The *material level* includes the appropriate use of herbs, eggs, water, candles, cupping, and animal products in making a diagnosis and treatment of Mexican American folk illnesses. The *spiritual level* includes knowledge on how to contact spirits by using crystal spheres, smudging, trances, and channeling as a spiritual medium. The *mental level* includes channeling positive thoughts to the patient and discussing stressful or anxiety-producing circumstances. This could also include the use of *barridas* or sweeping the body with herbs to cleanse the spirits from the body.

Other folk healers are also found in the Mexican American community (Arizaga, 1999). These include *sobadoras* (massage therapists), *senoras/abuelas* who foretell the future by reading cards, *yerberas* or herbalists who are trained in the use of medicinal herbs and plants, and *pateras* or midwives who are especially valuable in providing delivery and childcare services. Those whose conditions cannot be treated by a *senora/abuela* are usually referred to a *yerbero* (herbalist), *sobador* (massage therapist), or *partera* (midwife, who also treats problems with young children). If these specialists cannot handle the problem, the patient is referred to a *curandero* who may use multiple treatment modalities to treat the folk illness. Most *curanderos* know what they cannot handle and will refer severe health problems to the medical profession. Oftentimes, a patient will employ both biomedical and folk treatments to cure disease. Common Mexican American folk illnesses for which curanderos are sought include:

- *Mal de ojo* (evil eye): Young children are most susceptible, but all ages may suffer from *ojo*, which is thought to occur when a person with a "powerful" gaze glances or looks admiringly at a child without touching them. Symptoms include sudden onset of high fever, vomiting, headache, fainting, and sometimes convulsions. The diagnosis of *ojo* is made by consideration of the patient's symptoms and an examination of a fresh egg broken after being passed over the patient's body. A positive diagnosis is made when the egg appears cooked, or the yolk appears to have the image of an eye. The most effective treatment is to have the perpetrator touch the patient as soon as possible. When that is not an option, an alternative treatment is as follows: A fresh egg is passed over the patients' body; the egg is broken into a bowl/glass of water and covered by a cross of palm or straw and put under the head of the patient's bed; the patient is then put to bed for the night; and in the morning the egg is examined; if it is curdled, then that indicates that the *ojo* is cured and the egg is then disposed of.
- *Susto* (magical fright): This is a folk illness with strong psychological overtones, defined as a "fright sickness" and (literally) a loss of soul from the body. A more severe and potentially fatal form is called *espanto*. Susto is caused by a sudden frightening experience, such as an accident, a fall, witnessing a sudden death (especially a relative), or any other potentially dangerous event. Symptoms include nervousness, anorexia, insomnia, listlessness, despondency, involuntary muscle tics, and diarrhea. A diagnosis of susto is made by the associated symptoms and the history of a traumatic event. Treatment of susto includes oral remedies such as teas of orange blossom, Brazil wood, or cannabis. The most effective treatment is a ceremony known as a *barrida*, or "sweeping." Usually, a single barrida is not enough and is repeated every third day until the patient is healed (Rubel et al., 1991; Weller et al., 2008).
- *Empacho*: It literally means impacted stomach and mostly occurs with young children. *Empacho* is caused by adherence of soft food and difficult-to-digest substances to the stomach wall. Symptoms

include bloating, constipation, lethargy, anorexia, stomachache, vomiting, pain with diarrhea, and generalized abdominal fullness. A diagnosis of empacho is made by noting symptoms and checking for abdominal tenderness, feeling knots in the calves, and/or rolling a fresh chicken egg over the abdomen. *Empacho* is confirmed if the egg appears to stick to a particular area. Remedies include rubbing the stomach or back, cupping of the skin, and purgative teas of wormwood or chamomile. Lead (*azarcon*) or mercury (*greta*) powders are still occasionally given, which are extremely dangerous and should be avoided (Baer & Ackerman, 1988; Centers for Disease Control and Prevention, 1993; Flattery et al., 1994; Trotter, 1985).

- *Caida de mollera* (fallen fontanel) (see Figure 4.6). The actual etiology may be any severe illness resulting in a 10% loss of body weight in an infant such as bacterial or viral dysentery, meningitis, or sepsis. Etiology is believed to be mechanical in origin: the fontanel being pulled down by the soft palate when the nipple is pulled too suddenly out of the infant's mouth or by a sudden jolt, bump, or fall. Symptoms of *caida* include dehydration, crying, inability to achieve sufficient suction while nursing, fever, and diarrhea. *Caida* is diagnosed by noting the symptoms and observing the "sunken" appearance of the fontanel. Folk treatments are based on the mechanical nature of the illness and include pressing upward on the soft palate with thumbs or fingers, sucking the anterior fontanel, or holding the baby upside down over water with or without shaking or hitting the feet—all of which can prove dangerous and should not be performed! Other folk treatments include poultices that are applied to the fontanel with raw egg, oil, or liniment, and the hair is pulled up (so that the roots will raise the skin back up). This is the most challenging and potentially fatal pediatric folk illness because of the severe dehydration that accompanies it (Kay, 1993; Trotter et al., 1989).

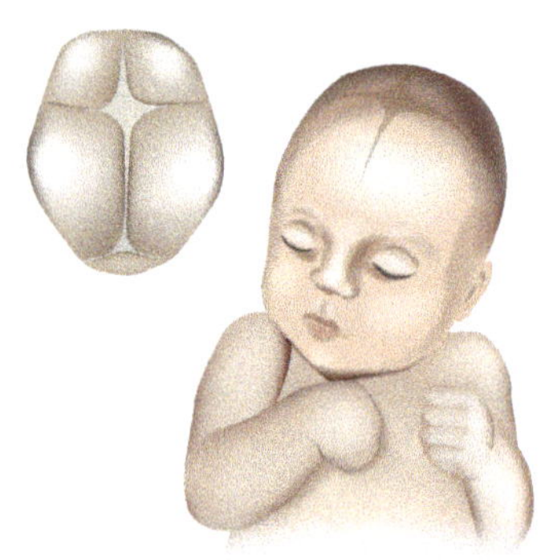

FIGURE 4.6 *Caida de Mollera* (Fallen Fontanelle)

Mexican American Cultural Values and Beliefs

Latinos of Mexican descent possess many traditional cultural values and beliefs that assist in framing interpersonal interactions (interfaces) with specific others in the social environment (Table 4.2). However, as one acculturates to non-Latino mainstream culture, some of these traditional cultural values and beliefs are lost or diminished (Padilla & Perez, 2003). As mentioned in our previous discussion of the Latino family, women are the primary source of cultural transmission to their children. Latino fathers and mothers play important roles in the socialization of gender roles as well, especially in the cultural scripts of *machismo* and *marianismo*.

For help-seeking behaviors, several Latino cultural values are important to consider (Cuellar et al., 1995a). Given the importance of family in Latino culture, *familismo*, or familism, are very important cultural values. Help-seeking is first sought within the family. Also, with chronic disease interventions like hypertension, diabetes, cancer, and heart disease, it is important to include the family of the individual. Alternatively, seeking assistance from the family first can delay medical attention (Lantz et al., 1994).

As with familism, many Latinos place a high value on *respeto*, a cultural value that frames or guides social interactions. It includes proper and differential behavior toward others as determined by their gender, social status, and especially age. For example, older Latino adults expect *respeto* from those who are younger. It is also important to use formal Spanish when interacting with older Latino adults or authority figures.

Fatalismo, or fatalism, is the belief that health and illness are up to the will of God and can determine whether a Latino goes to a physician in order to get well. The extent of fatalistic beliefs varies with acculturation level and perceived severity of the disease, especially diseases like cancer (Gallo et al., 2009; Perez-Stable et al., 1992; Ramirez, 2014; Ramirez et al., 2013).

The cultural scripts of *machismo* and *marianismo* may hinder help-seeking behaviors, and within chronic disease interventions they may influence whether risk reduction practices are adopted (Gallo et al., 2009). For more traditionally oriented Latinas, *marianismo* manifests in prioritizing others' needs above their own, which could affect delays in their own health care. Similarly, *machismo* for Latino males may mean delaying needed medical attention until symptoms become worse, fostering delays in diagnosis and treatment.

TABLE 4.2 Mexican American Cultural Values and Interfaces

	Interfaces		
Cultural values and beliefs	**Help-seeking behaviors**	**Patient–provider interactions**	**Risk reduction interventions**
Fatalismo: the belief that life events are up to the will of God.	x	x	x
Familism: the central importance of the family.	x	x	x
Spirituality/religiosity: the value of spirituality or religion in one's life.	x	x	x
Orgullo: a sense of pride.	x	x	x
Machismo: often seen as a male's prerogative.	x	x	x
Marianismo: exhibiting values and behaviors consistent with prescribed female gender roles.	x	x	x
Carino: demonstrating affection and caring.		x	x
Respeto: demonstrating respect for family structures and elders.		x	x

(*continued*)

TABLE 4.2 ***(continued)***

Cultural values and beliefs	Interfaces		
	Help-seeking behaviors	**Patient–provider interactions**	**Risk reduction interventions**
Dignidad: treating others with respect and dignity, especially elders.		x	x
Personalismo: exhibiting a personal rather than impersonal interaction with another person.		x	x
Confianza: demonstrating confidence and trust in another person.	x	x	x
Simpatia: nonconfrontational social interactions.	x	x	x
Cultural identity/ethnic pride: pride in ones' cultural or ethnic identification.			x
Communicacion: the way Latinos communicate with one another, including nonverbal cues, eye contact, and personal space.	x	x	x

Latino ethnic pride, Latino cultural identity, and positive aspects of orgullo can moderate the effects of acculturative stress and reduce depressive symptomatology (Jones et al., 2022; Kim et al., 2021; Mossakowski, 2003). Ethnic pride is an element of *ethnic identity,* which refers to an individual's self-concept comprised of a sense of belonging to a group, ethnic involvement with that group, and in-group positive attitudes (Phinney, 1996).

Simpatia is a term that denotes politeness and pleasantness and the avoidance of confrontation. Social interactions are guided by simpatia, and there is a reciprocity attached: One should receive as well as give simpatia. Similarly, *carino, dignidad, personalismo, confianza,* and *communicacion* are Latino cultural values that facilitate social interactions and personal space (Gallo et al., 2009a; Marin & Marin, 1991).

Latino cultural health beliefs serve many functions, including the etiology and potential source/cause of a disease, how the disease is defined or categorized, which remedies one will adhere to, and the use of traditional or biomedical treatments. They also serve the function of resocializing the individual to their family.

Latinos also see the Spanish language as a cultural value. According to the Pew Research Center (2021), 68% of Latinos speak Spanish at home, but that percentage decreases with each subsequent generation of Latinos born in the United States. Nevertheless, even with experiencing language discrimination for speaking Spanish, the language still conveys meaning and a sense of worth. There is a large body of research on language concordance and the use of Spanish translators and interpreters, with many

Spanish-speaking patients preferring bilingual providers (Diamond et al., 2019; Hsueh et al., 2021; Kanter et al., 2009; Villalobos et al., 2016).

Several studies (Diamond et al., 2019; Fernandez et al., 2011; Timmins, 2002; Jacobs et al., 2005; Parker et al., 2017; Portillo et al., 2021; Fox et al., 2020) have found that limited English proficient (LEP) patients:

- Receive less information about therapeutic regimens
- Understand less of the instructions related to medication
- Are less likely to keep subsequent appointments
- Are more likely to make emergency department visits
- Are less likely to receive preventive services
- May receive misdiagnoses due to lack of communication
- May receive poorer medical care
- May be prescribed inappropriate medications
- May perceive less quality in the medical care received

Horror stories abound in the use of nontrained translators, such as the use of janitorial or custodial staff to translate information or the use of the patient's relatives or children to assist in communication. The pitfalls of using these individuals include a lack of knowledge regarding medical terminology, and violation of cultural values regarding age and gender, and the use of strangers (*respeto* and *confianza*).

A study by González et al. (2010) showed that language congruence between physician and patient led to (a) a lower likelihood of confusion regarding medications and treatment; (b) less frustration in understanding; and (c) lower language-related poor-quality ratings and was positively associated with patient-reported higher quality of care.

Acculturation level is known to alter these traditional Latino cultural values and beliefs. Within Latino families, variation in acculturation level leads to familial conflict between parents and children (Dennis et al., 2010). In the following discussion, it is important to consider how these cultural values and beliefs form the basis of Cuellar's cognitive referents of acculturation because of their influences on affect, behaviors, and cognition, also known as the "ABCs of acculturation" (Cuellar et al., 1995a; Masgoret & Ward, 2006; Ward & Kagitcibasi, 2010).

The Culture of Western Medicine

The culture of Western medicine has deep historical roots in Galenic medicine and Roman philosophies of health and wellness. It wasn't until the Renaissance when Eastern knowledge and medical treatments were disseminated throughout Europe.

The primary focus of Western medicine is on pathology and curing disease using state-of-the-art techniques. Treatment should produce measurable positive outcomes in disease pathology. Medical practice is based on scientific theory and reductionism, and intervention should result in cure or management of disease (Cohen, 2018). Cultural disconnectedness begins with perceptions of cause and treatment. Western biomedical concepts of health and disease can conflict with more traditional folk beliefs of ethnic medicine. However, I have found that most Latinos of Mexican descent who utilize curanderos also utilize clergy and physicians, making sure that all avenues of cure are explore—from Western biomedicine, to talking with clergy, or seeing a curandero.

The differences in approach are dependent on the expectations of what the provider can do and for which aspects the patient is responsible—that is, one's worldview of health and healing within a cultural context (see Table 4.3).

TABLE 4.3 Western Medicine and Ethnic Medicine Values

Western medicine	Ethnic medicine
Meliorism: Make things better.	Accept the disease with grace.
Dominance over nature: Take control of the disease.	Achieve balance/harmony with nature.
Activism: Do something/act.	Wait and see what happens.
Timeliness: Do something sooner rather than later.	Use cautious deliberation.
Therapeutic aggressiveness: Stronger is better.	Take a gentle approach.
Future orientation: Plan. Newer is better.	Take life as it comes: Use "time-honored" approaches.
Standardization: Treat everyone the same.	Individualize: Recognize individual differences.

Familial Context and Cultural Transmission of Gender Roles and Expectations

Latinos of Mexican descent tend to live near extended, multigenerational families. Family unity is a cultural strength among Latinos of Mexican descent, who assist one another through difficult times. However, Latino nuclear families are increasing among third generation and higher, but they typically live close to one another and remain involved in extended families through *tias* (aunts), *tios* (uncles), and *primos* (cousins).

Respeto (respect) is highly valued within Mexican American families and is exhibited through deference to elderly family members, especially for nanas (grandmothers). Latino children are given much attention, as parents, grandparents, and godparents (*compadres/commadres*) usually spend a lot of time with them as they grow up. All relatives from both sides, the father's, and the mother's, are considered part of the family.

Traditionally, religion has played an important role in binding the Latino family together, however, there has been a steady decline of those who identify as Roman Catholic, from 67% in 2010 to 43% in 2023 (Krogstad et al., 2023). Nevertheless, ceremonies like christenings, quinceañeras, weddings, and funerals help Latino families connect and celebrate important life milestones together. For example, festivals like Día de los Muertos (Day of the Dead) celebrate the life and death of family ancestors. Traditions connected with the holiday include building private altars honoring the deceased using sugar skulls, marigolds, and the favorite foods and beverages of the departed and visiting gravesites with these as gifts. In traditional Mexican American families, the *quinceañera* is one of the most beloved days in the life of a Mexican American girl, which is celebrated on her 15th birthday. It marks her passage from girlhood to womanhood and is a very emotional tradition, as the father dances with his daughter (Santana, 2007).

More traditionally oriented Mexican American families have gender-specific roles that are transmitted via the family. Traditional gender roles for Latinas include being a wife, a mother, the caretaker of the family and extended family, and the primary cultural and religious resource in guiding the children. Cultural expectations for Latinas include being passive, submissive, secondary to men, virginal, nurturing, and family-oriented (Marin & Marin, 1991). Traditional gender roles for Latinos including being a good father, financial support, and role model for male children. Cultural expectations are the opposite of Latinas, and a double standard exists in relation to the number of sexual partners (Fugère et al., 2008). Within the Latino family, there is differential treatment of Latina girls and Latino boys:

- Privileging of boys in families with both sons and daughters
- Different household responsibilities based on gender
- Double standard in dating and sexuality
- Enforcement of stereotypically feminine behavior

Two gendered Latino cultural scripts are important to consider: *machismo* and *marianismo* (de la Torre & Estrada, 2015; Gallo et al., 2009a; Quintero & Estrada, 1998). In Latino culture, the term "macho" usually must be distinguished from that of "machismo" (Mirandé, 2018). *Macho* has different meanings in different social circumstances. Sometimes it refers simply to the male of a species, whether animal or plant; In other cultural contexts "to be macho" can have contradictory connotations: For older generations this may refer to something positive for men to emulate, so that a macho man is one who is responsible for the financial welfare of his family, whereas for younger men to be macho can refer to culturally stigmatized behavior like beating one's partner. *Machismo* is characterized by hyper-virility, or aggressive masculine behavior expected of males in Latino culture. Machos embody physical strength, courage, self-confidence, heightened sexual power, and bold advances toward women. Machos believe in the superiority of men over women and adhere to conservative gender role expectations. For example, men can seek extramarital affairs, while women are expected to be faithful.

Marianismo was originally a term used to examine women's gender identities and relationships within the context of inequality, by developing a model based on a religious icon (María), the quintessential expression of submissiveness and spiritual authority (Gil & Vazquez, 2014; Stevens, 1973). *Marianismo* expects women to model themselves after the Virgin Mary (mother of Jesus) and to accept their roles as mothers and wives. This means women should be pure, humble, emotional, kind, compliant, vulnerable, unassertive, and enduring of suffering. Women should live in the shadow of their husbands and children and should support them continuously. This kind of attitude involves the expectation that women should tolerate certain behavior of men, such as their aggressiveness, sexual infidelity, arrogance, stubbornness, and callousness. The expectations that a woman should be an ideal wife and mother require her to be spiritually superior to men.

Latino Ethnic Identity and Gender Socialization

Umaña-Taylor's theoretical model of ethnic identity formation suggests that adolescents' ethnic identity develops because of an individual's interactions with proximal and distal environmental factors (Umaña-Taylor & Fine, 2004). Umaña-Taylor's model suggests that a central component of adolescents' ethnic identity formation is the influence that family members have via familial ethnic socialization practices. *Familial ethnic socialization* refers broadly to parents:

- Talking with their children about their ethnic culture
- Practicing cultural traditions with their children at home
- Teaching their children about the traditions, culture, history, and holidays that are associated with their ethnic background

Several studies indicate that Mexican-origin parents' teaching about Mexican culture and teaching their children to speak Spanish at home were both positively associated with their children's ethnic identification as of Mexican origin. Additional evidence on socialization in ethnic minority families indicates that parents often feel it is important to teach their children about their ethnicity, instill in them a sense of ethnic pride, make them comfortable with being from an ethnic minority background, and help protect them from the harmful effects of discrimination.

Research shows that there are certain aspects of Latino culture that are of prime importance to parents. For example, these aspects often include the importance of the family unit and extended family, respect for elders, the maintenance of the Spanish language, and traditional gender roles, such as *machismo* and *marianismo* (Calzada et al., 2010; Grau et al., 2009; Cauce & Domenech-Rodriguez, 2002; Umaña-Taylor & Updegraff, 2013).

Latino families also face the pressure of *biculturalism* or being comfortable both in the native culture of origin and in the host or mainstream culture. Research on Latino families suggests (Umaña-Taylor & Updegraff, 2013: Calzada et al., 2010; Grau et al., 2009):

- These values are critical for familial ethnic socialization.
- Latino children's ethnic identity is related to their background and to what parents teach them about their culture.
- These cultural values can affect Latino children's performance in school settings.
- Latino parents would make an explicit attempt to pass these values on to their children because they are culturally important.

Research on Latino families has also shown that parental ethnic socialization influences what their children will learn about their cultures (Bernal et al., 1990; Knight et al., 1993a, 1993b; Romero et al., 2000). Socialization of children differs as a function of parents' sociocultural characteristics, such as generational status of family members, acculturation level, ethnic identity, language, and the cultural knowledge possessed by Latino parents. Additionally, it is important to examine differences in adolescents' ethnic socialization experiences based on parents' gender. Mothers, rather than fathers, tend to be more actively involved in socializing and talking to their children about intellectual and emotional aspects of life.

Gallegos & Ferdman (2007) identified several "lenses" through which Latino youth develop ethnic identities, including social institutions like the family, educational system, peer groups, and U.S. racial and cultural perceptions (see Table 4.4). These orientations are (Gallegos & Ferdman, 2007, p. 31):

- *Latino integrated*: understanding of racial constructs and ability to challenge them.
- *Latino identified*: acceptance of the races Latino and White and identification with Latino.
- *Subgroup identified*: identification of multiple Latino races and identification with a regional subgroup.
- *Latino as other*: identification as a generic Latino due to mixed heritage.
- *Undifferentiated*: colorblindness, adherence to dominant culture, and tendency to attribute failure to the individual rather than racial constructs.
- *White identified*: acceptance of White and Latino races and identification with White and rejection of Latino.

TABLE 4.4 Latina and Latino Racial Identity Orientations

Identity orientation	Lens	Identify as/prefer	Latinos are seen as	Whites are seen as	Framing of face
Undifferentiated/ denial	Closed	People	"Who are Latinos?"	Supposedly color-blind (accept dominant norms)	Denial, irrelevant, invisible
White-identified	Tinted	White	Negatively	Very positively	White/Black, either/or, one-drop or *mejorar la raza* (i.e., "improve the race")
Latino as other	External	Not White	Generically, fuzzily	Negatively	White/not White
Subgroup identified	Narrow	Own subgroup	My group OK, others maybe	Not central (could be barriers or blockers)	Not clear or central; secondary to nationality, ethnicity, culture

(continued)

TABLE 4.4 *(continued)*

Identity orientation	Lens	Identify as/prefer	Latinos are seen as	Whites are seen as	Framing of face
Latino-identified (racial/*raza*)	Broad	Latinos	Very positively	Distinct; could be barriers or allies	Latino/not Latino
Latino-integrated	Wide	Individuals in a group context	Positively	Complex	Dynamic, contextual, socially constructed

Source: Gallegos and Ferdman (2007, p.31)

Depending on the cultural orientation of the individual, Latinos can be perceived negatively, positively, or neutrally. One can also see the concept of colorism included in the "White-identified" orientation. Ultimately, the Latino-integrated individual holds an open and positive attitude toward oneself and others.

Cultural Competence and Cultural Humility

The field of medicine has embraced the concept of cultural competence only recently. The American Medical Association (1999) defined *cultural competence* as "the ability of physicians to provide patient-centered care by adjusting their attitudes and behaviors to account for the impact of emotional, cultural, social, and psychological issues on the main biomedical ailment" (p. viii). The AMA describes cultural competence as the fifth competence to be acquired by American physicians (the others being cognitive knowledge, technical skills, appropriate behaviors, and managerial competence).

However, the field of nursing has a substantive history of cultural competence implementation and practice. For example, Purnell and Paulanka (1998) define cultural competence as:

- Developing an *awareness* of one's own beliefs, sensations, and thoughts without letting them have an undue influence on those from other cultural backgrounds
- Demonstrating *knowledge* and *understanding* of the client's culture
- *Accepting* and *respecting* cultural differences
- *Adapting* care to be congruent with the client's culture

There are several terms used to express the inclusion of the client's culture in treatment: cultural sensitivity, cultural competence, cultural proficiency, and cultural humility. de la Torre and Estrada (2015, p. 145) have defined several of these terms, with the inclusion of a cultural competence continuum. The terms differ with respect to cultural inclusivity of the client and the extent of cultural adaptation by the provider. At minimum, *cultural sensitivity* includes the translation of materials from English to Spanish, the hiring of bilingual and/or bicultural personnel, whether the clinic, program, or access point is in the community (i.e., community-based), the extent to which providers are trained to recognize and respect cultural differences, and the creation of a culturally appropriate environment for the community. Cultural competence is like cultural sensitivity but differs by building the overall client interaction on cultural concepts, normative/cultural beliefs, or the essence of the culture itself. Cultural proficiency is a misnomer. Can anyone truly become proficient in another culture without experiencing their life struggles or accomplishments? Cultural proficiency is sometimes defined as implementing changes based upon cultural needs, but it is not clear if that is a consequence of proficiency or not.

The cultural competence continuum shown in Figure 4.7 has been used as a heuristic device to display various levels of the continuum, from cultural destructiveness (worst) to cultural proficiency (best) (de la Torre & Estrada, 2015, p. 145).

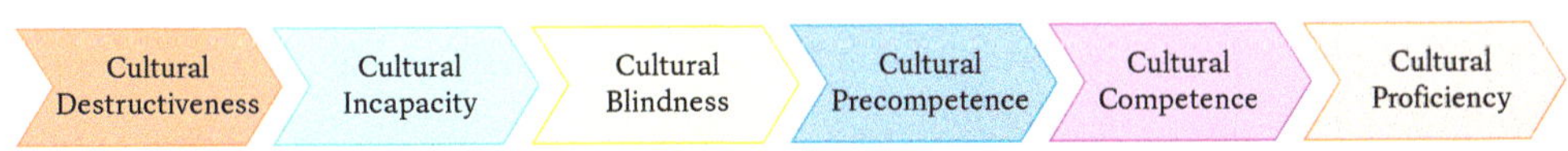

FIGURE 4.7 Cultural Competence Continuum

Source: Adapted from de la Torre and Estrada (2015)

- *Cultural destructiveness*: involves forced assimilation, subjugation, rights, and privileges for the dominant group only and uses power to exploit and destroy.
- *Cultural incapacity*: includes racism, creates negative stereotypes, discrimination, adopts paternalistic/maternalistic posture in dealing with other cultures, and supports segregation.
- *Cultural blindness*: cultural strengths ignored, "treat everyone the same," only meets the needs of dominant group, "blaming the victim," encourages assimilation to dominant culture.
- *Cultural pre-competence*: involves exploration of cultural strengths, commitment to change, assesses the diversity, equity, and inclusion (DEI) needs of agency, recognizes own weaknesses in serving different cultures.
- *Cultural competence*: recognizes and appreciates cultural differences, seeks concrete input from affected cultural groups, hires for diversity, equity, and inclusion, acknowledges cultural strengths.
- *Cultural proficiency*: implement and sustain changes to improve client-centered services based on cultural needs from community input, uses cultural strengths to empower people, advocates for cultural competence throughout the health care system.

Becoming culturally competent is a lifelong process and requires acknowledging one's own ethnocentrisms and racial or gender biases. There are, nevertheless, several essential elements for acquiring cultural competence: The first is to simply acknowledge that there are cultural differences in perceptions of health and to become aware of how they affect the delivery of health and mental health care services. Secondly, to fully appreciate cultural differences, we should recognize the influence of one's own culture on how we behave and think. We are rarely aware of how our implicit biases manifest in our perceptions of the world. Third, we must understand the "dynamics of difference" in the acquisition and delivery of services. The *dynamics of difference* are the social, historical, and economic foundations of historically marginalized populations that have influenced their health status. Fourth, make a conscious effort to understand the meaning of a client's behavior within their cultural context and include these elements in the development of productive cross-cultural interventions. Understanding traditional cultural values and beliefs can facilitate cross-cultural interactions and lead to beneficial health outcomes. Finally, seek out additional information that will add to one's repertoire of cultural interactions.

Like cultural competence, cultural humility is more practical in service-oriented professions. Cultural humility, like cultural competence, requires a lifelong practice of cultural engagement, appreciation, and understanding of other cultures (Foronda et al., 2016). According to Foronda et al. (2016), *cultural humility* is a process of openness, self-awareness, being egoless, and incorporating self-reflection and critique after interacting with individuals from diverse cultural backgrounds. The results of practicing cultural humility are mutual empowerment, respect, partnerships, optimal care, and the willingness to engage in lifelong learning (Agner, 2020; Kibakaya & Oyeku, 2022; Stubbe, 2020).

The need and rationale for cultural humility in health care is driven by demographic changes occurring in the U.S. population. For example, as discussed in Chapter 2, the Latino population continues to increase in size, which necessitates health care providers who can understand their cultural and socioeconomic circumstances. Additionally, the perception of health and disease and their causes varies by culture, and diverse belief systems exist related to health, healing, and wellness. It is also hoped that the elimination of persistent disparities in the health status of people of diverse racial, ethnic, and cultural backgrounds will be achieved by the implementation of culturally competent service. Also, cultural competency can improve the quality of health care services and health outcomes. The Office of Minority Health's National Standards for Culturally and Linguistically Appropriate Services in Health and Health Care incorporate many of the practices that would improve health services and health outcomes for Latinos and other historically marginalized populations.

Acculturation, Cognitive Referents, Acculturative Stress, and Cultural Buffers

This section explores the dynamic interaction between acculturation, cognitive referents of acculturation, acculturative stress, and cultural buffers that assist in mitigating stressful reactions among Latinos. Taken together, these cultural influences can enhance or decrease health care access and health status among Latinos.

Acculturation Among Latinos

One of the most frequently used concepts that examines intracultural variation among Latinos is acculturation level. Acculturation and assimilation studies have long documented changes in dietary practices among various ethnic groups. Health research among Latinos began using the concept of acculturation during the mid-1970s to help explain the prevalence of psychiatric disorders among Latinos and, by association, substance abuse prevalence and substance abuse disorders.

In general, *acculturation* is a term that signifies a process of learning about both cultures, in this case Mexican culture and American culture. Essentially, acculturation is a process of adaptation influenced by cultural norms, behavioral indicators, and cognitive appraisals (Berry, 2003, 2017; Padilla, 1980, 1987; Padilla & Perez, 2003).

Unidimensional and bidimensional acculturation models are widely used with Latino populations and others, with bidimensional or orthogonal models preferred (Andrews et al., 2013; Berry, 2017). Orthogonal models place individuals in quadrants of cultural affiliation, with "new culture" and "native culture" in opposite quadrants (see Figure 4.8).

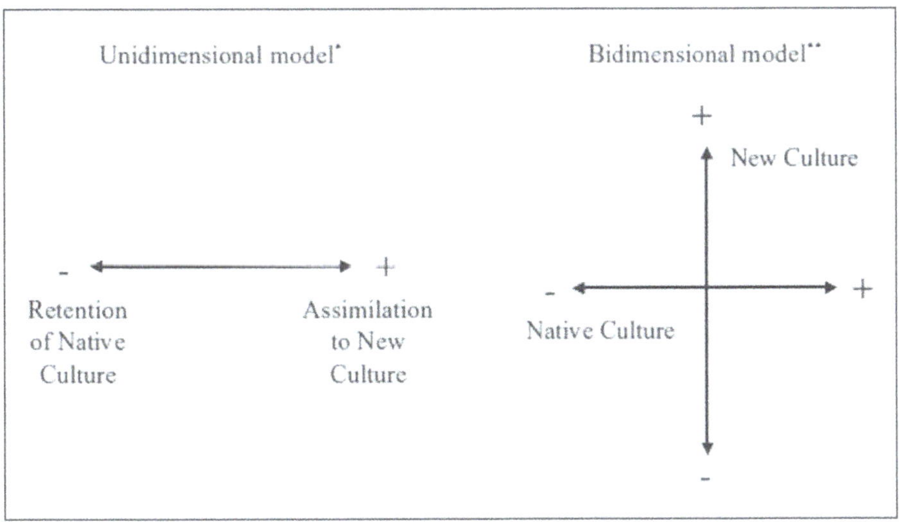

FIGURE 4.8 Unidimensional and Bidimensional Acculturation Models

One of the best-known orthogonal acculturation measures, which places Mexican and American ori entation into quadrants, is the ARSMA-II (Cuellar et al., 1995b). Rather than viewing acculturation on a continuum, these scholars view acculturation as adaptation to a new culture and retention of traditional culture (Figure 4.9).

Acculturation theorists have reached consensus on what changes during the adaptation from one culture to another. *Cultural accommodations* include value systems, child-development practices, social and gender roles, personal preferences, behavioral patterns, cultural norms, institutional adjustments, cultural awareness, and ethnic loyalty (Andrews et al., 2013; Padilla & Perez, 2003). Padilla's inclusion of several themes like social stigma (negative societal perceptions of one's culture), social identity (ethnic or cultural self-identity), and social cognitions (perceptions of the dominant group) extend theoretical formulations of acculturation among Latinos.

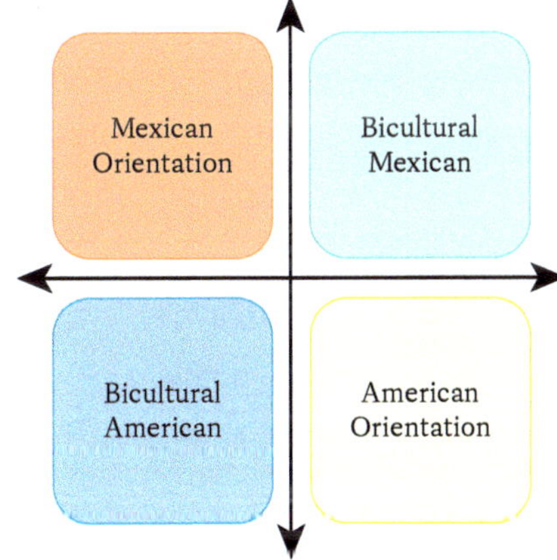

FIGURE 4.9 Acculturation Rating Scale for Mexican Americans-II (ARSMA-II)

Acculturation level influences the extent to which any of the Latino cultural values shown in Table 4.2 are shared and endorsed. Different members within the same family may have different levels of affiliation with any of the cultural values or health beliefs, especially those that are gender specific. Research has shown that as acculturation level increases, traditional cultural values and health beliefs decrease (Abraído-Lanza et al., 2005, 2016; Unger & Schwartz, 2012). Several studies on Latinos show that acculturation level is significantly associated with behavioral and health outcomes (Balcazar et al., 1996; Ebin et al., 2001;

Gorman et al., 2010; Vega et al., 1998). The importance of examining acculturation level among Latinos lies in understanding potential cultural influences at work in health risk behaviors (e.g., smoking, drug use); knowledge, attitudes, and beliefs related to health (e.g., etiology and treatment of disease); help-seeking behaviors (to whom one goes to for care); psychosocial well-being (e.g., rates of depression); and medication adherence, to name a few.

A plethora of acculturation measures have been used with Latinos and published in the literature. However, the usefulness of the concept has been questioned, especially in the U.S.-Mexico borderlands primarily because of the number of items that are language-related in most acculturation measures. At the simplest level, proxy measures are used to measure acculturation level among Latinos, primarily whether the research participant takes the interview in English or Spanish. At the most complex level, acculturation measures such as the Acculturation Rating Scale for Mexican Americans-II (ARSMA-II; Cuellar et al., 1995b) or the Los Angeles Epidemiologic Catchment Area study (LAECA; Hough, 1983) use more than 20 questions. By far, the most consistent item used in most, if not all, acculturation measures is language usage. Other items are sometimes included such as generation level, birthplace of parents and grandparents, social interactions with other racial/ethnic groups, preferred listening and viewing habits, types of Latino foods consumed, and participation in cultural activities, among others (Burnam et al., 1987; Marin, 1992; Wallace et al., 2010; Ward, 1999) (see Table 4.5).

There are many limitations in using acculturation level. For example, research conducted in the U.S.-Mexico border region, especially close to the international border, generally shows little variation in acculturation level, especially if language is used as a proxy measure, as the majority of Mexican Americans

TABLE 4.5 Common Areas in Latino Acculturation Measures

Area
• Language spoken
• Language thought
• Language reading/listening
• Ethnic identity—self • Ethnic identity—mother • Ethnic identity—father
• Birthplace—self • Birthplace—mother • Birthplace —father
• Language preferred (English or Spanish)
• Association with friends (White or Latino)
• Foods consumed (Latino or American)

in the region speak Spanish. Employing acculturation measures in Puerto Rico has similar limitations. Moving beyond language in acculturation measures is important to consider behavioral and cognitive aspects of the acculturation process.

Another limitation of acculturation measures is that they cannot provide meaningful cultural approaches to reducing chronic disease risk factors. As a former NIH grant reviewer, I have seen many applications that do not understand this limitation. It is more important to understand cognitive and behavioral changes that occur during the process of acculturation to acquire more knowledge on how culturally responsive interventions can be developed using Latino cultural values and beliefs like *familismo, respeto, marianismo,* and *machismo*, among others.

Cognitive Referents of Acculturation

Cuellar et al.'s (1995a) seminal work on the cognitive referents of acculturation has proven useful in understanding how cultural values and beliefs can shape Latinos' willingness to engage in protective health behaviors. Because the level of acculturation influences our thoughts (cognition), beliefs, values, and behaviors, it is important to acknowledge these cognitive referents of acculturation. Cuellar et al. validated several cognitive referents of acculturation, including familism, *personalismo*, fatalism, *machismo*, and folk beliefs. They also found that acculturation level was negatively associated with acculturation level, indicating that as one acculturates to non-Latino mainstream society cultural values, cognitive referents of acculturation are diminished. Similarly, Estrada et al. (2022) developed several cultural measures including *machismo*, traditionalism, and religiosity and found negative correlations with cognitive referents of acculturation. By extension, the cultural concept of *marianismo* would also be considered a cognitive referent of acculturation and should predictably diminish as Latinas acculturate.

How does the field get beyond measures of acculturation to get at the essence or substance of behavior change and, more importantly, to change risk behaviors? When an individual adapts or acculturates to mainstream society, there are changes that occur in cognition, values and beliefs, and behaviors through socialization processes, as noted by Padilla & Perez (2003). Moreover, the work of Cuellar and colleagues (1995a) is useful in examining cultural values and beliefs that change because of acculturation and that may be negative in terms of health behaviors (Figure 4.10).

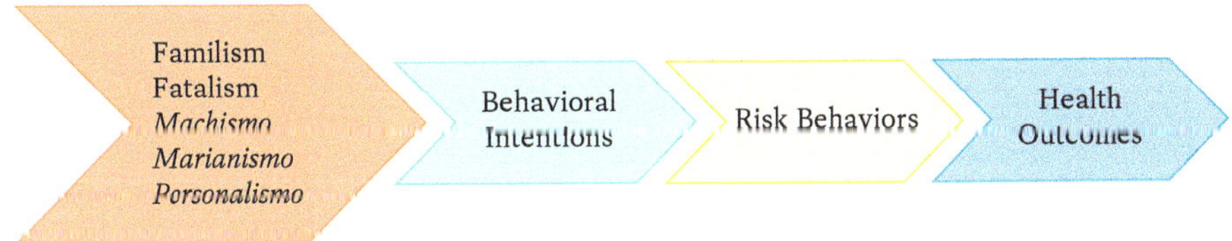

FIGURE 4.10 Cognitive Referents of Acculturation

Acculturative Stress

Is cultural adaptation to another culture stressful? If so, what personal and social adjustments must be made to successfully adapt? What elements of adaptation are more stressful than others? The research on acculturation and acculturative stress among Latinos and other groups has grown exponentially in the past 2 decades. The primary focus of acculturative stress research is on the experience of immigrants. As such, it is important to differentiate between psychosocial stressors experienced by new immigrants and second-generation or higher Latinos. Pressures to acculturate may be more pronounced among new immigrants, while ethnic/racial discrimination may be more pronounced among Latinos who are second generation or higher.

Cervantes et al. (2016) developed a revised version of the Hispanic Stress Inventory for both Latino immigrants and U.S.-born Latinos. The stressor domains were different for each Latino group. For Latino immigrants, 10 stressor domains were identified: parental, occupation and economic, marital, discrimination, immigration, marital acculturation gap, health, language, premigration stressors, and family stressors. For U.S.-born Latinos, seven stressor domains were identified: discrimination, marital, health, family, parental, occupation, and unemployment and economic stressors. The authors correctly address the need to continually revise measures of acculturative stress due to anti-immigrant sentiment and discrimination policies against Latinos.

Because acculturation is an adaptational process encompassing modifications in traditional cultural values, beliefs, and behaviors, many scholars have argued that acculturation causes psychological stress (Berry, 1995; Padilla, 1980, 1987; Padilla & Perez, 2003; Rudmin, 2003, 2009). The types of stress that a Latino of Mexican descent feels when living in a non-Latino majority (or different) culture could include learning another language; internalizing different mores, values, expectations, and understandings; exhibiting behaviors congruent with the majority culture; and differences in customs, foods, manners, dress, hairstyle, music, and personal space (Figure 4.11).

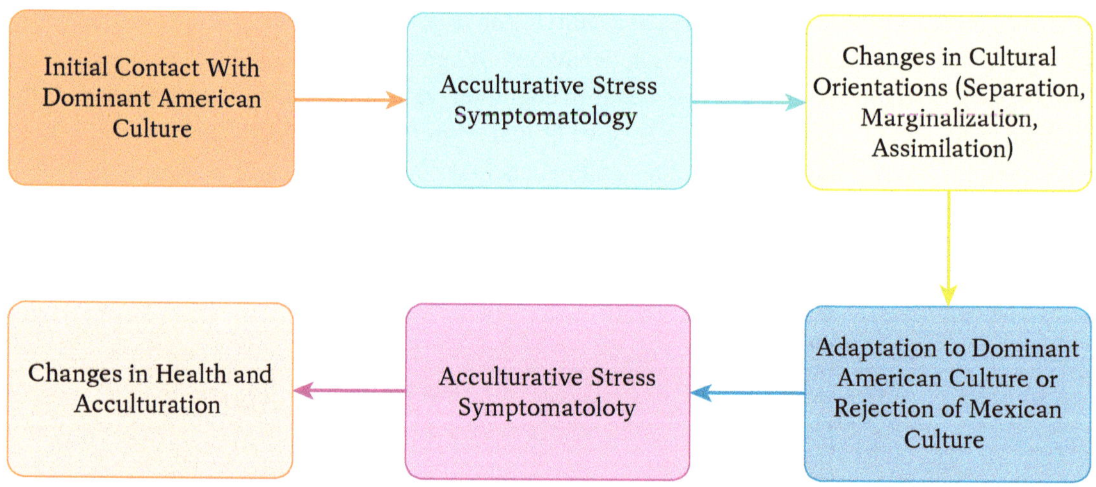

FIGURE 4.11 Simple Acculturative Stress Model

Adapted from Rudmin (2009)

Acculturation level is associated with socioeconomic status. Higher acculturated Latinos, those acculturated to American mainstream culture, also have higher educational attainment, higher incomes, and are more fluent in English. Although the benefits of increased acculturation are numerous (e.g., improved standard of living, better medical care, food, etc.), hidden negative effects can occur, including being politically alienated, pressures to acculturate or conform to American mainstream expectations, feelings of lack of belonging, feeling marginalized, losing control over children due to acculturation, and increased psychological adjustment leading to psychosocial stress.

Moreover, when Latinos acculturate to mainstream American culture, the protective quality of their traditional culture of origin decreases, including less supportive social supports, an increased risk for poor social interaction, an impaired self-image, feelings of inferiority, increased perception of poor life changes, increased discrimination, and deteriorating health practices.

Acculturative stress models discussed in the literature include (Berry, 2003, 2017; Doucerain et al., 2017):

- *Simple acculturation model*: Elements of a new culture are adopted. The acculturation process is not necessarily viewed as stressful.
- *Acculturative stress model*: The less acculturated, because of their values and behaviors, are not adequately equipped to deal with the dominant culture; therefore, they experience more stress.
- *Acculturative stress variant model*: The more acculturated have higher levels of stress due to (a) either giving up traditional culture or (b) adoption to the dominant culture and therefore experiencing more stress.
- *Bicultural model*: The complete relinquishing of traditional culture causes stress. Sharing elements of both cultures is seen as adaptive, therefore reducing stress.
- *Cultural marginality model*: The partially acculturated person, alienated from traditional culture but not yet integrated into the dominant culture, will experience the most stress.

Bidimensional stress models have also been developed in the literature that focus on the retention of a dual cultural orientation through successful adaptation across the life course (Doucerain et al., 2017; Romero & Pina-Watson, 2017; Schwartz et al., 2017). Bidimensional cultural stressors are characterized by their ability to create cognitive dissonance between behaviors and actions incongruent with living in two cultural contexts.

The successful acculturation to non-Latino dominant mainstream culture is a cognitive and emotional balancing act requiring the social skills and psychological resilience to overcome stress through active coping and social support (Cervantes & Castro, 1985). Research has shown that social support networks activated through familism and ethnic identity and cultural resilience through traditionalism and religiosity can moderate the stressful effects of acculturation and the negative effects of stereotyped discrimination of Latinos (Driscoll & Torres, 2013; Goebert, 2008; Maldonado et al., 2018; Torres, 2010; Torres et al., 2012).

Latino Cultural Buffers to Stressors

Recall from Chapter 1 that the social stress process articulated by Aneshensel and Avison (2015) includes several interdependent categories: life event and/or chronic stressors like poverty; resources that mitigate against life event and chronic stressors that can include internal personal coping resources (e.g., self-esteem and self-confidence); external resources like social support networks (e.g., family and friends); and cultural resources (e.g., biculturalism, ethnic self-identity). Also included were several types of stressors commonly experienced by Latinos, like anti-Latino sentiment and language discrimination (Bekteshi & Kang, 2020; Carvajal et al., 2013; Romero & Pina-Watson, 2017; Sanchez & Fernandez, 1993).

Differential exposure to social stressors can lead to various coping responses, ranging from passively ignoring them to active cognitive restructuring of their meaning and intent. Moreover, the intensity and continuity of a social stressor may exceed the internal and external coping capacity of the individual, which can then lead to "toxic stress," a physiological and psychological consequence of inadequate coping responses (Shern et al., 2016; Shonkoff et al., 2012, 2021).

Hypothetically, Latino cultural buffers should assist in mediating the response to stressors or moderating their negative effects on health. Latino cultural buffers to stressors include cultural identity, ethnic pride, social support networks, and religiosity.

One of the first conceptualizations of coping and stress among Mexican Americans was the work of Cervantes and Castro (1985). They conducted the first systematic literature review on the topic and provided a theoretical model of how internal and external coping mediated the consequences of stress on health outcomes: the stress-mediating-coping model (Cervantes & Castro, 1985, p. 11). The model consists of a potential stressor that is appraised by the individual as indeed stressful. The activation of both internal and external coping "mediators" elicits a coping response that could potentially have short-term and long-term health consequences. Feedback loops are included that focus on appraisal and reappraisal of the stressor experienced by the individual, with hypothesized reduction of the stressor's negative effect (see Figure 4.12).

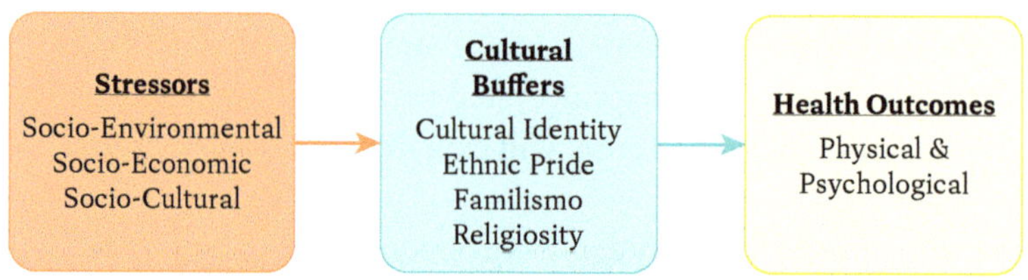

FIGURE 4.12 Stressors, Cultural Buffers, and Health Outcomes

Subsequent research has validated the major components of the model, but additional research findings on mediating (intervening) or moderating (lessening) influences are inconsistent (Driscoll & Torres, 2013; Goebert, 2008). Moreover, explicit cultural buffers (moderators or mediators) have not been examined systematically in relation to physical or psychological health outcomes. For example, hypothetical cultural buffers to stress like cultural identity or ethnic pride may have negative or positive effects on rates of depression or the experience of discrimination. Research continues to demonstrate that as Latinos acculturate to mainstream American society, they perceive more racism and discrimination directed toward their ethnic group (Bekteshi & Kang, 2020; Maldonado et al., 2018; Sanchez & Fernandez, 1993). For example, a positive cultural self-identity would hypothetically buffer the negative experience of discrimination, whereas a negative cultural self-identity would hypothetically be positively associated with perceived higher rates of discrimination.

An HIV/AIDS research program in the department of Mexican American Studies at the University of Arizona examined several cognitive referents of acculturation and their associations with behavioral intentions and self-efficacy to reduce HIV transmission risks among 406 Latinos who use drugs via injection (Estrada et al., 1999). The One-to-One HIV Intervention program used qualitative methods to identify and define cultural concepts with Latinos who use drugs via injection and quantitative methods to construct the cultural concepts. Several cultural (acculturation level, familism, traditionalism, and religiosity) and Latino subcultural concepts (e.g., *machismo*) were identified. All cultural constructs like *machismo* (11 items, alpha = .84), familism (6 items, alpha = .80), traditionalism (10 items, alpha = .79), religiosity (8 items, alpha = .86), and acculturation (13 items, alpha = .96) had good internal consistency as determined by Cronbach's alpha, a standard measure that assesses psychometric properties of scales, with values above .70 considered good measures of internal scale-item consistency. The cultural measures of familism, traditionalism, and religiosity were positively associated with positive behavioral intentions to reduce HIV risk behaviors and were all positively associated with self-efficacy to reduce HIV transmission risks. However, *machismo* was negatively associated with self-efficacy to reduce HIV transmission risks.

The added value of using Latino cultural concepts with measures of acculturation is that it provides an insight on how interventions can trigger behavioral change among Latinos at high risk for disease. Moving beyond acculturation level is necessary to develop Latino-focused interventions that are successful. Interventions designed to change risk behaviors should provide a contextual background that includes those cognitive referents of acculturation and not just acculturation per se. Understanding how to use culture to motivate behavior change goes far beyond placing individuals on an acculturation continuum.

Latino Cultural Resilience Models

Resilience is noted by scholars to be an interactive, dynamic process encompassing positive adaptation within the context of significant adversity and stress (Luthar & Cicchetti, 2000; Luthar et al., 2000; Rutter, 2006; Ungar, 2011).

The context in which resilience occurs can be at the personal or group level. Resilience is the capacity of the individual to successfully adapt and, over time, strengthens one's ability to adequately cope with stressful life events with improved internal and external coping resources (Gallo et al., 2009a, 2009b; Stewart et al., 1997). Resilience is a multidimensional concept that varies across age, gender, socioeconomic status, and cultural background. Studies have shown that individuals living in poverty or who are low income have less capacity for resilience than those with higher incomes, what Gallo and colleagues refer to as the *reserve capacity model,* suggesting that poverty depletes the reserve capacity of individuals (Gallo, 2009; Gallo et al., 2009a, 2009b).

Group resilience depends on their collective ability to withstand negative social environmental stressors like discrimination and racism directed toward them. *Cultural resilience* describes the extent to which cultural strengths promote individual and group well-being in the face of adversity (Clauss-Ehlers, 2004, 2008; Spence et al., 2016).

Cultural resilience models provide ways in which one can empower Latino individuals and communities through the enactment and instillation of positive cultural values and beliefs. Ongoing research shows that the inculcation of Latino cultural values among Latino youth and adolescents fosters resilience and cultural pride (Estrada et al., 2022; Piña-Watson et al., 2019). In addition, Latino cultural programs in U.S. prisons are found to have a positive effect on the well-being of participants (Castro et al., 2007).

Cultural resilience models developed for Latino youth include cultural stressors like discrimination, acculturative stress, perceptions of bias and economic stress, relational systems that include parenting and peer relationships, intrapersonal characteristics like depression and anxiety, and prosocial behaviors, including altruistic behaviors (Davis et al., 2021). Strengthening relational systems (social support networks) can moderate the impact of cultural stressors (discrimination, acculturative stress). Additionally, developing prosocial behaviors can lead to social integration and healthy behaviors.

Using Latino cultural strengths are especially important in developing prosocial behaviors and reducing health inequalities (see Table 4.2). Latino cultural values provide a foundational resiliency and survival for individuals and communities. The cultural values of *compadrazgo, familism, simpatia, respeto, confianza,* and religiosity are examples of cultural strengths that manifest in personal resiliency and community empowerment. These values come under the umbrella term "cultural wealth." *Cultural wealth* includes those tangible and intangible values, beliefs, and behaviors that enhance the well-being of Latinos. They assist in overcoming the ethnocentrism, racism, discrimination, prejudice, and other forms of oppression perpetrated upon Latinos by the Euro-American hegemony in the United States (Yosso, 2005).

Latino cultural wealth is viewed as an overarching protective factor for Latino communities and other historically disadvantaged groups (Acevedo & Solórzano, 2021). Acording to Yasso and Burciaga (2016), the interplay of cultural assets and resources yields a multidimensional view of Latino cultural wealth that comprises six dimensions:

- *Aspirational capital*: refers to the ability to maintain hopes and dreams for the future, even in the face of real and perceived barriers.
- *Linguistic capital*: includes the intellectual and social skills attained through communication in multiple languages and/or language styles (including communication through art, music, poetry, theatre, and dance).
- *Social capital*: can be understood as networks of people and community resources.
- *Navigational capital:* refers to skills in maneuvering through social institutions. This implies the ability to maneuver through institutions not created with historically marginalized and disadvantaged groups in mind.
- *Familial capital*: refers to cultural knowledge nurtured among familia that carry a sense of community history, memory, and cultural intuition.
- *Resistant capital*: refers to those knowledge and skills fostered through oppositional behavior that challenge inequality. (p. 4)

Together, the six cultural wealth dimensions facilitate the well-being of Latinos in the face of adversity and may mitigate the effects of psychosocial and cultural stressors in the social environment.

One of the dimensions noted above was linguistic capital, or the ability to communicate in English or Spanish. Many Latinos view the Spanish language as a cultural value. Its importance not only lies with the association between acculturation level and language spoken or preferred but additionally in one's sense of Latino identity: *Latinidad*. It is also playing an important role in social interactions with Latino elders, who convey cultural knowledge, customs, and *dichos*, or "sayings/stories," that connect to our cultural backgrounds.

Eliminating Health Inequalities Among Latinos

To eliminate health inequalities among Latinos of Mexican descent requires a fundamental knowledge of "upstream" and "downstream" factors in their etiology. It is important to examine the "causes of the causes," like historical and social factors that severely undermine the social determinants of health for Latinos and other historically marginalized populations. Understanding the origins of Latino health inequalities can assist in tracing them back to their historical and social root causes. Moreover, identifying the pathways of disease causation, from root causes to observed health differences, can facilitate interventions designed to reduce or eliminate fundamental causes of disease and mitigate their underlying pathways.

The Agency for Healthcare Research and Quality (Brach & Fraserirector, 2000) identified nine practices found in the literature on cultural competency that are used to reduce health inequalities among Latinos and other historically marginalized populations. These practices include:

- Interpreter services, either through phone or onsite personnel
- Recruitment and retention of patients/clients for follow-up
- Training health providers to become cognizant of cultural/linguistic differences
- Coordinating with traditional healers like curanderos or other folk healers
- Use of community health workers like *promotoras de salud* to reach the Latino community
- Culturally competent health romotion that focuses on cultural strengths
- Including family and/or community members in the practice of compadrazgo or familism
- Immersion in another culture/acquiring cultural humility
- Administrative and organizational accommodations for cultural humility (Brach & Fraserirector, 2000, p. 195)

Several of these areas have been implemented as stand-alone services, such as the use of interpreter services and programs aimed at improving recruitment and retention of patients. Language congruence enhances patient–provider communication, retention, and follow-up. Other practices have been the focus of interventions to increase medication adherence or the use of preventive services, like employing community health workers (promotoras de salud), or the inclusion of family members to assist the patient in understanding the importance of adhering to medications or reducing chronic disease risk behaviors. Less often used by health care facilities outside of Indian Health Service (IHS) is the coordination with traditional healers for aftercare and continued suppression of symptoms. Although medicine men are common referrals in Indian Country, there are no reported uses of curanderos for Latinos of Mexican descent. Cultural immersion is an important method for acquiring cultural competence that is used in the training of medical and mental health professionals.

Public health recommendations to eliminate health inequalities include developing new or improved approaches for:

- Detecting or diagnosing the onset or progression of disease and disabilities that contribute to health disparities (primary prevention)
- Preventing or delaying the onset or progression of disease or disabilities that contribute to health inequalities (secondary prevention)
- Treating diseases and disabilities that contribute to health inequalities (tertiary prevention)

Cultural humility practices are hypothesized to lead to changes in clinician and patient behavior through improved communication, enhanced trust, greater knowledge of differential epidemiology and treatment efficacy, and an expanded understanding of the patients' cultural behaviors and social environment (Brach & Fraserirector, 2000). These hypothesized changes in provider and patient behavior are expected to lead to the provision of culturally appropriate services, which in turn leads to positive health outcomes, including higher levels of health status, increased health and mental health functioning, improved patient and provider satisfaction, and ultimately a reduction in health inequalities.

CHAPTER SUMMARY

Cultural determinants of health include cultural beliefs, cultural values, and gender roles and expectations that are formed within the family or culture of origin and influenced by level of acculturation. Culture is a multidimensional concept that includes language preferences, communication styles, norms, values, and behaviors that can change over time.

Cultural determinants of health have not received as much attention as the social determinants of health in public health literature. For Latinos and other historically disadvantaged groups, cultural and social determinants coalesce to enhance or hinder help-seeking behaviors. Resiliency capacity research indicates that those who occupy the lower rungs of society have less capacity in the form of external and internal coping resources to successfully adapt to non-Latino mainstream society.

Latino health beliefs are a synthesis of Mesoamerican and Spanish worldviews regarding the well-being of the individual, family, and community. Integrating the physical, mental, and spiritual aspects of personal experiences contributes to the concept of "being healthy" or well-being. In addition, these health beliefs include a holistic approach that includes body, mind, and spirit.

Mesoamerican health beliefs merged with Spanish health beliefs to create a syncretic system of health beliefs that included concepts of "hot-cold" and "wet-dry" diseases and their treatment. Mexica cultural beliefs also included multiple souls (teyolia, tonnali, ihiyotl) that required a proper balance to maintain health.

The Mexican American health belief system of *curanderismo* is a blend of Indigenous, Spanish, and spiritual beliefs that have endured for centuries. *Curanderismo* provides the framework for cultural healing and defines the scope of practice for folk healers. Several common folk illnesses include *susto, empacho, mal de ojo,* and *caida de mollera* (fallen fontanel) that are cured or managed through folk treatments.

Mexican American cultural values and beliefs are critical in understanding how they may manifest in help-seeking behaviors, patient-provider interactions, and risk reduction interventions. Even though Spanish is a colonial language imposed on the Mexica and other populations of Mexico, Central America, and South America, many Latinos nevertheless perceive it as a cultural value, and it is important in cross-cultural communication. The culture of Western medicine can and does conflict with traditional or ethnic medicine with respect to etiology and treatment of disease and the expectations of the patient.

Family is very important to Latinos. It is the Latino cultural institution in which cultural transmission of gender roles and expectations occurs. Of importance are the gendered scripts of *machismo* and *marianismo,* which have been discussed in the context of hindering or facilitating help-seeking behaviors. The familial and social contexts of ethnic identity formation are important in orienting one's cultural and racial/ethnic affiliation.

Cultural humility is a preferred term over cultural competency. Rather than achieving specific benchmarks and communication skills, cultural humility embraces cultural understanding. The results of practicing cultural humility are mutual empowerment, respect, partnerships, optimal care, and the willingness to engage in lifelong learning.

Perhaps the most studied and complex concept is acculturation. It has proven useful as a measure of intracultural variation in attitudes, beliefs, and behaviors among Latinos. Acculturation level influences the extent to which any of the Latino cultural and beliefs values are endorsed. It is also known that as acculturation level increases, cultural beliefs, values, and behaviors deteriorate. Cognitive referents of acculturation are these important cultural beliefs, values, and behaviors that are associated with behavioral intentions and self-efficacy to reduce chronic risk behaviors.

Acculturative stress is another important consideration in the well-being of Latinos. Impediments to successful cultural adaptation can lead to stress, anxiety, and depression, as well as increased risk behaviors. One of the most reliable and validated acculturative stress measures is the Hispanic Stress Inventory that has been used with Latino adolescents and adults. Equally important are Latino cultural buffers to stress like familism and Latino ethnic/cultural identity.

Latino cultural resilience models include these cultural buffers and cognitive referents of acculturation that mitigate or moderate the effects of stress on physiological and psychological well-being. Eliminating health inequalities among Latinos requires attention to both upstream and downstream influences on health and integrating cultural determinants that can facilitate positive health outcomes.

QUESTIONS TO CONSIDER

1. What are some important Latino cultural values that are related to help-seeking behaviors, patient-provider interactions, and risk reduction interventions?
2. Define curanderismo, and describe the folk healers commonly found in Mexican American communities. What are their levels of expertise? Is there a place for curanderismo in modern medical practice with Mexican-origin Hispanics?
3. What is acculturation and acculturative stress? Why are they considered important influences on the health status of Hispanics/Latinos?
4. What are cognitive referents of acculturation?
5. Define cultural competency and cultural humility as they are related to health care. Why are they important? What are some ways that one can practice cultural humility?
6. What is cultural resiliency and cultural wealth? How might cultural strengths be used to assist positive changes in health behaviors?

SUGGESTED READINGS

Abraído-Lanza, A. F., Chao, M. T., & Flórez, K. R. (2005). Do healthy behaviors decline with greater acculturation? Implications for the Latino mortality paradox. *Social Science & Medicine*, *61*(6), 1243–1255.

Berry, J. W. (2017). Theories and models of acculturation. In S. J. Schwartz & J. B. Unger (Eds.), *The Oxford handbook of acculturation and health* (pp. 15–28). Oxford University Press.

Cervantes, R. C., Fisher, D. G., Padilla, A. M., & Napper, L. E. (2016). The Hispanic Stress Inventory Version 2: Improving the assessment of acculturation stress. *Psychological Assessment, 28*(5), 509.

Clauss-Ehlers, C. S. (2008). Sociocultural factors, resilience, and coping: Support for a culturally sensitive measure of resilience. *Journal of Applied Developmental Psychology, 29*(3), 197–212.

Cuellar, I., Arnold, B., & Gonzalez, G. (1995). Cognitive referents of acculturation: Assessment of cultural constructs in Mexican Americans. *Journal of Community Psychology, 23*(4), 339–356.

Marin, G., & Marin, B. V. (1991). *Research with Hispanic populations*. SAGE.

Ortiz de Montellano, B. R. (1990). *Aztec medicine, health, and nutrition*. Rutgers University Press.

Padilla, A. M., & Perez, W. (2003). Acculturation, social identity, and social cognition: A new perspective. *Hispanic Journal of Behavioral Sciences, 25*(1), 35–55.

Rudmin, F. (2009). Constructs, measurements and models of acculturation and acculturative stress. *International Journal of Intercultural Relations, 33*(2), 106–123.

Stubbe, D. E. (2020). Practicing cultural competence and cultural humility in the care of diverse patients. *Focus, 18*(1), 49–51.

Torres, L., Driscoll, M. W., & Voell, M. (2012). Discrimination, acculturation, acculturative stress, and Latino psychological distress: A moderated mediational model. *Cultural Diversity and Ethnic Minority Psychology, 18*(1), 17.

Yosso, T. J. (2005). Whose culture has capital? A critical race theory discussion of community cultural wealth. *Race Ethnicity and Education, 8*(1), 69–91.

REFERENCES

Abraído-Lanza, A. F., Chao, M. T., & Flórez, K. R. (2005). Do healthy behaviors decline with greater acculturation? Implications for the Latino mortality paradox. *Social Science & Medicine, 61*(6), 1243-1255.

Abraído-Lanza, A. F., Echeverría, S. E., & Flórez, K. R. (2016). Latino immigrants, acculturation, and health: Promising new directions in research. *Annual Review of Public Health, 37*, 219–236.

Abril, I. F. (1977). Mexican American folk beliefs: How they affect health care. *The American Journal of Maternal/Child Nursing, 2*(3), 168–173.

Acevedo, N., & Solórzano, D. G. (2021). An overview of community cultural wealth: Toward a protective factor against racism. *Urban Education, 58*(7).

Agner, J. (2020). Moving from cultural competence to cultural humility in occupational therapy: A paradigm shift. *The American Journal of Occupational Therapy, 74*(4), 7404347010p1–7404347010p7.

Ailinger, R. L., & Causey, M. E. (1995). Health concept of older Hispanic immigrants. *Western Journal of Nursing Research, 17*(6), 605–613.

American Medical Association. (1999). *Cultural competence compendium*.

Andrews, A. R., III, Bridges, A. J., & Gomez, D. (2013). A multi-study analysis of conceptual and measurement issues related to health research on acculturation in Latinos. *Journal of Transcultural Nursing, 24*(2), 134–143.

Aneshensel, C. S., & Avison, W. R. (2015). The stress process: An appreciation of Leonard I. Pearlin. *Society and Mental Health, 5*(2), 67–85. https://doi.org/10.1177/2156869315585388

Arizaga, G. (1999). Curanderismo as holistic medicine. In G. Cajete (Ed.), *A people's ecology: Explorations in sustainable living* (pp. 209–222). Clear Light Publishers.

Baer, R. D., & Ackerman, A. (1988). Toxic Mexican folk remedies for the treatment of empacho: The case of azarcon, greta, and albayalde. *Journal of Ethnopharmacology, 24*(1), 31–39.

Balcazar, H., Peterson, G., & Cobas, J. A. (1996). Acculturation and health-related risk behaviors among Mexican American pregnant youth. *American Journal of Health Behavior, 20*(6), 425.

Bekteshi, V., & Kang, S. W. (2020). Contextualizing acculturative stress among Latino immigrants in the United States: A systematic review. *Ethnicity & Health, 25*(6), 897–914.

Bernal, M. E., Knight, G. P., Garza, C. A., Ocampo, K. A., & Cota, M. K. (1990). The development of ethnic identity in Mexican-American children. *Hispanic Journal of Behavioral Sciences, 12*(1), 3–24.

Berry, J. W. (2003). Conceptual approaches to acculturation. In K. M. Chun, P. B. Organizta, & G. Mar (Eds.), *Acculturation: Advances in theory, measurement, and applied research* (pp.17–37). American Psychological Association.

Berry, J. W. (2017). Theories and models of acculturation. In S. J. Schwartz & J. B. Unger (Eds.), *The Oxford handbook of acculturation and health* (pp. 15–28). Oxford University Press.

Brach, C., & Fraserirector, I. (2000). Can cultural competency reduce racial and ethnic health disparities? A review and conceptual model. *Medical Care Research and Review, 57*(Suppl. 1), 181–217.

Burnam, M. A., Telles, C. A., Karno, M., Hough, R. L., & Escobar, J. I. (1987). Measurement of acculturation in a community population of Mexican Americans. *Hispanic Journal of Behavioral Sciences, 9*(2), 105–130.

Calzada, E. J., Fernandez, Y., & Cortes, D. E. (2010). Incorporating the cultural value of respeto into a framework of Latino parenting. *Cultural Diversity and Ethnic Minority Psychology,* 16(1), 77.

Carvajal, S. C., Rosales, C., Rubio-Goldsmith, R., Sabo, S., Ingram, M., McClelland, D. J., Redondo, F., Torres, E., Rombero, A. J., Oleary A. O., Sanchez, Z., & De Zapien, J. G. (2013). The border community and immigration stress scale: A preliminary examination of a community responsive measure in two Southwest samples. *Journal of Immigrant and Minority Health, 15*(2), 427–436.

Castro, F. G., Nichols, E., & Kater, K. (2007). Relapse prevention with Hispanic and other racial/ethnic populations: Can cultural resilience promote relapse prevention? In K. Witkiewitz & G. Alan Marlatt (Eds.), *Therapist's guide to evidence-based relapse prevention* (pp. 259–292). Academic Press.

Cauce, A. M., & Domenech-Rodriguez, M. (2002). Latino families: Myths and realities. *Latino children and families in the United States: Current research and future directions,* 3–25.

Centers for Disease Control and Prevention. (1993, July 16). Lead poisoning associated with use of traditional ethnic remedies—California, 1991–1992. *Morbidity and Mortality Weekly Report, 42*(27), 484–524.

Cervantes, R. C., & Castro, F. G. (1985). Stress, coping, and Mexican American mental health: A systematic review. *Hispanic Journal of Behavioral Sciences, 7*(1), 1–73.

Cervantes, R. C., Fisher, D. G., Padilla, A. M., & Napper, L. E. (2016). The Hispanic Stress Inventory Version 2: Improving the assessment of acculturation stress. *Psychological Assessment, 28*(5), 509–522.

Clauss-Ehlers, C. S. (2004). Re-inventing resilience: A model of "culturally focused resilient adaptation." In C. S. Clauss-Ehlers & M. D. Weist (Eds.), *Community planning to foster resilience in children* (pp. 27–41). Kluwer Academic Publishers.

Clauss-Ehlers, C. S. (2008). Sociocultural factors, resilience, and coping: Support for a culturally sensitive measure of resilience. *Journal of Applied Developmental Psychology, 29*(3), 197–212.

Cohen, K. S. (2018). *Honoring the medicine: The essential guide to Native American healing.* Ballantine Books.

Colson A. B., & de Armellado C. (1983). An Amerindian derivation for Latin American Creole illnesses and their treatment. *Social Science & Medicine, 17*(17), 1229–1248.

Cuellar, I., Arnold, B., & Gonzalez, G. (1995a). Cognitive referents of acculturation: Assessment of cultural constructs in Mexican Americans. Journal of Community Psychology, *23*(4), 339–356.

Cuellar, I., Arnold, B., & Maldonado, R. (1995b). Acculturation rating scale for Mexican Americans-II: A revision of the original ARSMA scale. *Hispanic Journal of Behavioral Sciences, 17*(3), 275–304.

Currier, R. L. (1966). The hot-cold syndrome and symbolic balance in Mexican and Spanish-American folk medicine. *Ethnology, 5*(3), 251–263.

Davis, A. N., Carlo, G., & Maiya, S. (2021). Towards a multisystem, strength-based model of social inequities in U.S. Latinx youth. *Human Development, 65*(4), 204–216.

Davis, R. E., Lee, S., Johnson, T. P., & Rothschild, S. K. (2019). Measuring the elusive construct of personalismo among Mexican American, Puerto Rican, and Cuban American adults. *Hispanic Journal of Behavioral Sciences, 41*(1), 103–121.

de la Fuente, J., & de la Fuente, J. (1949). *Yalalag: Una villa zapoteca serrana* (Vol. 1). Museo Nacional de Antropología.

de la Torre, A., & Estrada, A. L. (2015). *Sana! Sana! Mexican Americans and health* (2nd ed.). The University of Arizona Press.

Dennis, J., Basanez, T., & Farahmand, A. (2010). Intergenerational conflicts among Latinos in early adulthood: Separating values conflicts with parents from acculturation conflicts. *Hispanic Journal of Behavioral Sciences, 32*(1), 118–135.

Diamond, L., Izquierdo, K., Canfield, D., Matsoukas, K., & Gany, F. (2019). A systematic review of the impact of patient-physician non-English language concordance on quality of care and outcomes. *Journal of General Internal Medicine, 34,* 1591–1606.

Doucerain, M., Segalowitz, N., & Ryder, A. G. (2017). Acculturation measurement: From simple proxies to sophisticated tool-kit. In S. J. Schwartz & J. B. Unger (Eds.), *The Oxford handbook of acculturation and health* (pp. 97–117). Oxford University Press.

Driscoll, M. W., & Torres, L. (2013). Acculturative stress and Latino depression: the mediating role of behavioral and cognitive resources. *Cultural Diversity and Ethnic Minority Psychology, 19*(4), 373–382.

Ebin, V. J., Sneed, C. D., Morisky, D. E., Rotheram-Borus, M. J., Magnusson, A. M., & Malotte, C. K. (2001). Acculturation and interrelationships between problem and health-promoting behaviors among Latino adolescents. *Journal of Adolescent Health, 28*(1), 62–72.

Estrada, A. L., Estrada, B. D., & Quintero, G. (1999). *The influence of cultural values on self-efficacy in reducing HIV risk behaviors.* Mexican American Studies & Research Center.

Estrada, A. L., Jasso, R., & Estrada, B. D. (2022). Fostering Latino cultural self-identity among Mexican American adolescents. *Advances in Preventive Medicine and Health Care, 5,* 1036.

Fernandez, A., Schillinger, D., Warton, E. M., Adler, N., Moffet, H. H., Schenker, Y., ... & Karter, A. J. (2011). Language barriers, physician-patient language concordance, and glycemic control among insured Latinos with diabetes: the Diabetes Study of Northern California (DISTANCE). *Journal of General Internal Medicine,* 26, 170–176.

Flattery, J., Gambatese, R., Schlag, R., Goldman, L., Bartzen, M., Reyes, J., Martinez, A. Derry, M., Fuller, L., Moore, P., Chase, C., Giboyeaux, S., Lampkin, K., Adams, H., Meyers, K., Peterson, R., Rao, T., Barber, V., Ranshaw, C., ... Sandel, C. (1994). Lead poisoning associated with use of traditional ethnic remedies: California, 1991 through 1992. *Ethnicity & Disease, 4*(1), 95–97.

Foronda, C., Baptiste, D. L., Reinholdt, M. M., & Ousman, K. (2016). Cultural humility: A concept analysis. *Journal of Transcultural Nursing, 27*(3), 210–217.

Foster, G. M. (1953). Relationships between Spanish and Spanish-American folk medicine. *The Journal of American Folklore, 66*(261), 201–217.

Foster, G. M. (1987). On the origin of humoral medicine in Latin America. *Medical Anthropology Quarterly, 1,* 355–393. https://doi.org/10.1525/maq.1987.1.4.02a00020

Fox, M. T., Godage, S. K., Kim, J. M., Bossano, C., Muñoz-Blanco, S., Reinhardt, E., ... & DeCamp, L. R. (2020). Moving from knowledge to action: improving safety and quality of care for patients with limited English proficiency. *Clinical Pediatrics,* 59(3), 266–277.

Fugère, M. A., Escoto, C., Cousins, A. J., Riggs, M. L., & Haerich, P. (2008). Sexual attitudes and double standards: A literature review focusing on participant gender and ethnic background. *Sexuality & Culture, 12,* 169–182.

Gallegos, P. V., & Ferdman, B. M. (2007). Identity orientations of Latinos in the United States. *The Business Journal of Hispanic Research, 1*(1), 26–41.

Gallo, L. C. (2009). The reserve capacity model as a framework for understanding psychosocial factors in health disparities. *Applied Psychology: Health and Well-Being, 1*(1), 62–72.

Gallo, L. C., Penedo, F. J., Espinosa de los Monteros, K., & Arguelles, W. (2009a). Resiliency in the face of disadvantage: do Hispanic cultural characteristics protect health outcomes? *Journal of Personality, 77*(6), 1707–1746.

Gallo, L. C., de Los Monteros, K. E., & Shivpuri, S. (2009b). Socioeconomic status and health: What is the role of reserve capacity? *Current Directions in Psychological Science, 18*(5), 269–274.

García-Hernández, K. Y., Vibrans, H., Colunga-GarcíaMarín, P., Vargas-Guadarrama, L. A., Soto-Hernández, M., Katz, E., & Luna-Cavazos, M. (2021). Climate and categories: Two key elements for understanding the Mesoamerican hot-cold classification of illnesses and medicinal plants. *Journal of Ethnopharmacology, 266,* Article 113419.

Gil, R. M., & Vazquez, C. I. (2014). *The Maria paradox: How Latinas can merge old world traditions with new world self-esteem.* Open Road Media.

Goebert, D. (2008). Social support, mental health, minorities, and acculturative stress. In S. Loue & M. Sajatovic (Eds.), *Determinants of minority mental health and wellness* (pp. 1–24). Springer.

González, H. M., Vega, W. A., & Tarraf, W. (2010). Health care quality perceptions among foreign-born Latinos and the importance of speaking the same language. *The Journal of the American Board of Family Medicine, 23*(6), 745–752.

Gorman, B. K., Read, J. N. G., & Krueger, P. M. (2010). Gender, acculturation, and health among Mexican Americans. *Journal of Health and Social Behavior, 51*(4), 440–457.

Grau, J. M., Azmitia, M., & Quattlebaum, J. (2009). Latino families. *Handbook of US Latino psychology: Developmental and community-based perspectives,* 153.

Guerra, F. (1966). Aztec medicine. *Medical History, 10*(4), 315–338.

Hough, R. (1983). The Los Angeles Epidemiologic Catchment Area research program and the epidemiology of psychiatric disorders among Mexican Americans. *Journal of Operational Psychiatry, 14*(1), 42–51.

Hsueh, L., Hirsh, A. T., Maupomé, G., & Stewart, J. C. (2021). Patient-provider language concordance and health outcomes: A systematic review, evidence map, and research agenda. *Medical Care Research and Review, 78*(1), 3–23.

Jacobs, E. A., Karavolos, K., Rathouz, P. J., Ferris, T. G., & Powell, L. H. (2005). Limited English proficiency and breast and cervical cancer screening in a multiethnic population. *American Journal of Public Health, 95*(8), 1410–1416.

Jones, B. L., Grendell, M. K., Bezzant, J. M., Russell, K. A., Williams, B. W., Jensen, L., Peterson, C., Pyper, B., Muh, J., & Taylor, Z. E. (2022). Stress and health outcomes in midwestern Latinx youth: The moderating role of ethnic pride. International *Journal of Environmental Research and Public Health, 19*(24), 16966.

Kanter, M. H., Abrams, K. M., Carrasco, M. R., Spiegel, N. H., Vogel, R. S., & Coleman, K. J. (2009). Patient-physician language concordance: A strategy for meeting the needs of Spanish-speaking patients in primary care. *The Permanente Journal, 13*(4), 79–84.

Kay, M. A. (1993). Fallen fontanelle: Culture-bound or cross-cultural? *Medical Anthropology, 15*(2), 137–156.

Keeler, A. R., Siegel, J. T., & Alvaro, E. M. (2014). Depression and help seeking among Mexican-Americans: The mediating role of familism. *Journal of Immigrant and Minority Health, 16*, 1225–1231.

Kibakaya, E. C., & Oyeku, S. O. (2022). Cultural humility: A critical step in achieving health equity. *Pediatrics, 149*(2), Article 35098316.

Kim, S., Rodríguez-Guzmán, V. M., Hamm, T., & Nugent, N. R. (2021). Childhood trauma and the role of ethnic pride and interpersonal relationships among Latina mothers. *Psychological Trauma: Theory, Research, Practice, and Policy, 13*(1), 26–34.

Knight, G.P., Bernal, M.E., Cota, M.K., Garza, C.A., & Ocampo, K.A. (1993a). Family socialization and Mexican American identity and behavior. In G.P. Knight & M.E. Bernal (Eds.), *Ethnic identity*. Albany, NY: State University of New York Press.

Knight, G. P., Cota, M. K., & Bernal, M. E. (1993b). The socialization of cooperative, competitive, and individualistic preferences among Mexican American children: The mediating role of ethnic identity. *Hispanic Journal of Behavioral Sciences, 15*(3), 291–309.

Krogstad, J.M., Alvarado, J. & Mohamed, B. (2023). Among U.S. Latinos, Catholicism continues to decline but is still the largest faith. Pew Research Center, April 17, 2024. Accessed from https://www.pewresearch.org/religion/2023/04/13/among-u-s-latinos-catholicism-continues-to-decline-but-is-still-the-largest-faith/

Lantz, P. M., Dupuis, L., Reding, D., Krauska, M., & Lappe, K. (1994). Peer discussions of cancer among Hispanic migrant farm workers. *Public Health Reports, 109*(4), 512–520.

Lopez Austin, A. (1980). *Cuerpo humano e ideologia: Las concepciones de los antiguos Nahuas*. Universidad Nacional Autonoma de Mexico. Mexico.

Luthar, S. S., & Cicchetti, D. (2000). The construct of resilience: Implications for interventions and social policies. *Development and Psychopathology, 12*, 857–885.

Luthar, S. S., Cicchetti, D., & Becker, B. (2000). The construct of resilience: A critical evaluation and guidelines for future work. *Child Development, 71*, 543–562.

Maduro, R. (1983). Curanderismo and Latino views of disease and curing. *Western Journal of Medicine, 139* (6), 868–874.

Maldonado, A., Preciado, A., Buchanan, M., Pulvers, K., Romero, D., & D'Anna-Hernandez, K. (2018). Acculturative stress, mental health symptoms, and the role of salivary inflammatory markers among a Latino sample. *Cultural Diversity and Ethnic Minority Psychology, 24*(2), 277–283.

Marin, G. (1992). Issues in the measurement of acculturation among Hispanics. In K. F. Geisinger (Ed.), *Psychological testing of Hispanics* (pp. 235–251). American Psychological Association.

Marín, G., & Gamba, R. J. (2003). Acculturation and changes in cultural values. In K. M. Chun, P. Balls Organista, & G. Marín (Eds.), *Acculturation: Advances in theory, measurement, and applied research* (pp. 83–93). American Psychological Association.

Marin, G., & Marin, B. V. (1991). *Research with Hispanic populations*. SAGE.

Masgoret, A. M., & Ward, C. (2006). Culture learning approach to acculturation. In D. L. Sam & J. W. Berry (Eds.), *The Cambridge handbook of acculturation psychology* (pp. 58–77). Cambridge University Press.

Messer, E. (1987). The hot and cold in Mesoamerican Indigenous and Hispanicized thought. *Social Science and Medicine, 25*(4), 339–346.

Mirandé, A. (2018). *Hombres y machos: Masculinity and Latino culture*. Routledge.

Mossakowski, K. N. (2003). Coping with perceived discrimination: Does ethnic identity protect mental health? *Journal of Health and Social Behavior, 44*(3), 318–331.

Ortiz de Montellano, B. R. (1990). *Aztec medicine, health, and nutrition*. Rutgers University Press.

Padilla, A. M. (1980). The role of cultural awareness and ethnic loyalty in acculturation. In A. M. Padilla (Ed.), *Acculturation: Theory, models and some new findings* (pp. 47–84). Westview

Padilla, A. M. (1987). Acculturation and stress among immigrants and later generation individuals. In D. Frick (Ed.), *The quality of urban life: Social, psychological, and physical conditions* (pp. 101–120). Walter de Gruyter.

Padilla, A. M., & Perez, W. (2003). Acculturation, social identity, and social cognition: A new perspective. *Hispanic Journal of Behavioral Sciences, 25*(1), 35–55.

Padilla, R., Gomez, V., Biggerstaff, S. L., & Mehler, P. S. (2001). Use of curanderismo in a public health care system. *Archives of Internal Medicine, 161*(10), 1336–1340.

Parker, M. M., Fernández, A., Moffet, H. H., Grant, R. W., Torreblanca, A., & Karter, A. J. (2017). Association of patient-physician language concordance and glycemic control for limited-English proficiency Latinos with type 2 diabetes. *JAMA Internal Medicine, 177*(3), 380–387.

Perez-Stable, E. J., Sabogal, F., Otero-Sabogal, R., Hiatt, R. A., & McPhee, S. J. (1992). Misconceptions about cancer among Latinos and Anglos. *JAMA, 268*(22), 3219–3223.

Portillo, E. N., Stack, A. M., Monuteaux, M. C., Curt, A., Perron, C., & Lee, L. K. (2021). Association of limited English proficiency and increased pediatric emergency department revisits. *Academic Emergency Medicine, 28*(9), 1001–1011.

Purnell, L., & Paulanka, B. (1998). *Transcultural health care: A culturally competent approach*. F. A. Davis.

Phinney, J. S. (1996). Understanding ethnic diversity: The role of ethnic identity. *American Behavioral Scientist, 40*(2), 143–152.

Piña-Watson, B., Gonzalez, I. M., & Manzo, G. (2019). Mexican-descent adolescent resilience through familismo in the context of intergeneration acculturation conflict on depressive symptoms. *Translational Issues in Psychological Science, 5*(4), 326.

Quintero, G. A., & Estrada, A. L. (1998). Cultural models of masculinity and drug use: "Machismo," heroin, and street survival on the U.S.-Mexico border. *Contemporary Drug Problems, 25*, 147–168.

Ramírez, A. S. (2014). Fatalism and cancer risk knowledge among a sample of highly acculturated Latinas. *Journal of Cancer Education, 29*, 50–55.

Ramírez, A. S., Rutten, L. J. F., Oh, A., Vengoechea, B. L., Moser, R. P., Vanderpool, R. C., & Hesse, B. W. (2013). Perceptions of cancer controllability and cancer risk knowledge: The moderating role of race, ethnicity, and acculturation. *Journal of Cancer Education, 28*, 254–261.

Romero, A. J., Cuéllar, I., & Roberts, R. E. (2000). Ethnocultural variables and attitudes toward cultural socialization of children. *Journal of Community Psychology, 28*(1), 79–89.

Romero, A., & Pina-Watson, B. (2017). Acculturative stress and bicultural stress: Psychological measurement and mental health. In S. J. Schwartz & J. B. Unger (Eds.), *The Oxford handbook of acculturation and health* (pp. 119–133). Oxford University Press.

Rubel, A. J., O'Nell, C. W., & Collado-Ardon, R. (1991). *Susto: A folk illness* (Vol. 12). University of California Press.

Rudmin, F. (2009). Constructs, measurements and models of acculturation and acculturative stress. *International Journal of Intercultural Relations, 33*(2), 106–123.

Rudmin, F. W. (2003). Critical history of the acculturation psychology of assimilation, separation, integration, and marginalization. *Review of General Psychology, 7*(1), 3–37.

Rutter, M. (2006). Implications of resilience concepts for scientific understanding. *Annals of the New York Academy of Sciences, 1094*(1), 1–12.

Sanchez, J. I., & Fernandez, D. M. (1993). Acculturative stress among Hispanics: A bidimensional model of ethnic identification. *Journal of Applied Social Psychology, 23*(8), 654–668.

Santana, K. (2007). The Quinceñera rising: Self-discoveries on the heels of city and rural town. *Human Architecture: Journal of the Sociology of Self-Knowledge, 5*(2).

Schwartz, S. J., & Unger, J. B. (2017). Acculturation and health: state of the field and recommended directions. In S. J. Schwartz and J. B. Unger (Eds.), *Oxford Handbook of Acculturation and Health* (pp. 1–14). Oxford University Press.

Shern, D. L., Blanch, A. K., & Steverman, S. M. (2016). Toxic stress, behavioral health, and the next major era in public health. *American Journal of Orthopsychiatry, 86*(2), 109.

Shonkoff, J. P., Garner, A. S., Committee on Psychosocial Aspects of Child and Family Health, Committee on Early Childhood, Adoption, and Dependent Care, and Section on Developmental and Behavioral Pediatrics, Siegel, B. S., Dobbins, M. I., Earls, M. F., Garner, A. S., McGuinn, L., Pascoe, J., & Wood, D. L. (2012). The lifelong effects of early childhood adversity and toxic stress. *Pediatrics, 129*(1), e232–e246.

Shonkoff, J. P., Slopen, N., & Williams, D. R. (2021). Early childhood adversity, toxic stress, and the impacts of racism on the foundations of health. *Annual Review of Public Health, 42*, 115–134.

Spence, N. D., Wells, S., Graham, K., & George, J. (2016). Racial discrimination, cultural resilience, and stress. *The Canadian Journal of Psychiatry, 61*(5), 298–307.

Stein, G. L., Cupito, A. M., Mendez, J. L., Prandoni, J., Huq, N., & Westerberg, D. (2014). Familism through a developmental lens. *Journal of Latina/o Psychology, 2*(4), 224.

Stevens, E. (1973). Machismo and marianismo. *Society, 10*, 57–63.

Stewart, M. J., Hirth, A. M., Klassen, G., Makrides, L., & Wolf, H. (1997). Stress, coping, and social support as psychosocial factors in readmissions for ischemic heart disease. *International Journal of Nursing Studies, 34*(2), 151–163.

Stubbe, D. E. (2020). Practicing cultural competence and cultural humility in the care of diverse patients. *Focus, 18*(1), 49–51.

Timmins, C. L. (2002). The impact of language barriers on the health care of Latinos in the United States: a review of the literature and guidelines for practice. *Journal of Midwifery & Women's Health*, 47(2), 80–96.

Torres, L. (2010). Predicting levels of Latino depression: acculturation, acculturative stress, and coping. *Cultural Diversity and Ethnic Minority Psychology, 16*(2), 256–263.

Torres, L., Driscoll, M. W., & Voell, M. (2012). Discrimination, acculturation, acculturative stress, and Latino psychological distress: A moderated mediational model. *Cultural Diversity and Ethnic Minority Psychology, 18*(1), 17–25.

Trotter, R. (1985). Greta and azarcon: A survey of episodic lead poisoning from a folk remedy. *Human Organization, 44*(1), 64–72.

Trotter, R. T., de Montellano, B. O., & Logan, M. H. (1989). Fallen fontanelle in the American Southwest: Its origin, epidemiology, and possible organic causes. *Medical Anthropology, 10*(4), 211–221.

Umaña-Taylor, A. J., & Fine, M. A. (2004). Examining ethnic identity among Mexican-origin adolescents living in the United States. *Hispanic Journal of Behavioral Sciences, 26*(1), 36–59.

Umaña-Taylor, A. J., & Updegraff, K. A. (2013). Latino families in the United States. In *Handbook of marriage and the family* (723–747). Boston, MA: Springer US.

Ungar, M. (Ed.). (2011). *The social ecology of resilience: A handbook of theory and practice.* Springer Science & Business Media.

Unger, J. B., & Schwartz, S. J. (2012). Conceptual considerations in studies of cultural influences on health behaviors. *Preventive Medicine, 55*(5), 353–355.

Vega, W. A., Alderete, E., Kolody, B., & Aguilar-Gaxiola, S. (1998). Illicit drug use among Mexicans and Mexican Americans in California: The effects of gender and acculturation. *Addiction, 93*(12), 1839–1850.

Villalobos, B. T., Bridges, A. J., Anastasia, E. A., Ojeda, C. A., Hernandez Rodriguez, J., & Gomez, D. (2016). Effects of language concordance and interpreter use on therapeutic alliance in Spanish-speaking integrated behavioral health care patients. *Psychological Services, 13*(1), 49–59.

Wallace, P. M., Pomery, E. A., Latimer, A. E., Martinez, J. L., & Salovey, P. (2010). A review of acculturation measures and their utility in studies promoting Latino health. *Hispanic Journal of Behavioral Sciences, 32*(1), 37–54.

Ward, C. (1999). Models and measurements of acculturation. In. W. J. Lonner, D. L. Dinnel, D. K. Fograys, & S. A. Hayes (Eds.), *Merging past, present and future in cross cultural psychology* (pp. 221–230). CRC Press.

Ward, C., & Kagitcibasi, C. (2010). Introduction to "Acculturation theory, research and application: Working with and for communities." *International Journal of Intercultural Relations, 34*(2), 97–100.

Weller, S. C., Baer, R. D., Garcia de Alba Garcia, J., & Salcedo Rocha, A. L. (2008). Susto and nervios: Expressions for stress and depression. *Culture, Medicine, and Psychiatry, 32*, 406–420.

Yosso, T. J. (2005). Whose culture has capital? A critical race theory discussion of community cultural wealth. *Race Ethnicity and Education, 8*(1), 69–91.

Yosso, T. J. (2006). *Critical race counterstories along the Chicana/Chicano educational pipeline.* Routledge.

Yosso, T. J. & Burciaga, R. (2016, June). *Reclaiming our histories, recovering community cultural wealth.* Center for Critical Race Studies.

Yosso, T. J., & García, D. G. (2007). "This is no slum!": A critical race theory analysis of community cultural wealth in Culture Clash's Chavez Ravine. *Aztlan: A Journal of Chicano Studies, 32*(1), 145–179.

Figure Credits

Fig. 4.2a: John Walker, "Full Moon," https://commons.wikimedia.org/wiki/File:Penumbral_lunar_eclipse_Aug_6_2009_John_Walker.gif, 2009.

Fig. 4.2b: Copyright © by Luc Viatour (CC BY-SA 3.0) at https://commons.wikimedia.org/wiki/File:Man_in_the_Moon.jpg.

Fig. 4.2c: Copyright © 2018 Depositphotos/kwasny222.

Fig. 4.2d: Copyright © 2018 Depositphotos/kwasny222.

Fig. 4.3a: Copyright © by Gerbil (CC BY-SA 3.0) at https://commons.wikimedia.org/wiki/File:Rabbit_(agouti)_03.jpg.

Fig. 4.3b: Copyright © by James Heilman, MD (CC by 3.0) at https://commons.wikimedia.org/wiki/File:Cleftlipandpalate.JPG.

Fig. 4.4: Copyright © by Wellcome Trust (CC by 4.0) at https://commons.wikimedia.org/wiki/File:Antiquities_of_Mexico,_1831;_Aztec_zodiac_man_Wellcome_L0020862.jpg.

Fig. 4.5: Copyright © 2017 Depositphotos/celiafoto.

Fig. 4.6: Copyright © 2021 Depositphotos/Sakurra.

Fig. 4.8: Arthur R. Andrews III, Ana J. Bridges, and Debbie Gomez, "Unidimensional and Bidimensional Acculturation Models," *Journal of Transcultural Nursing*, vol. 24, no. 2, p. 14. Copyright © 2013 by SAGE Publications.

Fig. 4.9: Israel Cuellar, Bill Arnold, and Roberto Maldonado, "Acculturation Rating Scale for Mexican Americans II," *Hispanic Journal of Behacioral Sciences*. Copyright © 1995 by SAGE Publications.

CHAPTER 5

Paradigms and Paradoxes

Theories of Health Inequalities Among Mexican Americans

LEARNING OBJECTIVES

- Discuss the conceptual differences between health disparities and health inequalities.
- Describe several social justice applications in public health.
- Evaluate the efficacy of several important areas of investigation within socioenvironmental theories of health inequalities.
- Assess important areas of investigation within psychosocial/behavioral theories of health inequalities and their application to Mexican Americans.
- Argue some of the pros and cons of the Mexican American mortality paradox.
- Explain genetic and physiological theories of health inequalities. Do they move beyond theories of inherent racial bias? Are any applicable to Mexican Americans?

A fundamental understanding of the health paradigms associated with theories or hypotheses of health inequalities is important in understanding the potential underlying mechanisms that lead to increased incidence and prevalence of disease in historically marginalized and disenfranchised populations in the United States. This chapter highlights several health paradigms and hypotheses relevant to Latino health. Readers will gain an appreciation of their utility in developing theory-driven risk reduction interventions commonly used in implementation science with Latinos.

Health Disparities or Health Inequalities?

What is the difference, if any, between a health disparity and a health inequality? Is one more organic than the other? Do the terms "disparity" and "inequality" accurately describe the underlying factors that may contribute to each together or separately?

The National Institutes of Health (2002) defined *health disparities* as "differences in incidence, prevalence, mortality, and burden of diseases and other adverse health conditions that exist among specific population groups in the United States" (p. 7).

It's not too difficult to understand incidence and prevalence, but does the definition refer to premature mortality or mortality in general? *Premature mortality* or "years of life lost" have known underlying sociocultural factors (e.g., poverty) as well as physiological contributors in the social and built environment (e.g., psychosocial stressors, exposure to environmental pollution). Additionally, what is meant by "burden of diseases and other adverse conditions"? The *burden of diseases* refers to the cumulative effects of higher disease incidence, prevalence, disability, and mortality associated with low-SES and historically marginalized populations, who carry a heavier burden of chronic and infectious diseases. *Adverse health conditions* arise from socioeconomic inequities, age-related injuries, lack of access to quality health care, and living environments that increase exposure to hazardous substances.

Health inequalities derive from the complex interplay of historical, social, geopolitical, and biological exposure to toxic environments, both physical and psychosocial. *Health inequalities* are defined as the systematic, avoidable, and unjust differences in the health and well-being of historically marginalized and disenfranchised populations. The perpetuation of unequal access to resources is seen as the fundamental cause of health inequalities (LaVeist, 2011). From this perspective, health inequalities are *created* by the social environment, while health disparities simply *exist.* One of the major goals of public health is to eliminate health inequalities through the practice and application of social justice. *Social justice* in public health seeks to enhance physical health and mental well-being through corrective (and collective) action focused on sociocultural health determinants. Examples include the use of *promotoras de salud* (community health workers) to foster health promotion and disease prevention among Latinos who lack access to health care (Pérez & Martinez, 2008).

Health equity is a value defined by the American Public Health Association (n.d.) that occurs when "everyone has the opportunity to attain their highest level of health" (para. 1). It would be better to eliminate barriers to attaining one's highest level of health in addition to providing opportunities to achieve it. Health equity and health equality differ in that one seeks to eliminate barriers to health in one instance while the other seeks to provide opportunities (supports) to achieve it.

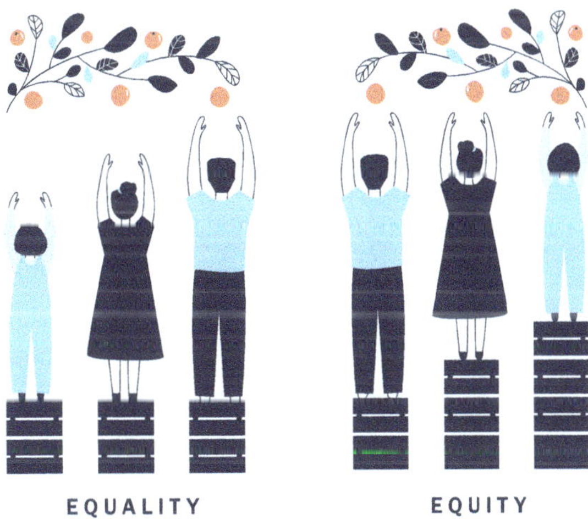

FIGURE 5.1 Equality Versus Equity

In Figure 5.1, equality and equity are compared. *Equality* signifies the provision of the same support for everyone: Everyone is being treated equally but not equitably. Equity addresses systemic barriers and advocates for their removal so that everyone has the same access. Focusing attention on those barriers in the physical, social, and cultural environment that are amenable to change can foster and develop opportunities for everyone to attain their highest level of physiological and psychological well-being (Braveman et al., 2011).

Theories of Health Inequalities Among Historically Marginalized Populations

Grounded within the social determinants of health (SDOH) framework, several theories of health inequalities call critical attention to examining how social disadvantage, racism and discrimination, and gene-environment interactions initiate, converge, and persist to produce disease. Three general types of health inequality theories or paradigms have been proposed in the scientific literature that examine the "root causes" of health inequalities, including socioenvironmental theories of health inequalities, psychosocial or behavioral theories of health inequalities, and genetic and physiological theories of health inequalities (LaVeist, 2011) (Table 5.1). Context and place are crucial in many of these theories, where the interaction of race, gender, socioeconomic status (SES), and age create oppressive cycles of health inequalities.

TABLE 5.1 Paradigms and Paradoxes—Theories of Health Inequalities

Socioenvironmental theories of health inequalities	Psychosocial/behavioral theories of health inequalities	Genetic and physiological theories of health inequalities
Racial/ethnic segregation	Racial discrimination and prejudice (biopsychosocial racism model)	Biological or genetic differences among racial/ethnic groups (BRCA1 & 2)
Risk exposure theory "riskscapes"	Immigration and acculturation hypotheses	Biogenetic-environment interactions (epigenetic clocks and aging)
Resource deprivation theory	Latino epidemiologic paradox and related hypotheses	Socio-epigenetic processes (intergenerational trauma)

Adapted from LaVeist (2011, p. 133)

Socioenvironmental Theories of Health Inequalities

Social disadvantage is the main driver of socioenvironmental theories of health inequalities among historically marginalized populations in the United States. *Social disadvantage* includes many of the SDOH discussed in previous chapters, like poverty, low educational attainment, racial and ethnic segregation, environmental pollution, and disordered neighborhoods. Social disadvantage contributes to health inequalities through restricting equitable health care access and perpetuating social exclusion, urban isolation and decay, rural pockets of persistent poverty, and limited financial opportunities. According to the U.S. Code of Federal Regulations:

> Socially disadvantaged individuals are those who have been subjected to racial or ethnic prejudice or cultural bias within American society because of their identities as members of groups and without regard to their individual qualities. The social disadvantage must stem from circumstances beyond their control. (13 C.F.R. § 124.103)

This definition includes Latinos, non-Latino Black Americans, Native Americans, and certain Asian and Pacific Islander populations. Increased vulnerability to disease is enhanced by poor living environments and undermining the social determinants of historically marginalized populations through policies of deceit, misappropriation, racism, and discrimination. In general, concentrated, and persistent poverty is associated with poorer health outcomes among Latinos, especially those residing in the U.S.-Mexico border region. But cultural resiliency inclusive of familism, *respeto*, and religiosity appears to moderate the deleterious effects on physical health and psychological well-being among Latinos of Mexican descent (Ruiz et al., 2013; Andrade et al., 2021).

Racial and Ethnic Segregation

Racial and ethnic segregation is primarily de facto in the United States and occurs regularly through restriction of affordable housing. As noted in previous chapters, "place" is a powerful social determinant of health. Place can have both positive and enhancing influences on SDOH or negative and detrimental influences on the health of individuals and populations.

Toxic stress is defined as a high allostatic load produced through the biopsychosocial response to psychosocial stress and stressors (Shonkoff & Garner, 2012; Shanks & Robinson, 2013; McEwen, 2022). The inability to adequately cope with external psychosocial stressors leads to high allostatic load and, inevitably, toxic stress.

Massey and colleagues provide a useful conceptual model on how residential segregation and socio-economic inequality increases allostatic load (i.e., toxic stress) and chronic illnesses like coronary heart disease among low-SES and residentially segregated communities (Massey 2004; Massey & Wagner, 2018, Massey et al., 2018).

The *biosocial model of racial stratification* (*BMRS*) hypothesizes that the persistence and duration of living in a stressful environment (e.g., in areas where there is concentrated and persistent poverty and residential segregation), coupled with a disorganized social environment, increases allostatic load, culminating in negative physiological and psychological effects on the individual, especially over the long term (Araújo & Borell, 2006; Massey & Wagner, 2018) (see Figure 5.2).

Some research suggests that similar socioenvironmental stressors exist in the U.S.-Mexico border region with high prevalence rates of depression, anxiety, fear of deportation and family separation, and constant surveillance by Homeland Security (Carvajal et al., 2013; Sabo et al., 2014). However, more research is necessary to confirm if there is a causal link between exposure to this specific regional environment and higher rates of psychological disorders and cerebrovascular disease.

Numerous studies have confirmed that racial and ethnic segregation among non-Latino Black Americans creates unequal access to needed goods and services, including health care, healthy food, and safe

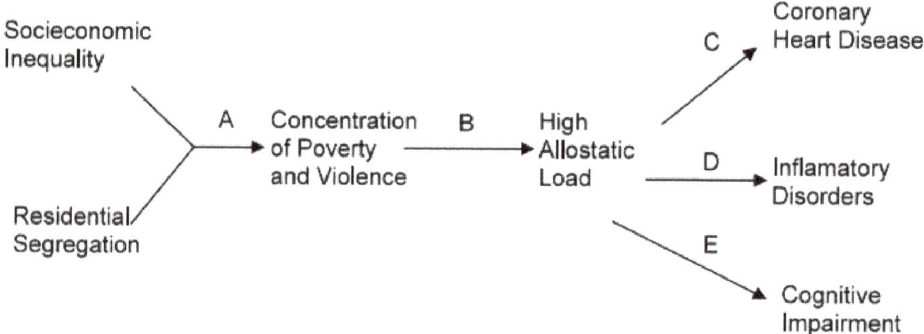

FIGURE 5.2 Massey's Biosocial Model of Racial Stratification (BMRS)

living environments (Arnett et al., 2016; Gaskin et al., 2009, 2014; Kramer & Hogue, 2009, LaVeist & Issac, 2012; LaVeist et al., 2011; White & Borrell, 2011; Xiao & Graham, 2019; Yang et al., 2017). For example, Gaskin et al. (2009) suggests that disparities in health care utilization are related to both individuals' racial and ethnic identity and the racial and ethnic composition of their communities. Ethnic composition is not necessarily the same as ethnic segregation: The first looks at the proportion of racial/ethnic mix in a neighborhood, while the second looks at spatial differences across neighborhoods among racial/ethnic groups (Lee et al., 2014; Yang et al., 2020). Most of the research on racial/ethnic segregation is focused on Black-White differences in health outcomes, with relatively little attention focused on the systematic investigation of Latino segregation and physical or psychological well-being (Acevedo-Garcia et al., 2003).

Demographic data indicates that Latinos have become increasingly segregated since 1980, with higher concentrations of Latinos than other racial/ethnic groups (see Chapter 3). Findings suggest that Latino-White segregation is complex and different from Black-White segregation with more informal structural supports, social cohesion, traditional food consumption, and overall cultural wealth (Yang et al., 2017). According to the *Latino immigrant social ties theory* (Viruell-Fuentes et al., 2013), Latino immigrants choose to live in closer proximity to one another to maximize their social capital and capitalize on their collective cultural wealth. Health outcomes associated with segregation, then, may be qualitatively different for Latinos than for non-Latino Black Americans.

Alternatively, racial, and ethnic enclaves can hinder the consumption of healthier foods and increase food insecurity (Grigsby-Toussaint et al., 2010). For example, a study conducted by Grigsby-Toussaint et al. (2010) found that neighborhood stores in which most residents were non-Latino Black or Latino were more likely to carry fresh fruits and vegetables that were culturally relevant. However, most neighborhood stores had less than 50% of the commonly consumed or culturally specific fruits and vegetables, which limited access to a healthier diet.

Findings from studies investigating the association between segregation, ethnic density, and health among Latinos are mixed. For example, Plascak et al. (2016) found that self-rated health status among Latinos residing in Washington state improved with increased Latino segregation and decreased with increased non-Latino integration. Other studies have found that health effects vary within Latino subgroups, with Latinos of Puerto Rican descent showing some of the more negative effects of segregation and high density, while Latinos of Mexican descent, especially second generation and higher, have better health outcomes with increasing ethnic segregation (Bécares, 2014; Eshbach et al., 2004; Franzini & Spears, 2003; Hong et al., 2014; Inagami et al., 2006; Nelson, 2013; Ostir et al., 2003; Patel et al., 2003). However, Eshbach et al. (2004) found that living in Latino ethnic enclaves within 50 miles of the U.S.-Mexico border increased mortality among older Mexican Americans.

Taken together, the available empirical evidence suggests a complex interaction between ethnicity, generational status, years lived in the United States, and place among Mexican Americans. Racial segregation appears to have a strong negative health impact among non-Latino Black Americans, but the same cannot be said for some Latino subgroups. In fact, Latino ethnic enclaves appear to have a more positive health impact among Latinos in the context of higher ethnic segregation and lower income—a paradoxical finding. Cultural wealth, including community empowerment, cultural resilience, and social capital, are important factors that may partially explain some of the observed differences in health outcomes between non-Latino Black Americans and Mexican Americans (i.e., the Latino mortality paradox; Abraido-Lanza et al. 1999; Andrade et al., 2021; Arellano-Morales et al. 2015; Cobb et al., 2021).

Risk Exposure Theory—"Riskscapes"

Risk exposure theory proposes that historically marginalized populations encounter more physical and psychosocial environmental stressors than non-Latino White Americans by virtue of the geospatial environments in which they live. Intersectionality and critical race theory (CRT) assess the cumulative and interactional effects of race, ethnicity, gender, and SES in producing differential negative health outcomes. There is no question that "place" is the confluence of these oppressive identities that converge to create potentially life-threatening environments.

As noted previously, residential segregation confers both physical and psychosocial neighborhood risks. A term coined by Morello-Frosch et al. (2001) aptly describes these neighborhoods and community environments as *riskscapes* (i.e., those neighborhood environments that have a higher-than-normal distribution of traffic congestion, air pollution, waste management sites, EPA Superfund sites, increased crime, and other forms of social disorder). Morello-Frosch et al. (2011) hypothesize that there are four key concepts that highlight the importance of *riskscapes* among historically marginalized populations:

- Several types of chronic diseases (e.g., diabetes mellitus, heart disease) are linked to social disadvantage and poor physical environments.
- Exposure to environmental risks are persistent and are linked to negative health outcomes.
- Intrinsic biological and physiological factors can modify the effects of environmental factors and independently contribute to variations in the frequency and severity of diseases related to the social and physical environment.
- Extrinsic social vulnerability factors at the individual and community level may amplify the negative effects of socioenvironmental hazards and contribute to health inequalities found among historically marginalized populations. (p. 880)

Historically marginalized populations are more likely than others to live in environments that expose them to psychosocial stressors and environmental risks (Hajat et al., 2015; LaVeist et al., 2009; Pratt et al., 2015; Woo et al., 2019). A study by Chambliss et al. (2021) found higher concentrations of air pollutants in Latino and non-Latino Black residential areas than in non-Latino White residential areas, sometimes 8–30 times higher than the population average. Similarly, Jones et al. (2014) found that living in majority non-Latino White neighborhoods was associated with lower air pollution exposures, while living in majority Latino neighborhoods was associated with higher air pollution exposures. Environmental studies clearly show that higher concentrations of air pollution are associated with increased upper respiratory diseases, heart disease, and cancer.

The most comprehensive examination of place and risk exposure are the suite of studies from the Multi-Ethnic Study of Atherosclerosis (MESA), a prospective, longitudinal study of men and women in Los Angeles County, California; St. Paul, Minnesota; Chicago, Illinois; Forsyth County, North Carolina; Baltimore, Maryland; and New York, New York (Kaiser et al., 2016). Examination of incident hypertension, carotid artery health, coronary artery calcium, overall cardiovascular health, overall cardiovascular disease with neighborhood composition (segregation), neighborhood stressors, identified differential results in relation to Geographic Information System (GIS) data available to the study (a data system with information on density of food stores and recreational resources in the community). For hypertension, after adjusting for individual characteristics (i.e., age, sex, income, race, etc.), survey-based healthy food availability and walking environment were found to be predictors of hypertension risk, whereas GIS-based food environment and physical activity environment scores were not (Kaiser et al., 2016). The incidence of hypertension was found to be highest for non-Latino White Americans (39%), followed by non-Latino Black Americans (26.1%), and Latino Americans (22.7%).

In another study using MESA data (Mujahid et al., 2011), the prevalence of hypertension was found to be 59.5% for non-Latino Black Americans, 43.9% for Latinos, and 42.0% for non-Latino White Americans. Several chronic stressors were examined including chronic life stressors, perceived major discrimination, everyday discrimination, and neighborhood stressors in relation to the prevalence of hypertension. They found that the chronic stressors affected non-Latino White Americans the least, non-Latino Black Americans moderately, and Latino Americans the most. However, non-Latino Black Americans reported more perceived major and everyday discrimination versus non-Latino White Americans, whereas Latino Americans reported levels of major and everyday discrimination similar to non-Latino White Americans (Mujahid et al., 2011).

In the examination of carotid artery health and air pollution, a study by Jones et al. (2014) found that living in majority Latino (> 60%) neighborhoods was associated with 8% higher PM2.5 (parts/million larger than 2.5mm) and 31% higher nitrous oxide (NOX) exposures than that in neighborhoods with less than 25% Latino population. A study by Kershaw et al. (2015) related to cardiovascular disease and neighborhood segregation found significant differences between non-Latino White Americans and non-Latino Black Americans in the prevalence of cardiovascular disease (CVD). Each unit increase in non-Latino Black segregation was associated with a 12% increase in CVD hazard, even after adjusting for age, sex, and study site. They found that the association did not diminish after additional adjustments for individual SES, physical neighborhood characteristics, social environment, or traditional CVD risk factors. There was no evidence for a link between segregation and CVD incidence in Latinos, however.

Environmental pollution and psychosocial stress foster *riskscapes* that have an undue burden of disease on historically marginalized populations, especially for Latino Americans and non-Latino Black Americans. A complex picture again emerges for Latinos, who appear to benefit from tangible and intangible aspects of social capital, which may modify the effects of environmental and psychosocial stressors on health in the Latino community.

Resource Deprivation Theory—Unequal Access to Resources

Racial/ethnic segregation and areas of heightened risk (real or appraised) that increase susceptibility and vulnerability to disease are integral to understanding how limited resources are differentially allocated and invested. Studies reviewed have shown that residential segregation and social disadvantage limit access to goods and services necessary for physical health and psychological well-being. A large body of research exists on the uneven distribution of resources through processes of social stratification, racism, and discrimination (see Chapter 3). Residential segregation and the creation of *riskscapes* are the consequence of inferior and marginalized social status conferred upon historically marginalized populations by the majority non-Latino White society.

According to LaVeist (2011, p. 141) *Resource deprivation theory* hypothesizes that restricted access to resources increases the probability of negative health outcomes for these populations. It is a historical fact that Mexican Americans have had less access to health care and are more socioeconomically disadvantaged than non-Latino White Americans (see Chapter 3). Latinos are more segregated than non-Latino Black Americans, and a significant proportion of Mexican American children and older adults are exposed to hazardous living environments.

Food insecurity is linked to non-insulin-dependent diabetes mellitus (type 2 diabetes) among Latinas (Fitzgerald et al., 2011). A study by Potochnick et al. (2019) found a very high prevalence of food insecurity among Latino adolescents (42%), compounding their increased risk for developing type 2 diabetes. In 2021, approximately 10.2% of the U.S. population were food insecure, another symptom of unequal access to resources among historically marginalized populations (Coleman-Jensen et al., 2022). Coincidentally, the U.S. Department of Agriculture's Economic Research Service (Rabbitt & Coleman-Jensen, 2017) assessed the effect of interview language on Latinos contrasted with non-Latinos and found no differences in the statistical properties of the food security measure.

An analysis by the Brookings Institution conducted in late June 2020 found that 27.5% of households with children were food insecure, meaning some 14 million children lived in a household characterized by child food insecurity (Bauer et al., 2020). A separate analysis by Schanzenbach and Pitts (2020) found insecurity had more than tripled among households with children to 29.5% during the COVID-19 pandemic. They found that in March and April 2020, food insecurity among U.S. residents more than tripled, to 38% of the population (see Figure 5.3). Overall, food insecurity was highest among non-Latino Black Americans, followed by Latino Americans. Moreover, among adults with income less than 250% of the 2020 poverty level, 44% of all households were food insecure, with the highest rates among Latino households (52%) and non-Latino Black households (48%).

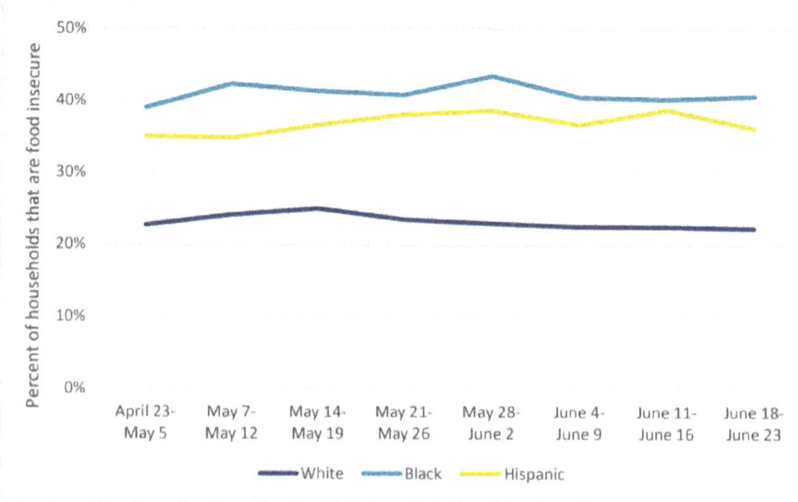

FIGURE 5.3 Food Insecurity in the United States, 2020

Food insecurity had been decreasing since the Great Recession (2009) and prior to the COVID-19 pandemic. According to Coleman-Jensen et al. (2022), in 2021, non-Latino Black Americans and Latino Americans had higher rates of food insecurity than non-Latino White Americans (Table 5.2). The researchers used the U.S. Department of Agriculture's definitions for "low" and "very low" food security. Overall, low, and very low food insecurity among Latinos was twice the rate as non-Latino White Americans (10.7% and 5.5%, compared to 4.4% and 2.6%, respectively).

TABLE 5.2 Food Insecurity by Race/Ethnicity, United States, 2021

	Food insecurity		
Race/ethnicity of households	**All (%)**	**Low food security (%)**	**Very low food security (%)**
Non-Latino White	7.0	4.4	2.6
Non-Latino Black	19.8	11.9	7.9
Latino	16.2	10.7	5.5

Source: Coleman-Jensen et al. (2022)

Food swamps, those places that have an overabundance of poor food options, also contribute to increased morbidity among historically marginalized populations. For example, Bevel and colleagues (2023) analyzed 3,038 U.S. counties and found a dose-response relationship between food swamps and obesity-related cancer mortality among non-Latino Black Americans, with approximately 3 times the rate in high obesity-related cancer mortality counties compared to low obesity-related cancer mortality counties. High-mortality counties had a higher percentage of non-Latino Black residents, a higher percentage of persons older than 65 years, higher poverty rates, higher adult obesity rates, and higher adult diabetes rates compared to counties with low obesity-related cancer mortality. These high-prevalence counties also had higher percentages of persons residing in food deserts and food swamps compared with counties with low obesity-related cancer mortality. Paradoxical findings were obtained for Latino Americans and non-Latino White Americans, however. Findings showed that Latino Americans and non-Latino White Americans had lower obesity related mortality rates in the high-mortality counties and higher obesity-related cancer mortality in lower prevalence counties (see Table 5.3).

TABLE 5.3 Prevalence of Obesity-Related Cancer Mortality in High- and Low-Prevalence Counties by Race/Ethnicity

	Age-adjusted obesity-related cancer mortality rates	
Race/ethnicity	**Low (%)**	**High (%)**
Non-Latino White	86.11	82.85
Non-Latino Black	1.77	3.26
Latino	3.69	2.34

Source: Bevel et al. (2023)

Most research to date shows equivocal results regarding resource deprivation theories and Latinos of Mexican descent. More research is needed on the presumed positive moderating effects of social capital and/or cultural wealth in segregated neighborhoods and their negative health outcomes among Latinos.

Psychosocial/Behavioral Theories of Health Inequalities

In Chapter 1, we discussed the biopsychosocial stress response and the social stress process where psychosocial stress can manifest in psychological symptoms and even modify underlying physiological processes that cause chronic disease within the context of place, like structural discrimination in the form of residential segregation and social stratification (Massey, 2004; Massey & Wagner, 2018).

In this section we examine other theories, like individual and internalized racial discrimination and prejudice (Clark's biopsychosocial racism model), immigration and acculturation theory (Abraido-Lanza et al., 2006, 2016; Alegria et al., 2007, 2008; Lara et al., 2005; Vega et al., 2004; Viruell-Fuentes et al., 2013), and findings related to the Latino mortality paradox (Abraido-Lanza et al., 1999; Elo et al., 2004; Palloni & Arias, 2004; Scriber, 1996; Turra & Elo, 2008; Turra & Goldman, 2007).

Racial and ethnic discrimination is a complex social phenomenon. For example, Brondolo et al. (2009a, 2009b, 2009c) acknowledge several different forms of discrimination, such as personal or group discrimination, as well as several different contexts in which discrimination can be enacted (e.g., school, employment, medical settings). Additionally, personal phenotypic characteristics can lead to the experience of ethnic or racial discrimination. Moreover, racial and ethnic stereotypes can take on a life of their own, which can lead to internalized racism. All these forms of racial and ethnic discrimination are associated with negative physical health status and psychological well-being (Araújo & Borrell, 2006).

Health behaviors are also negatively impacted by racial and ethnic discrimination. The lack of adequate coping resources can manifest in unhealthy coping behaviors, like drug and alcohol use and other risk-taking behaviors that lead to overall poorer health (Cervantes & Castro, 1985).

Racial Discrimination and Prejudice: Biopsychosocial Racism Model (BPRM)

Clark et al. (1999, 2013) provides a theoretical model (the BPRM) on how perceived racism among Non-Latino Black Americans is linked to poor health outcomes (see Figure 5.4). Empirical support for the BPRM among Non-Latino Black Americans substantiates the stress and coping processes involved (Calvin et al., 2003; Cuevas et al., 2014). The experience of discriminatory and racial stressors requires the individual to enable internal and external coping resources. If coping responses are successful, the perception of stress is no longer toxic. If coping responses are unsuccessful, then harmful behaviors and adverse disease outcomes become more prevalent (Pieterse & Powell, 2016).

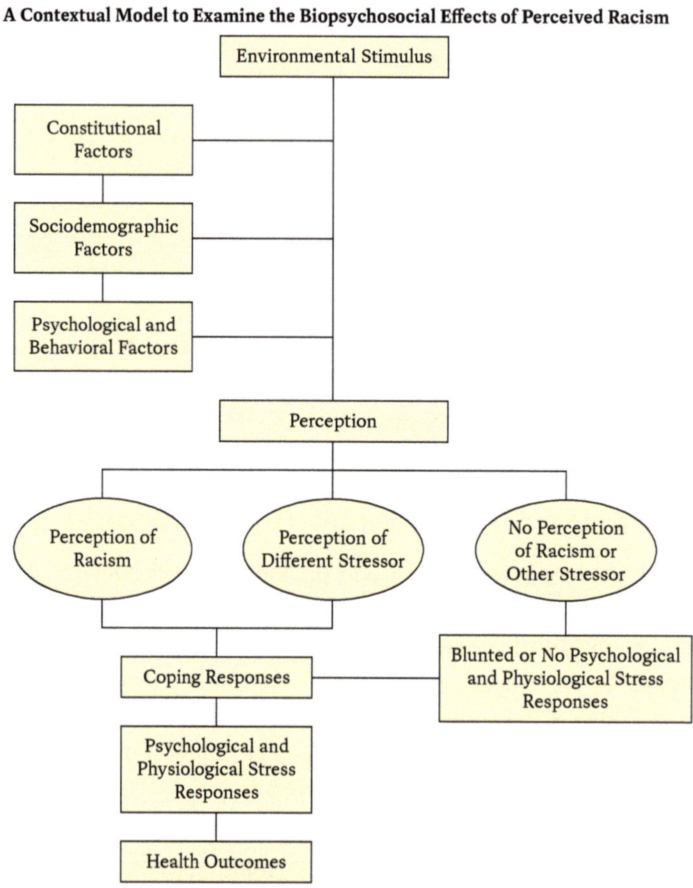

FIGURE 5.4 Clark's Biopsychosocial Racism Model

However, some research with Mexican Americans suggests that the model may not be as applicable to them (Molina et al., 2013). Individually perceived discrimination and racism may be less important than perceiving group discrimination. Molina et al. (2019) found that higher perceived personal discrimination was directly associated with poorer physical health quality of life. Additionally, higher levels of perceived group discrimination were positively associated with ethnic group identity. They suggest that perceiving group discrimination contributes to stronger group identification, which in turn is protective of psychological well-being. However, studies have shown that perceived personal discrimination is associated with poorer overall self-rated health, physical health (Molina et al., 2013), and mental health outcomes among Mexican Americans (Perreira et al., 2015).

Similarly, there is some Latino research that indicates ethnic density is protective against the stress or discrimination and racism through increased neighborhood cohesion, one component of cultural wealth (see Figure 5.5). Bécares (2014) hypothesizes that Latino ethnic solidarity and culture are important mediators in the perception of personal racism and discrimination.

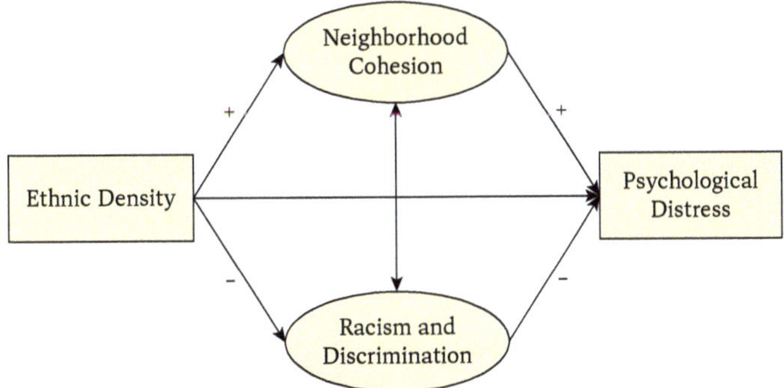

FIGURE 5.5 Latino Ethnic Density and Psychological Distress

Pascoe and Richman's (2009) model of perceived discrimination and health also shows a direct pathway to mental and physical health status (see Figure 5.6). Additionally, perceived discrimination increases stress and negative health behaviors (e.g., drug and alcohol as coping strategies). Other research has confirmed the mediating effects of social support (extrinsic) and active coping (intrinsic) on pathways leading from perceived discrimination to heightened stress response and health behaviors (Allen, 2019; Flores et al., 2010). Research on negative health behaviors also shows that they are implicated in mental and physical health (Jackson & Knight, 2006). Moreover, research on psychosocial stress and adverse mental and physical health has shown this pathway to be a viable source of health inequalities among historically marginalized populations, especially Latinos of Mexican descent.

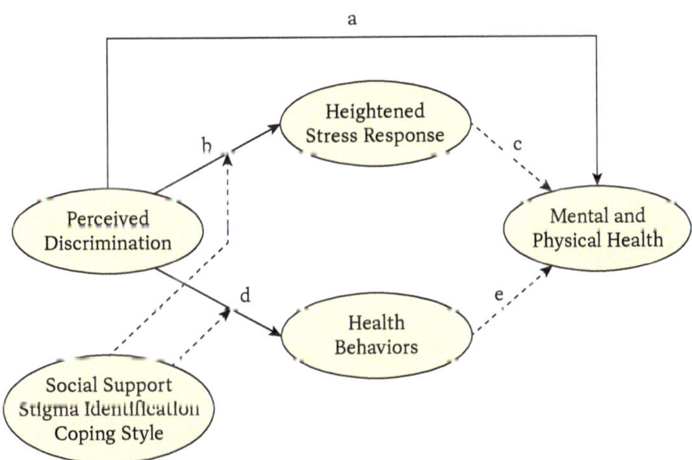

FIGURE 5.6 Pathways Showing Perceived Discrimination and Health Outcomes

Anti-Mexican sentiment reached a peak when Donald Trump, then a candidate for 45th president of the United States, said, "When Mexico sends its people, they're not sending their best. They're sending people that have lots of problems. They're bringing drugs. They're bringing crime. They're rapists. And some, I assume, are good people" (Trump, 2015). After he was no longer president, he made the statement "Migrants are poisoning the blood of our country" (Trump, 2023).

These microaggression-filled attacks were only the latest within a 180-year time span of hate directed toward Latinos of Mexican descent. As previously discussed, Mexicans were seen as inferior both culturally and intellectually to non-Latino White Americans. The spillover effect of anti-immigrant legislation and rhetoric has led to increased psychological distress among Latinos of Mexican descent (Ayón & Becerra, 2013; Sabo & Lee, 2015; Viruell-Fuentes et al., 2012).

Kessler et al. (1999) reported results on the prevalence of racial discrimination among Non-Latino Black Americans. They found that non-Latino Black Americans reported higher rates of discrimination (71.3%) than non-Latino White Americans (23.7%). An examination of the prevalence of racial discrimination and its social correlates was conducted by Pérez et al. (2008) using data from the National Latino and Asian American Study (NLAAS; Alegria et al., 2004). Findings showed that Puerto Ricans reported the highest rate of discrimination (40%), followed by Mexicans and "other" Latinos (both at 34.4%) with Cubans reporting the lowest rate of discrimination (16.4%). Important social correlates included higher levels of acculturation and a weak ethnic identity, which were associated with higher rates of discrimination. Interestingly, the study found that speaking English was associated with twice the rate of reporting everyday discrimination, compared to Spanish-speaking Cubans, Mexicans, Puerto Ricans, and "other" Latinos. Similarly, several studies have found that increasing acculturation level among Latinos is associated with increased experiences of personal and group discrimination, possibly due to more interaction with non-Latino White Americans.

Another study that used a large national sample of Latinos to examine the prevalence of discrimination was conducted by Almeida et al. (2016). Using the 2008 National Latino Health Care Survey, they found significant variation among Latino subgroups. Puerto Ricans reported the highest prevalence of perceived discrimination (80.7%), followed by Mexicans (67.6%), with Cubans reporting the lowest rate of perceived discrimination (45.8%). The overall prevalence of perceived discrimination was 68.4%, which is similar to the prevalence reported by Non-Latino Black Americans (Kessler et al., 1999). Moreover, their findings indicate that more anti-immigrant policies are associated with a higher perception of discrimination among Latinos of Cuban and Mexican descent, especially in those states with more anti-immigrant policies. Alternatively, they found that Puerto Ricans living in states with more anti-immigrant policies had a lower probability of perceived discrimination. There were also generational effects, with third-generation Latinos compared to first- and second-generation Latinos reporting higher rates of perceived discrimination.

Arellano-Morales et al. (2015) used data from the Hispanic Community Health Study/Study of Latinos Sociocultural Ancillary Study (HCHS/SOL) consisting of over 5,000 Latino respondents with adequate samples of Central Americans, Cubans, Dominicans, Mexicans, Puerto Ricans, and South Americans. Overall, the prevalence of experiencing at least one episode of discrimination was 79.5%. Variation was observed across Latino subgroups, with South Americans reporting the highest rate (94%), followed by Central Americans (92.1%), Puerto Ricans (86%), Dominicans (86%), Cubans (69.1%), and Mexicans (64.9%), who reported the lowest rate of discrimination, which is like the rates reported by Almeida et al. (2016)

for Latinos of Mexican descent. Variation in discrimination among Latino subgroups was also reported by Held and Lee (2017), with Latinos of Mexican and Puerto Rican descent having a higher likelihood of having a psychiatric disorder.

Cobb et al. (2021) examined the prevalence of perceived and recurrent discrimination among Latinos using datasets from 2004/2005 and 2012/2013. The experience of "any" discrimination among Latinos increased from about 25.1% to 39.9% over this 8-year period. In addition, the experience of recurrent discrimination among Latinos increased from 15.1% to 23.7%. Foreign-born Latinos experienced the highest rates of discrimination (22.4%–40.7%, respectively) compared to U.S.-born Latinos (28.4%–39.1%, respectively) and recurrent discrimination (13.8%–25.1% among foreign-born Latinos and 16.8%–22.2% among U.S.-born Latinos).

Variation in skin tone among Latinos may also lead to the experience of discrimination. As noted in Chapter 3, colorism is a colonial legacy that is present in Mexican and Latin American societies. Some research has shown that Latinos with darker skin experience more discrimination than Latinos with lighter skin (Hunter, 2005, 2012). Tezler & Garcia (2009) found that immigrant Latinas with darker skin tended to have poorer self-perceptions than their U.S.-born counterparts, including lower self-esteem, lower feelings of attractiveness, and a desire to change their skin color to be lighter. U.S.-born Latinas did not show any negative associations between skin color and self-perceptions. Codina and Montalvo (1994) found that U.S.-born Mexican men with darker skin had higher levels of depression, as measured by the CES-D, than Mexican-born men with lighter skin and U.S.-born Mexican women, inferring that darker skinned Mexicans experience more discrimination that leads to higher levels of depression.

Although Latinos experience varying rates of discrimination by subgroup, overall perceived discrimination rates are lower than those experienced by non-Latino Black Americans. The few research findings among Latinos indicate that discrimination is consistently associated with greater stress and higher rates of depression (Araújo & Borrell, 2006).

Latino Immigration and Acculturation Hypotheses

Several epidemiological studies have demonstrated that length of residence in the United States is associated with decreasing physical and mental health status among Latinos, especially those of Mexican descent (Alderete et al., 2000; Vega et al., 2004). Reasons proposed for this finding include increasing acculturation effects with the loss of cultural protective resources and the experience of psychosocial stressors (Finch & Vega, 2003; Vega et al., 2004).

According to a Pew Research Center report by Gonzales-Barrera (2021), between 1965 and 2015, Mexican immigrants constituted one of the largest mass migrations in modern history when more than 16 million Mexican immigrants migrated to the United States—more than from any other country. During this period, Mexican immigration peaked in 2007, with an estimated 12.8 million Mexicans residing in the United States. Gonzales-Barrera found that during this period, 25% of immigrants to the United States were born in Mexico. An estimated 62% of foreign-born Mexicans have been in the United States for over 20 years, and 35% of foreign-born Mexicans are U.S. citizens. The fact is not all Mexicans residing in the United States are immigrants, with about 75% second generation or higher. The preponderance of literature on Latino immigrants appears to be misplaced and should be refocused on the generations of Latinos born in the United States. This is the Latino population most at risk for developing chronic diseases that are linked to the social determinants of heath.

The immigration and acculturation hypotheses, then, are pertinent only to newly arrived Latino immigrants who are in the process of adapting to mainstream U.S. society or older Latinos, immigrant or not, who have retained more of their traditional cultural upbringing. Comparisons between foreign-born and U.S.-born Latinos and Latino immigrants and non-immigrants provides some insight into nativity differences and perhaps a stronger association with traditional ways of living.

The association between the social determinants of health and level of acculturation among Latinos is unequivocal. Acculturation level is associated with economic stability, access to quality education, community and neighborhood characteristics, access to quality health care, and exposure to elements within the built environment (Abraido-Lanza et al., 2006; Finch & Vega, 2003). The cumulative body of research shows that higher levels of acculturation are associated with higher income levels, higher educational attainment, higher levels of health insurance coverage, and increased access to health care. Paradoxically, however, higher acculturation is also associated with poorer dietary practices (Ayala et al., 2008), higher prevalence rates of obesity (Guerra et al., 2022), metabolic syndrome (Vella et al., 2011), diabetes mellitus (Lara et al., 2005), alcohol and drug abuse (Castro et al., 2010), and HIV knowledge and risk behaviors (Marin & Marin, 1990; Diaz et al., 2020). In fact, Latinos who are third generation and higher have similar prevalence rates of some chronic diseases as do their non-Latino White counterparts (Abraido-Lanza et al., 2016; Portes & Zhou, 1993). This is consistent with acculturation theory wherein Latinos adapt to non-Latino White attitudes and behaviors over time.

Acculturation level is of course associated with immigration status among Latinos. As generational status and years lived in the United States increases, acculturation level also increases. Immigrant Latinos are less acculturated due to their lack of interaction with non-Latino mainstream society. The *immigrant selection hypothesis* suggests that immigrants are generally healthier both physically and psychologically than those who do not immigrate (Alegria et al., 2007). There is a growing body of research that confirms this hypothesis. However, once immigrated, research also shows that traditional values and behaviors begin to erode over time, with immigrants adapting to their new social and cultural environments (Allen et al., 2014).

The complexity of the relationship between length of time in the United States and physical and psychological well-being is shown by the intersecting factors like age of arrival, prevalence of chronic and psychiatric disorders in the sending country, gender, and relative poverty status (Alegria et al., 2007, 2008). Because of differential outcomes, it is also worthwhile to separate discussions related to physical health status like cardiovascular disease and obesity from those related to psychiatric disorders, like substance use disorders and depression.

Physical Health Status

Acculturation level among Latinos has been shown to be associated with higher prevalence rates of obesity and cardiovascular disease risks (Ai et al., 2018; Isasi et al., 2015). Allen et al. (2014) provides a useful conceptual model outlining the major pathways between acculturation and health behaviors. Research shows that acculturation level is associated with several demographic characteristics producing significant interactions with income, education, age, and gender. Studies have also shown that social support and social ties moderate the effects of perceived stress and material hardship (Viruell-Fuentes et al., 2013).

The model shows the hypothetical relationship between perceived stress and health behaviors, which has also been confirmed by the research literature (see Chapter 2).

The direct effect of acculturation on health behaviors has also been reported in the research literature, as noted above, with higher levels of acculturation being more risk inducing than lower levels (see Figure 5.7). Moreover, findings related to segmented assimilation, the intersection of acculturation and U.S. societal economic integration, show differential influences on health behaviors and health risks (Castro et al., 2010; Lara et al., 2005; Portes & Zhou, 1993; Valdez, 2006). For example, Flórez and Abraído-Lanza (2019) examined whether segmented assimilation trajectories, derived from cluster analyses, were associated with obesity among Latinos. They found partial support for the theory, with second- and third-generation patterns 1.73 and 2.01 times, respectively, more likely to be obese compared to the segmented assimilation group.

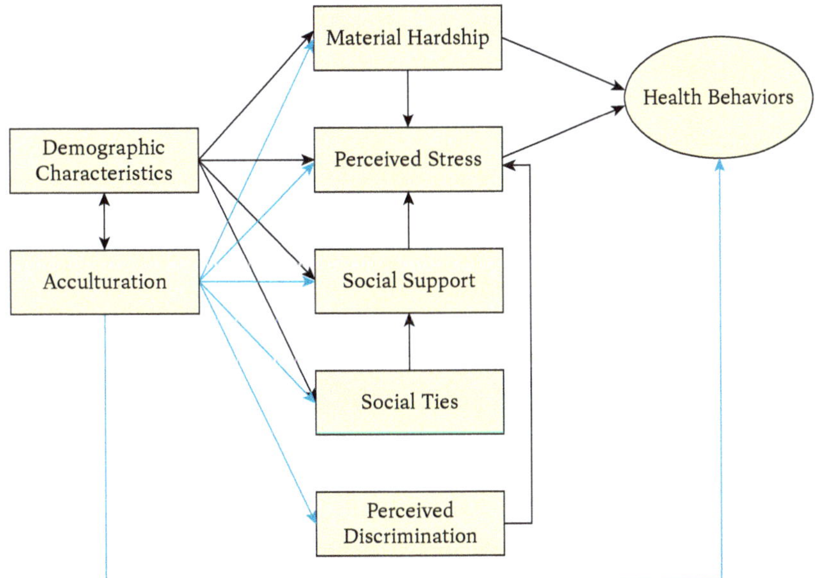

FIGURE 5.7 Hypothesized Pathways Between Acculturation and Health Behaviors

Isasi et al. (2015) found that prolonged socioenvironmental exposure was a stronger predictor of obesity among Latinos, with length and place of residence associated with a higher prevalence of obesity and extreme obesity. However, most of the research on obesity and acculturation among Latinos is associated with dietary practices, physical activity, and food insecurity (Ayala et al., 2008). Studies are relatively consistent in their finding that healthy diets and food security are strongly associated with increased acculturation but are also linked to gender and socioeconomic status in complex ways. Thus, acculturation processes would appear to be more associated with factors that limit healthy behaviors, like lower socioeconomic status, than directly linked to obesity-related behaviors (Ai et al., 2018; Buscemi et al., 2011; Fitzgerald, 2010; Guerra et al., 2022). Acculturation and cardiovascular disease among Latinos show similar results as obesity. Acculturation influences dietary habits and physical exercise among Latinos (Alegria et al., 2022; Cuy Castellanos, 2015; Peréz-Escamilla & Putnix, 2007). These factors increase the risk for obesity, which increases the risk of diabetes mellitus, which then increases the risk for cardiovascular disease (Lutsey et al., 2008).

Mental Health Status

Specific components of acculturation, like length of residence in the United States and place of birth, have been found to be more consistently related to psychological well-being among Latinos. Long-term residence in the United States significantly increases rates in mental disorders, with particularly profound increases in the rates of substance use disorders (Vega et al., 1998). Additionally, the prevalence of psychiatric and substance use disorders significantly increases with each subsequent generation of Latinos in the United States (Alegria et al., 2007).

This finding has been replicated in research on substance use disorders among Cubans and other Latino groups, which has given rise to the immigrant hypothesis (Alegría et al., 2008) and the acculturation hypothesis (Rogler et al., 1991). In addition, there is accumulating evidence that indicates that the transition to high risk for substance use disorder begins quickly among immigrants: Those who arrive as children have a higher risk for substance use disorder than immigrants who arrive in the United States as adolescents or adults and a lower risk for substance use disorder than U.S.-born Latinos (Borges et al., 2011).

The *immigrant hypothesis* suggests that foreign nativity protects against psychiatric, and substance use disorders, somehow inoculating immigrants who migrate to the United States as adults but not necessarily subsequent generations that are born in the United States. The *acculturation hypothesis* suggests that the acculturation process is stressful for immigrants and subsequent generations of Latinos with increasing rates of substance use and psychiatric disorders.

According to a study conducted by Grant et al. (2004), compared to foreign-born Mexican Americans, U.S.-born Mexican Americans were 2.1 times more likely to have any psychiatric disorder, 2.6 times more likely to have any alcohol use disorder, 7.5 times more likely to have any drug use disorder, and 8.6 times more likely to have any drug dependence. They also found that compared to Mexicans born in Mexico, Mexicans born in the United States had significantly higher prevalence rates of any mood disorder and any anxiety disorder.

Alegria et al. (2007) documented results showing that U.S.-born Latinos have higher rates of any lifetime psychiatric disorder than foreign-born Latinos (36.7% compared to 23.7%, respectively). Alegría et al. (2008) also showed that lifetime prevalence rates of any psychiatric disorder where significantly higher among Latinos of Mexican descent, with those born in the United States having much higher rates than immigrants, then similar cohorts of Puerto Ricans, Cubans, and "other" Latinos. Similarly, lifetime prevalence rates of any substance disorder were higher for U.S.-born than immigrants, with Latinos of Mexican descent having higher rates than their immigrant peers.

Borges et al. (2011) examined place of birth and age of migration among a sample of Latinos of Mexican descent. They found that those Latinos of Mexican descent who were U.S.-born with one parent who was also U.S.-born had the highest prevalence rates of lifetime drug use (53.87%), lifetime alcohol abuse/dependence (20.3%), and any lifetime drug abuse/dependence (10.9 %). Those Latinos of Mexican descent who were born in Mexico and migrated to the United States at 13 years of age or older had the lowest prevalence of lifetime drug use (17.1%) and any lifetime drug abuse/dependence (1.87%). For lifetime alcohol abuse/dependence, this group was one fourth as likely as U.S.-born Mexicans with one U.S.-born parent (5.8% compared to 20.3%).

Available evidence from research studies consistently shows the dynamic interplay between acculturation and immigration, with years of residence in the United States having a profound negative effect on the psychological well-being of Latinos, especially those of Mexican descent.

Paradox Found, Paradox Lost, Paradox Found Again!

A *paradox* is a phenomenon that runs contrary to expectations of how it should behave. The fact that Latinos of Mexican descent have lower economic stability and lack access to quality education and health care compared to non-Latino White Americans yet have better mortality outcomes is a paradox because research shows that low income and education are often correlated with higher mortality rates.

One of the first mentions of an "epidemiologic paradox" among Latinos of Mexican descent was research conducted by Jaco (1961) on the incidence of mental illness in Texas. He (and others) found that given the high incidence of mental illness among Mexicans, there was not a concomitant increase in mental health utilization rates (Karno & Edgerton, 1969; Lopez, 1981). Markides & Coriel (1986), however, are recognized as the first scholars to link the epidemiologic paradox to Latino health outcomes and coined the term "Hispanic paradox." They examined infant mortality rates, life expectancy, cancer mortality, cardiovascular disease mortality, diabetes mellitus, and functional health and concluded that Latinos of Mexican descent have a health advantage on several health indicators relative to non-Latino White Americans, apart from diabetes mellitus and some infectious diseases. Markides & Coriel (1986) hypothesized that several other factors are involved in the mortality paradox including selective migration, cultural practices, social ties, dietary practices, and genetics (primarily Native American ancestry).

The Latino epidemiologic paradox became a paradigm shift in 1990s in examining the health and mental health status of Latinos, not restricted to those of Mexican descent, with numerous studies conducted over the past 3 decades (Abraido-Lanza et al., 1999; Ruiz et al., 2013; Sorlie et al., 1993; Turra & Elo, 2008). Why would Latinos have better mortality rates relative to non-Latino White Americans given their lower socioeconomic status (SES), when it is known that SES is linked to an excess of chronic diseases and increased mortality? Additionally, although the evidence is equivocal, acculturation level is associated with better access to health care and better nutrition, as noted previously. Reasons for this apparent paradox have focused on cultural factors, lifestyle characteristics, immigration, and inherent resiliency factors among Latinos of Mexican descent (Ruiz et al., 2013).

For example, two hypotheses have been advanced to account for Latino mortality differences: the "salmon bias" hypothesis and the "immigrant selection" hypothesis. The *salmon bias hypothesis* held that the apparent differences in mortality were due to terminally ill persons returning to their home country, and thus their data was not reported in U.S. death rates (Abriado-Lanza et al. 1999; Aguila et al., 2013; Diaz et al., 2016). The *immigrant selection hypothesis* suggests that due to migrants' better health, they stay inoculated against risk behaviors that may increase mortality risk and that migrants may be healthier initially (Bostean, 2013; Dubowitz et al., 2010).

To date, there is some empirical support for both hypotheses, but conceptual and methodological limitations in the research render the findings equivocal. Neither hypothesis fully explains observed mortality differences between Latinos and non-Latino White people living in the United States or between immigrant and nonimmigrant Latinos (Bostean, 2013, Dubowitz et al., 2010, Palloni & Arias, 2004, Ruiz et al., 2013; Viruell-Fuentes & Schulz, 2009). For instance, misclassification of race or ethnicity on death certificates could lead to erroneous findings related to the salmon bias hypothesis. Linkages of health assessments in the sending country to the receiving country are inherently complicated for individuals in ensuring identification of the same person. Nevertheless, support for the selective migration hypothesis is developing (Martinez-Cardoso & Geronimus, 2021).

Palloni and Arias (2004) provided one of the most comprehensive modeling approaches to examine the Latino paradox. Using National Health Interview Survey data, they found strong support for a return migration effect, primarily among foreign-born Mexicans and foreign-born other Latinos but not for Puerto Ricans and Cubans. They found no support for a cultural hypothesis associated with a mortality advantage among Latinos. Their finding that foreign-born Mexicans and other Latinos experience mortality rates that are 35%–47% lower than those experienced by non-Latino White Americans translates into approximately 5–8 years of additional life expectancy at age 45 (Palloni & Arias, 2004, p. 409). Their analyses underscore the importance of examining mortality rates among Latino subgroups rather than aggregating them into a homogenous group. This makes sense given the various historical, social, and geopolitical interactions with American society and government.

If the Latino mortality paradox exists, does it hold for mortality rates among various demographic subgroups? A review of mortality rates for Latino infants and adolescents as well as pre-COVID-19 overall mortality rates and post-COVID-19 overall mortality rates may show differential mortality outcomes.

Latino Infant Mortality Rates

In 2019, national data do not show a mortality advantage for Latinos' infant mortality rates in the United States (Figure 5.8). Latino infant mortality is slightly higher than non-Latino White infant mortality but half as much as non-Latino Black infant mortality.

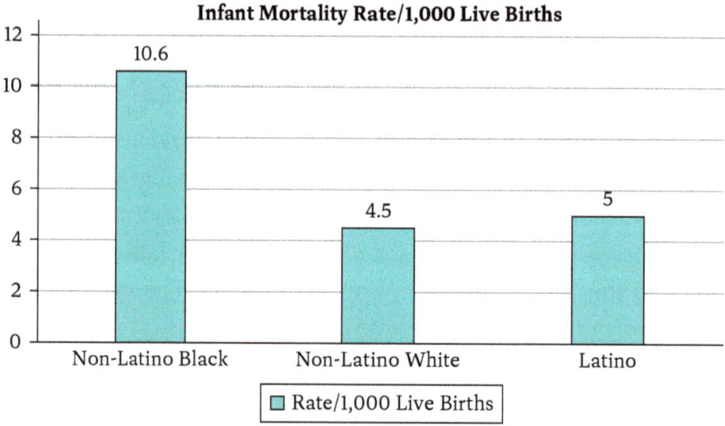

FIGURE 5.8 Infant Mortality Rates by Race/Ethnicity, United States, 2019

Data From the Period Linked Birth/Infant Death File

There are significant differences in infant mortality rates among infants born to teenagers 15–19 years old (Woodall & Driscoll, 2020). In 2017-2018, infants of teenagers aged 15-19 had the highest mortality rates (8.77 deaths per 1,000 live births) compared with infants of women aged 20 and over (see Figure 5.9).

Moreover, infants born to Latina teenagers had the lowest mortality rates for all five leading causes of death except maternal complications of pregnancy (35.69 per 1,000 compared with 28.51 among non-Latino White and 68.18 among non-Latino Black teenagers). Mortality rates were highest for infants of non-Latino Black teenagers (12.54) compared with infants of non-Latino White (8.43) and Latino (6.47) teenagers.

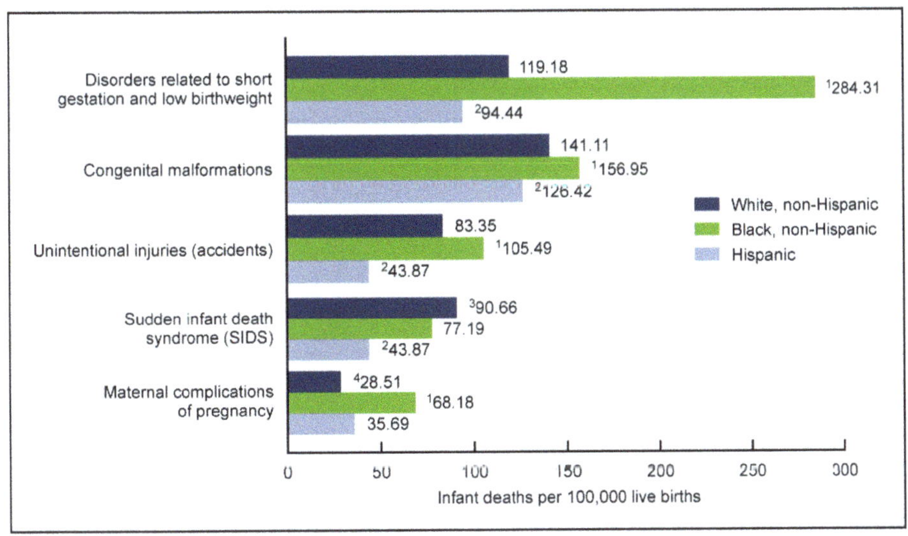

[1]Significantly higher than non-Hispanic white and Hispanic rates ($p < 0.05$).
[2]Significantly lower than non-Hispanic white and non-Hispanic black rates ($p < 0.05$).
[3]Significantly higher than non-Hispanic black and Hispanic rates ($p < 0.05$).
[4]Significantly lower than non-Hispanic black and Hispanic rates ($p < 0.05$).
NOTES: Causes of death are ranked according to number of deaths. Data table for Figure 3 includes number of deaths for leading causes. Access data table for Figure 3 at: https://www.cdc.gov/nchs/data/databriefs/db371-tables-508.pdf#3.
SOURCE: National Center for Health Statistics, National Vital Statistics System, Linked birth/infant death file.

FIGURE 5.9 Infant Mortality Rates for the Five Leading Causes of Death Among Infants Born to Mothers Aged 15–19, by Maternal Race and Latino Origin, United States, 2017–2018

Maternal Mortality Rates Among Latinas

According to Hoyert (2023), maternal mortality rates for Latinas were lower than non-Latina White and non-Latina Black women from 2018–2020 (see Table 5.4). In 2021, however, the maternal mortality advantage for Latinas disappears relative to non-Latina White women (28.0 compared to 26.6 per 100,000 live births). Maternal mortality rates are significantly higher among African American women than for other groups during 2018–2021.

TABLE 5.4 Maternal Mortality Rates 2018–2021 per 100,000 Live Births

Race/ethnicity	2018	2019	2020	2021
Non-Latino Black	37.3	44.0	55.3	69.9
Non-Latino White	14.9	17.9	19.1	26.6
Latino	11.8	12.6	18.2	28.0

Source: Hoyert (2023)

Latino Adolescent/Young Adult Mortality Rates

Young Latino males have slightly higher mortality rates than Latinas (women) (Rogers et al., 2017). The leading causes of mortality among this age group include motor vehicle fatalities, suicide, and homicide or assault. Latino youth have higher motor vehicle mortality rates than non-Latino White Americans (36% and 20%, respectively).

According to Curtin and Garnett (2023), there were no statistically significant trends in suicide or homicide rates from 2001–2007, then a significant increasing trend from 2007–2021 (Figure 5.10). Suicide rates were significantly lower than the rates for homicide from 2001–2009 and then significantly higher from 2011–2019. There were no statistically significant trends for homicides from 2001–2006, then there was a significant decreasing trend from 2006–2014, and then a significant increasing trend from 2014–2021.

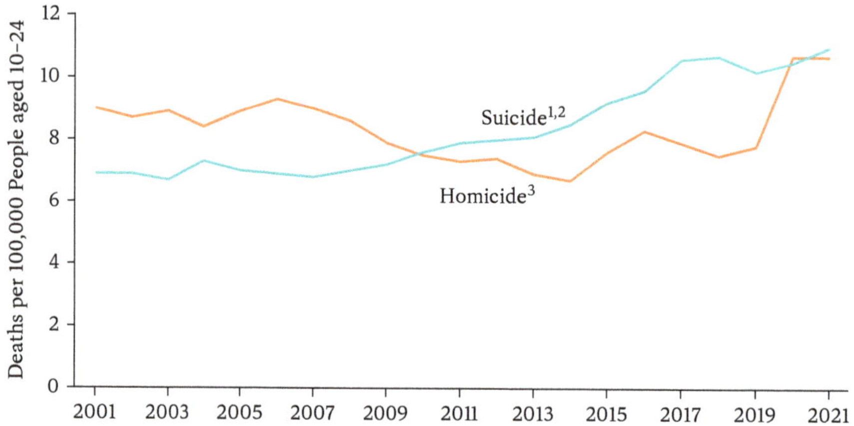

[1]No statistically significant trend from 2001–2007, then significant increasing trend from 2007–2021 ($p < 0.05$).
[2]Rate significantly lower than the rates for homicide from 2001–2009 and significantly higher from 2011–2019 ($p < 0.05$).
[3]No statistically significant trend for homicides from 2001–2006, then significant decreasing trend from 2006–2014, and a significant increasing trend from 2014–2021 ($p < 0.05$). The rate in 2021 was not significantly different than the rate in 2020 ($p < 0.05$).
NOTES: Suicides are identified with International Classification of Diseases, 10th Revision codes U03, X60–X84, and Y87.0, and homicides with codes U01–U02, X85–Y09, and Y87.1. Access data table for Figure 1 at: https://www.cdc.gov/nchs/data/databriefs/db471-tables.pdf#1.
Source: National Center for Health Statistics, National Vital Statistics System, Mortality data file.

FIGURE 5.10 Suicide and Homicide Rates Among Persons 10–24, United States, 2001–2021

Firearm-related pediatric (0–19 years of age) homicides show major differences by race and ethnicity (Roberts et al., 2023). In 2021, non-Latino Black Americans had the highest crude death rate of firearm-related homicides at 18.9/100,000 which was more than 3 times the rate for non-Latino White Americans (3.6/100,000). Latino Americans compared to non-Latino Americans showed lower crude death rates (4/100,000 compared to 6.4/100,000, respectively) (see Figure 5.11).

Xu et al. (2021) found that suicide rates were substantially higher among males than females across ethnic/racial groups, as shown in Table 5.5. Latina males and females have lower suicide mortality rates than their non-Latino White and non-Latino Black counterparts.

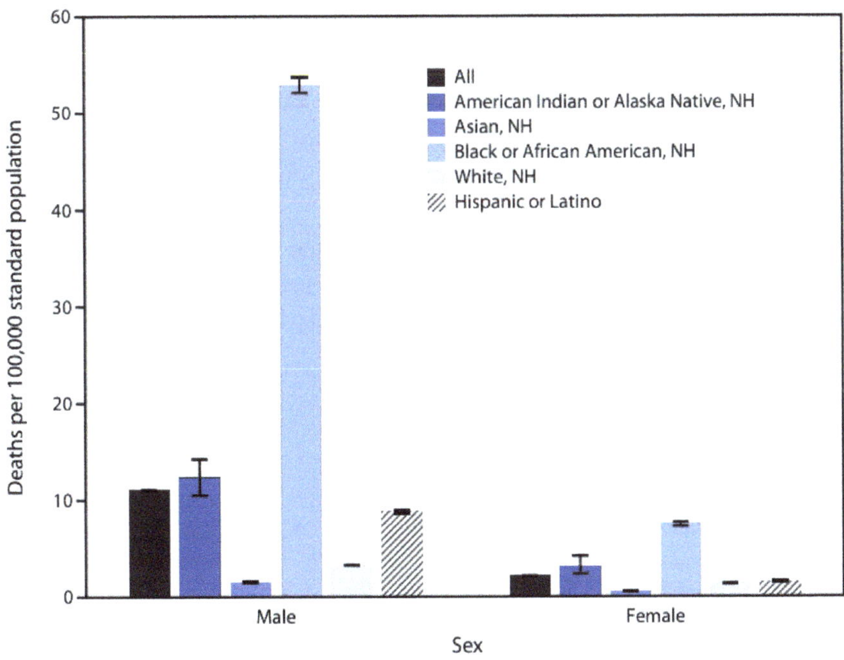

Abbreviation: NH = non-Hispanic.

* Deaths per 100,000 population are age-adjusted to the 2000 U.S. standard population, with 95% CIs indicated by error bars. In 2021, the age-adjusted rate of firearm-related homicide was 11.1 deaths per 100,000 standard population for males and 2.1 for females.

† Firearm-related homicides were identified using *International Classification of Diseases, Tenth Revision* underlying cause-of-death codes U01.4 and X93–X95.

§ Race groups are non-Hispanic; persons of Hispanic origin can be of any race. Native Hawaiian or other Pacific Islander persons are not shown separately because of small numbers. All includes all race and Hispanic origin groups including those not shown. Death rates for Asian, American Indian or Alaska Native, and Hispanic or Latino (Hispanic) persons might be affected by misclassification of race and Hispanic origin on death certificates. https://www.cdc.gov/nchs/data/series/sr_02/sr02_172.pdf

FIGURE 5.11 Age-Adjusted Rates of Firearm-Related Homicide by Race, Hispanic Origin, and Sex—National Vital Statistics System, United States, 2021

TABLE 5.5 Suicide Rates Among 15- to 24-Year-Olds by Gender and Race/Ethnicity, United States, 2019

Race/ethnicity	Rate per 100,000
Non-Latino White males	25.6
Non-Latino White females	6.1
Non-Latino Black males	18.3
Non-Latino Black females	4.4
Latino males	16.6
Latino females	4.4

Source: Adapted from Xu et al. (2021)

Pre-COVID-19 Overall Mortality Rates

In 2018, Latino Americans had lower age-adjusted mortality rates than non-Latino White Americans for diseases of the heart (200.3/100,000 vs. 67.7/100,000, respectively), cancer (183.2/100,000 vs. 70.3/100,000, respectively), and diabetes mellitus (28.1/100,000 vs. 15.7/100,000) (Murphy et al., 2020). Additionally, Latino Americans had significantly lower mortality rates than non-Latino Black Americans for these chronic diseases (Murphy et al., 2020).

Mortality trends for adults aged 25 and over showed that Latino Americans had lower mortality rates than both non-Latino White Americans and non-Latino Black Americans (Curtin & Arias, 2019) (Figure 5.12). This was the case for each age cohort examined (25–44, 45–65, and 65+).

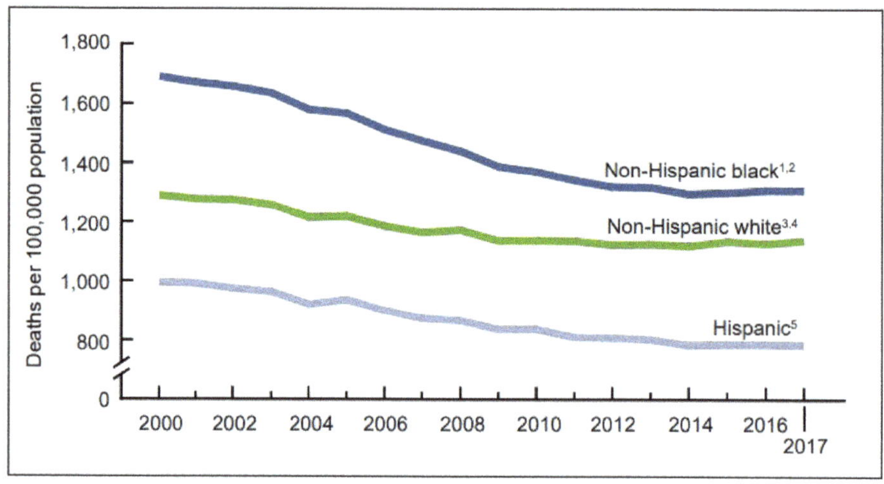

[1]Significant decreasing trend for 2000–2012 with different rates of change over time; stable trend for 2012–2017; $p < 0.05$.
[2]Rate significantly higher than the rate for non-Hispanic white and Hispanic persons, $p < 0.05$.
[3]Significant decreasing trend for 2000–2011; stable trend for 2011–2017, $p < 0.05$.
[4]Rate significantly higher than the rate for Hispanic persons, $p < 0.05$.
[5]Significant decreasing trend for 2000–2017 with different rates of change over time; $p < 0.05$.
NOTE: Access data table for Figure 1 at: https://www.cdc.gov/nchs/data/databriefs/db342_tables-508.pdf#1.
SOURCE: NCHS, National Vital Statistics System, Mortality.

FIGURE 5.12 U.S. Mortality Trends, 2000–2017

Prior to the COVID-19 pandemic, data clearly showed that Latino Americans experienced a higher life expectancy than non-Latino White Americans and non-Latino Black Americans (Arias & Xu, 2022a): 79.1 years compared to 76.5 and 71.8, respectively, for men and 83.8 compared to 81.2 and 78.1, respectively, for women. Between 2018 and 2019, life expectancy at birth increased by 0.1 year for men (76.2 to 76.3) and by 0.2 years for women (81.2 to 81.4). The life expectancy for Latinos was 81.9 years, followed by 78.8 years for the non-Latino White population and 74.8 years for the non-Latino Black population. Also, between 2018 and 2019, life expectancy increased 0.2 years for non-Latino White populations and by 0.1 year for Latino and non-Latino Black populations (Xu & Arias, 2022b). In 2019, the overall expectation of life at birth was 78.8 years, increasing from 78.7 in 2018 (Figure 5.13).

National data clearly showed an overall mortality advantage for Latinos. Researchers examining the Latino subgroup differences found that the mortality advantage appeared to hold mostly for Latinos of Mexican descent (Bostean, 2013; Dubowitz et al., 2010; Fenelon et al., 2017; Palloni & Arias, 2004; Ruiz et al., 2013).

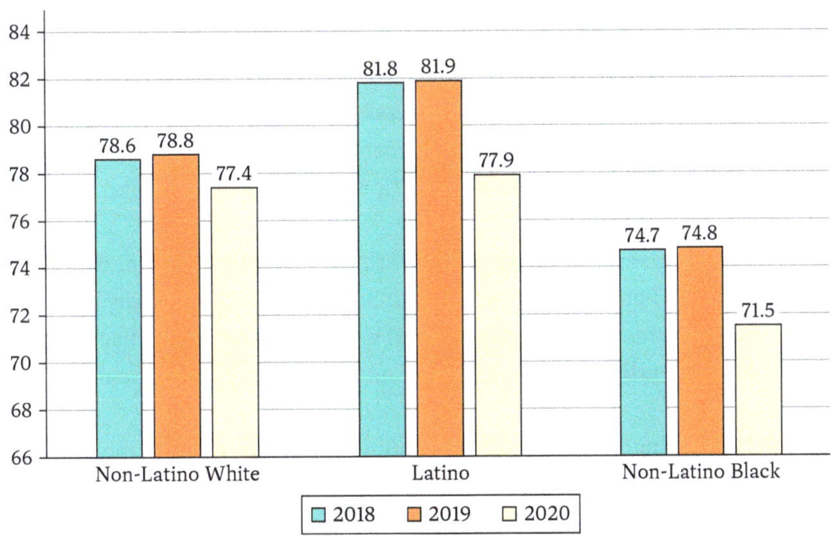

FIGURE 5.13 Life Expectancy at Birth by Latino Origin and Race, 2018–2020

Unintentional injuries are one of the leading causes of death in the United States, and rates vary significantly by race and ethnicity. The National Safety Council (n.d.) provides analyses on unintentional and intentional injuries in the United States. In 2021, poisoning, accidental falls, and motor vehicle accidents were the leading causes of unintentional mortality, accounting for 86% of all preventable injury related deaths. The overall preventable death rate per 100,000 population increased 10% among non-Latino White Americans but increased by 15% among Latinos. Similarly, preventable poisoning increased by 13% among non-Latino White Americans but 20% among Latinos. In 2021, the motor-vehicle death rate per 100,000 population increased among all groups: 9% among non-Latino White Americans and 13% among Latinos.

Intentional injuries that are addressed by the National Safety Council (n.d.) include suicide and homicide/assault. Intentional self-harm includes suicide and attempted suicide resulting from purposely self-inflicted poisoning or injury. The most common methods of suicide are firearms, hanging, strangulation and suffocation, and poisoning. Suicide accounted for 45,979 deaths, or 17% of all injury-related deaths in 2020. Assault includes homicide and injuries inflicted by another person with intent to injure or kill. The most common means of homicide are firearms, sharp objects, and hanging, strangulation, and suffocation. Assault deaths totaled 24,576 in 2020, or 9% of all injury-related deaths.

Premature mortality is an indicator of many adverse conditions that are influenced by social and cultural determinants of health (CDC, 1986). Years of potential life lost (YPLL) is a widely used measure of the rate and distribution of premature mortality. Measuring premature mortality, rather than overall mortality, focuses attention on deaths that might have been prevented. YPLL emphasizes deaths of younger persons, whereas statistics that include all mortality are dominated by deaths of older adults. For example, using YPLL-75, a death at age 55 counts twice as much as a death at age 65, and a death at age 35 counts eight times as much as a death at age 70.

Studies have consistently shown that despite their socioeconomic disadvantages, Latinos residing in the United States have lower premature mortality rates than do non-Latino White populations (McDonald & Paulozzi, 2019). McDonald and Paulozzi (2019) examined age-adjusted mortality rates for 113 causes of death for Latinos and non-Latino White Americans during 1999–2015. All-cause, age-adjusted mortality rates per 100,000 were 581.1/100,000 for Latino Americans and 788.8/100,000 for non-Latino White Americans. Lower Latino mortality from cancer, heart disease, and respiratory disease accounted for almost all the all-cause mortality gap. Latino rates were higher than non-Latino rates for cancers of the stomach, liver, and cervix, diabetes mellitus, liver disease, and homicide, which is similar to findings reported by others (Chen et al., 2020; Shiels, 2017).

Prior to the COVID-19 pandemic, Shiels et al. (2017) found that premature mortality decreased significantly across all age groups in Latino Americans (up to 3.2% per year), and Non-Latino Black Americans (up to 3.9% per year), mainly because of declines in HIV, cancer, and heart disease deaths, resulting in an estimated 112,000 fewer deaths in Latino Americans and 311,000 fewer deaths in Non-Latino Black Americans aged 25–64 years.

Fenelon et al. (2017) examined mortality rates among Latino subgroups, including foreign-born and U.S.-born Mexicans, Puerto Ricans, Cubans, Dominicans, Central/South Americans, and other Latinos, compared to non-Latino White Americans. They found that among Latino adults aged 25–64, several subgroups experience a mortality *disadvantage* relative to non-Latino White adults, which they suggest reflects socioeconomic disadvantage. When the researchers adjusted for socioeconomic covariates (e.g., education and poverty), they found that SES mediates the disadvantage of these groups, suggesting that younger adult Mexicans and Puerto Ricans experience a mortality disadvantage as a function of socioeconomic disadvantage. They also found that only foreign-born Central/South Americans and other Latinos experience lower mortality risks in this age group. Among Latino adults 65 years old and above, nearly all Latino subgroups experience lower adult mortality risks than non-Latino White adults, with wide variation across subgroups. The most favorable outcomes occur for foreign-born Mexicans, Central/South Americans, and Dominicans. This finding held for both men and women.

Nevertheless, although nationally aggregated data show a Latino mortality advantage vis-à-vis non-Latino White Americans, state-level data is inconsistent in supporting the Latino mortality paradox. For example, Latinos in Arizona have higher premature mortality rates than their non-Latino White counterparts (Arizona Health Status and Vital Statistics, 2020). In 2020, the median age at death for non-Latino White Americans was 78 years, while for Latino Americans it was 69 years. Percent of deaths before expected years of life reached (77 years for U.S. residents) was significantly higher for non-Latino White Americans compared to Latino Americans (46.1% compared to 65.0%, respectively), which means, on average, that 65% of Latino Americans die prematurely in Arizona.

Data from the Arizona Department of Health and Vital Statistics (2020) show that age-adjusted mortality rates over a 20-year period show that Latinos in Arizona, primarily of Mexican descent, have a better mortality trend than non-Latino White Americans, non-Latino Black Americans, and American Indians (Figure 5.14). However, the Latino mortality advantage disappears in 2020, with Latinos showing higher mortality rates than non-Latino White Americans (871.7/100,000 compared to 794.6/100,000, respectively).

An examination of mortality rates in Arizona (Arizona Health Status and Vital Statistics, 2020) found both advantages and disadvantages among Latinos, primarily of Mexican descent, using state data available in 2015. In Arizona, Latino Americans have higher mortality rates than non-Latino White Americans for diabetes mellitus, chronic liver disease and cirrhosis, primary hypertension, cerebrovascular diseases, kidney disease, and cervical cancer. Latinos have lower mortality rates than their non-Latino White counterparts for cardiovascular disease, diseases of the heart, coronary heart disease, all site cancer, lung cancer, breast cancer, colorectal cancer, prostate cancer, Alzheimer's disease, and chronic lower respiratory disease. However, there was no adjustment for socioeconomic covariates.

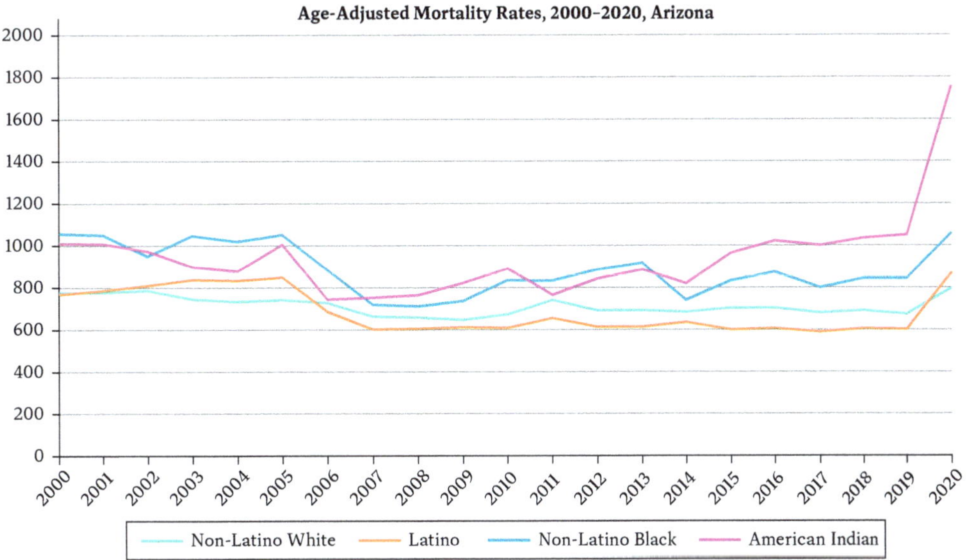

FIGURE 5.14 Age-Adjusted Mortality Rates by Race and Ethnicity, Arizona, 2000–2020

Arias et al. (2020) found that Latino adults experience lower mortality than non-Latino Black Americans and American Indians and Alaska Natives, and that the difference between non-Latino White Americans and Latino Americans may be mediated by nativity and race in the United States. A recent study by Montanez-Valverde et al. (2021) found no support for the Latino mortality paradox in relation to cardiovascular disease (CVD). They found that the age-adjusted CVD rate in men was significantly higher in Latinos, with 9.2% compared to non-Latino Black Americans (8.1%) and non-Latino White Americans (7.6%). In women, the age-adjusted CVD rate was significantly higher among non-Latino Black Americans (7.7%) compared to Latino Americans (6.1%) and non-Latino White Americans (3.9%). Both Latinos (men) and Latinas (women) had higher age-adjusted CVD rates than their non-Latino counterparts.

All-Cause Mortality Rates in the U.S.–Mexico Border Region

The U.S.–Mexico border region represents a significantly large population of Latinos of Mexican descent. An examination of mortality rates may provide insight on selective migration and the salmon bias hypotheses. For example, Latinos living in the U.S.–Mexico border region have lower age-adjusted all-cause mortality rates than non-Latino White Americans and non-Latino Black Americans living in the same region (CDC, 2021a). Interestingly, Latinos and non-Latino White Americans have lower all-cause mortality than their counterparts not living in the U.S.–Mexico border region. Non-Latino Black Americans have higher mortality in the U.S.–Mexico border region than their counterparts living in other parts of the United States (Figure 5.15).

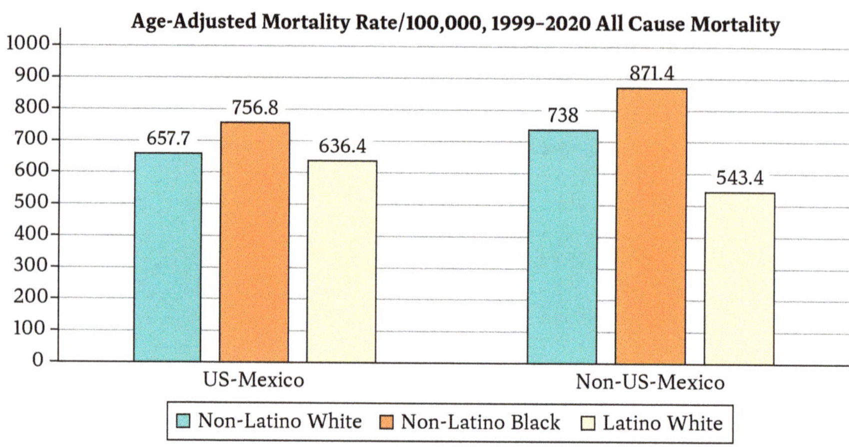

FIGURE 5.15 Age-Adjusted Mortality Rates, U.S.-Mexico Border Region, 1999–2020

Likewise, cancer mortality the rates are lower in the U.S.-Mexico border region compared to the non-border region (CDC, 2021b) (Figure 5.16). Cancer mortality rates are lower among Latino Americans compared to non-Latino White Americans and non-Latino Black Americans residing in the U.S.-Mexico border region but higher than their non-border Latino counterparts. Non-Latino White Americans and non-Latino Black Americans have lower cancer mortality in the U.S.-Mexico Border Region than their respective counterparts living in non-border regions.

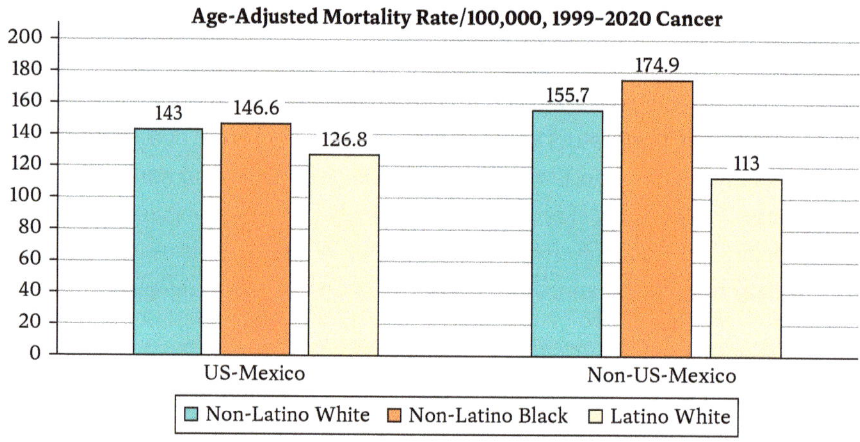

FIGURE 5.16 Age-Adjusted Cancer Mortality, U.S.-Mexico Border Region, 1999–2020

All-cause mortality and cancer mortality rates differ in the U.S.-Mexico border region from the non- border region. Latinos, primarily of Mexican descent, have higher all-cause mortality compared to Latinos living in non-border regions. Additionally, cancer mortality is higher for Latinos in the U.S.-Mexico border region than it is for Latinos in non-border regions. Given the proximity to Mexico, the return migration of terminally ill Mexicans does not appear to be an underlying reason for the mortality rate differences observed.

Post-COVID-19 Mortality Rates

In 2020, after the first full year of the COVID-19 pandemic, life expectancy across all groups decreased (Arias et al., 2021). According to Arias et al. (2021) from 2019 to 2020, life expectancy at birth decreased by 1.8 years for men (76.3 to 74.5) and by 1.2 years for women (81.4 to 80.2). Life expectancy decreased by 3.7 years for Latino males, 2.0 years for Latina women, 3.3 years for male non-Latino Black Americans 2.4 years for female non-Latino Black Americans, 1.3 years for male non-Latino White Americans, and 1.1 years for female non-Latina White Americans. Still, the Latino mortality paradox with respect to life expectancy is evident post-COVID-19 (Arias & Xu, 2022b). According to Arias and Xu (2022a), the mortality gap between the Latino and non-Latino White populations decreased by 83.4% from 2019 (3.1) to 2020 (0.5), which is remarkable given that the mortality advantage had been reported by Palloni & Arias (2004) as 35%–47% higher than non-Latino White Americans.

The Latino population *lost* most of the mortality advantage it had experienced relative to the non-Latino White population due primarily to excess deaths attributed to COVID-19, a health inequality that will be discussed in Chapter 7. Among racial and ethnic groups, the smallest average percentage increase in numbers of COVID-19 attributable deaths compared with previous years occurred among non-Latino White Americans (11.9%) and was the largest for Latinos (53.6%), with Non-Latino Black Americans intermediate (Rossen et al., 2020). Only Latinos exhibited a bimodal distribution of COVID-19 mortality rates during the pandemic.

Garcia and Sáenz (2023) found evidence that the Latino mortality paradox persisted through the COVID-19 pandemic. They analyzed deaths related to COVID-19, non-COVID-19, and overall mortality. Indeed, for COVID-19 mortality, the Latino health advantage disappeared in 2020. However, the paradox continued for non-COVID-19-related mortality. They examined 13 states with the largest Latino populations and found that for most states the paradox continued, but for three states—Arizona, California, and Colorado—the paradox disappeared across all age groups assessed (45–85+). For non-COVID-19 mortality, they found that Latinos had significantly lower rates than non-Latino White Americans across all age categories in both 2020 and 2021. They found that Latinos died from non-COVID-19 deaths at rates ranging from 23% lower among adults 65–74 years old to 31% lower among those in the 45–54 age group in 2021. The persistence of the Latino paradox among non-COVID-19 deaths was generally consistent across almost all 13 states apart from Colorado, New Mexico, and Arizona.

Bassett et al. (2020) found that for all U.S. racial/ethnic groups compared to non-Latino White Americans, there were excess COVID-19 deaths across all ages. However, although for all racial/ethnic groups, most deaths occurred at older ages, there was also substantial loss of life at younger ages, before age 65, among Latino Americans and Non-Latino Black Americans. More years of life were lost before 65 years among the non-Latino Black Americans and Latinos, despite the smaller size of these groups, than among the non-Latino White population. They also found that for young adults into midlife, non-Latino Black Americans, Latinos, and non-Latino American Indian or Alaska Natives had a much higher risk of death from COVID-19 than the non-Latino White population.

Mortality data from 2021 shows that both Latino males and female Americans had lower mortality rates than non-Latino White Americans and non-Latino Black Americans, respectively (Xu et al., 2022). Through 2021, Latinos still show a mortality paradox vis-à-vis their non-Latino White counterparts (Figure 5.17).

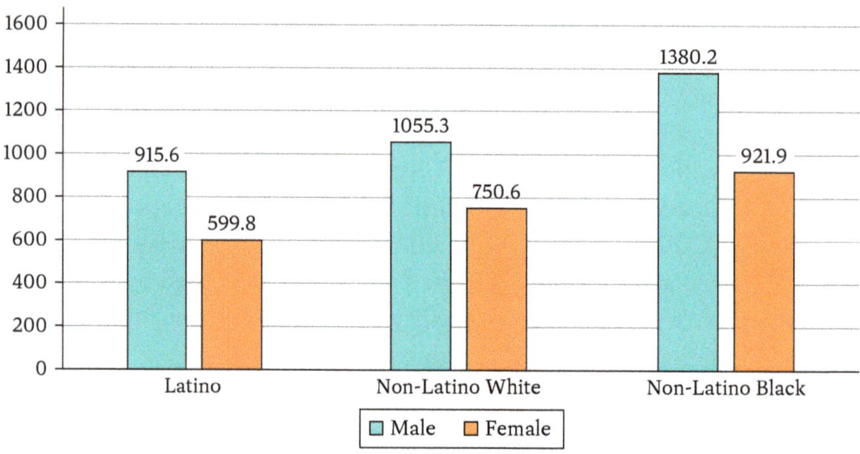

FIGURE 5.17 Mortality Rates by Race/Ethnicity and Gender (per 100,000 Population), United States, 2021

Limitations of the Latino Mortality Paradox

Problems with the Latino mortality paradox as an explanation for better health outcomes for Latinos are noted, especially among younger Latinos and Latina pregnancy outcomes (Acevedo-Garcia, 2005). Hayes-Bautista and others call attention to the increase in premature mortality rates among Latino adolescents, especially those who are U.S.-born, and the increase in motor vehicle fatalities and homicides (Hayes-Bautista et al., 2002; Vaca et al., 2011). Studies on low birth weight (LBW) among Latinas shows that increasing acculturation is associated with higher risk for LBW infants, and that immigrant Latinas have lower infant mortality rates than U.S.-born Latinas (Acevedo-Garcia et al., 2005). Acevedo-Garcia et al. (2005) found that Mexican immigrant women were 20% less likely than other Latino subgroups to have LBW infants.

Recent research on the Latino mortality and morbidity paradox notes the complex and interacting effects of the sending country, receiving country, socioeconomic status, generation status, nativity, and gender (Arias et al., 2020; Garcia & Reyes, 2017; Garcia et al., 2017, 2018; Markides & Rote, 2019). The trend is support for the selection immigrant hypothesis over other factors associated with return migration or Latino cultural factors (Martinez-Cardoso & Geronimus, 2021).

Taken together, support for the Latino mortality paradox is strongly linked to socioeconomic status—primarily higher poverty rates and lower educational attainment—and not necessarily to cultural protective factors. However, one cannot ignore the impact of dietary changes among Latino immigrants with length of stay in the United States. Little support to date is found for cultural factors, other than increasing acculturation level, and a Latino mortality advantage. However, when SES covariates are statistically controlled, the statistical strength of the association between acculturation level and health attenuates or disappears altogether.

Notwithstanding the abundance of research in support of the Latino epidemiologic paradox, there are serious conceptual and methodological problems with the theory as presently formulated. Several major problems have been noted in the literature: Latino subgroups and applicability of the paradox beyond Mexicans, misclassification of Latinos on death certificates, data collection issues, the absence of cultural measures apart from acculturation measures and familism, and lack of longitudinal studies.

Genetic and Physiological Theories of Health Inequalities

Genetic and physiological theories of health inequalities focus on biological, genetic, epigenetic, and gene-environment interactions to examine differences between non-Latino White Americans and Latino Americans in mortality and morbidity. Most biological or physiological theories related to differences in intelligence have been thoroughly refuted. Those theories that have gained support are associated with cancer, diabetes mellitus, and obesity.

Biological or Genetic Differences and Cancer Among Latinos

Cervical cancer inequalities are observed for Latina Americans compared to non-Latino White Americans, with higher incidence and mortality rates. Genetic research has uncovered possible causative agents: the breast cancer susceptibility genes BRCA1 and BRCA2. Oncological prevalence studies have found that the prevalence of these genetic mutations is about 20% in Latinas (John et al., 2007; Vogel et al., 2007; Weitzel et al., 2013). These mutations may be inherited (germline) or arise because of a combination of genetic and environmental factors (somatic; Pinney & Simmons, 2010).

Specific subgroups have been identified as having a higher proportion of individuals who carry a BRCA mutation, including those who have been diagnosed with triple-negative breast cancer (TNBC) and those from different ethnic groups, including Latino and Black populations and those of Ashkenazi Jewish heritage (Greenup et al., 2013). The risk for BRCA mutation carriers to develop breast cancer varies from 57% by age 70 years to 85% lifetime risk among high-risk clinic patients, with lower risks reported from population-based studies. They also have a 20%–50% risk for ovarian cancer (Antoniou et al., 2003; Ford et al., 1998). Weitzel et al. (2013) found a prevalence rate of 25% for BRCA1 among Latinas of Mexican descent. The linkage to Ashkenazi Jewish ancestry was also confirmed. One might think this is surprising, but it is widely known that *conversos*, those Spanish Jews who converted to Christianity, were among the first conquistadores in the Americas, which is why it is called the Mexican founder mutation, which represents 10%–12% of all BRCA 1 mutations in clinic- and population-based cohorts in the United States (Weitzel et al., 2013). However, their research suggests that the genetic mutation arose 1,480 years ago, predating Spanish colonization, revealing a complex genetic and environmental interaction.

John et al. (2007) reported on the prevalence of BRCA 1 in the United States. They found that rates of women with breast cancer diagnosed at age 65 or younger with pathogenic BRCA1 mutations were highest in Ashkenazi Jewish patients (8.3%), followed by Latino patients (3.5%), non-Latino White patients (2.2%), non-Latino Black patients (1.3%), and Asian American patients (0.5%). In young patients diagnosed before age 35 years, the prevalence was remarkably high in Non-Latino Black Americans (16.7%) and next highest among Latinas (8.9%). However, among those women aged 35–64, Latinas had the highest prevalence rate of 3.0%, compared to Non-Latino Black Americans (0.5%). Non-Ashkenazi Jewish White women aged 35–64 had a prevalence of 1.9%, compared to Ashkenazi Jewish White women ages 35–65 who had the highest prevalence of 6.4%.

Biogenetic–Environment Interactions

Environmental toxins are known to cause genetic mutations in humans (Perla et al., 2015). Also, a balanced diet with ample nutritional ingredients can enhance immunological function and resistance to disease. Thus, biogenetic–environment interactions can increase and decrease the risk for disease. The application of this theory focuses on the built environment and increased exposure to environmental toxins.

Individuals living in low-income neighborhoods are often exposed to chemical and nonchemical stressors: physical (e.g., noise pollution, lack of green space) and psychosocial (e.g., food desert, violence or threat of violence, discrimination, residential segregation, and psychosocial stress). Health inequalities may arise not only because of higher levels of exposure to environmental hazards among minority groups but also because of the synergistic effect of exposure to multiple environmental hazards and psychosocial stressors (Appleton et al., 2016; Münzel & Daiber, 2018; Payne-Sturges et al., 2018).

The Flint water crisis exposed the problems with the built environment and exposure to contaminates (Sadler et al., 2017). Increased exposure to environmental pollutants is not randomly distributed in the United States but rather is disproportionately higher in communities where historically marginalized and disenfranchised populations reside (Shim et al., 2017). The overwhelming burden of exposure to metal toxins like lead (Pb), mercury (Hg), cadmium (Cd), and arsenic (As) is concentrated in these communities (Moody & Grady, 2021; Perla et al., 2015; Sadler et al., 2017). A study by Perla et al. (2015), using data from the National Health and Nutrition Examination Survey (NHANES) from 1999 to 2008, found that Mexican Americans had higher levels of dichlorodiphenyldichloroethylene (a result of DDT exposure), lead, and cadmium compared to other groups.

Epigenetics and Social Epigenetics

The term *epigenetics* refers to the heritable, but modifiable, regulation of genetic functions that are mediated through non-DNA-encoded mechanisms. The epigenome can mark DNA in two ways, both of which play a role in turning genes on or off: The first occurs when certain chemical tags called *methyl groups* attach to CpG sites in the DNA molecule; the second occurs when a variety of chemical tags attach to the tails of histones, which are spool-like proteins that package DNA neatly into chromosomes. This action affects how tightly DNA is wound around the histones.

Epigenetic alterations may be induced spontaneously, in response to environmental factors, through accumulation over the lifespan, or may simply be part of a person's genetic background. To date, most epigenetic research has focused on alterations associated with cancer (Biswas & Rao, 2017). Methylated genes have been identified in biogenesis and signaling of genetic pathways to cancer.

Epigenetics focuses on processes that regulate how and when certain genes are turned on and turned off. *Epigenomics* pertains to the analysis of epigenetic changes across many genes in a cell or entire organism. Epigenetic processes control normal growth and development, and this process is deregulated in diseases such as cancer. Diet and exposure to environmental toxins throughout all stages of human development, among other factors, can cause epigenetic changes that may turn on or turn off certain genes. Changes in genes that would normally protect against a disease, as a result, could make people more susceptible to developing that disease later in life.

Epigenetics and Psychosocial Stress

There is a growing body of recent research suggesting that psychosocial stress can induce long-lasting epigenetically based changes in gene regulation that are linked to changes in behavior and physiology (Linnér & Almgren, 2020; Weaver et al., 2017). There is additional evidence that these epigenetic changes can be transmitted across generations (Keverne & Curley, 2008; Nagy & Turecki, 2015). These changes occur through at least two interrelated epigenetic processes: addition of a methyl group to CpG dinucleotides, which are special regions in DNA bases where gene activity can be silenced when methyl groups are attached, and removal of acetyl groups from histone tails, which stops the gene activity of the DNA bases wrapped around the histone, causing the DNA to coil up tightly and be silenced.

Perhaps the best available evidence that there are epigenetic changes associated with psychosocial stress are the findings from the Detroit Neighborhood Health Study (DNHS) reported by Uddin et al. (2010). The study assessed posttraumatic stress disorder (PTSD) and the correlation between the number of potential traumatic events and methylation of CpG sites. Compared to PTSD-unaffected individuals, PTSD-affected individuals showed higher levels of DNA unmethylation (gene expression = risk for PTSD). They also found that genes whose methylation levels were significantly and negatively correlated with traumatic burden showed a similar strong signal of immune function among PTSD affected individuals. These findings strongly suggest that epigenetic processes are mediators of social environmental influences on psychiatric disorders, including PTSD.

Social epigenetics attempts to identify classes of genes and/or specific signaling pathways through which social factors might influence mechanisms through which social environments might alter gene expression and affect minority health and health inequalities. Psychosocial stressors may affect health status through epigenomic modifications of various biological pathways. Studies on adverse childhood experiences (ACEs) have also shown ties to epigenetic changes affecting genes related to mental health, drug addiction, and obesity (Felitti, 2009; Rubin, 2016).

Adverse social and environmental experiences early in life may predispose an individual to dysfunctional physiological responses and to future stressors in adulthood (Ling & Groop, 2009; Pinney & Simmons, 2010; Ravelli et al., 1998). Exposure to emotional or physical abuse or neglect might alter DNA methylation levels, creating an epigenetic signature, which in turn might influence risk of cardiovascular disease, cancer, cerebrovascular disease, and psychiatric illnesses (Felitti et al., 2019). The prevalence of adverse childhood experiences (ACEs) among Latinos was reported by Llabre et al. (2017). They found a prevalence of 77.2% for reporting experiencing at least one ACE, and 28.7% reported experiencing four or more ACEs. Research has demonstrated a dose-response relationship between the number of ACEs experienced and adverse health outcomes. In their Latino sample, they also found that ACEs were associated with depressive symptoms, body mass index, smoking, alcohol use, cancer, coronary heart disease, and chronic obstructive pulmonary disease. They did not find associations with asthma, diabetes mellitus, or stroke. We will examine ACEs and health outcomes among Latinos in Chapter 6.

Epigenetics and Diabetes Mellitus and Obesity

Several factors are known to influence the incidence of diabetes mellitus: obesity, poor nutrition, lack of exercise, insulin resistance and sensitivity, and a family history (Sterns et al., 2014). For example, Sterns et al. (2014) theorize that diabetes mellitus is an interaction of the social environment, the intrauterine environment, genetics, and epigenetic modifications. (Figure 5.18).

Evidence supporting the development of diabetes mellitus (DM) and obesity linked to epigenetic modification has been increasing over the past decade. Several studies have noted the contribution of the intrauterine environment and maternal nutrition, discussed in the literature as metabolic programming, to increasing rates of offspring born with DM (Drong et al., 2012; Hales & Barker, 1992). Similarly, studies documenting the incidence and prevalence of DM among Pima Indians in Arizona note the high incidence of female infants with DM associated with maternal DM, which suggests epigenetic transmission across generations (Pettitt et al., 1983, 1988). According to Drong et al. (2012), however, "There are no convincing estimates of the extent to which individual differences in the risk of DM and obesity reflect epigenetic variation" (p. 711).

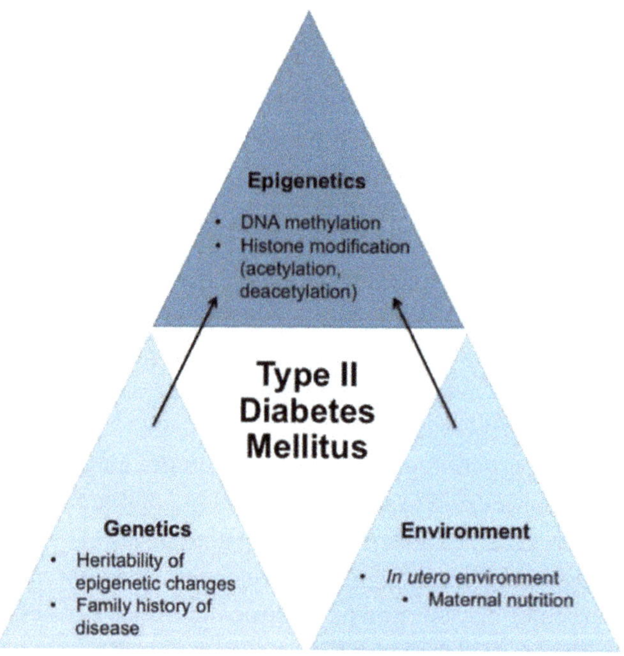

FIGURE 5.18 Factors Related to Diabetes Mellitus

Epigenetics and Life Expectancy Among Latinos

Life expectancy has been shown to be longer among Mexican Americans than non-Latino White Americans prior to the COVID-19 pandemic. An association between aging and epigenetic modifications is noted in the literature, with increasing age associated with increased DNA methylation, which has been associated with cognitive impairment, cancer, and increased mortality rates (Dhingra et al., 2018).

Horvath (2013) measured the epigenetic age of tissue samples by combining the DNA methylation levels of multiple dinucleotide markers, known as *cytosine-phosphate-guanines* (*CpGs*) to develop an "epigenetic clock" to measure age, known as *DNA methylation age* or *epigenetic age*. This technique was confirmed by Hannum et al. (2013) for the capability of assessing ageing in humans. Using this DNA epigenetic clock, Horvath et al. (2016) found that Latinos age more slowly because they are more resistant to natural processes that interfere with cell repair and development as people grow older. The biological clock measured Latina's (women) "genetic age" as 2.4 years younger than non-Latino women of the same actual age after menopause. The findings suggest that genetic or environmental factors linked to Latino ethnicity may influence how quickly a person ages and how long they live (Horvath & Raj, 2018). The utility of the epigenetic clock method using various tissues and organs has been demonstrated in applications surrounding Alzheimer's disease, centenarian status, development, Down syndrome, frailty, HIV infection, Huntington's disease, obesity, lifetime stress, menopause, osteoarthritis, and Parkinson's disease (Quach et al., 2017).

The complex interaction of heredity, epigenetic mechanisms, and the social and physical environment explains the incidence and prevalence of diabetes mellitus among Latinos of Mexican descent, Puerto Ricans, and others (Figure 5.19).

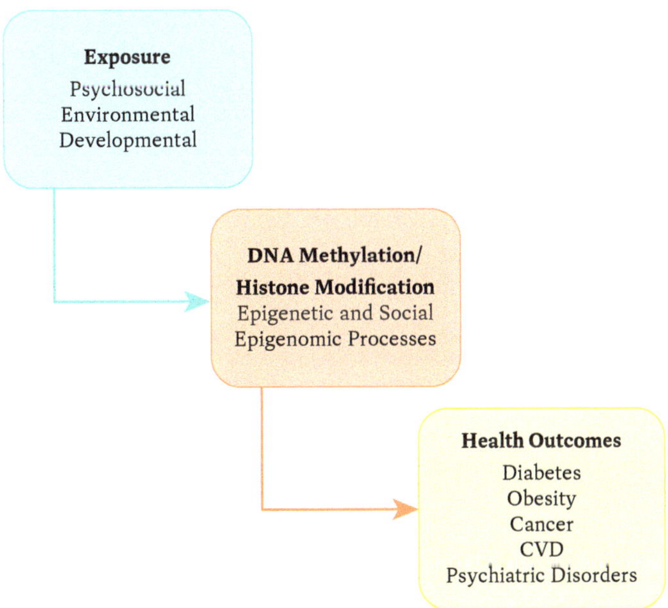

FIGURE 5.19 Pathways to Disease

Implementation science has emerged as a novel approach for integrating health paradigms and prevention of disease using the sociocultural context of populations to enhance the adoption of risk-protective behaviors. Eccles and Mittman (2006) have defined *implementation science* as "the scientific study of methods to promote the systematic uptake of research findings and other evidence-based practices into routine practice, and, hence, to improve the quality and effectiveness of health services" (p. 1). The focus is typically on health organizations and personnel to use research findings in everyday practice. However, we should take this definition one step further by including the populations under examination and including cultural practices that enhance study findings and their applicability. Moreover, using culture to recruit, enroll, maintain, and empower Latinos can increase healthy behaviors and strengthen intervention designs.

Results from studies that have examined acculturation, length of residence, generation status, and the Latino mortality paradox can be used to strengthen operationalization of cultural concepts, research design, data collection methods, and statistical controls that can facilitate the elucidation of important sociocultural factors that enhance research findings and their utilization.

Given that most Latinos residing in the United States are U.S.-born, there is an overabundance of studies investigating the Latino epidemiological paradox and Latino immigrant health, with less attention given to the sociocultural dynamics of Latinos who are second generation and higher. The focus on immigrant health further perpetuates the stereotype that all Latinos are immigrants, which obscures important etiological factors and differences among U.S.-born Latinos that are inextricably linked to historical, geopolitical, and social factors present in the United States. More systematic health research is needed on U.S.-born Latinos to fully understand socioeconomic and sociocultural influences on health inequalities that exist with length of residence and exposure in non-Latino White mainstream society (Hummer et al., 2007).

Equivocal findings regarding health paradigms and Latinos are the norm. This situation has more to do with varying definitions of concepts, different research methods, sample size, an overreliance on cross-sectional studies, and the inclusion of Latino subgroups. There is an urgent need for longitudinal population-based studies that can disentangle sociodemographic and sociocultural factors correlated over time with disease outcomes.

CHAPTER SUMMARY

The intersection of race, ethnicity, socioeconomic status, gender, age, and place contributes to health inequalities in the United States among historically excluded population groups, like non-Latino Black Americans and Mexican Americans. The relationships between and among sociodemographic characteristics and adverse health outcomes is made more complex by the introduction of cultural factors, including acculturation level, length of residence in the United States, and immigration status, and protective factors, like familism and cultural resiliency or cultural wealth.

Health inequalities require social justice policies and interventions for their elimination. There are several community-based interventions that utilize cultural strengths through promotoras de salud to maximize health promotion and disease prevention among Latinos. Theoretically driven interventions that incorporate cultural measures beyond level of acculturation can inform implementation strategies.

Theories of health inequalities among historically marginalized populations cover three broad categories: socioenvironmental theories (e.g., segregation, resource deprivation), psychosocial and behavioral theories (e.g., acculturation theory, Latino mortality paradox), and genetic, epigenetic, and physiological theories (e.g., BRCA 1&2, psychiatric illnesses). Each of these theories include specific hypotheses regarding how risk exposure is associated with negative social and environmental influences that promote negative health status.

Several of these theories or paradigms are relevant for Latino health and have been discussed, especially immigration and acculturation hypotheses, the Latino epidemiological paradox, and potential epigenetic mechanisms underlying longevity, cancer, psychiatric illnesses, and diabetes mellitus among Latinos. In Chapter 6, we will discuss more aspects of "upstream" causes, including epigenetics and ACEs and their hypothesized link to intergenerational trauma. Latinos experience a high level of ACEs that are associated with several chronic diseases and risk behaviors.

Latino ethnic density/ethnic enclaves have been proposed as modifying the effects of racism and discrimination, contrary to research among Non-Latino Black Americans. This observation has prompted some researchers to examine positive aspects of Latino enclaves, including social cohesion, social networks, and cultural wealth. The built manmade environment, also called *riskscapes*, also contributes to psychosocial and environmental stressors. Food insecurity is a major problem in the United States, and rates are highest among non-Latino Black Americans. In 2020, Latinos had almost twice the rate of food insecurity as non-Latino White Americans. Interestingly, an apparent paradox was observed for higher rates of obesity-related cancers among Latino Americans in lower prevalence counties.

Discrimination is linked to poorer health status among historically marginalized populations, like non-Latino Black Americans. Perceived discrimination is very high among Latino Americans and varies with each subgroup, with Latinos of Puerto Rican descent reporting higher rates of perceived discrimination, followed by Mexicans. Studies have shown that perceived discrimination is consistently associated with higher rates of depression and psychiatric disorders among Latinos. The link between discrimination and physical health is less clear.

Literally hundreds of research articles, reviews, and commentaries have been published since the first mention of the Latino epidemiologic paradox in the mid-1980s. Additionally, hundreds of research articles have been published on the topic of Latino acculturation and health. Despite the substantial amount of evidence accumulated on these topics, consensus has been elusive. Nevertheless, there are more consistent findings related to (a) length of residence in the United States and risk for psychiatric disorders and (b) acculturation and the adoption of unhealthy behaviors.

Acculturation level has been found to be linked to dietary practices, risk behaviors, obesity, and cardiovascular disease among Latinos, with some variation seen between men and women. These findings, however, may be associated with confounding factors like socioeconomic status and length of residence in the United States. Two related hypotheses have sought to account for these differences—the acculturation hypothesis and the immigrant hypothesis—with varying levels of empirical support found for each.

Much of the research on the Latino mortality paradox has used national data to examine mortality rates among Latinos and non-Latinos. Many scholars would argue that the Latino mortality paradox is empirically supported and settled. National findings, however, belie regional and state-level findings on the Latino mortality paradox where residence in some U.S.–Mexico border states and elsewhere show higher mortality rate in Latino Americans compared to non-Latino White Americans. Nevertheless, across all age groups, except for Latino adolescents, the mortality paradox is apparent. For Latino adolescents, homicides and motor vehicle accidents are higher than those for non-Latino White adolescents. The COVID-19 pandemic significantly reduced the Latino mortality paradox in 2020, but it rebounded in 2021. Still, if there is a mortality paradox, then what factors account for the apparent resiliency of Latinos of Mexican descent? More research into cultural resiliency and health among Latinos is necessary, again coupled with longitudinal research designs to help disentangle socioeconomic and cultural influences.

The cause of disease in Latino and other populations is multifactorial, with intersecting relationships among important antecedents like epigenetic risks and social determinants of health. Knowledge of health inequality theories and Latino health paradigms are integral to developing culturally responsive interventions for Latinos of Mexican descent.

QUESTIONS TO CONSIDER

1. How well do the theories of health inequalities model risk for exposure and subsequent illness among historically marginalized populations?
2. Does the concept of "*riskscapes*" adequately encompass risk of exposure and death in urban and rural areas?
3. Does the Latino epidemiological paradox include cultural and social factors that might help explain mortality differences between Latinos of Mexican descent and non-Latino Black Americans or between Latinos of Mexican descent and non-Latino White Americans?
4. Describe the epigenetic basis for diabetes mellitus among Latinos and the possibility for intergenerational transmission.
5. Discuss the efficacy of genetic and genetic-environmental interactions related to increased longevity and the risk for breast cancer among Latinos of Mexican descent.

SUGGESTED READINGS

Abraido-Lanza, A. F., Dohrenwend, B. P., Ng-Mak, D. S., & Turner, J. B. (1999). The Latino mortality paradox: A test of the "salmon bias" and healthy migrant hypotheses. *American Journal of Public Health, 89*, 1543–1548.

Antoniou, A., Pharoah, P. D., Narod, S., Risch, H. A., Eyfjord, J. E., Hopper, J. L., Loman, N., Olsson, H., Johannsson, O., Borg, A., Pasini, B., Radice, P., Manoukian, S., Eccles, D. M., Tang, N., Olah, E., Anton-Culver, H., Warner, E., Lubinski, J., ... Easton, D. (2003). Average risks of breast and ovarian cancer associated with BRCA1 or BRCA2 mutations detected in case series unselected for family history: A combined analysis of 22 studies. *The American Journal of Human Genetics, 72*(5), 1117–1130.

Braveman, P. A., Kumanyika, S., Fielding, J., LaVeist, T., Borrell, L. N., Manderscheid, R., & Troutman, A. (2011). Health disparities and health equity: The issue is justice. *American Journal of Public Health, 101*(Suppl. 1), S149–S155.

Eschbach, K., Ostir, G. V., Patel, K. V., Markides, K. S., & Goodwin, J. S. (2004). Neighborhood context and mortality among older Mexican Americans: Is there a barrio advantage? *American Journal of Public Health, 94*(10), 1807–1812.

Fenelon, A., Chinn, J. J., & Anderson, R. N. (2017). A comprehensive analysis of the mortality experience of Hispanic subgroups in the United States: Variation by age, country of origin, and nativity. *SSM Population Health, 3*, 245–254.

Garcia, M. A., & Reyes, A. M. (2017). Prevalence and trends in morbidity and disability among older Mexican Americans in the Southwestern United States, 1993–2013. *Research on Aging, 40*(4), 311–339. https://doi.org/10.1177/0164027517697800

Morello-Frosch, R., Pastor, M., & Sadd, J. (2001). Environmental justice and Southern California's "riskscape" the distribution of air toxics exposures and health risks among diverse communities. *Urban Affairs Review, 36*(4), 551–578.

Nelson, K. A. (2013). Does residential segregation help or hurt? Exploring differences in the relationship between segregation and health among U.S. Hispanics by nativity and ethnic subgroup. *The Social Science Journal, 50*(4), 646–657.

Palloni A., & Arias E. (2004). Paradox lost: Explaining the Hispanic adult mortality advantage. *Demography, 41*(3), 385–415.

Pascoe, E. A., & Richman, L. S. (2009). Perceived discrimination and health: A Meta-analytic review. *Psychological Bulletin, 135*(4), 531–554. https://doi.org/10.1037/a0016059.

Rubin, L. P. (2016). Maternal and pediatric health and disease: Integrating biopsychosocial models and epigenetics. *Pediatric Research, 79*(1), 127–135.

Viruell-Fuentes, E. A., Morenoff, J. D., Williams, D. R., & House, J. S. (2013). Contextualizing nativity status, Latino social ties, and ethnic enclaves: An examination of the "immigrant social ties hypothesis." *Ethnicity & Health, 18*(6), 586–609.

REFERENCES

Abraido-Lanza, A.F., Armbrister, A.N., Florez, K. R., & Aguirre, A. N. (2006). Toward a theory-driven model of acculturation in public health research. *American Journal of Public Health, 96*, 1342–1346

Abraido-Lanza, A. F., Dohrenwend, B. P., Ng-Mak, D. S., & Turner, J. B. (1999). The Latino mortality paradox: A test of the "salmon bias" and healthy migrant hypotheses. *American Journal of Public Health, 89*, 1543–1548.

Abraído-Lanza, A. F., Echeverría, S. E., & Flórez, K. R. (2016). Latino immigrants, acculturation, and health: Promising new directions in research. *Annual Review of Public Health, 37*, 219–236.

Acevedo-Garcia, D., Lochner, K. A., Osypuk, T. L., & Subramanian, S. V. (2003). Future directions in residential segregation and health research: A multilevel approach. *American Journal of Public Health, 93*(2), 215–221.

Acevedo-Garcia, D., Soobader, M. J., & Berkman, L. F. (2005). The differential effect of foreign-born status on low birth weight by race/ethnicity and education. *Pediatrics, 115*(1), e20–e30.

Aguila, E., Escarce, J., Leng, M., & Morales, L. (2013). Health status and behavioral risk factors in older adult Mexicans and Mexican immigrants to the United States. *Journal of Aging and Health, 25*(1), 136–158.

Ai, A. L., Appel, H. B., & Lee, J. (2018). Acculturation factors related to obesity of Latino American men nationwide. *American Journal of Men's Health, 12*(5), 1421-1430.

Alderete, E., Vega, W. A., Kolody, B., & Aguilar-Gaxiola, S. (2000). Effects of time in the United States and Indian ethnicity on *DSM-III-R* psychiatric disorders among Mexican Americans in California. *The Journal of Nervous and Mental Disease, 188*(2), 90–100.

Alegria, K., Fleszar-Pavlović, S., Hua, J., Ramirez Loyola, M., Reuschel, H., & Song, A. V. (2022). How socioeconomic status and acculturation relate to dietary behaviors within Latino populations. *American Journal of Health Promotion, 36*(3), 450–457.

Alegría, M., Canino, G., Shrout, P. E., Woo, M., Duan, N., Vila, D., Torres, M., Chen, C.-N., & Meng, X. L. (2008). Prevalence of mental illness in immigrant and non-immigrant U.S. Latino groups. *American Journal of Psychiatry, 165*(3), 359–369.

Alegria, M., Sribney, W., Woo, M., Torres, M., & Guarnaccia, P. (2007). Looking beyond nativity: The relation of age of immigration, length of residence, and birth cohorts to the risk of onset of psychiatric disorders for Latinos. *Research in Human Development, 4*(1–2), 19–47.

Alegria, M., Takeuchi, D., Canino, G., Duan, N., Shrout, P., Meng, X.-L., Vega, W., Zane, N., Vila, D., Woo, M., Vera, M., Guarnaccia, P., Aguilar-gaxiola, S., Sue, S., Escobar, J., Lin, K.-M., & Gong, F. (2004). Considering context, place and culture: The National Latino and Asian American Study. *International Journal of Methods in Psychiatric Research, 13*(4), 208–220.

Allen, J. D., Caspi, C., Yang, M., Leyva, B., Stoddard, A. M., Tamers, S., Tucker-Seeley, R. D., & Sorensen, G. C. (2014). Pathways between acculturation and health behaviors among residents of low-income housing: The mediating role of social and contextual factors. *Social Science & Medicine, 123*, 26–36.

Allen, E. (2019). Perceived discrimination and health: Paradigms and prospects. *Sociology Compass, 13*(8), Article e12720.

Almeida, J., Biello, K. B., Pedraza, F., Wintner, S., & Viruell-Fuentes, E. (2016). The association between anti-immigrant policies and perceived discrimination among Latinos in the U.S.: A multilevel analysis. *SSM-Population Health, 2*, 897–903.

Amaro, H., & de la Torre, A. (2002). Public health needs and scientific opportunities in research on Latinas. *American Journal of Public Health, 92*(4), 525–529.

American Public Health Association. (n.d.). *Health equity*. Retrieved June 2, 2023, from https://apha.org/Topics-and-Issues/Health-Equity#:~:text=Creating%20health%20equity%20is%20a,their%20highest%20level%20of%20health

Andrade, N., Ford, A. D., & Alvarez, C. (2021). Discrimination and Latino health: A systematic review of risk and resilience. *Hispanic Health Care International, 19*(1), 5–16.

Antoniou, A., Pharoah, P. D., Narod, S., Risch, H. A., Eyfjord, J. E., Hopper, J. L., Loman, N., Olsson, H., Johannsson, O., Borg, A., Pasini, B., Radice, P., Manoukian, S., Eccles, D. M., Tang, N., Olah, E., Anton-Culver, H., Warner, E., Lubinski, J., ... Easton, D. (2003). Average risks of breast and ovarian cancer associated with BRCA1 or BRCA2 mutations detected in case series unselected for family history: A combined analysis of 22 studies. *The American Journal of Human Genetics, 72*(5), 1117–1130.

Appleton, A. A., Holdsworth, E. A., & Kubzansky, L. D. (2016). A systematic review of the interplay between social determinants and environmental exposures for early-life outcomes. *Current Environmental Health Reports, 3*, 287–301.

Araújo, B., & Borrell, L. (2006). Understanding the link between discrimination, mental health outcomes, and life chances among Latinos. *Hispanic Journal of Behavioral Sciences, 28*, 245–266. https://doi.org/10.1177/0739986305285825

Arellano-Morales, L., Roesch, S. C., Gallo, L. C., Emory, K. T., Molina, K. M., Gonzalez, P., Penedo, F. J., Navas-Nacher, E. L., Teng, Y., Deng, Y., Isasi, C. R., Schneiderman, N., & Brondolo, E. (2015). Prevalence and correlates of perceived ethnic discrimination in the Hispanic Community Health Study/Study of Latinos Sociocultural Ancillary Study. *Journal of Latina/o Psychology, 3*(3), 160–176.

Arias, E., Johnson, N. J., & Vera, B. T. (2020). Racial disparities in mortality in the adult Hispanic population. *SSM-Population Health, 11*, Article 100583.

Arias, E., Tejada-Vera, B., Ahmad, F., Kochanek, K.D. (2021, July). *Provisional life expectancy estimates for 2020. Vital Statistics Rapid Release; no 15.* Hyattsville, MD: National Center for Health Statistics. DOI: https://dx.doi.org/10.15620/cdc:107201.

Arias, E., & Xu, J. Q. (2022a). United States life tables, 2019. *National Vital Statistics Reports*, 70(19). https://doi.org/10.15620/cdc:113096

Arias, E., & Xu, J. Q. (2022b). United States life tables, 2020. *National Vital Statistics Reports*, 71(1). https://doi.org/10.15620/cdc:118055

Arizona Health Status and Vital Statistics. (2020). *Patterns of premature mortality.* https://pub.azdhs.gov/health-stats/report/ahs/ahs2020/pdf/text2d.pdf

Arnett, M. J., Thorpe, R. J., Jr., Gaskin, D. J., Bowie, J. V., LaVeist, T. A. (2016). Race, medical mistrust, and segregation in primary care as usual source of care: Findings from the Exploring Health Disparities in Integrated Communities Study. *Journal of Urban Health, 93*(3), 456–467. https://doi.org/10.1007/s11524-016-0054-9

Ayala, G. X., Baquero, B., & Klinger, S. (2008). A systematic review of the relationship between acculturation and diet among Latinos in the United States: Implications for future research. *Journal of the American Dietetic Association, 108*, 1330–1344

Ayón, C., & Becerra, D. (2013). Mexican immigrant families under siege: The impact of anti-immigrant policies, discrimination, and the economic crisis. *Advances in Social Work, 14*, 206–228.

Bassett, M. T., Chen, J. T., & Krieger, N. (2020). Variation in racial/ethnic disparities in COVID-19 mortality by age in the United States: A cross-sectional study. *PLoS Medicine, 17*(10), Article e1003402.

Bauer, L, Pitts, A., Ruffini, K., & Schanzenbach, D. W. (2020). *The effect of pandemic EBT on measures of food hardship.* The Hamilton Project, Brookings.

Bécares, L. (2014). Ethnic density effects on psychological distress among Latino ethnic groups: An examination of hypothesized pathways. *Health & Place, 30*, 177–186.

Bevel, M. S., Tsai, M. H., Parham, A., Andrzejak, S. E., Jones, S., & Moore, J. X. (2023). Association of food deserts and food swamps with obesity-related cancer mortality in the U.S. *JAMA Oncology, 9*(7), 909–916.

Biswas, S., & Rao, C. M. (2017). Epigenetics in cancer: fundamentals and beyond. *Pharmacology & Therapeutics, 173*, 118–134.

Borges, G., Breslau, J., Orozco, R., Tancredi, D. J., Anderson, H., Aguilar-Gaxiola, S., & Mora, M. E. M. (2011). A cross-national study on Mexico-U.S. migration, substance use and substance use disorders. *Drug and Alcohol Dependence, 117*(1), 16–23.

Bostean, G. (2013). Does selective migration explain the Hispanic paradox? A comparative analysis of Mexicans in the U.S. and Mexico. *Journal of Immigrant and Minority Health, 15*, 624–635.

Braveman, P. A., Kumanyika, S., Fielding, J., LaVeist, T., Borrell, L. N., Manderscheid, R., & Troutman, A. (2011). Health disparities and health equity: The issue is justice. *American Journal of Public Health, 101*(Suppl. 1), S149–S155.

Brondolo, E., Beatty, D. L., Cubbin, C., Pencille, M., Saegert, S., Wellington, R., Tobin, J., Cassells, A., & Schwartz, J. (2009c). Sociodemographic variations in self-reported racism in a community sample of Blacks and Latino(a)s. *Journal of Applied Social Psychology, 39*(2), 407–429.

Brondolo, E., Brady ver Halen, N., Pencille, M., Beatty, D., & Contrada, R. J. (2009b). Coping with racism: A selective review of the literature and a theoretical and methodological critique. *Journal of Behavioral Medicine, 32*, 64–88.

Brondolo, E., Gallo, L. C., & Myers, H. F. (2009a). Race, racism and health: Disparities, mechanisms, and interventions. *Journal of Behavioral Medicine, 32*, 1–8.

Buscemi, J., Beech, B. M., & Relyea, G. (2011). Predictors of obesity in Latino children: Acculturation as a moderator of the relationship between food insecurity and body mass index percentile. *Journal of Immigrant and Minority Health, 13*, 149–154.

Calvin, R., Winters, K., Wyatt, S. B., Williams, D. R., Henderson, F. C., & Walker, E. R. (2003). Racism and cardiovascular disease in African Americans. *The American Journal of the Medical Sciences, 325*(6), 315–331.

Carvajal, S. C., Rosales, C., Rubio-Goldsmith, R., Sabo, S., Ingram, M., McClelland, D. J., Redondo, F., Torres, E., Romero, A. J., Oleary, A. O., Sanchez, Z., & De Zapien, J. G. (2013). The border community and immigration stress scale: A preliminary examination of a community responsive measure in two southwest samples. *Journal of Immigrant and Minority Health, 15*(2), 427–436.

Castro, F. G., Marsiglia, F. F., Kulis, S., Kellison, J. G. (2010). Lifetime segmented assimilation trajectories and health outcomes in Latino and other community residents. *American Journal of Public Health, 100*, 669–676.

Centers for Disease Control and Prevention. (1986). Premature mortality in the United States: Public health issues in the use of years of potential life lost. *Morbidity and Mortality Weekly Report, 35*(Suppl. 2), 1S–11S.

Centers for Disease Control and Prevention. (2021a). *CDC WONDER Online Database, released 2021. Age-Adjusted Mortality Rates, all cause mortality,1999–2020, US-Mexico Border Region.* Retrieved on October 3, 2023, from: https://wonder.cdc.gov/controller/datarequest/D141

Centers for Disease Control and Prevention. (2021b). CDC WONDER Online Database, released 2021. Age-Adjusted Cancer Mortality, 1999–2020, US-Mexico Border Region. Retrieved on October 3, 2023 from: https://wonder.cdc.gov/controller/datarequest/D141

Cervantes, R. C., & Castro, F. G. (1985). Stress, coping, and Mexican American mental health: A systematic review. *Hispanic Journal of Behavioral Sciences, 7*(1), 1–73.

Chambliss, S. E., Pinon, C. P., Messier, K. P., LaFranchi, B., Upperman, C. R., Lunden, M. M., Robinson, A. L., Marshall, J. D., & Apte, J. S. (2021). Local-and regional-scale racial and ethnic disparities in air pollution determined by long-term mobile monitoring. *Proceedings of the National Academy of Sciences, 118*(37), Article e2109249118.

Chen, Y., Freedman, N. D., Rodriquez, E. J., Shiels, M. S., Napoles, A. M., Withrow, D. R., Spillane, S., Sigle, B., Perez-Stable, E. J., & de González, A. B. (2020). Trends in premature deaths among adults in the United States and Latin America. *JAMA Network Open, 3*(2), e1921085–e1921085.

Clark, R., Anderson, N. B., Clark, V. R., & Williams, D. R. (1999). Racism as a stressor for African Americans: A biopsychosocial model. *American Psychologist, 54*(10), 805–816.

Clark, R., Anderson, N. B., Clark, V. R., & Williams, D. R. (2013). Racism as a stressor for African Americans: A biopsychosocial model. In T. A. LaVeist & L. A. Isaac (Eds.), *Race, ethnicity, and health: A public health reader* (2nd ed., pp. 79–103). Jossey-Bass/Wiley.

Cobb, C. L., Salas-Wright, C. P., John, R., Schwartz, S. J., Vaughn, M., Martínez, C. R., Jr., Awad,, G., Pinedo, M., & Cano, M. Á. (2021). Discrimination trends and mental health among native-and foreign-born Latinos: Results from national surveys in 2004 and 2013. *Prevention Science, 22*, 397–407.

Codina, G. E., & Montalvo, F. F. (1994). Chicano phenotype and depression. *Hispanic Journal of Behavioral Sciences, 16*(3), 296–306.

Coleman-Jensen, A., Rabbitt, M. P., Gregory, C. A., & Singh, A. (2022, September). *Household food security in the United States in 2021.* U.S. Department of Agriculture, Economic Research Service

Cuevas, A. G., Reitzel, L. R., Adams, C. E., Cao, Y., Nguyen, N., Wetter, D. W., Watkins, K. L., Regan, S. D., & McNeill, L. H. (2014). Discrimination, affect, and cancer risk factors among African Americans. *American Journal of Health Behavior, 38*(1), 31–41.

Curtin, S. C., & Arias, E. (2019). *Mortality trends by race and ethnicity among adults aged 25 and over, 2000–2017.* National Center for Health Statistics.

Curtin, S. C., & Garnett, M. F. (2023). *Suicide and homicide death rates among youth and young adults aged 10–24: United States, 2001–2021.* National Center for Health Statistics. https://doi.org/10.15620/cdc:12842

Cuy Castellanos, D. (2015). Dietary acculturation in Latinos/Hispanics in the United States. *American Journal of Lifestyle Medicine, 9*(1), 31–36.

Dhingra, R., Nwanaji-Enwerem, J. C., Samet, M., & Ward-Caviness, C. K. (2018). DNA methylation age—environmental influences, health impacts, and its role in environmental epidemiology. *Current Environmental Health Reports, 5*, 317–327.

Diaz, C. J., Koning, S. M., & Martinez-Donate, A. P. (2016). Moving beyond salmon bias: Mexican return migration and health selection. *Demography, 53*(6), 2005–2030.

Diaz, J. E., Schrimshaw, E. W., Tieu, H. V., Nandi, V., Koblin, B. A., & Frye, V. (2020). Acculturation as a moderator of HIV risk behavior correlates among Latino men who have sex with men. *Archives of Sexual Behavior, 49*, 2029–2043.

Drong, A. W., Lindgren, C. M., & McCarthy, M. I. (2012). The genetic and epigenetic basis of type 2 diabetes and obesity. *Clinical Pharmacology & Therapeutics, 92*(6). http://www.nature.com/doifinder/doi:10.1038/clpt.2012.149

Dubowitz, T., Bates, L. M., & Acevedo-Garcia, D. (2010). The Latino health paradox. In C. E. Bird, A. M. Fremont, & S. Timmermans (Eds.), *Handbook of medical sociology* (pp. 106–123). Vanderbilt University Press.

Eccles, M., & Mittman, B. (2006). Welcome to implementation science. *Implementation Science, 1*, Article 1.

Elo, I. T., Turra, C. M., Kestenbaum, B., & Ferguson, B. R. (2004). Mortality among elderly Hispanics in the United States: Past evidence and new results. *Demography, 41*(1), 109–128

Engel, C., & Fischer, C. (2015). Breast cancer risks and risk prediction models. *Breast Care, 10*(1), 7–12. https://doi.org/10.1159/000376600

Eschbach, K., Ostir, G. V., Patel, K. V., Markides, K. S., & Goodwin, J. S. (2004). Neighborhood context and mortality among older Mexican Americans: Is there a barrio advantage? *American Journal of Public Health, 94*(10), 1807–1812.

Felitti, V. J. (2009). Adverse childhood experiences and adult health. *Academic Pediatrics, 9*(3), 131–132.

Felitti, V. J., Anda, R. F., Nordenberg, D., Williamson, D. F., Spitz, A. M., Edwards, V., Koss, M. P., & Marks, J. S. (2019). Relationship of childhood abuse and household dysfunction to many of the leading causes of death in adults: The Adverse Childhood Experiences (ACE) Study. *American Journal of Preventive Medicine, 14*(4), 245–258.

Fenelon, A., Chinn, J. J., & Anderson, R. N. (2017). A comprehensive analysis of the mortality experience of Hispanic subgroups in the United States: Variation by age, country of origin, and nativity. *SSM Population Health, 3*, 245–254.

Finch, B. K., & Vega, W. A. (2003). Acculturation stress, social support, and self-rated health among Latinos in California. *Journal of Immigrant Health, 5*, 109–117.

Fitzgerald, N. (2010). Acculturation, socioeconomic status, and health among Hispanics. *Napa Bulletin, 34*(1), 28–46.

Fitzgerald, N., Hromi-Fiedler, A., Segura-Pérez, S., & Pérez-Escamilla, R. (2011). Food insecurity is related to increased risk of type 2 diabetes among Latinas. *Ethnicity & Disease, 21*(3), 328–334.

Flores, E., Tschann, J. M., Dimas, J. M., Pasch, L. A., & de Groat, C. L. (2010). Perceived racial/ethnic discrimination, posttraumatic stress symptoms, and health risk behaviors among Mexican American adolescents. *Journal of Counseling Psychology, 57*(3), 264–273.

Flórez, K. R., & Abraído-Lanza, A. (2017). Segmented assimilation: An approach to studying acculturation and obesity among Latino adults in the United States. *Family & Community Health, 40*(2), 132–138.

Ford, D., Easton, D. F., Stratton, M., Narod, S., Goldgar, D., Devilee, P., Bishop, D. T., Weber, B., Lenoir, G., Chang-Claude, J., Sobol, H., Teare, M. D., Stuewing, J., Arason, A., Scherneck, S., Peto, J., Rebbeck, T. R., Tonin, P., Neuhausen, S., ... Zelada-Hedman, M. (1998). Genetic heterogeneity and penetrance analysis of the BRCA1 and BRCA2 genes in breast cancer families. *The American Journal of Human Genetics, 62*(3), 676–689.

Franzini, L., & Spears, W. (2003). Contributions of social context to inequalities in years of life lost to heart disease in Texas, USA. *Social Science & Medicine, 57*(10), 1847–1861.

Garcia, M. A., Garcia, C., Chiu, C. T., Raji, M., & Markides, K. S. (2018). A comprehensive analysis of morbidity life expectancies among older Hispanic subgroups in the United States: Variation by nativity and country of origin. *Innovation in Aging, 2*(2), Article igy014.

Garcia, M. A., & Reyes, A. M. (2017). Prevalence and trends in morbidity and disability among older Mexican Americans in the southwestern United States, 1993–2013. *Research on Aging, 40*(4), 311–339. https://10.1177/0164027517697800

Garcia, M. A., & Sáenz, R. (2023). Latino mortality paradox found (again): COVID-19 mortality a tale of two years. *Journal of Aging and Health*. Advance online publication.

Garcia, M. A., Valderrama-Hinds, L. M., Chiu, C.-T., Mutambudzi, M. S., Chen, N.-W., & Raji, M. (2017). Age of migration life expectancy with functional limitations and morbidity in Mexican Americans. *Journal of the American Geriatrics Society, 65*(7), 1591–1596. https://doi.org/10.1111/jgs.14875

Gaskin, D. J., Price, A., Brandon, D. T., & LaVeist, T. A. (2009). Segregation and disparities in health services use. *Medical Care Research and Review, 66*(5), 578–589.

Gaskin, D. J., Thorpe, R. J., Jr., McGinty, E. E., Bower, K., Rohde, C., Young, J. H., LaVeist, T. A., & Dubay, L. (2014). Disparities in diabetes: The nexus of race, poverty, and place. *American Journal of Public Health, 104*(11), 2147–2155.

Gonzalez-Barrera, A. (2021, July 9). *Before COVID-19, more Mexicans came to the U.S. than left for Mexico for the first time in years*. Pew Research Center. https://www.pewresearch.org/short-reads/2021/07/09/before-covid-19-more-mexicans-came-to-the-u-s-than-left-for-mexico-for-the-first-time-in-years/

Grant, B. F., Stinson, F. S., Hasin, D. S., Dawson, D. A., Chou, S. P., & Anderson, K. (2004). Immigration and lifetime prevalence of *DSM-IV* psychiatric disorders among Mexican Americans and non-Hispanic Whites in the United States: Results from the National Epidemiologic Survey on Alcohol and Related Conditions. *Archives of General Psychiatry, 61*(12), 1226–1233.

Greenup, R., Buchanan, A., Lorizio, W., Rhoads, K., Chan, S., Leedom, T., King, R., McLennan, J., Crawford, B., Marcom, P. K., & Hwang, E. S. (2013). Prevalence of BRCA mutations among women with triple-negative breast cancer (TNBC) in a genetic counseling cohort. *Annals of Surgical Oncology, 20*(10), 3254–3258. https://doi.org/10.1245/s10434-013-3205-1

Grigsby-Toussaint, D. S., Zenk, S. N., Odoms-Young, A., Ruggiero, L., & Moise, I. (2010). Availability of commonly consumed and culturally specific fruits and vegetables in African-American and Latino neighborhoods. *Journal of the American Dietetic Association, 110*(5), 746–752.

Guerra, Z. C., Moore, J. R., Londoño, T., & Castro, Y. (2022). Associations of acculturation and gender with obesity and physical activity among Latinos. *American Journal of Health Behavior, 46*(3), 324–336.

Hajat, A., Hsia, C., & O'Neill, M. S. (2015). Socioeconomic disparities and air pollution exposure: A global review. *Current Environmental Health Reports, 2*, 440–450.

Hales, C. N., & Barker, D. J. (1992). Type 2 (non-insulin-dependent) diabetes mellitus: The thrifty phenotype hypothesis. *Diabetologia, 35*, 595–601.

Hannum, G., Guinney, J., Zhao, L., Zhang, L. I., Hughes, G., Sadda, S., Klotzle, B., Bibikova, M., Fan, J.-B., Gao, Y., Deconde, R., Chen, M., Rajapakse, I., Friend, S., Ideker, T., & Zhang, K. (2013). Genome-wide methylation profiles reveal quantitative views of human aging rates. *Molecular Cell, 49*(2), 359–367.

Hayes-Bautista, D. E., Hsu, P., Hayes-Bautista, M., Iniguez, D., Chamberlin, C. L., Rico, C., & Solorio, R. (2002). An anomaly within the Latino epidemiological paradox: The Latino adolescent male mortality peak. *Archives of Pediatrics & Adolescent Medicine, 156*(5), 480–484.

Held, M. L., & Lee, S. (2017). Discrimination and mental health among Latinos: Variation by place of origin. *Journal of Mental Health, 26*(5), 405–410.

Hong, S., Zhang, W., & Walton, E. (2014). Neighborhoods and mental health: Exploring ethnic density, poverty, and social cohesion among Asian Americans and Latinos. *Social Science & Medicine, 111*, 117–124.

Horvath, S. (2013). DNA methylation age of human tissues and cell types. *Genome Biology, 14*(10), 1–20.

Horvath, S., Gurven, M., Levine, M. E., Trumble, B. C., Kaplan, H., Allayee, H., Ritz, B. R., Chen, B., Lu, A. T., Rickabuagh, T. M., Jamieson, B. D., Sun, D., Li, S., Chen, W., Quintana-Murci, L., Fagny, M., Kobor, M. S., Tsao, P. S., Reiner, A. P., & & Assimes, T. L. (2016). An epigenetic clock analysis of race/ethnicity, sex, and coronary heart disease. *Genome Biology, 17*(1), 1–23.

Horvath, S., & Raj, K. (2018). DNA methylation-based biomarkers and the epigenetic clock theory of ageing. *Nature Reviews Genetics, 19*(6), 371–384.

Hoyert, D. (2023). *Maternal mortality rates in the United States, 2021.* Centers for Disease Control, National Center for Health Statistics. https://www.cdc.gov/nchs/data/hestat/maternal-mortality/2021/maternal-mortality-rates-2021.pdf

Hummer, R. A., Powers, D. A., Pullum, S. G., Gossman, G. L., & Frisbie, W. P. (2007). Paradox found (again): Infant mortality among the Mexican-origin population in the United States. *Demography, 44*(3), 441–457.

Hunter, M. (2012). The consequences of colorism. In R. E. Hall (Ed.), *The melanin millennium: Skin color as 21st century international discourse* (pp. 247–256). Springer Netherlands.

Hunter, M. L. (2005). *Race, gender, and the politics of skin tone.* Routledge.

Inagami, S., Borrell, L. N., Wong, M. D., Fang, J., Shapiro, M. F., & Asch, S. M. (2006). Residential segregation and Latino, Black and White mortality in New York City. *Journal of Urban Health, 83*, 406–420.

Isasi, C. R., Ayala, G. X., Sotres-Alvarez, D., Madanat, H., Penedo, F., Loria, C. M., Elder, J. P., Daviglus, M. L., Barnhart, J., Siega-Riz, A.M., Van Horn, L., & Schneiderman, N. (2015). Is acculturation related to obesity in Hispanic/Latino adults? Results from the Hispanic Community Health Study/Study of Latinos. *Journal of Obesity*, Article 186276. https://doi.org/10.1155/2015/186276

Jackson, J. S., & Knight, K. M. (2006). Race and self-regulatory health behaviors: The role of the stress response and the HPA axis in physical and mental health disparities. In K. Warner Schaie & L. L. Carstensen (Eds.), *Social structures, aging, and self-regulation in the elderly* (pp. 189–239). Springer.

Jaco, E. G. (1960). *The social epidemiology of mental disorders.* Russell Sage.

John, E. M., Miron, A., Gong, G., Phipps, A. I., Felberg, A., Li, F. P., West, D. W., & Whittemore, A. S. (2007). Prevalence of pathogenic BRCA1 mutation carriers in 5 U.S. racial/ethnic groups. *JAMA, 298*(24), 2869–2876.

Jones, M. R., Diez-Roux, A. V., Hajat, A., Kershaw, K. N., O'Neill, M. S., Guallar, E., Post, W. S., Kaufman, J. D., & Navas-Acien, A. (2014). Race/ethnicity, residential segregation, and exposure to ambient air pollution: The Multi-Ethnic Study of Atherosclerosis (MESA). *American Journal of Public Health, 104*(11), 2130–2137.

Kaiser, P., Diez Roux, A. V., Mujahid, M., Carnethon, M., Bertoni, A., Adar, S. D., Shea, S., McClelland, R., & Lisabeth, L. (2016). Neighborhood environments and incident hypertension in the Multi-Ethnic Study of Atherosclerosis. *American Journal of Epidemiology, 183*(11), 988–997.

Karno, M., & Edgerton, R. B. (1969). Perception of mental illness in a Mexican-American community. *Archives of General Psychiatry, 20*, 233–238.

Kershaw, K. N., Osypuk, T. L., Do, D. P., De Chavez, P. J., & Diez Roux, A. V. (2015). Neighborhood-level racial/ethnic residential segregation and incident cardiovascular disease: The Multi-Ethnic Study of Atherosclerosis. *Circulation, 131*(2), 141–148.

Kessler, R. C., Mickelson, K. D., & Williams, D. R. (1999). The prevalence, distribution, and mental health correlates of perceived discrimination in the United States. *Journal of Health and Social Behavior, 40*(3), 208–230.

Keverne, E. B., & Curley, J. P. (2008). Epigenetics, brain evolution and behaviour. *Frontiers in neuroendocrinology, 29*(3), 398–412.

Kochanek, K. D., Murphy, S. L., Xu, J., & Tejada-Vera, B. (2016, June 30). Deaths: Final data for 2014. *National Vital Statistics Reports, 65*(4), 1–122.

Kramer, M. R., & Hogue, C. R. (2009). Is segregation bad for your health? *Epidemiologic Reviews, 31*(1), 178–194.

Lara, M., Gamboa, C., Kahramanian, M. I., Morales, L. S., & Hayes Bautista, D. E. (2005). Acculturation and Latino health in the United States: A review of the literature and its sociopolitical context. *Annual Review of Public Health, 26*, 367–397.

LaVeist, T. A. (2011). *Minority populations and Health: An introduction to health disparities in the United States*. John Wiley & Sons.

LaVeist, T. A., & Isaac, L. A. (Eds.). (2012). *Race, ethnicity, and health: A public health reader* (Vol. 26). John Wiley & Sons.

LaVeist, T., Pollack, K., Thorpe Jr, R., Fesahazion, R., & Gaskin, D. (2011). Place, not race: Disparities dissipate in southwest Baltimore when Blacks and Whites live under similar conditions. *Health Affairs, 30*(10), 1880–1887.

LaVeist, T. A., Thorpe, R. J., Galarraga, J. E., Bower, K. M., & Gary-Webb, T. L. (2009). Environmental and socio-economic factors as contributors to racial disparities in diabetes prevalence. *Journal of General Internal Medicine, 24*, 1144–1148.

Lee, B. A., Iceland, J., & Farrell, C. R. (2014). Is ethnoracial residential integration on the rise? Evidence for metropolitan and micropolitan America since 1980. In J. Logan (Ed.), *Diversity and disparities: America enters a new century* (pp. 415–456). Russell Sage Foundation.

Ling, C., & Groop, L. (2009). Epigenetics: A molecular link between environmental factors and type 2 diabetes. *Diabetes, 58*, 2718–2725. https://doi.org/10.2337/db09-1003

Linnér, A., & Almgren, M. (2020). Epigenetic programming—The important first 1000 days. *Acta Paediatrica, 109*(3), 443–452.

Liu, G. S., Nguyen, B. L., Lyons, B. H., Sheats, K. J., Wilson, R. F., Betz, C. J., & Fowler, K. A. (2023). Surveillance for Violent Deaths—National Violent Death Reporting System, 48 states, the District of Columbia, and Puerto Rico, 2020. *MMWR Surveillance Summary, 72*(Suppl. 5), 1–38.

Llabre, M. M., Schneiderman, N., Gallo, L. C., Arguelles, W., Daviglus, M. L., Franklyn Gonzalez, II., Isasi, C. R., Perreira, K. M., & Penedo, F. J. (2017). Childhood trauma and adult risk factors and disease in Hispanics/Latinos in the U.S.: Results from the Hispanic Community Health Study/Study of Latinos (HCHS/SOL) Sociocultural Ancillary Study. *Psychosomatic Medicine, 79*(2), 172–180.

Lopez, S. (1981). Mexican-American usage of mental health facilities: Underutilization reconsidered. In A. Baron Jr. (Ed.), *Explorations in Chicano psychology* (pp. 139–164). Praeger.

Lutsey, P. L., Diez Roux, A. V., Jacobs Jr, D. R., Burke, G. L., Harman, J., Shea, S., & Folsom, A. R. (2008). Associations of acculturation and socioeconomic status with subclinical cardiovascular disease in the Multi-Ethnic Study of Atherosclerosis. *American Journal of Public Health, 98*(11), 1963–1970.

Marin, B. V., & Marin, G. (1990). Effects of acculturation on knowledge of AIDS and HIV among Hispanics. *Hispanic Journal of Behavioral Sciences, 12*(2), 110–121.

Markides, K. S., & Coreil, J. (1986). The health of Hispanics in the southwestern United States: An epidemiologic paradox. *Public Health Reports, 101*(3), 253.

Markides, K. S., & Rote, S. (2019). The healthy immigrant effect and aging in the United States and other western countries. *The Gerontologist, 59*(2), 205–214.

Martinez-Cardoso, A. M., & Geronimus, A. T. (2021). The weight of migration: Reconsidering health selection and return migration among Mexicans. *International Journal of Environmental Research and Public Health, 18*(22), 12136.

Massey, D. S. (2004). Segregation and stratification: A biosocial perspective. *Du Bois Review: Social Science Research on Race, 1*(1), 7–25.

Massey, D. S., & Wagner, B. (2018). Segregation, stigma, and stratification: A biosocial model. In. B. Major, J. F. Dovidio, & B. G. Link (Eds.), *The Oxford handbook of stigma, discrimination, and health* (pp. 142–162). Oxford University Press.

Massey, D. S., Wagner, B., Donnelly, L., McLanahan, S., Brooks-Gunn, J., Garfinkel, I., Mitchell, C., & Notterman, D. A. (2018). Neighborhood disadvantage and telomere length: results from the fragile families study. *RSF: The Russell Sage Foundation Journal of the Social Sciences, 4*(4), 28–42.

McDonald, J. A., & Paulozzi, L. J. (2019). Parsing the paradox: Hispanic mortality in the U.S. by detailed cause of death. *Journal of Immigrant and Minority Health, 21*(2), 237–245.

McEwen, B. S., & Lasley, E. N. (2002). *The end of stress as we know it*. Joseph Henry Press.

McEwen, C. A. (2022). Connecting the biology of stress, allostatic load and epigenetics to social structures and processes. *Neurobiology of Stress, 17*, 100426.

Molina, K. M., Alegría, M., & Mahalingam, R. (2013). A multiple-group path analysis of the role of everyday discrimination on self-rated physical health among Latina/os in the USA. *Annals of Behavioral Medicine*, 45(1), 33–44.

Molina, K. M., Alegria, M., Mahalingam, R., Alegría, M., & Mahalingam, R. (2013). A multiple-group path analysis of the role of everyday discrimination on self-rated physical health among Latina/os in the USA. *Annals of Behavioral Medicine, 45*, 33–44. https://doi.org/10.1007/s12160-012-9421-2.

Molina, K. M., Estrella, M. L., Durazo-Arvizu, R., Malcarne, V. L., Llabre, M. M., Isasi, C. R., Ornelas, I. J., Perreira, K. M., Penedo, F. J., Brondolo, E., Gallo, L., & Daviglus, M. L. (2019). Perceived discrimination and physical health-related quality of life: The Hispanic Community Health Study/Study of Latinos (HCHS/SOL) Sociocultural Ancillary Study. *Social Science & Medicine, 222*, 91–100.

Montanez-Valverde, R. A., Zucher, S., Isasi, R., McCauley, J., & Carrasquillo, O. (2021). The Latino epidemiological paradox in cardiovascular disease in The All of Us Research Program. *Journal of the American College of Cardiology, 77*(18 Suppl. 1), 1464–1464.

Moody, H. A., & Grady, S. C. (2021). Lead emissions and population vulnerability in the Detroit Metropolitan Area, 2006–2013: Impact of pollution, housing age and neighborhood racial isolation and poverty on blood lead in children. *International Journal of Environmental Research and Public Health, 18*(5), 2747.

Morello-Frosch, R., Pastor, M., & Sadd, J. (2001). Environmental justice and Southern California's "riskscape" the distribution of air toxics exposures and health risks among diverse communities. *Urban Affairs Review, 36*(4), 551–578.

Morello-Frosch, R., Zuk, M. Jerret, M., Shamasunder, B., & Kyle, A. D. (2011). Understanding The cumulative impacts of inequalities in environmental health: Implications for policy. *Health Affairs*, 30(5), 879–887. https://doi.org/10.1377/hlthaff.2011.0153

Mujahid, M. S., Roux, A. V. D., Cooper, R. C., Shea, S., & Williams, D. R. (2011). Neighborhood stressors and race/ethnic differences in hypertension prevalence (the Multi-Ethnic Study of Atherosclerosis). *American Journal of Hypertension, 24*(2), 187–193.

Münzel, T., & Daiber, A. (2018). Environmental stressors and their impact on health and disease with focus on oxidative stress. *Antioxidants & Redox Signaling, 28*(9), 735–740.

Murphy, S.L., Xu, J.Q., Kochanek, K.D., Arias, E., & Tejada-Vera, B. (2020). Deaths: Final data for 2018. *National Vital Statistics Reports, 69*(13). Hyattsville, MD: National Center for Health Statistics. 2020.

Nagy, C., & Turecki, G. (2015). Transgenerational epigenetic inheritance: an open discussion. *Epigenomics*, 7(5), 781–790.

National Institutes of Health. (2002). *Strategic research plan and budget to reduce and ultimately eliminate health disparities: Vol. 1. Fiscal years 2002–2006*. U.S. Department of Health and Human Services. https://www.nimhd.nih.gov/docs/2002_2006__vol1_031003ed_rev.pdf

National Safety Council. (n.d.). *Deaths by demographics: Race and ethnicity*. Retrieved June 22, 2023, from https://injuryfacts.nsc.org/all-injuries/deaths-by-demographics/race-and-ethnicity/data-details/

Nelson, K. A. (2013). Does residential segregation help or hurt? Exploring differences in the relationship between segregation and health among U.S. Hispanics by nativity and ethnic subgroup. *The Social Science Journal, 50*(4), 646–657.

Office of Minority Health. (2021). *Minority Health Social Vulnerability Index Overview*. https://stacks.cdc.gov/view/cdc/117536

Ostir, G. V., Eschbach, K., Markides, K. S., & Goodwin, J. S. (2003). Neighbourhood composition and depressive symptoms among older Mexican Americans. *Journal of Epidemiology & Community Health, 57*(12), 987–992.

Palloni, A., & Arias, E. (2004). Paradox lost: Explaining the Hispanic adult mortality advantage. *Demography, 41*(3), 385–415.

Pascoe, E. A., & Richman, L. S. (2009). Perceived discrimination and health: A meta-analytic review. *Psychological Bulletin, 135*(4), 531–554. https://doi.org/10.1037/a0016059

Patel, K. V., Eschbach, K., Rudkin, L. L., Peek, M. K., & Markides, K. S. (2003). Neighborhood context and self-rated health in older Mexican Americans. *Annals of Epidemiology, 13*(9), 620–628.

Payne-Sturges, D. C., Scammell, M. K., Levy, J. I., Cory-Slechta, D. A., Symanski, E., Carr Shmool, J. L., Laumbach, R., Linder, S., & Clougherty, J. E. (2018). Methods for evaluating the combined effects of chemical and nonchemical exposures for cumulative environmental health risk assessment. *International Journal of Environmental Research and Public Health, 15*(12), Article 2797.

Pérez, D. J., Fortuna, L., & Alegria, M. (2008). Prevalence and correlates of everyday discrimination among U.S. Latinos. *Journal of Community Psychology, 36*(4), 421–433.

Pérez, L. M., & Martinez, J. (2008). Community health workers: social justice and policy advocates for community health and well-being. *American Journal of Public Health, 98*(1), 11–14.

Pérez-Escamilla, R., & Putnik, P. (2007). The role of acculturation in nutrition, lifestyle, and incidence of type 2 diabetes among Latinos. *The Journal of Nutrition, 137*(4), 860–870.

Perla, M. E., Rue, T., Cheadle, A., Krieger, J., & Karr, C. K. (2015). Population-based comparison of biomarker concentrations for chemicals of concern among Latino-American and non-Hispanic White children. *Journal of Immigrant and Minority Health, 17*, 802–819.

Perreira, K. M., Gotman, N., Isasi, C. R., Arguelles, W., Castañeda, S. F., Daviglus, M. L., Giachello, A. L., Gonzalez, P., Penedo, F. J., Salgado, H., & Wassertheil-Smoller S. (2015). Mental health and exposure to the United States. *Journal of Nervous and Mental Disease, 203*, 670–678.

Pettitt, D. J., Aleck, K. A., Baird, H. R., Carraher, M. J., Bennett, P. H., & Knowler, W. C. (1988). Congenital susceptibility to NIDDM: Role of intrauterine environment. *Diabetes, 37*, 622–628.

Pettitt, D. J., Baird, H. R., Aleck, K. A., Bennett, P. H., & Knowler, W. C. (1983). Excessive obesity in offspring of Pima Indian women with diabetes during pregnancy. *New England Journal of Medicine, 308*, 242–245.

Pieterse, A., & Powell, S. (2016). A theoretical overview of the impact of racism on people of color. In A. N. Alvarez, C. Liang, & H. A. Neville (Eds.), *The cost of racism for people of color: Contextualizing experiences of discrimination* (pp. 11–30). Amerian Psychological Association.

Pinney, S. E., & Simmons, R. (2010). Epigenetic mechanisms in the development of type 2 diabetes. *Trends in Endocrinology and Metabolism, 21*, 223–229. https://doi.org/10.1016/j.tem.2009.10.002

Plascak, J. J., Molina, Y., Wu-Georges, S., Idris, A., & Thompson, B. (2016). Latino residential segregation and self-rated health among Latinos: Washington state behavioral risk factor surveillance system, 2012–2014. *Social Science & Medicine, 159*, 38–47.

Portes, A., & Zhou, M. (1993). The new second generation: Segmented assimilation and its variants. *Annals of the Amerian Academy of Political and Social Science, 530*(1), 74–96

Potochnick, S., Perreira, K. M., Bravin, J. I., Castañeda, S. F., Daviglus, M. L., Gallo, L. C., & Isasi, C. R. (2019). Food insecurity among Hispanic/Latino youth: Who is at risk and what are the health correlates? *Journal of Adolescent Health, 64*(5), 631–639.

Pratt, G. C., Vadali, M. L., Kvale, D. L., & Ellickson, K. M. (2015). Traffic, air pollution, minority and socio-economic status: Addressing inequities in exposure and risk. *International Journal of Environmental Research and Public Health, 12*(5), 5355–5372.

Quach, A., Levine, M. E., Tanaka, T., Lu, A. T., Chen, B. H., Ferrucci, L., Ritz, B., Bandinelli, S., Neuhouser, M. L., Beasley, J. M., Snetselaar, L., Wallace, R. B., Tsao, P. S., Absher, D., Assimes, T. L., Stewart, J. D., Li, Y., Hou, L., Baccarelli, A. A., Whisel, E. A., & Horvath, S. (2017). Epigenetic clock analysis of diet, exercise, education, and lifestyle factors. *Aging (Albany NY), 9*(2), 419–446.

Rabbitt, M. P., & Coleman-Jensen, A. (2017). Rasch analysis of the standardized Spanish translation of the U.S. Household Food Security Survey Module. *Journal of Economic and Social Measurement, 42*(2), 171–197.

Ramírez, A. S., Wilson, M. D., & Miller, L. M. S. (2022). Segmented assimilation as a mechanism to explain the dietary acculturation paradox. *Appetite, 169*, Article 105820.

Ravelli, A. C., van der Meulen, J. H., Michels, R. P., Osmond, C., Barker, D. J., Hales, C. N., & Bleker, O. P. (1998). Glucose tolerance in adults after prenatal exposure to famine. *Lancet, 351*, 173–177. https://doi.org/10.1016/S0140-6736(97)07244-9

Roberts, B. K., Nofi, C. P., Cornell, E., Kapoor, S., Harrison, L., & Sathya, C. (2023). Trends and disparities in firearm deaths among children. *Pediatrics, 152*(3).

Rogers, R. G., Lawrence, E. M., Hummer, R. A., & Tilstra, A. M. (2017). Racial/ethnic differences in early-life mortality in the United States. *Biodemography and Social Biology, 63*(3), 189–205.

Rogler, L. H., Cortes, D. E., & Malgady, R. G. (1991). Acculturation and mental health status among Hispanics: Convergence and new directions for research. *American Psychologist, 46*(6), 585–597.

Rossen, L. M., Branum, A. M., Ahmad, F. B., Sutton, P., & Anderson, R. N. (2020). Excess deaths associated with COVID-19, by age and race and ethnicity—United States, January 26–October 3, 2020. *Morbidity and Mortality Weekly Report, 69*, 1522–1527. http://doi.org/10.15585/mmwr.mm6942e2

Rubin, L. P. (2016). Maternal and pediatric health and disease: Integrating biopsychosocial models and epigenetics. *Pediatric Research, 79*(1), 127–135.

Ruiz, J. M., Steffen, P., & Smith, T. B. (2013). Hispanic mortality paradox: A systematic review and meta-analysis of the longitudinal literature. *American Journal of Public Health, 103*(3), e52–e60.

Sabo, S., & Lee, A. E. (2015). The spillover of U.S. immigration policy on citizens and permanent residents of Mexican descent: How internalizing "illegality" impacts public health in the borderlands. *Frontiers in Public Health, 3*, Article 155.

Sabo, S., Shaw, S., Ingram, M., Teufel-Shone, N., Carvajal, S., De Zapien, J. G., Rosales, C., Redondo, F., Garcia, G., & Rubio-Goldsmith, R. (2014). Everyday violence, structural racism and mistreatment at the U.S.-Mexico border. *Social Science & Medicine, 109*, 66–74.

Sadler, R. C., LaChance, J., & Hanna-Attisha, M. (2017). Social and built environmental correlates of predicted blood lead levels in the Flint water crisis. *American Journal of Public Health, 107*(5), 763–769.

Schanzenbach, D. W., & A. Pitts. (2020, July 9). *Food Insecurity during COVID-19 in households with children: Results by racial and ethnic groups.* Institute for Policy Research Rapid Research Report. https://www.ipr.northwestern.edu/documents/reports/ipr-rapid-research-reports-pulse-hh-data-9-july-2020-by-race-ethnicity.pdf

Scribner, R. (1996). Paradox as paradigm-the health outcomes of Mexican Americans [editorial]. *American Journal of Public Health, 86*, 303–305.

Shanks, T. R. W., & Robinson, C. (2013). Assets, economic opportunity and toxic stress: A framework for understanding child and educational outcomes. *Economics of Education Review, 33*(1), 154–170.

Shiels, M. S., Chernyavskiy, P., Anderson, W. F., Best, A. F., Haozous, E. A., Hartge, P., Rosenberg, P. S., Thomas, D., Freedman, N. D., & de Gonzalez, A. B. (2017). Trends in premature mortality in the USA by sex, race, and ethnicity from 1999 to 2014: An analysis of death certificate data. *The Lancet, 389*(10073), 1043–1054.

Shim, Y. K., Lewin, M. D., Ruiz, P., Eichner, J. E., & Mumtaz, M. M. (2017). Prevalence and associated demographic characteristics of exposure to multiple metals and their species in human populations: The United States NHANES, 2007–2012. *Journal of Toxicology and Environmental Health, 80*(9), 502–512.

Shonkoff, J. P., & Garner, A. S. (2012). The lifelong effects of early childhood adversity and toxic stress. *American Academy of Pediatrics*, 129 (1), e232–e246.

Sorlie, P. D., Backlund, E., Johnson, N. J., & Rogot, E. (1993). Mortality by Hispanic Status in the United States. *Journal of the American Medical Association, 270*, 2464–2468.

Sterns, J. D., Smith, C. B., Steele, J. R., Stevenson, K. L., & Gallicano, G. I. (2014). Epigenetics and type II diabetes mellitus: Underlying mechanisms of prenatal predisposition. *Frontiers in Cell and Developmental Biology, 2*, 15.

Telzer, E. H., & Garcia, H. A. V. (2009). Skin color and self-perceptions of immigrant and U.S.-born Latinas: The moderating role of racial socialization and ethnic identity. *Hispanic Journal of Behavioral Sciences, 31*(3), 357–374. https://doi.org/10.1177/0739986309336913

Trump, Donald. (2015, June 16). Presidential announcement speech. *Washington Post.* https://www.washingtonpost.com/news/post-politics/wp/2015/06/16/full-text-donald-trump-announces-a-presidential-bid/

Trump, Donald. (2023, December 16). *New Hampshire rally.* NBC News. https://www.nbcnews.com/politics/2024-election/trump-says-immigrants-are-poisoning-blood-country-biden-campaign-liken-rcna130141

Turra, C. M., & Elo, I. T. (2008). The impact of salmon bias on the Hispanic mortality advantage: New evidence from social security data. *Population Research and Policy Review, 27*, 515–530.

Turra, C. M., & Goldman, N. (2007). Socioeconomic differences in mortality among U.S. adults: Insights into the Hispanic paradox. *The Journals of Gerontology Series B: Psychological Sciences and Social Sciences, 62*(3), S184–S192.

Uddin, M., Aiello, A. E., Wildman, D. E., Koenen, K. C., Pawelec, G., de Los Santos, R., Goldmann, E., & Galea, S. (2010). Epigenetic and immune function profiles associated with posttraumatic stress disorder. *Proceedings of the National Academy of Sciences, 107*(20), 9470–9475.

Vaca, F. E., Anderson, C. L., & Hayes-Bautista, D. E. (2011). The Latino adolescent male mortality peak revisited: attribution of homicide and motor vehicle crash death. *Injury Prevention, 17*(2), 102–107.

Valdez, Z. (2006). Segmented assimilation among Mexicans in the Southwest. *The Sociological Quarterly, 47*(3), 397–424.

Vega, W. A., Sribney, W. M., Aguilar-Gaxiola, S., & Kolody, B. (2004). 12-month prevalence of *DSM-III-R* psychiatric disorders among Mexican Americans: Nativity, social assimilation, and age determinants. *The Journal of Nervous and Mental Disease, 192*(8), 532–541.

Vella, C. A., Ontiveros, D., Zubia, R. Y., & Bader, J. O. (2011). Acculturation and metabolic syndrome risk factors in young Mexican and Mexican-American women. *Journal of Immigrant and Minority Health, 13*, 119–126.

Viruell-Fuentes, E. A. (2007). Beyond acculturation: Immigration, discrimination, and health research among Mexicans in the United States. *Social Science & Medicine, 65*, 1524–1535.

Viruell-Fuentes, E. A., Miranda, P. Y., & Abdulrahim, S. (2012). More than culture: Structural racism, intersectionality theory, and immigrant health. *Social Science & Medicine, 75*(12), 2099–2106.

Viruell-Fuentes, E. A., Morenoff, J. D., Williams, D.R., & House, J. S. (2013). Contextualizing nativity status, Latino social ties, and ethnic enclaves: an examination of the "immigrant social ties hypothesis." *Ethnicity & Health, 18*, 586–609.

Viruell-Fuentes, E. A., & Schulz, A. J. (2009). Toward a dynamic conceptualization of social ties and context: Implications for understanding immigrant and Latino health. *American Journal of Public Health, 99*(12), 2167–2175.

Vogel, K. J., Atchley, D. P., Erlichman, J., Broglio, K. R., Ready, K. J., Valero, V., Amos, C. I., Hortobagyi, G. N., Lu, K. H., & Arun, B. (2007). BRCA1 and BRCA2 genetic testing in Hispanic patients: Mutation prevalence and evaluation of the BRCAPRO risk assessment model. *Journal of Clinical Oncology, 25*(29), 4635–4641.

Weaver, I. C., Korgan, A. C., Lee, K., Wheeler, R. V., Hundert, A. S., & Goguen, D. (2017). Stress and the emerging roles of chromatin remodeling in signal integration and stable transmission of reversible phenotypes. *Frontiers in Behavioral Neuroscience, 11*, 41.

Weitzel, J. N., Clague, J., Martir-Negron, A., Ogaz, R., Herzog, J., Ricker, C., Jungbluth, C., Cina, C., Duncan, P., Unzeitig, G., Saldivar, J. S., Beattie, M., Feldman, N., Sand, S., Port, D., Barragan, D. I., John, E. M., Neuhausen, S. L., & Larson, G. P. (2013). Prevalence and type of BRCA mutations in Hispanics undergoing genetic cancer risk assessment in the southwestern United States: A report from the Clinical Cancer Genetics Community Research Network. *Journal of Clinical Oncology, 31*(2), 210–216.

White, K., & Borrell, L. N. (2011). Racial/ethnic residential segregation: Framing the context of health risk and health disparities. *Health & Place, 17*(2), 438–448.

Woo, B., Kravitz-Wirtz, N., Sass, V., Crowder, K., Teixeira, S., & Takeuchi, D. T. (2019). Residential segregation and racial/ethnic disparities in ambient air pollution. *Race and Social Problems, 11*, 60–67.

Woodall, A. M., & Driscoll, A. K. (2020). *Racial and ethnic differences in mortality rate of infants born to teen mothers: United States, 2017–2018*. National Center for Health Statistics.

Xiao, Y. Y., & Graham, G. (2019). Where we live: The impact of neighborhoods and community factors on cardiovascular health in the United States. *Clinical Cardiology, 42*(1), 184–189.

Xu, J.Q., Murphy, S.L., Kochanek, K.D., & Arias, E. (2021). *Deaths: Final data for 2019. National Vital Statistics Reports*; *70*(8). Hyattsville, MD: National Center for Health Statistics. 2021. DOI: https://dx.doi.org/10.15620/cdc:106058

Yang, T. C., Park, K., & Matthews, S. A. (2020). Racial/ethnic segregation and health disparities: Future directions and opportunities. *Sociology Compass, 14*(6), Article e12794.

Yang, T. C., Zhao, Y., & Song, Q. (2017). Residential segregation and racial disparities in self-rated health: How do dimensions of residential segregation matter? *Social Science Research, 61*, 29–42.

Figure Credits

Fig. 5.1: Copyright © 2020 Depositphotos/Vectorbox.

Fig. 5.2: Douglas Massey, "Massey's Biosocial Model of Racial Stratification (BMRS)," Segregation and Stratification: A Biosocial Perspective, p. 15. Copyright © 2004 by Cambridge University Press.

Fig. 5.3: Diane Schanzenbach and Abigail Pitts, "Food Insecurity in the United States, 2020," https://www.ipr.northwestern.edu/documents/reports/ipr-rapid-research-reports-pulse-hh-data-9-july-2020-by-race-ethnicity.pdf, p. 2. Copyright © 2020 by Northwestern University.

Fig. 5.4: Rodney Clark, Norman B. Anderson, Vanessa R. Clark, and David R. Williams, "Clark's Biopsychosocial Racism Model," https://psycnet.apa.org/record/1999-11644-001?doi=1. Copyright © 1999 by American Psychological Association.

Fig. 5.5: Copyright © by Laia Bécares (CC by 3.0) at https://www.sciencedirect.com/science/article/pii/S1353829214001403.

Fig. 5.6: Elizabeth A. Pascoe and Laura Smart Richman, "Pathways showing Perceived Discrimination and Health Outcomes," *Perceived Discrimination and Health: A Meta-Analytic Review*. Copyright © 2009 by American Psychological Association.

Fig. 5.7: Jennifer Dacey Allen, Caitlin Caspi, Bryan Leyva, Anne M. Stoddard, Sara Tamers, Reginald D. Tucker-Seeley, and Glorian C. Sorensen, "Hypothesized Pathways between Acculturation and Health Behaviors," https://www.sciencedirect.com/science/article/pii/S0277953614006807?via%3Dihub, pp. 27. Copyright © 2014 by Elsevier B.V.

Fig. 5.10: Sally C. Curtin and Matthew F. Garnett, "Suicide and Homicide Rates Among Persons 10-24: US, 2001-2021," https://www.cdc.gov/nchs/products/databriefs/db471.htm, 2023.

Fig. 5.11: National Center for Health Statistics, "Age-Adjusted Rates of Firearm-Related Homicide by Race, Hispanic Origin, and Sex," https://www.cdc.gov/mmwr/volumes/72/wr/pdfs/mm7226-H.pdf, p. 737, 2023.

Fig. 5.12: Centers for Disease Control and Prevention, "US Mortality Trends, 2000–2017," https://stacks.cdc.gov/view/cdc/80172#tabs-2, p. 1, 2019.

Fig. 5.18: Copyright © by J. David Sterns, Colin B. Smith, John R. Steele, Kimberly L. Stevenson, and G. Ian Gallicano (CC by 3.0) at https://www.ncbi.nlm.nih.gov/pmc/articles/PMC4207047/.

CHAPTER 6

Causes of the Causes

LEARNING OBJECTIVES

- Analyze how social epigenetics influence health inequalities among historically disadvantaged populations.
- List two of the primary mechanisms by which the epigenome is modified.
- Explain whether epigenetic modifications are heritable.
- Describe how prenatal and maternal stress contributes to the risk for disease in adulthood.
- Explain the role of fetal programming in the development of disease risk.
- Discuss the relation between Fetal Origins of Adult Disease (FOAD) and Developmental Origins of Health and Disease (DoHAD).
- Examine the prevalence of ACEs among the general U.S. population and Latino subgroups.
- Define historical trauma and intergenerational trauma.
- Identify the mechanisms involved in the intergenerational transmission of disease risk.

In this chapter, we discuss the contributions of several convergent theories that document the "causes of the causes" of health inequalities among historically marginalized populations like non-Latino Black Americans, Native Americans, and Latino Americans. Each of the theories contributes to a wholistic perspective of epigenetic and social environmental interactions that can cause disease in vulnerable and susceptible populations through physiological mechanisms associated with psychosocial stress (e.g., poverty, racism, discrimination, stressful life events, early childhood adversity, prenatal and maternal stress). Commonly referred to in the public health literature as *developmental origins of health and disease* (*DOHaD*), the practical applications to health inequalities among Latinos lies in developing techniques that can accurately assess risk for disease early in life and potentially modify these risks through novel therapies.

USEFUL EPIGENETIC TERMINOLOGY

- Genome
- Epigenome
- Genotype
- Phenotype
- Chromatin
- Histones
- CpG dinucleotide sites

Health Inequalities and Social Epigenetics

One of the major theories of health inequalities is a focus on gene–environment interactions, in particular social epigenetic processes that may be involved in the intergenerational transmission of vulnerability and susceptibility to disease (Fox et al., 2015; Taouk & Schulkin, 2016). Several authors note that structural racism has created and maintained health inequalities in the United States, negatively impacting non-Latino Black Americans, Latino Americans, and Native Americans (Bowleg & Landers, 2023; Phillips-Beck et al., 2019).

The term *epigenetics* refers to the heritable but modifiable regulation of genetic functions that are mediated through non-DNA-encoded mechanisms. The epigenome can mark DNA in two ways, both of which play a role in expressing or silencing genes. The first occurs when certain chemical tags called *methyl groups* attach to CpG sites in the DNA molecule (see Useful Epigenetic Terminology). The second occurs when a variety of chemical tags attach to the tails of histones, which are spool-like proteins that package DNA into chromosomes. This action affects how tightly wound DNA is around the histones (MacDonald & Roskams, 2009).

To date, most epigenetic research has focused on alterations associated with cancer (e.g., epigenetic silencing of tumor suppressor genes; Esteller, 2008). Epigenetics focuses on processes that regulate how and when certain genes are expressed or silenced. *Epigenomics* pertains to the analysis of epigenetic changes across many genes in a cell or entire organism. Epigenetic processes control normal growth and development, and this process is deregulated in diseases such as cancer. Diet and exposure to environmental toxins throughout all stages of human development, among other factors, can cause epigenetic changes that may turn on or turn off certain genes. Changes in genes that would normally protect against a disease, as a result, could make people more susceptible to developing that disease later in life. It has been demonstrated that some epigenetic changes can be passed on from generation to generation, referred to as *intergenerational transmission* or *historical trauma*, where the past social environment manifests in the present or future generations through epigenetic signatures (Fox et al., 2015; Mulligan et al., 2012; Oyama & Terry, 2016).

A famous example of how epigenetic processes can lead to illness in future generations is the Dutch famine experience (Roseboom et al., 2006). During World War II, Nazi Germany blocked food to the Dutch in the winter of 1944. Calorie consumption among the population dropped from 2,000 per day to 500 per day for 4.5 million people. Children born or raised during this time were small, short in stature, and had many diseases, including edema, anemia, diabetes, and depression. The Dutch Famine Birth Cohort Study showed that women living during this time had children 20–30 years later with the same problems despite being conceived and born during a normal dietary period (De Rooij et al., 2022).

The burgeoning field of social epigenomics has now linked epigenetic changes with social factors (Banaudha et al., 2018; Oblak et al., 2021). Scientists can identify classes of genes and/or specific signaling pathways through which social factors might influence the mechanisms through which social environments might alter gene expression and affect historically marginalized groups and health disparities and social stressors that may negatively affect health status through epigenomic modifications of various biological pathways. Studies on adverse childhood experiences (ACEs) have also shown ties to epigenetic changes affecting genes related to mental health, drug addiction, and obesity (Dube et al., 2003; Hughes et al., 2017).

It is well known that individuals living in low-income neighborhoods are often exposed to chemical and nonchemical stressors: physical (e.g., noise pollution, lack of green space) and psychosocial (e.g., food desert, violence or threat of violence, discrimination, residential segregation, and psychosocial stress). Therefore, health disparities may arise not only because of higher levels of exposure to environmental hazards among historically marginalized racial and ethnic groups but also because of the synergistic effect of exposure to multiple environmental hazards and social stressors that may be prolonged.

Adverse social and environmental experiences early in life may predispose an individual to dysfunctional physiological responses and to future stressors in adulthood (Kuzawa & Sweet, 2009; Metz et al., 2015). Exposure to emotional or physical abuse or neglect might alter DNA methylation levels, creating an epigenetic signature, which in turn might influence risk of cardiovascular disease, cancer, cerebrovascular disease, and psychiatric disorders (see Figure 6.1).

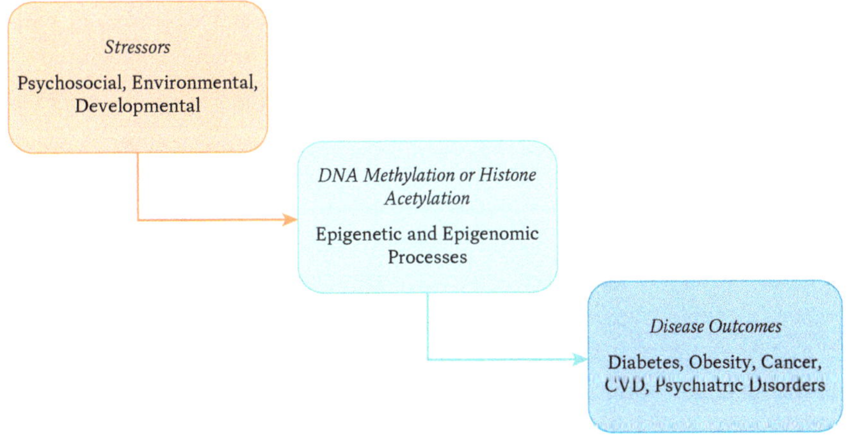

FIGURE 6.1 Hypothesized Social Epigenetic Process

The human genome is in the nucleus of every cell in the body, except for red blood cells. The human genome includes 25,000 genes. The *epigenome* is another layer of information that assists in the regulation gene expression (Esteller, 2008). *Chromatin* is the DNA itself, comprised of histones and other proteins that make up chromosomes. *Histones* are the main protein component of chromatin, which is like a spool of thread around which DNA winds itself. Histones help regulate the structure of chromatin and gene expression. *CpG dinucleotide sites* are cytosine-guanine nucleotide sites that comprise DNA and are typically the areas associated with epigenetic modifications (Biswas & Rao, 2017).

The epigenome can mark DNA in several ways that play a role in turning genes on or off (gene expression). The two DNA markers that are most often examined are DNA methylation and histone modification. The first occurs when certain chemical tags called *methyl groups* attach to CpG sites in the DNA molecule. The second occurs when a variety of chemical tags attach to the tails of histones, the spool-like proteins that package DNA neatly into chromosomes (Jones & Takai, 2001). This action affects how tightly DNA is wrapped around the histones, again influencing gene transcription. When DNA CpG sites are methylated (adding a methyl group), it leads to transcriptional gene silencing. When these CpG sites are demethylated (removing a methyl group), it leads to gene expression. In humans, approximately 50%–70% of all CpG sites are methylated. Similarly, histone modification occurs through the addition or removal of acetyl groups. Acetylation of histones leads to transcriptional gene expression, while deacetylation leads to transcriptional gene silencing (Kristensen et al., 2009).

Social epigenetics is the study of genes and/or specific pathways through which social factors might influence epigenetic mechanisms that alter gene expression and affect the health of non-Latino Black Americans, Latinos, and Native Americans (Bagby et al., 2019; Loi et al., 2013; Martin et al., 2022). Studies on ACEs have also shown ties to epigenetic changes affecting genes related to mental health, drug addiction, and metabolic syndrome/obesity (Anda et al., 2006; Gilbert et al., 2015). Social epigenetic research has also demonstrated that accelerated epigenetic aging is associated with adverse health outcomes, including all-cause mortality (Crimmins et al., 2021; Horvath, 2013; Marioni et al., 2015; Ryan et al., 2020). Recall from Chapter 5 that Horvath (2013) found that DNA methylation was associated with epigenetic aging (the epigenetic clock) and that accelerated aging among non-Latinos White Americans was higher than found among Latinos. Moreover, a literature review conducted by Martin et al. (2022) found that ACEs, prenatal and maternal stress (e.g., prenatal exposure to maternal psychosocial stressors, cumulative stressors), socioeconomic position (i.e., income, education, unemployment), perceived racism and discrimination, the neighborhood and the social environment (e.g., concentrated and persistent poverty, violence, social disorder), and toxic stress were all associated with accelerated epigenetic aging and all-cause mortality.

The role of social epigenetics as a major contributing factor in the etiology of disease among historically marginalized populations has been theorized by several researchers (Salas et al., 2021; Thayer & Kuzawa, 2011; Vick & Burris, 2017). As well, there is some research that examines the synergistic effects of ACEs on DNA methylation among Native Americans (Brockie et al., 2013). It is plausible that repeated exposure to adverse life events triggers epigenetic modifications resulting in increased *risk* for disease as well as increased disease *incidence*. Vick & Burris (2017) hypothesize that differential exposure to various environmental toxins (e.g., air pollution, smoking, and psychosocial stress) increases the odds of DNA methylation, which is associated with cardiovascular disease, preterm birth, and cancer.

Mamtani et al. (2016) found that DNA methylation in two genes, *CPT1A* and *ABCG1*, which are involved in fatty acid and triglyceride metabolism, respectively, were significantly associated with hyper triglyceridemic waist (HTGW) phenotype (fat distribution around the waist) among Latinos of Mexican descent and remained significant after adjusting for metabolic syndrome. The study also found that this phenotype is highly heritable among Latinos of Mexican descent, with 26% of persons in their sample expressing the HTGW phenotype. Because Latinos of Mexican descent have a very high prevalence of metabolic syndrome (insulin resistance), the authors suggest that the identification of these DNA methylated genes could be a marker for increased risk for type 2 diabetes and cardiovascular disease among Latinos of Mexican descent. The epigenetic association with type 2 diabetes among Latinos of Mexican descent also demonstrates heritable non-DNA-encoded signatures contributing to increased risk in subsequent generations (intergenerational transmission; Grant et al., 2017; Kim et al., 2022). A contrary argument to heritable risk for disease through epigenetic mechanisms is heritable non-DNA-encoded income, wealth, and higher socioeconomic status, which are highly correlated with advantages in physical and mental health status but are not biologically transmitted (Mackenbach, 2005; Will & Wang, 2021). The causal linkages between psychosocial stress, epigenetic modification, and poor health may in fact be synergistic, including socioeconomic status (Crimmins et al., 2021).

A comprehensive examination of 13 epigenetic clocks was conducted by Crimmins et al. (2021) to study the effects of socioeconomic status and epigenetic aging. They found that epigenetic aging varied with gender and socioeconomic characteristics, with women having slower age acceleration compared to men and individuals with lower levels of education having faster age acceleration than those with higher levels of education. Among racial/ethnic groups, Black Americans had faster age acceleration than White Americans, and Mexican Americans had slower age acceleration than White Americans. This finding confirms results obtained by Horvath and others indicating that Latinos of Mexican descent have slower age acceleration, suggesting a higher life expectancy and better overall mortality outcomes, as indicated by research examining the Latino epidemiologic paradox. Thus, epigenetic characteristics of Latinos of Mexican descent may be at the foundation of the observed mortality paradox.

Recent advances in epigenetics research have also led to novel discoveries of the processes by which non-DNA-encoded genetic mechanisms influence the regulation of several genomic functions, including gene expression and gene silencing (Banaudha et al., 2018; MacDonald & Roskams, 2009). An example of applied epigenetic research are cancer treatments that target these epigenetic processes (Esteller, 2008). Epigenetic processes control normal growth and development. When this process is interrupted, diseases such as cancer develop. Diet and exposure to environmental toxins throughout all stages of human development, among other factors, can also cause epigenetic changes that interrupt signaling pathways related to gene expression or silencing (Coker et al., 2018; Dube et al., 2003; Hughes et al., 2017). For example, Coker et al. (2018) found that neighborhood poverty and DNA methylation among Latinos of Mexican descent was mediated by maternal diet during pregnancy. They found no support for early-life socioeconomic environment and DNA methylation in Latino infants.

Several studies have found that negative socioenvironmental experiences early in life may predispose an individual to dysfunctional physiological responses and to future stressors in adulthood (Anda et al., 2006; Felitti & Anda, 2003; Felitti et al., 1998a). Additionally, exposure to emotional or physical abuse or neglect might alter DNA methylation levels, creating an epigenetic signature, which in turn might influence risk of for cardiovascular disease, certain types of cancers, cerebrovascular disease, and psychiatric disorders among socially disadvantaged populations (Akinyemiju et al., 2018; Martin et al., 2022).

From a social epidemiological perspective and through the lens of critical race theory and intersectionality theory, the fundamental causes of health inequalities among Mexican Americans and non-Latino Black Americans are based in the sociohistorical foundation and development of a race-conscious U.S. society where racial and ethnic demarcations matter and become manifest in the oppression, discrimination, racism, social injustice, and health inequalities among Mexican Americans, non-Latino Black Americans, and Native Americans (Bagby et al., 2019). Multiple stressors can lead to physiological stress responses through the biopsychosocial stress process, increasing the risk for chronic and communicable diseases. Moreover, persistent stress can lead to epigenetic modifications that increase the risk for disease. Together, both processes can induce fundamental changes to the epigenome leading to increased vulnerability and susceptibility to disease.

To be sure, biological, and nutritional deficiencies were present in the Indigenous populations of the Americas and may have initiated epigenetic modifications prior to European contact (Steckel, 2005; Storey, 1986). Parasitic diseases, like amebic dysentery; infectious diseases, like hepatitis A, tuberculosis, and pertussis; nutritional deficiencies, like iron-deficiency anemia; and musculoskeletal disorders, like osteoarthritis and injuries, and perhaps syphilis (though still controversial) were common pre-Columbian conditions (Harper et al., 2011; Schultz et al., 2007; Tampa et al., 2014). Research also shows that childhood mortality was also very high prior to European contact. Certainly, these harsh conditions contributed to epigenetic modification in subsequent generations.

Additionally, environmental climactic changes occurred in the southwestern states and northern Mexico around 1130 CE, with chronic climactic instability, including a series of severe droughts that struck the region between 1250 and 1450. Recall that the Mexica began their journey to the south from Aztlan around 1100 CE. These environmental changes forced Indigenous populations to adapt and often led to insufficient diets lacking in protein, carbohydrates, and essential amino acids. Thus, Puebloan and Mexica ancestors' diets and physical environments caused fundamental changes in our human genome (i.e., the inheritable and epigenetic characteristics that are the causes of the causes). The phrase "You are what your grandmother ate" is more apt than we sometimes realize.

Prenatal and Maternal Stress (PMS)

Prenatal and maternal stress (*PMS*) refers to the stress—physical or psychosocial—that a pregnant woman and her fetus experience during pregnancy, fetal development, and postpartum depression (DiPietro, 2004; Witt et al., 2014). Much of the research on PMS focuses on the social environment of the mother and its association with antenatal, prenatal, and postnatal stress (DiPietro et al., 2002; Van den Bergh et al., 2005). The physiological response to stress and stressors is activated through the hypothalamic-pituitary-adrenal axis (HPA) and sympathetic-adrenomedullary (SAM) system. The HPA is responsible for stress responses, energy metabolism, and neuropsychiatric functioning (Miller, 2018) and the SAM secretes noradrenaline and norepinephrine in the presence of stressors (Godoy et al., 2018). This activation causes the production and release of stress hormones that influence neuroendocrine, metabolic, and immune function. Transplacental transmission of these stress hormones to the developing fetus can cause physical, psychological, and mental health problems later in life (Burris & Hacker, 2017; Kinsella & Monk, 2009; O'Donnell et al., 2009).

A conceptual model developed to examine inequalities in Black-White birth outcomes could be adapted to Latinos as well (see Figure 6.2). The model includes discrimination, income inequality, and educational achievement gaps, which are stressors experienced by Latinos as well. As we have discussed previously, residential segregation in Latino neighborhoods or census tracts have both positive and negative influences on the health of Latinos (see Chapter 5). Ethnic enclaves provide social support, informal social control, and cultural capital. Alternatively, these same neighborhoods lack access to health care and are characterized as food swamps and deserts (Joassart-Marcelli et al., 2017; MacNell et al., 2017). The influence of acculturation can also be detrimental to positive health behaviors during pregnancy, increasing the risk for negative health behaviors like smoking and alcohol consumption (Bethel & Schenker, 2005; Hoggatt et al., 2012; Zemore, 2007). For example, a study by Hoggatt et al. (2012) found that level of acculturation was associated with low birth weight (LBW) infants among both foreign-born and U.S.-born Latinas.

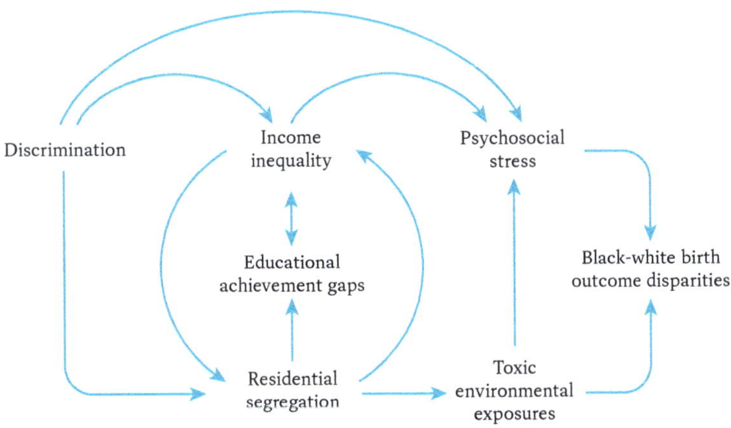

FIGURE 6.2 Conceptual Model of Socioenvironmental Factors That Lead to Psychosocial Stress and Black-White Birth Outcomes

Approximately 20% of U.S. women experience a stressful life event (SLE) prior to conception (Witt et al., 2014). Witt et al. (2014) confirmed the link between SLEs and LBW infants, with a possible dose-response relationship. Paradoxically, they found that Latinas experienced fewer SLEs than non-Latina White women and had fewer LBW infants. The authors also confirmed the hypothesis that the type and timing of stressful events—that is, the kind of stressful event and whether it occurred prior to conception, within 1 year of conception, or cumulative across the women's lifespan—is an important contributor to adverse birth outcomes, childhood development, and a potentially cause of diseases later in life (Barker, 2007; Khashan et al. 2008, 2009; Witt et al., 2014). Type of stressors experienced by pregnant women was examined by Lu & Chen (2005). They found that pregnant Latinas and non-Latina Black women experienced more "traumatic stressors" before and during pregnancy than pregnant non-Latina White women. Studies have also shown that relational and financial stressors are more common among Latina and non-Latina Black pregnant women than non-Latina White pregnant women and are related to depressed affect (Liu et al., 2016).

Research shows there are several psychosocial stressors that commonly affect women during pregnancy and fetal development. These include stressful life events (exits and entrances), anxiety and depression, inadequate material resources, unfavorable employment conditions, family and household responsibilities, strain in intimate relationships, intimate partner violence, and biological complications during pregnancy (Beydound & Saftlas, 2008; Foss et al., 2023).

Dunkel Schetter & Tanner (2015) examined the association between affective states and the experience of anxiety, depression, and racism on fetal development during pregnancy. Their review highlights the effects these stressors have on adverse maternal and child health outcomes resulting in LBW infants and neurological development of the fetus and preterm birth. The research strongly indicates that anxiety, depression, major life events, pregnancy anxiety, and racism are precursors to preterm birth and LBW, with more distal outcomes related to the infant, mother, and family. Moreover, *maternal trauma*—defined as the experience of intimate partner violence (IPV) and other physically or psychologically damaging events that women may experience during pregnancy— is known to have negative influences on the developing fetus and infant (Foss et al., 2023).

Foss and colleagues (2023) found that maternal trauma was directly related to lower infant physiological regulation and indirectly related with lower levels of both infant behavioral and physiological regulation via higher maternal anxiety during pregnancy. The authors suggest that maternal stress could potentially contribute to children displaying maladaptive stress responses, which have been associated with poorer behavioral, cognitive, and academic outcomes among children. This may be especially true for mothers who experienced IPV and other forms of trauma during their pregnancy. "IPV" and "domestic violence" are used synonymously to describe abusive behavior by one person upon another. "Intimate partner" includes current and former spouses or dating partners. Approximately 15%–45% of Latina women report an experience of IPV during their lifetime (Gonzalez et al., 2020; Klevens, 2007; Sabina et al., 2015). A study conducted by Bonomi et al. (2009) found that the prevalence of IPV for Latina versus non-Latina women was 44.6% versus 44%, respectively, for lifetime occurrence; 20.1% and 14.5%, respectively, for the past 5 years; and 11.5% and 7.8%, respectively, for the past year. Moreover, Rodriguez et al. (2008) found that among pregnant Latinas, IPV was significantly associated with depression and PTSD.

Previous research has demonstrated that historically disenfranchised populations experience more psychosocial stressors than non-Latino White Americans, and particularly during the COVID-19 pandemic (Almeida et al., 2016; Cobb et al., 2021; McKnight-Eily et al., 2021; Menselton et al., 2008; Torres et al., 2012). For example, Cobb et al. (2021) found a dose-response relationship between experiencing discrimination across multiple domains with increased likelihood of mood, anxiety, and substance use disorders among Latinos.

The differential effects of stressors were discussed in Chapter 1, with responses through the hypothalamic-pituitary-adrenal axis (HPA) resulting in a biopsychosocial stress response that affects several physiological mechanisms, which can lead to toxic stress, the result of high allostatic load (Bosquet Enlow et al., 2017; Braveman et al., 2010; Liu et al., 2016). For example, Campbell et al. (2020) found that among Latinas, posttraumatic stress influenced the association between PMS and higher negative affectivity among infants. Prior research has demonstrated that negative affectivity (emotional reactivity) in childhood increases the risk for psychological disorders later in life (Spry et al., 2020). Additional research around ACEs lends support to the association between emotional reactivity and subsequent psychological disorders later in life (Anda et al., 2006; Felitti & Anda, 2003; Ryznar et al., 2021; Campbell et al., 2020).

Myers (2009) has provided a detailed reciprocal and recursive conceptual model that examines the direct and indirect influences on adverse health outcomes among historically disadvantaged populations (see Figure 6.3).

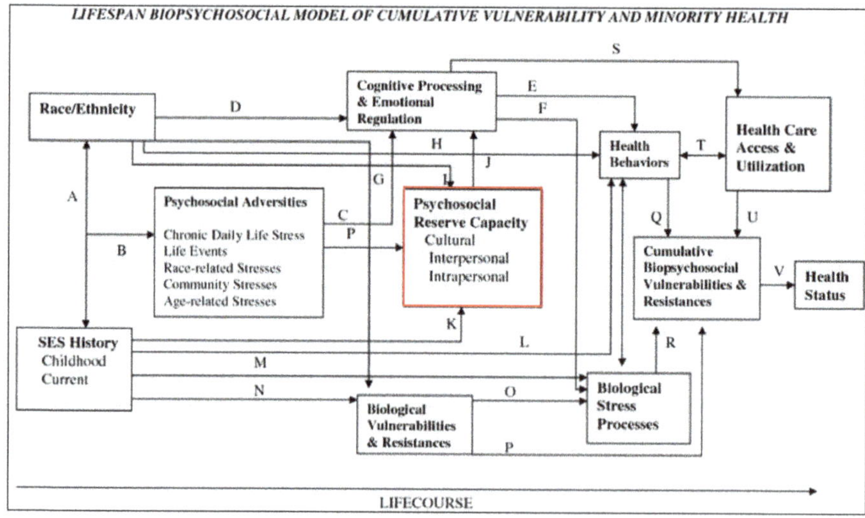

FIGURE 6.3 Myers's Conceptual Model of Cumulative Vulnerability

One of the more important components in the hypothesized model is psychosocial reserve capacity, including cultural, interpersonal, and intrapersonal factors (highlighted in red in figure 6.3). For Latinos, this component is associated with resiliency when confronted with adversity. I believe this helps explain the relationship between stressors and health outcomes, with Latinos of Mexican descent having a cultural advantage that buffers the adverse effects on mortality rates.

Latina Epidemiologic Paradox Redux

The Latino epidemiological paradox has become the predominant paradigm to examine morbidity and mortality advantages among Latinos. Latino immigrants typically show better health status, measured in several different ways, than their U.S.-born counterparts. For example, much of the research on Latina immigrants and Mexican-origin immigrant women show similar or better birth outcomes compared to non-Latina White Americans or U.S.-born Latinas (Flores et al., 2012).

The *Latina birth outcome paradox* refers to the observation that despite socioeconomic disadvantages, Latina mothers in the United States have a similar or lower risk for delivering a low birth weight (LBW) infant compared to non-Latina White mothers (Hoggatt et al., 2012; Gonzalez-Quintero et al., 2020). However, research findings are mixed, depending on study design, study population, and region. For example, a study conducted in New York among Latinas from different subgroups showed that Puerto Rican women had the highest rates of adverse birth outcomes compared to Mexican-origin women (Rosenbeg et al., 2005). Moreover, they found that Mexican-born women had lower LBW prevalence than U.S.-born Mexican women (5.1% compared to 8.4%, respectively). In a study conducted in California, Latinas had worse birth outcomes (preterm births and LBW infants) than non-Latina White women (Sanchez-Vaznaugh et al., 2016), suggesting no health advantage for Latinas with respect to adverse birth outcomes (i.e., no support for a Latina birth outcome paradox).

Macro influences on prenatal and maternal stress are grounded in the unequal distribution of resources necessary for human and fetal development, particularly those associated with critical social determinants of health. Economic stability, the built environment, neighborhood context, and access to adequate health care provide the social and cultural context that can adversely affect maternal, infant, and child health. In addition, maternal exposure to extreme stress can result in increased risk of mental disorders among children, including autism, depression, ADHD, anxiety disorders, and schizophrenia (Campbell et al., 2020; Spry et al., 2020).

Fetal Programming and Maternal Stress

Increased psychosocial stress, anxiety, and depression during pregnancy is associated with elevated secretion of cortisol and other hormones that are transmitted to the fetus through the placenta. Cortisol exposure during this period has a direct effect on fetal brain development and mediates the link between prenatal stress/anxiety and infant outcomes. Early exposure may "program" certain systems, suggesting long-term effects on behavior (e.g., fear), immune system modulation, and stress physiological reactions.

The human fetus shows 8 times more cell divisions before birth compared with cell divisions during the remainder of life (Barker, 1998). With this tremendous activity, the fetus is susceptible to influences that can alter the fetal developmental trajectory with lasting influences on health. These influences on the fetus have been described as "programming" or "fetal programming" (Beydoun & Saftlas, 2008; Kapoor et al., 2006; Kwon & Kim, 2017). *Fetal programming* (also called *prenatal programming*) is the hypothesis that during development of the embryo and fetus, important physiological characteristics can be reset epigenetically by environmental events. This epigenetic resetting can endure into adulthood and even affect the following generation to produce a transgenerational nongenetic disorder (Coker et al., 2018; Conching & Thayer, 2019). Assaults on local fetal cellular environments can change gene expression during the developmental construction of tissues and organs. These changes can result in long-range consequences for the function of those tissues and organs during childhood and adulthood.

The first 2 months of pregnancy are the most sensitive to prenatal stress (Barker, 1995; De Boo & Harding, 2006). *Neurogenesis*—when new neurons are generated from neural stem cells and progenitor cells—occurs around the 10th week of fetal development when the brain produces approximately 250,000 new neurons every minute (Kostović et al., 2019). During weeks 24 through 30 of fetal development, new cell connections are occurring called *synaptogenesis*, when the formation between synapses and neurons begins to develop.

Exposure to extreme stress during these critical periods of pregnancy will influence which developing structures are affected and therefore determine the physical, cognitive, or behavioral outcome of the person:

- Physical: Recent research findings have demonstrated that obstetrical complications, low birth weight, and delayed physical development may all be influenced by prenatal maternal stress.
- Cognitive: Several recent human research findings have shown that acute prenatal stress affects children's cognition (their ability to think).
- Behavioral: There is consistent evidence demonstrating that prenatal maternal stress affects the behavior of children. Children exposed to this stress may show difficulties with paying attention and have aggressive attitudes. (Buitelaar et al., 2003; Cao Lei et al., 2016; Charil et al., 2010; DiPietro, 2004)

These complex micro and macro interactions are also congruent with the concept of fetal onset of adult diseases (FOAD) championed by Barker's and his colleagues' research (Barker, 1998, 1999a, 1999b).

Fetal Onset of Adult Diseases (FOAD)

An extension of fetal programming—and sometimes used interchangeably with it—is the fetal onset of adult disease (FOAD) hypothesis, also known as the "Barker hypothesis." The *Barker hypothesis* states that adverse influences early in fetal development, particularly during intrauterine life, can result in permanent changes in physiology and metabolism, which result in increased disease risk in adulthood (De Boo & Harding, 2006). The importance of FOAD has been recognized by the World Health Organization (2006) in the following statement: "The global burden of death and disability because of impaired fetal development is huge. Although the burden is particularly high in developing countries, it is also a significant concern in developed countries" (pp. 1–2).

David Barker proposed FOAD as an explanatory hypothesis on how adult diseases originate during the embryonic fetal development stage (Barker, 1995, 1999a, 1999b, 2007). Research has conclusively linked several chronic diseases, such as low birth weight (LBW), coronary heart disease, cardiovascular disease, hypertension, type 2 diabetes, and cancer, to intrauterine fetal development. FOAD is based on the premise of *developmental plasticity*, which refers to when a single genotype, influenced by specific intrauterine events, has the capability to produce different phenotypes. This hypothesis relies on the fact that there exist specific developmental periods whereby an organism is "plastic" or "sensitive" to its intrauterine environment. Using LBW and preterm births as proxy measures for fetal and adult health, researchers have found that these adverse birth outcomes are associated with a host of chronic diseases ranging from coronary artery disease, obesity, diabetes mellitus, cancer, and osteoporosis to various psychiatric illnesses like schizophrenia and bipolar disorder (see Table 6.1). Given the higher prevalence of obesity-related diseases, including type 2 diabetes, among Mexican Americans compared to non-Latino White Americans, it is important to conduct additional research on the influence of socioenvironmental interactions on intrauterine development and across the life course (Scott Yoshizawa, 2012).

TABLE 6.1 Chronic Diseases Associated With FOAD

Diabetes mellitus
Obesity
Dyslipidemia
Hypertension
Coronary artery disease
Stroke
Kidney failure
Liver failure
Lung abnormalities—bronchopulmonary dysplasia, reactive airway disease
Immune dysfunction
Reduced bone mass
Alzheimer's disease
Depression, anxiety, bipolar disorder, schizophrenia
Cancer

Adapted from: Calkins and Devaskar (2011)

Adverse Childhood Experiences (ACEs) Inequalities Among Latinos

Adverse childhood experiences (*ACEs*) are the cumulative effect of severe biological and/or psychosocial stressors that begin in childhood and occur across a person's lifespan (Anda et al., 2006; Felitti et al., 1998b;) Examples of ACEs include but are not limited to victimization, violence, abuse (physical, emotional, and sexual), neglect (physical and emotional), dysfunctional households, bullying (personal and cyber), forced separation from parents, detention of minors, racism, discrimination, and homelessness (Felitti, 2019). Scientists believe that ACEs can create a burden of psychological stress that influences behavior, cognitions, emotions, and physical functioning in ways that promote health problems and illness in adult life (Felitti et al., 1998a). Research has also shown that ACEs lead to depression and posttraumatic stress disorder (PTSD), which in turn can lead to substance abuse, sleep disorders, physical inactivity, immunosuppression, inflammatory responses, and inconsistent health care utilization, which can potentially lead to other medical conditions later in life (Crouch et al., 2019; Gilbert et al., 2015).

Research also shows that especially for younger children, the recurrent experience of or exposure to ACEs can significantly affect brain development (Sheridan & McLaughlin, 2014; Herzog & Schmahl, 2018). Early negative life conditions, such as prenatal undernutrition and stress or maternal stress during pregnancy, can modify developmental biology in offspring that then increases their risk of developing diseases like diabetes mellitus, hypertension, and cardiovascular disease as adults. Additionally, some research shows that children born under these conditions can be more sensitive to social environmental stressors, experiencing greater stress (Bosquet-Enlow et al., 2017; Campbell et al., 2020; Spry et al., 2020).

ACEs are common in the United States. The Centers for Disease Control and Prevention (CDC; 2023) estimate that approximately 64% of persons aged 18 and older have experienced at least one ACE, and about 17% have experienced four or more ACEs. Not everyone who has experienced an ACE or even those who have experienced four or more ACEs will develop a disease or health condition. The type, frequency, and intensity of ACEs, as with other psychosocial stressors, are causally associated with the odds of developing disease. The type of ACEs used in the original 1998 CDC-Kaiser study are shown in Table 6.2.

For example, the classic Felitti et al. study (1998a) found that persons who had experienced four or more ACEs had a 4–12 times increased risk of drug abuse, alcoholism, depression, and suicide attempts; a 2–4 times increased risk of poor self-rated health, being a smoker, ever having a STI, or having multiple sexual partners; and a 1.4–1.6 times increase in physical inactivity and severe obesity. Felitti et al. found that 56% of persons in the study with no ACEs had none of the health risk behaviors, whereas only 14% of those with four or more ACEs had no health risk behaviors.

TABLE 6.2 ACE Definitions, CDC-Kaiser ACE Study, 1998

Emotional abuse: A parent, stepparent, or adult living in your home swore at you, insulted you, put you down, or acted in a way that made you afraid that you might be physically hurt.
Physical abuse: A parent, stepparent, or adult living in your home pushed, grabbed, slapped, threw something at you, or hit you so hard that you had marks or were injured.
Sexual abuse: An adult, relative, family friend, or stranger who was at least 5 years older than you touched or fondled your body in a sexual way, made you touch his/her body in a sexual way, or attempted to have any type of sexual intercourse with you.
Mother treated violently: Your mother or stepmother was pushed, grabbed, slapped, had something thrown at her, kicked, bitten, hit with a fist, hit with something hard, repeatedly hit for over at least a few minutes, or threatened or hurt by a knife or gun by your father (or stepfather) or mother's boyfriend.
Household substance abuse: A household member was a problem drinker or alcoholic or a household member used street drugs.

(continued)

Mental illness in household: A household member was depressed or mentally ill or a household member attempted suicide.	
Parental separation or divorce: Your parents were separated or divorced.	
Criminal household member: A household member went to prison.	
Emotional neglect: Someone in your family did not help you feel important or special, you felt unloved, people in your family did not look out for each other and did not feel close to each other, and your family was not a source of strength and support.	
Physical neglect: There wasn't someone to take care of you, protect you, and take you to the doctor if you needed it. You didn't have enough to eat, your parents were too drunk or too high to take care of you, and you had to wear dirty clothes.	

Source: Boullier and Blair (2018, p. 133)

ACE Prevalence in the United States

The CDC-Kaiser Permanente Adverse Childhood Experiences Study (Felitti et al., 1998a, 1998b) was one of the largest investigations of childhood abuse and neglect and later-life health and well-being (Anda et al., 2006). The original ACE Study was conducted at Kaiser Permanente from 1995 to 1997 with two waves of data collection (Felitti, 2019). Over 17,000 health maintenance organization (a type of insurance plan) members from Southern California receiving physical exams completed confidential surveys regarding their childhood experiences and current health status and behaviors (via patient recall). The study found that ACEs are common: Almost two thirds of study participants reported at least one ACE, and more than 1 in 5reported three or more ACEs (Felitti et al., 1998a, 1998b).

Felitti et al. (1998a, p. 251) were the first to identify a "strong dose-response relationship" between ACEs and negative health and well-being outcomes across the life course. *Dose-response* describes the change in an outcome (e.g., alcoholism) associated with differing levels of exposure (or doses) to a stressor (e.g., ACEs). A graded dose-response means that as the dose of the stressor increases the intensity of the outcome also increases. Anda et al. (2006) demonstrated that this graded dose-response relationship was strong for 18 health outcomes (Table 6.3). Additionally, using a subset of the first wave sample (n = 8,708), they found very strong relationships between four or more ACEs and prevalence and risk for memory impairment, high level of perceived stress, difficulty controlling anger, and risk of perpetrating IPV.

TABLE 6.3 Prevalence and Odds Ratio for Four or More ACES and Health Outcomes in U.S. Sample Population (N = 17,337)

Health outcomes	Percent of sample	Adjusted odds ratio (OR) and confidence interval
Panic reactions	20.9	2.5 (2.2–2.9)
Depressed affect	49.0	3.6 (3.2–4.0)

(*continued*)

TABLE 6.3 ***(continued)***

Health outcomes	Percent of sample	Adjusted odds ratio (OR) and confidence interval
Anxiety	19.0	2.4 (2.1–2.8)
Hallucinations	4.0	2.7 (1.9–3.7)
Sleep disturbance	56.1	2.1 (1.9–2.4)
Severe obesity	11.9	1.9 (1.6–2.2)
Multiple somatic symptoms	13.9	2.7 (2.3–3.2)
Smoking	14.5	1.8 (1.5–2.1)
Alcoholism	15.3	7.2 (5.9–8.9)
Illicit drug use	35.2	4.5 (3.9–5.2)
Injected drug use	3.7	11.1 (6.2–19.9)
Early intercourse	14.2	6.6 (5.3–8.2)
Promiscuity (≥30 partners)	10.8	3.6 (3.0–4.4)
Sexual dissatisfaction	32.3	2.0 (1.8–2.2)

Source: Anda et al. (2006)

The highest odds ratio in Table 6.3 is for injected drug use, with those persons having four or more ACEs having an 11.1-fold risk. The ORs for alcoholism, early sexual intercourse, and illicit drug use are also very high for those persons having four or more ACEs.

ACE Prevalence Among Latinos

A study by Gilbert et al. (2015) using Behavioral Risk Factor Surveillance System (BRFSS) data from 10 states and the District of Columbia shows the prevalence of ACES to be about 60%, which is about 4% lower than reported by Felitti et al. (1998a, 1998b). The types of ACEs reported by the large sample (*N* = 53,998) included emotional abuse (35.1%), physical abuse (16.0%) and sexual abuse (10.9%). The number of ACEs varied by gender, age, race or ethnicity, education, and income level. For example, women reported more ACEs than men, persons 18–24 years of age reported more ACEs than older age groups, persons with lower educational attainment reported more ACEs than those with higher levels of education, and those with lower incomes reported more ACEs than those with higher incomes. The study also found a dose-response relationship between the number of ACEs reported and several health conditions, including ratings of fair or poor health, frequent mental distress, type 2 diabetes, myocardial infarction, coronary heart disease, stroke, asthma, and disability.

Looking specifically at race/ethnicity, Gilbert et al. (2015) found that non-Latino Black Americans and Latinos had a higher frequency of ACEs than non-Latino White Americans. They also found that Latinos and non-Latino Black Americans reported higher rates of experiencing four or more ACEs (21.8%, 21.2%, and 14.5%, respectively). Moreover, 41.5% of non-Latino White participants did not experience any ACEs, compared to 30.3% for non-Latino Black and 31.1% for Latino participants (see Figure 6.4).

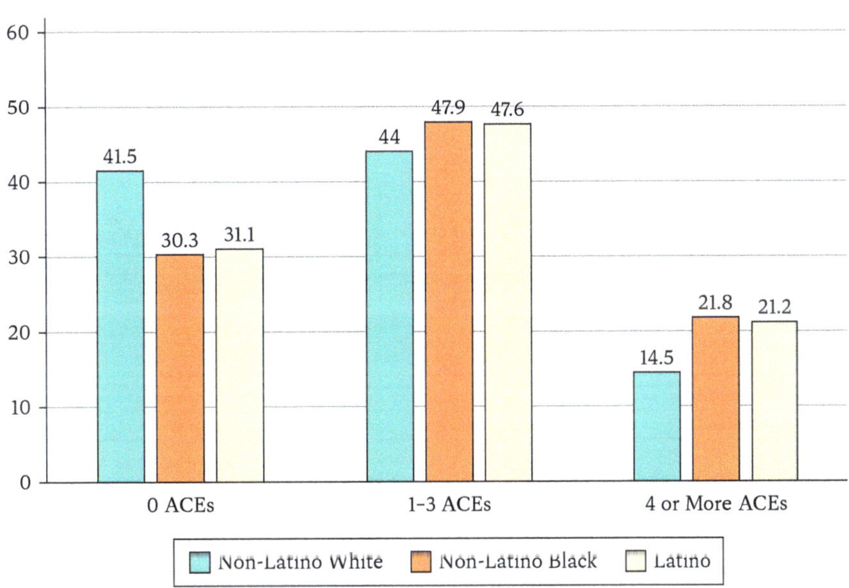

FIGURE 6.4 Percentage of Adults Reporting ACEs by Race and Latino Origin

Crouch and colleagues (2019) studied the prevalence of ACEs among U.S. children between the ages 0 and 17, using the 2016 National Survey of Childrens Health (NSCH). Findings showed that Latino children reported higher rates than non-Latino White children for parental divorce (26% vs. 22%, respectively), economic hardship (28.9% vs. 21.5%, respectively), and exposure to violence in the home or neighborhood

(7.9% vs. 6.2%, respectively). Living in a disrupted household was the same for Latino children and non-Latino White children at 17%, almost identical to results derived from the national BRFSS reported by Gilbert et al. (2015).

A more recent study of ACEs among Latinos shows relatively high prevalence rates. Swedo et al. (2023) examined BRFSS data from 2011–2020. Overall, 63.9% of U.S. adults reported at least one ACE, and 17.3% reported four or more ACEs, results very consistent with previous studies. Experiencing four or more ACEs was most more common among women (19.2%), adults aged 25–34 years (25.2%), non-Latino American Indian or Alaska Native adults (32.4%), non-Latino multiracial adults (31.5%), adults with less than a high school education (20.5%), and those who were unemployed (25.8%) or unable to work (28.8%). Although the prevalence of ACEs was high, they were differentially distributed in the U.S. population by race and ethnicity, income level, gender, and educational status.

The distribution of ACEs by race and Latino origin is presented in Figure 6.5. Among Latinos in the Swedo et al. (2023) study, 65.4% experienced at least one ACE, a slightly higher prevalence than non-Latino White respondents. Additionally, Latino Americans had a higher prevalence than non-Latino White Americans for four or more ACEs. Previous research (i.e., Felitti & Anda, 2003; Felitti et al., 1998a, 1998b; Gilbert et al., 2015) has demonstrated that those persons who experience four or more ACES are at increased risk for developing disease and other adverse health outcomes.

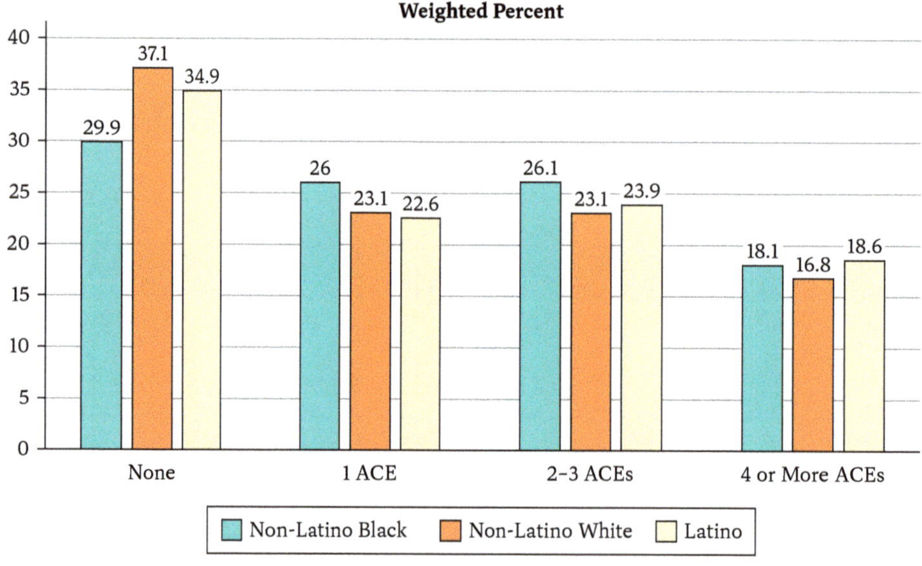

FIGURE 6.5 Adverse Child Experience Scores by Race and Latino Origin

Caballero et al. (2017) examined the prevalence of ACEs among Latino immigrant and U.S.-native Latino children. They found that 30% of children in U.S.-native families reported high ACEs, compared with only 16% of children in Latino immigrant families. Additionally, children in immigrant families had significantly lower odds of ACE exposure despite their higher prevalence of poverty. This study suggests that cultural buffers modify the experience and effect of ACEs in Latino immigrant families. Another study conducted by Mersky and Janczewski (2018) showed that Latino Americans had significantly lower

ACE scores than non-Latino White Americans and non-Latino Black Americans. For example, non-Latino White participants reported the highest prevalence of any abuse or neglect (61.6%). Non-Latino White participants also reported the highest rates of physical abuse (43.6%), sexual abuse (30.1%), and emotional abuse (33.6%). Latinos in their study were less likely than non-Latino White Americans to report physical abuse, emotional abuse, and emotional neglect, but they were more likely to report physical neglect.

An examination of ACE scores among violent-offending and non-violent-offending Latinos using data from the National Epidemiologic Survey on Alcohol and Related Conditions (NESARC-III; $N = 6{,}866$ Latino adults) was conducted by Powers and colleagues (2022). They found that first-generation Latino offenders were more at risk for adverse health outcomes than native-born or second-generation Latinos. Native-born U.S. Latinos reported the highest overall ACEs ($M = 1.86$, $SD = 1.98$) followed by second-generation ($M = 1.37$, $SD = 1.72$) and first-generation ($M = 1.28$, $SD = 1.61$) Latinos. Moreover, among violent offenders, first-generation Latinos had significantly higher prevalence of parental drug or alcohol use, but second-generation Latinos had significantly higher prevalence of physical abuse, emotional abuse, and sexual abuse. Among nonviolent offenders, second-generation Latinos had higher prevalence of parental death and physical abuse. First-generation Latinos had a higher prevalence of sexual abuse.

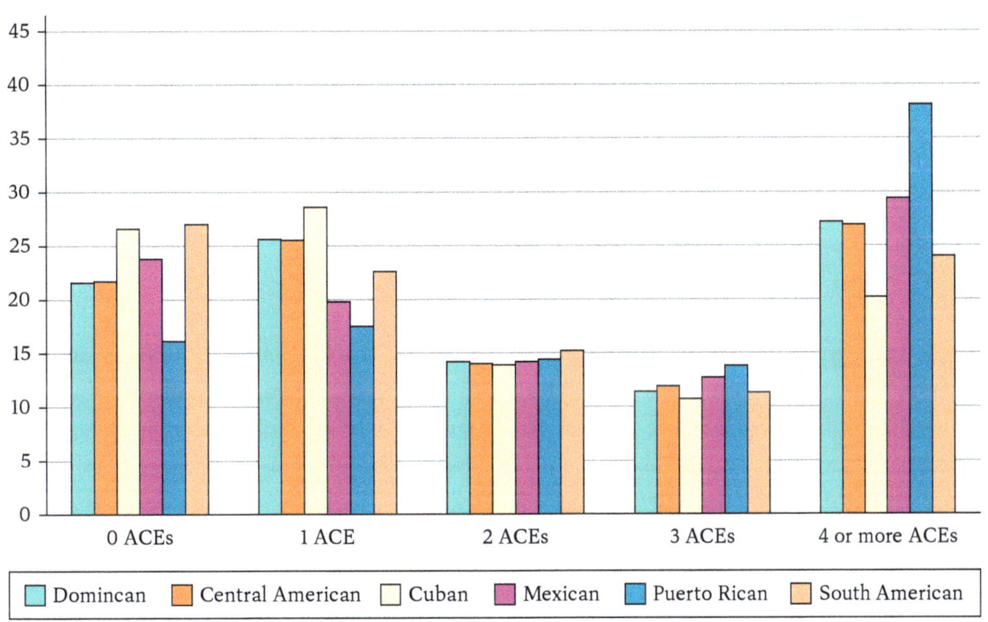

FIGURE 6.6 Prevalence of ACEs Among Latino Subgroups

Most ACE studies focused on Latinos, though few, consistently show that about 1 in 5 Latinos report experiencing four or more ACEs. However, a study by Llabre et al. (2017) using the landmark Hispanic Community Health Study/Study of Latinos (HCHS/SOL) reported much higher ACE scores among Latinos than previously reported. Their findings are presented in Figure 6.6.

In Llabre et al.'s (2017) study, the highest prevalence of no ACEs was among South Americans (27%), followed by Cubans (26.6%) and Mexicans (23.8%). The highest prevalence of experiencing four or more

ACEs (the highest at-risk group) was found among Puerto Ricans (38.1%), followed by Mexicans (29.4%). The study used the same ACE scale that had been previously used by the CDC-Kaiser ACE study, so the findings cannot be due to the difference in ACE items. The study also found that U.S.-born Latinos experienced a significantly higher prevalence of four or more ACEs than foreign-born Latinos (37.6% vs. 26.3%, respectively; see Figure 6.7).

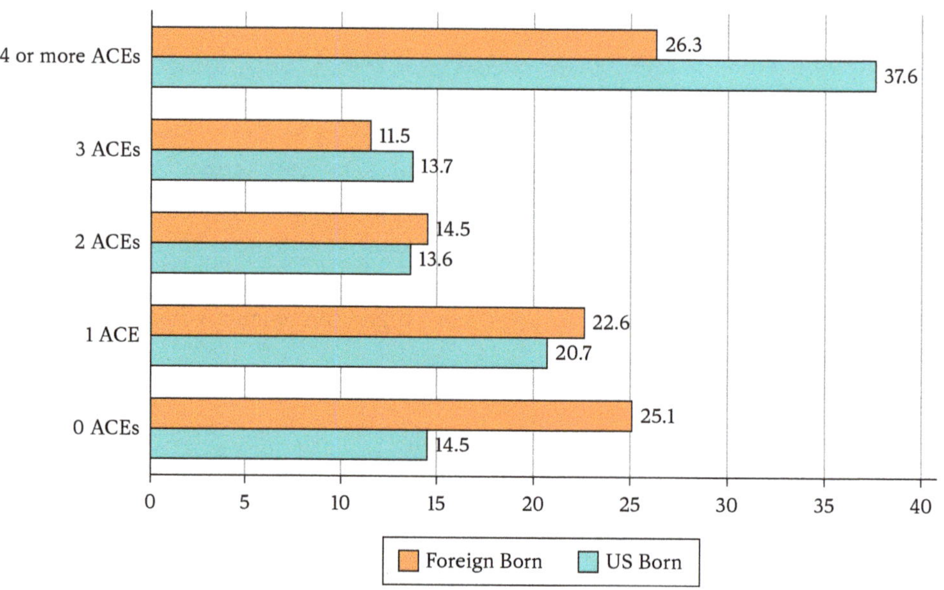

FIGURE 6.7 Prevalence of ACES and Place of Birth Among Latinos

Moreover, and consistent with the research literature on the association between ACE scores and health risk behaviors, the Llabre et al. (2017) study found that ACEs were significantly associated with depressive symptoms, body mass index (BMI), smoking, and use of alcohol. With respect to disease, ACEs were associated with coronary heart disease, chronic obstructive pulmonary disease (COPD), and cancer even after controlling for demographics and risk factors. ACEs were not associated with asthma, type 2 diabetes, or stroke among Latinos in their study.

The future development of ACEs in Latino children is of great concern given the recent anti-immigrant and anti-Latino sentiment in the United States. Recent Department of Homeland Security (DHS) policy on family separation and detention has led to the forced removal of Latino children from their parents. Many children born to Latino immigrants are U.S. citizens and therefore deserve some measure of protection under the law. Latino children separated from their parents display fear, confusion, and grief that trigger depression and anxiety affecting their emotional and physical well-being (Dreby, 2012; Vargas & Ybarra, 2017). Brabeck & Xu (2010) found that Latino immigrant parents believed that the impact of their deportation would have negative effects on their children's emotional well-being and academic performance. Additionally, Allen et al. (2015) found that Latino children with a deported parent were more likely to demonstrate elevated levels of internalizing and externalizing problems than Latino children without a deported parent.

When DHS officials forcibly remove and detain Latino children, they are exposing them to several adverse childhood experiences. Media reports of Latino children detained in "cages" will undoubtedly add to their experiences of trauma. What types of adverse experiences are Latino immigrant children reporting? Reports have included maltreatment, lack of a nurturing physical and social environments, isolation, depression, anxiety, PTSD, constant crying, unresolved grief, and poor cognitive and social development. Time will tell the effects of these ACEs on the adult lives of Latino immigrant children who have experienced removal and detention.

According to the ACE Interface website (https://www.aceinterface.com), the population attributable risk (PAR), or the proportion of a disease that can be attributed to a specific cause, is very high, ranging from 14%–78% (Figure 6.8). Felitti & Anda (2003) reported on the association between PAR and ACEs for women, finding that the PAR was 48% for depression and suicide, 52% for domestic violence, and 62% for sexual assault. The authors conclude that ACEs and, importantly, the number and type determine the probability of mortality from the 10 most common causes of death.

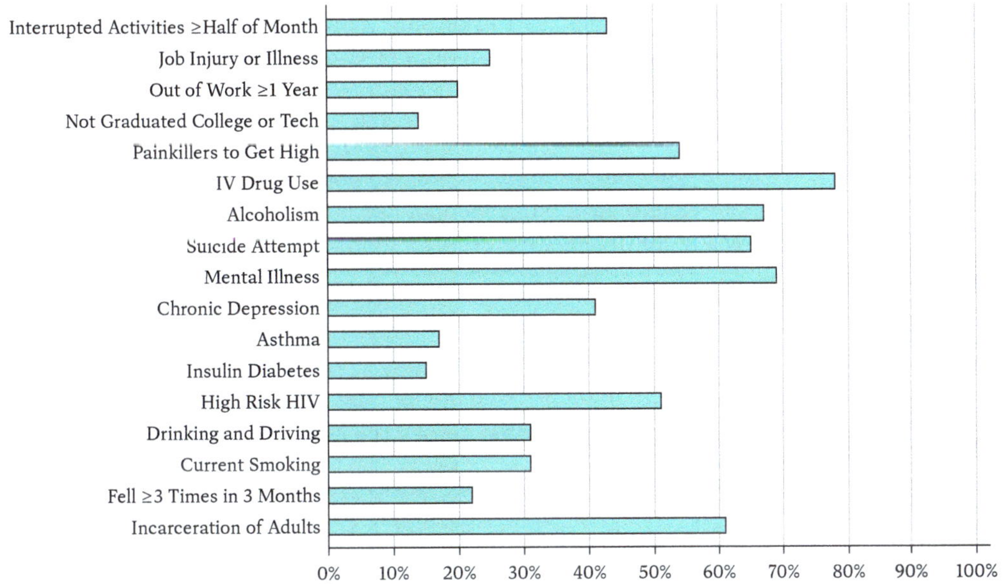

FIGURE 6.8 Population Attributable Risk, ACEs, and Health

Extant research on ACEs has clearly established a graded dose-response relationship, with those persons reporting an ACE score of zero having few risk factors for disease compared to those persons reporting four or more ACEs who have multiple risk factors for disease or have the disease itself. Adjusted odds ratios provided in Table 6.3 show the profound level of risk associated with experiencing four or more ACEs.

ACEs and the Development of Psychiatric Disorders

Several studies have shown that the interactions between genetics and socioenvironmental stressors contribute to the incidence and prevalence of psychiatric disorders (Gatt et al., 2015; Leaune et al., 2019; López-León et al., 2008, Tsuang et al., 1999). For example, research on identical twins shows the genetic contribution of schizophrenia to be as high as 83%. Twin studies of other psychiatric disorders generally show much lower genetic contributions between 31% and 42% for major depressive disorders, 30% and 40% for PTSD, 56% and 86% for anorexia nervosa, and 50% and 60% for alcohol dependence and drug abuse disorders.

Perhaps the best available evidence for social epigenetic changes associated with psychosocial stress are the findings from the Detroit Neighborhood Health Study (DNHS; Kessler & Wang, 2008; Uddin et al., 2010). For example, Uddin et al. (2010) assessed PTSD and the correlation between the number of potential traumatic events and DNA methylation levels at over 27,000 CpG sites covering more than 14,000 genes. They found that compared to PTSD-unaffected individuals, PTSD-affected individuals showed higher levels of DNA demethylation (gene expression). Additional research on the DNHS suggests that, as with major depressive disorders, DNA methylation of the serotonin transporter gene (SLC6A4) plays an important role in risk for PTSD. These findings and others strongly suggest that social epigenetic processes contribute to gene expression in the development of psychiatric disorders.

According to McCance-Katz (2019), using data from the 2018 National Survey on Drug Use and Health (NSDUH), approximately 20.3 million people aged 12 or older had a substance use disorder related to their use of alcohol or illicit drugs in the past year, including 14.8 million people who had an alcohol use disorder and 8.1 million people who had an illicit drug use disorder. They also found that compared to the national average, Latino adults have lower rates of alcohol use, higher rates of binge alcohol use, and lower rates of illicit drug use in the past month. Also, among adults aged 18–25, Latinos of the same age were found to have lower rates of alcohol use, binge alcohol use, and illicit drug use in the past month. Compared to the national average of adult women, Latinas had lower rates of alcohol use, binge alcohol use, and illicit drug use in the past month. Compared to the national average of adult men, Latino men had lower rates of alcohol use, higher rates of binge alcohol use, and lower rates of illicit drug use in the past month. However, there were differences related to nativity and Latino subgroups. Compared to non-U.S.-born Latinos, U.S.-born Latinos were found to have higher rates of alcohol use, binge alcohol use, and illicit drug use in the past month. The study found that among the Latino subgroups, Cubans have higher rates of alcohol use, Puerto Ricans have higher rates of binge alcohol use, and they have higher rates of illicit drug use in the past month.

The identification of risk factors associated with increasing rates of psychiatric and substance use disorders include nativity (individual and parents), number of years lived in the United States, and generation status (Alegría et al., 2007, 2008). The common element among these risk factors is the potential for subsequent generations to inherit predispositions for psychiatric and substance use disorders. Another important element is the social environment and its impact on developmental trajectories for risk of psychiatric and substance use disorders in utero and among those Latino youth who experience a high number of ACEs, as well as maternal and prenatal stressors.

Together, these potential gene–environment interactions, expressed through complex epigenetic processes, may confer an increased risk for psychiatric and substance use disorders among subsequent generations of U.S.-born Latinos, like physical health. According to a model suggested by Wong et al. (2011), these inherited predispositions, what they term *differentially methylated regions* (*DMRs*), are affected by a triggering event, like toxic stress, that can cause epigenetic changes (DNA methylation or histone acetylation) that modifies chromatin that either silences or expresses genes. In turn, this process influences one's susceptibility to substance use disorders that can lead to intergenerational transmission (see Figure 6.9).

If epigenetic modifications are a consequence of social environmental influences, either through the experience of maternal and prenatal stress, fetal programming, or vulnerability and susceptibility to the adverse and cumulative effects of multiple ACEs, are they a more direct "cause of the causes"? Moreover, given what is known about the intergenerational transmission of these effects, isn't it plausible to theorize that these effects could be transmitted to subsequent generations, which could then increase their risk and susceptibility to disease?

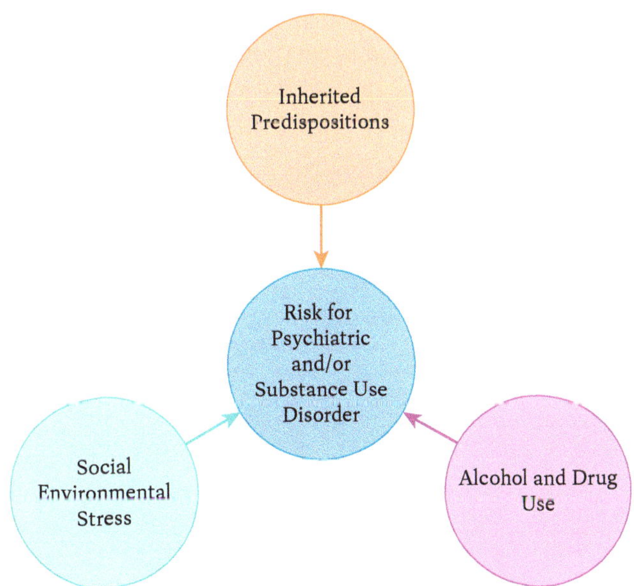

FIGURE 6.9 Risk for Psychiatric and/or Substance Use Disorders

Intergenerational Transmission/Historical Trauma and Latinos

Research on the intergenerational transmission of vulnerability and susceptibility to disease encoded in non-DNA structures is gaining increasing support. Heijmans et al. (2008) were among the first to provide epidemiologic evidence that changes in epigenetic processes in humans might arise from fetal exposures and persist into adulthood using the data from the Dutch famine of 1945–1946. The research study obtained blood from 112 participants 60 years later and analyzed DNA methylation of the insulin-like growth factor II gene (IGF2), an imprinted gene with a well-defined DMR that helps regulate expression. They found that women in the study who were exposed to famine during the periconceptional period (n = 60) had significantly lower methylation of the IGF2 DMR compared to their siblings. The periconceptional period is a 5- to 6-month period in women when significant epigenetic modifications to chromatin occur that correspond with normal development (Steegers-Theunissen et al., 2013).

Several researchers argue that epigenetic modifications can be transmitted intergenerationally, placing not only the first but subsequent generations of offspring at risk for disease (Ryznar et al., 2021). Epigenetic research suggests that the impact of stress on the epigenome can be transmitted across generations through several plausible biological processes: transmission of epigenetic markers through reproduction, maternal and prenatal stressors that influence fetal programming, and parental transmission to children of increased risk for experiencing both social stressors and developing disease (Conching & Thayer, 2019; Cunliffe, 2015, 2016).

The epigenome is a combination of histones and methyl-chemical compounds formed by a person's nutritional status (i.e., the foods that are consumed). Epigenetic modifications are central to understanding the cumulative and complex causes of disease associated with the fetal programming and FOAD hypotheses. Epigenetic research has shown that histone acetylation influences signaling pathways for gene expression or silencing through DNA methylation at DNA CpG sites (Ryan et al., 2020; Vick & Burris, 2017). Histone tails are chemically tagged, allowing gene transcription (see Figure 6.10).

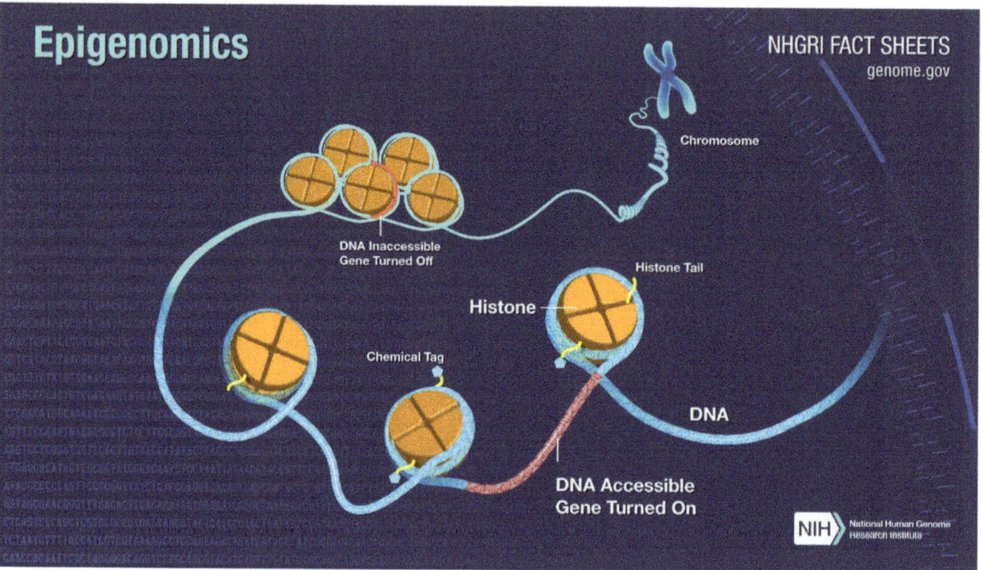

FIGURE 6.10 A Diagram of DNA Epigenomics

Epigenetic modifications encompassing the epigenome can be relatively stable while transmitting from one cell generation to the next. DNA methylation, histone modifications, genomic imprinting, chromatin remodeling, and non-coding RNA are all mechanisms for epigenetic modifications. DNA methylation of cytosine bases and histone modifications cause specific changes in chromatin structure and therefore regulate gene expression patterns (Ryznar et al., 2021).

The causal link between epigenetic modification and fetal programming is based on prenatal and maternal interactions with their intrauterine, social, and physical environments (Mancilla et al., 2020; Salas et al., 2021). The National Genome Research Institute (NHGRI) is at the forefront of groundbreaking research that will advance the understanding of the complex interplay between these environments and disease expression (Mars et al., 2022; Gunn et al., 2022; Sapkota et al., 2022; Breast Cancer Association Consortium et al., 2021).

Social epigenetics can potentially identify classes of genes or specific signaling pathways through which socioenvironmental factors might alter gene expression and affect Latino health and health inequalities (e.g., type 2 diabetes) or identify social stressors that affect health through epigenetic modifications of various biological pathways (Fox et al., 2015). Research has already demonstrated that early life experiences can cause epigenetic changes related to mental health, drug addiction, obesity, and other chronic diseases. Several authors now suggest that health inequalities arise not only because of higher levels of exposure to environmental hazards among historically disadvantaged and marginalized populations but also because of the synergistic effect of exposure to multiple environmental hazards and social stressors (Bagby et al., 2019; Hughes et al., 2017; Lu & Chen, 2004; Martin et al., 2022; Taouk & Schulkin, 2016; Wong et al., 2011).

Intergenerational trauma is a term used to describe the trauma experiences passed from generation to generation. The type of trauma can include physical abuse, sexual abuse, addictions to alcohol, tobacco, and other drugs, gang violence, homelessness, and poor nutrition/dietary patterns experienced in childhood (Felitti et al., 1998a; Powers et al., 2022; Swedo et al., 2023). How these experiences are passed from generation to generation is thought to occur through complex social epigenetic processes. Understanding these complex genetic processes provides insight into how intergenerational trauma is potentially transmitted from one generation to the next (see Figure 6.11).

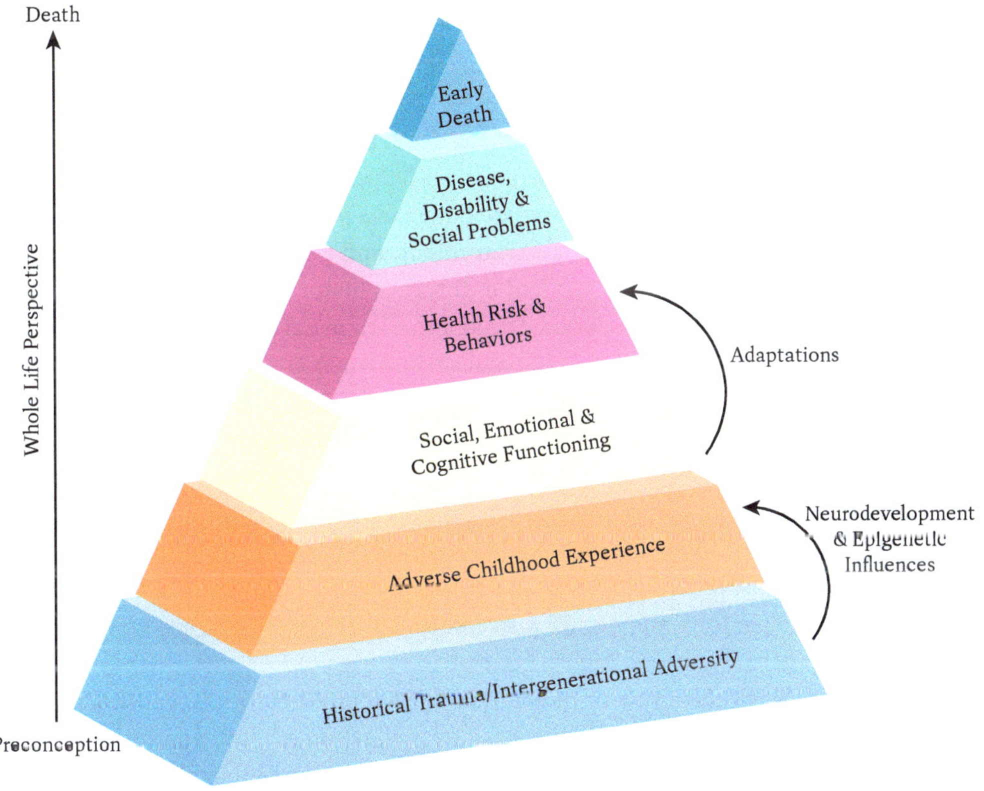

FIGURE 6.11 Pyramidic Influences of Intergenerational Trauma

Sotero (2006) developed a conceptual model of historical trauma that includes a mass trauma experience such as that experienced by the Mexica during the time of the Spanish conquest through the Spanish colonial period. According to the theory, the oppression and subjugation of the Indigenous populations of the Southwest resulted in segregation, displacement, physical and psychological violence, economic destruction, and cultural dispossession eliciting a "trauma response" in the first generation and subsequent generations, which includes physical responses, social responses, and psychological responses that are intergenerationally transmitted.

Physical responses include nutritional stress, a compromised immune system, biochemical abnormalities like increased triglycerides, endocrine impairment, adrenal maladaptation, and gene impairment or expression resulting in higher rates of malnutrition, type 2 diabetes, hyperglycemia, infectious disease, heart disease, hypertension, and cancer. Social responses to historical trauma include increased suicide rates, intimate partner violence, unemployment, low educational attainment, poverty, substance abuse, and child abuse resulting in the erosion or breakdown of community and family structures, social support networks, and loss of cultural capital. Psychological responses include an increased risk for PTSD, depression, anxiety, panic and anxiety disorders, substance use disorders, and other addictive disorders resulting in increased anger, aggression, social isolation, loss of self-worth, and addiction. Additionally, sleep disturbances, loss of concentration, and internalized shame can result as a response to historical trauma. Estrada (2009) proposed several health status implications for Latinos, including lack of health insurance coverage, lack of access to care, cultural and institutional barriers, and lack of culturally competent physicians. Health outcomes could also include metabolic syndrome and severe obesity.

There is little research to date on the application of historical or intergenerational trauma to the health status of Latinos. Some researchers (e.g., Cerdeña et al., 2021) argue that given the heterogeneity of the Latino population, there wasn't an explicit mass trauma event as articulated by Sotero (2006) and Estrada (2009). Certainly, there is a commonality of experience with Spanish colonialism, but it was manifested in various and unique ways throughout the New World. Indigenous populations of Mexico and the Southwest experienced oppression, cultural subjugation, enslavement, and political and land disenfranchisement. Latinos of Cuban and Puerto Rican descent had a different historical and political relationship with Spanish colonialism and with the United States. The length of time Latinos of Mexican descent have been exposed to the deleterious elements of Spanish colonialism and American neocolonialism has facilitated the development of physiological protective factors, also known as *biological resiliency*, among this population.

Fox et al. (2015) proposes an integration of fetal programming and maternal acculturation as a potential pathway to intergenerational transmission of disease risk. The authors provide a persuasive biological and epigenetic argument that maternal acculturation influences fetal programming and development. These epigenetic and acculturative signatures are then passed down through subsequent generations. The effect is increased risk and prevalence of disease with each generation of Latinos, resulting in the decline of a Latino epidemiologic paradox and higher prevalence of disease and higher mortality rates among third-generation, fourth generation, and higher Latinos.

I have argued that Latinos of Mexican descent have had a unique historical, political, and social experience different from other Latino groups that makes the application of intergenerational trauma a better fit. Structural and institutional violence toward Latinos of Mexican descent have persisted for almost 200 years in the United States. Consider the legacy of Spanish colonialism and the destruction of religious icons and native languages, replacing them with Catholicism and Spanish. So thoroughly have Latinos become colonized that we think Spanish is our native tongue! The Spanish colonial legacy was compounded by Euro-American neocolonialism with the establishment of an internal colonial model in the Southwest. Moreover, deficit models promulgated by social scientists to explain the "inferior culture" of Mexicans and Mexican Americans resulted in negative internalized attitudes of their culture and themselves. Nevertheless, there is cumulating evidence that suggests that Latinos of Mexican descent have inherited epigenetic resiliency characteristics that are protective of both stress and the development of disease.

Latino Cultural Resiliency

Given the negative influences on birth outcomes and adult disease associated with maternal and prenatal stress, fetal programming, and ACEs, one would expect to see higher rates of disease among Latinos and, in particular, Mexican Americans, than among non-Latino White Americans. Empirical evidence supports a dose–response relationship between stress and increased allostatic load with the odds of developing at-risk behaviors and increasing prevalence of disease with each generation of Latinos (Fox et al., 2015). Additionally, research shows that as the number of years lived in the United States increases, so does the risk of engaging in negative health behaviors, morbidity, and mortality, substantiating the selective migration hypothesis over the salmon bias hypothesis, both of which contribute to the Latino epidemiologic paradox (Abraído-Lanza et al., 1999, 2005; Scribner, 1996).

The fact that not all individuals exposed to adverse stressful life events or ACEs develop stress-related disorders clearly implies that socioenvironmental factors interact with genetic attributes and, together, affect resilience. The possibility also exists that epigenetic signatures that enhance resilience to stressful life experiences may be heritable.

Although the research literature on resilience, its meaning, and its potential buffering effects against disease is still burgeoning, the concept is not new to Latinos. Cultural resilience is an important characteristic of Latino culture, through Latino cultural beliefs and the closeness of Latino families. The cultural values discussed in Chapter 4, including familism, *respeto,* fatalism, and religiosity, are examples of active coping: an adaptive response to adversity that enables Latinos to overcome negative life experiences in their lives. Resilience embodies a strong sense of cultural identity and pride, self-confidence and self-esteem and being responsible and accountable for one's actions. It also includes aspects of community and collective resilience using interpersonal relationships in families, communities, and wider social networks. Latino cultural activities associated with fostering resilience among adolescents and adults include cultural immersion, cultural reawakening, emphasis on cultural strengths (i.e., familism, *compadrazgo,* religiosity, *respeto*), strengthening social support networks, and emphasizing cultural capital through community empowerment (see Chapter 4).

Compared to non-Latino White Americans, Mexican Americans have lower levels of the life-enhancing social determinants of health: lower levels of economic stability, less access to health care, less access to quality education, adverse risk exposure within the built environment, segregated and lower income neighborhoods, and the experience of racism and discrimination. Nevertheless, within Latino communities, cultural capital, including social support networks and informal social control, often mitigate against community and social stressors. Gallo and colleagues (2003, 2009) proposed the *reserve capacity model* (*RCP*) as a framework for understanding how psychosocial risk and resiliency may contribute to health inequalities among Latinos. The RCP is a product of the cultural strengths of Latinos, including familism and religiosity, that are relied upon when faced with stressful life events.

Two major spheres of influence on health risks and outcomes are the sociocultural context and psychosocial risk and resiliency factors, as depicted in Figure 6.12. Within the sociocultural contextual sphere are socioeconomic status characteristics (e.g., social mobility and cumulative deprivation) and cultural factors (e.g., ethnic identity, acculturation, generational status, etc.). Psychosocial risk and resiliency factors include two aspects: risk-inducing factors like stressful life events (positive and negative), positive or negative affect, and risk resiliency (referred to as "reserve capacity" in the model). Gallo and colleagues' (2003, 2009) model includes instrumental and monetary resources (i.e., tangible resources), interpersonal resources, intrapersonal resources, and culture-specific resources.

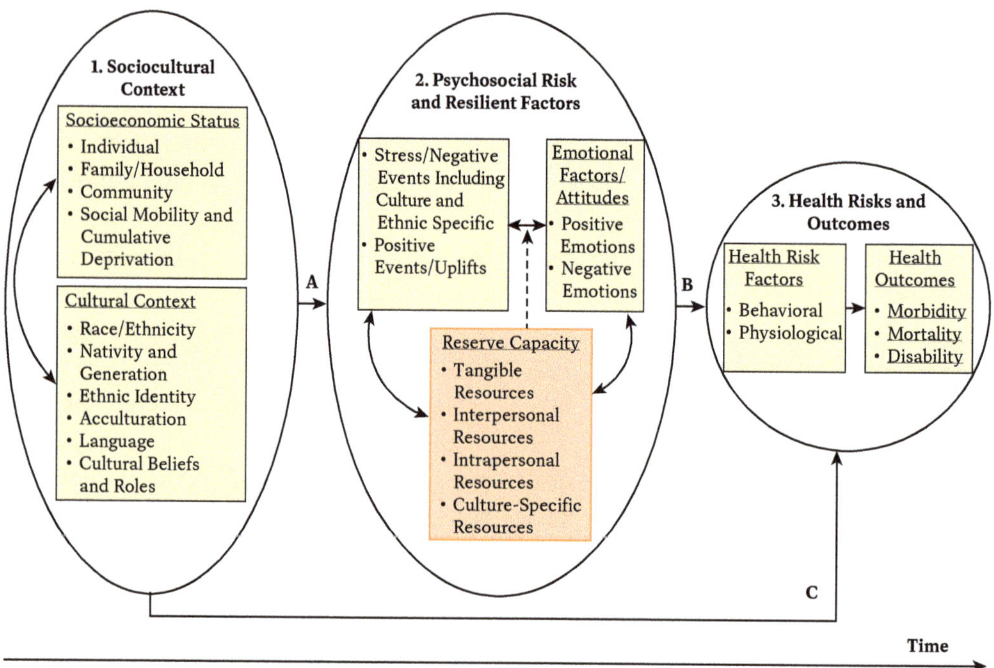

FIGURE 6.12 The Reserve Capacity Model (RCM)

Although the model is useful in illustrating the major antecedents of health risks and outcomes, the buffering or mediating effects of cultural capital or reserve capacity on health risks and health outcomes are not fully delineated. Reserve capacity directly influences (mitigates or buffers) health risks, which directly influence health outcomes. Nevertheless, the RCM is one of the first models to explicitly include a Latino cultural context and what has been termed in this book as "Latino cultural strengths" and the nurturing environment of the Latino family that fosters interdependency, collective achievement, and ethical and moral development.

Shevell and Denov (2021) suggest that historically marginalized populations have a reduced capacity to build adequate resiliency reserves because of the frequent stresses they experience. It is these "multiple layers of risk that interact to reduce the potency of available resilient resources. In contexts of inequality, it is not that some groups are simply not resilient, but rather that they face added barriers, vulnerabilities and/or risks that undermine opportunities for resilience" (Shevell & Denoy, 2021, p.3). Their conceptualization of intergenerational resilience is the cumulative and learned adaptation to severe circumstances built upon the previous generation that are culturally transmitted.

The convergence of epigenetics, neurobiology, and psychology has fueled interest in identifying whether resilience, as an adaptive human response to stressors, is encoded within the human genome and thereby passed to subsequent generations (McEwen, 2016; Zannas & West, 2014). Several studies have identified candidate genes that contribute to resiliency in the response to stress and trauma (Wu et al., 2013). For example, Donner et al. (2012) identified neuropeptide Y gene (NPY), which increased susceptibility to anxiety disorders after the experience of childhood adversity. Similarly, Heinz & Smoka (2006) and Skelton et al. (2012) identified the catechol-O-methyltransferase gene (COMT), which influences the risks of developing PTSD and deficits in stress response and emotional resilience. Other genes related to resilience are shown in Table 6.4.

TABLE 6.4 Genes Associated With Psychological and Emotional Resilience

Central nervous system actions	Genes related to resilience	Influences of polymorphisms on resilience	References
NPYergic	Neuropeptide Y gene (NPY)	Increased susceptibility to anxiety disorders after childhood adversity	Donner et al. (2012)
HPA Axis	CRH receptor 1 gene (CRHR1)	Affected the likelihood of developing adult depressive symptoms from child abuse	Bradley et al. (2008)
	FK506-binding protein 5 gene (FKBP5)	Predicted severity of adult PTSD symptoms and onset of depression in individuals with childhood trauma.	Binder et al. (2008); Zimmerman et al. (2011)
Noradrenegic and dopaminergic	Catechol-O-methyltransferase gene (COMT)	Influenced the risks of developing PTSD and deficits in stress response and emotional resilience	Heinz & Smolka (2006); Skelton et al. (2012)
Dopaminergic	Dopamine transporter gene (DAT1)	Contributed to susceptibility to PTSD with a history of trauma	Segman et al. (2002)
	Dopamine receptor genes (e.g., DRD2, DRD4)	Induced differential emotional processing and variability in brain responses to emotional stimuli; influenced vulnerability to stress and trauma and risk of developing PTSD	Blasi et al. (2009); Ptacek et al. (2011)

(continued)

TABLE 6.4 (*Continued*)

Central nervous system actions	Genes related to resilience	Influences of polymorphisms on resilience	References
Serotonergic	Promoter region of serotonin transporter gene (5-HTTLPR)	Short allele strongly associated with increased stress sensitivity and risk for depression upon stress exposure, especially early life stress	Karg et al. (2011)
	Serotonin receptor genes (e.g., HTR1A, HTR3A, HTR2C)	Interacted with environment to mediate stress response and to predict susceptibility to depression	Gatt et al. (2010); Kim et al. (2011a); Brummett et al. (2012)
BDNF	Brain-derived neurotrophic factor gene (BDNF)	Interacted with early life stress to predict syndromal depression and anxiety; no clear evidence of association between the valine and methionine polymorphism and anxiety disorders	Frustaci et al. (2008); Gatt et al. (2009)

Copyright © by Gang Wu, Adriana Feder, Hagit Cohen, Joanna J. Kim, Solara Calderon, Dennis S. Charney and Aleksander A. Mathe (CC by 3.0) at https://www.frontiersin.org/articles/10.3389/fnbeh.2013.00010/full.

Epigenetic research has shown that histone modification and DNA methylation regulate gene expression and stress response, as discussed previously regarding risk for psychiatric disorders and physical health conditions. The possibility of the intergenerational transmission of epigenetic signatures, coupled with DNA encoded responses to stress, may confer increased susceptibility and vulnerability to stress and stress-related diseases via the psychobiological stress response and the HPA axis (McEwen, 2016; Rutten et al., 2013; Roberts et al., 2015; Zannas & West, 2014).

The convergence of epidemiological, neurological, and DOHaD research findings provides a strong case for the potential intergenerational transmission of risk for physical and mental illness among Latinos of Mexican descent. Epigenetic signatures have been associated with type 2 diabetes, severe obesity, mental health, and metabolic syndrome among this population group. Additionally, some studies examining early child adversity show that Latinos report higher rates of experiencing ACEs than non-Latino White Americans, which are associated with several chronic diseases.

A conceptual model of the convergent influences on intergenerational transmission of increased risk for chronic and communicable diseases is presented in Figure 6.13. The arrows represent intergenerational transmission. Causes of the causes include prenatal maternal stress, fetal programming, ACEs, and epigenetic modifications that contribute to increased risk for disease. Latino resiliency is a product of positive epigenetic changes that confer protection through modification of signaling pathways by DNA methylation of histone acetylation. All components in the model are related to the developmental origins of adult disease.

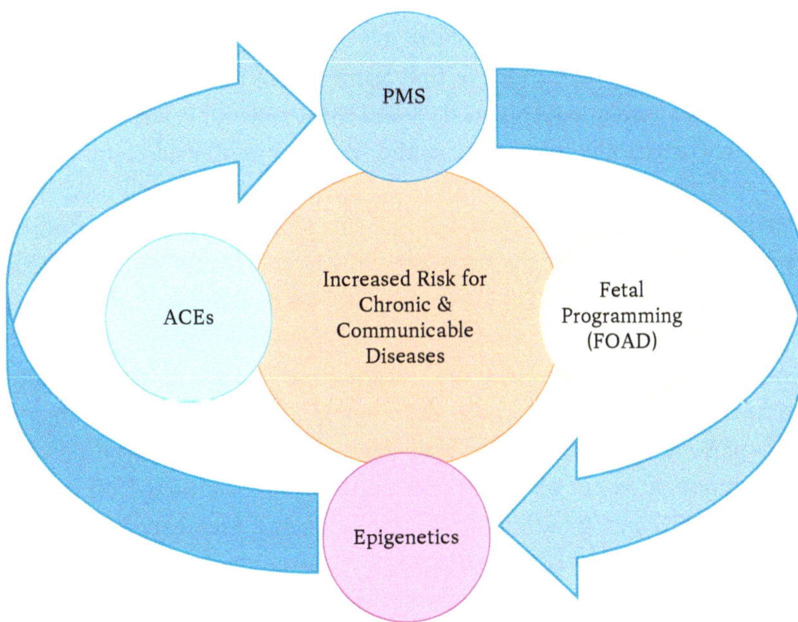

FIGURE 6.13 Conceptual Model of Convergent Influences and Intergenerational Transmission of Increased Risk for Chronic and Communicable Disease

CHAPTER SUMMARY

While the examination of the cultural and social influences on disease are important, the identification of the "causes of the causes" provides a psychobiological and epigenetic grounding that influences the susceptibility and vulnerability to disease processes. Moreover, recent studies suggest that epigenetic risk and protective factors can be transmitted to subsequent generations of offspring. Previous research has documented how stress and stressors trigger the psychobiological stress response that leads to increased stress hormone production (ACTH, glucocorticoids) that then stimulates physiological changes that initiate disease processes.

Gene-environment interactions influence epigenomic processes that signal genes to turn "on" or "off," thus causing disease. The epigenome accomplishes this process through either DNA methylation or histone acetylation at CpG dinucleotide sites. Epigenetic modification contributes to disease expression or gene silencing, as well as accelerated aging. Studies show that Mexican Americans have slower aging processes than non-Latino White Americans, contributing to increased longevity, and perhaps is associated with the Latino mortality paradox.

Prenatal and maternal stress is an important contributor to the etiology of health inequalities. External stress on pregnant women can cause increased stress hormone production that is trans-placentally delivered to the developing fetus, causing significant changes in brain developmental structures and health problems later in life. Acculturation level is implicated in the prevalence of low birth weight and preterm infants, with Latinas higher in acculturation level showing higher rates of low birth weight and preterm infants than lower acculturated Latinas. Maternal trauma (i.e., IPV) can also negatively affect the developing fetus and infant.

Fetal programming and fetal origins of adult disease is another important contributor to the etiology of health inequalities. It is well known that the first trimester of fetal development is crucial for brain development—neurogenesis and synaptogenesis—and influences physical, cognitive, and behavioral development in children. Historically referred to as the "Barker hypothesis," fetal programming and fetal origins of adult disease is an explanatory hypothesis on how diseases in adulthood originate during fetal development. A host of diseases have been linked to this developmental origin's hypothesis, including type 2 diabetes, obesity, hypertension stroke, liver disease, cancer, and psychological disorders.

Adverse childhood experiences (ACEs) are widely accepted as markers for adult disease. The population attributable risk for ACEs is exceptionally high for mental illnesses and substance abuse later in life. Research has also demonstrated a strong dose-response relationship between the number of ACEs and many negative health outcomes, with those experiencing four or more ACEs having higher rates of disease than those experiencing no ACEs. The prevalence of experiencing at least one ACE in the U.S. adult population is common, at about 63%. The prevalence of ACEs among Latinos is reported to be as high as 38% (Llabre et al., 2017), with Latinos of Puerto Rican and Mexican descent experiencing higher rates of four or more ACEs than other Latino subgroups in the study.

Historical trauma and the intergenerational transmission of trauma to subsequent generations of Latinos are important new avenues of research that may identify epigenetic signatures that cause or prevent disease. The research on epigenetic aging continues to show that Latinos have increased longevity and lower mortality than non-Latino White Americans; that is, the detrimental effects of aging are slower. There are several chronic health conditions that are prevalent among Latinos of Mexican descent that also have an epigenetic basis: type 2 diabetes, severe obesity, insulin resistance, and overall higher prevalence of metabolic syndrome. There is also evidence that living in the United States for an extended period (length of residence) has detrimental effects on health behaviors, risk profiles for disease, psychological well-being, and chronic health conditions.

Latino cultural resiliency is both socially constructed an epigenetically transmitted. Cultural resilience embodies cultural identity and pride, self-confidence, and self-esteem. If adverse life events in childhood can initiate disease processes later in life, then positive life events should confer the opposite. Evidence for positive epigenetic modifications can be determined by the slower aging process found in Latinos of Mexican descent, which in turn supports the Latino epidemiologic paradox. The confluence of research in the fields of social epidemiology, neurobiology, psychology, and sociocultural influences clearly demonstrates that health inequalities originated in the lived experiences of our ancestors, including our grandparents and parents. The evolution of epigenetic mechanisms over time allowed adaptation to stressful life conditions, and these positive adaptations are transmitted intergenerationally. Negative adaptations are also transmitted, increasing the risk of type 2 diabetes and other obesity-related health conditions.

QUESTIONS TO CONSIDER

1. Why is it important to examine the developmental origins of health and disease?
2. Do social epigenetic processes increase the risk for disease among historically marginalized populations like Latinos of Mexican descent?

3. What is the role of prenatal and maternal stress in exposing the developing fetus to increased risk for disease in adulthood?
4. How does the intergenerational transmission of risk for disease occur?
5. Synthesize the theoretical and empirical underpinnings for advancing research into the developmental origins of health and disease as causes for health inequalities.

USEFUL EPIGENETIC TERMINOLOGY

- Genome: in the nucleus of every cell in the body, except for red blood cells, which have no nuclei. It includes 25,000 genes.
- Epigenome: a second layer of information that regulates several genomic functions, including when and where genes are turned on (expressed) or off (silenced).
- Genotype: the genetic makeup of a person.
- Phenotype: the physical manifestation of a genotype in the form of a trait or disease.
- Chromatin: the complex of DNA, histones, and other proteins that make up chromosomes.
- Histones: a main protein component of chromatin that acts as a spool around which DNA winds. Histones regulate the structure of chromatin and gene expression.
- CpG dinucleotide sites: regions of DNA where a cytosine nucleotide is followed by a guanine nucleotide.

SUGGESTED READINGS

Conching, A. K. S., & Thayer, Z. (2019). Biological pathways for historical trauma to affect health: A conceptual model focusing on epigenetic modifications. *Social Science & Medicine, 230*, 74–82.

De Boo, H. A., & Harding, J. E. (2006). The developmental origins of adult disease (Barker) hypothesis. *Australian and New Zealand Journal of Obstetrics and Gynaecology, 46*(1), 4–14.

DiPietro, J. A. (2004). The role of prenatal maternal stress in child development. *Current Directions in Psychological Science, 13*(2), 71–74.

Dube, S. R., Felitti, V. J., Dong, M., Giles, W. H., & Anda, R. F. (2003). The impact of adverse childhood experiences on health problems: Evidence from four birth cohorts dating back to 1900. *Preventive Medicine, 37*(3), 268–277. https://doi.org/10.1016/s0091-7435(03)00123-3

Estrada, A. L. (2009). Mexican Americans and historical trauma theory: A theoretical perspective. *Journal of Ethnicity in Substance Abuse, 8*(3), 330–340.

Felitti, V. J., Anda, R. F., Nordenberg, D., Williamson, D. F., Spitz, A. M., Edwards, V., & Marks, J. S. (1998). Relationship of childhood abuse and household dysfunction to many of the leading causes of death in adults: The Adverse Childhood Experiences (ACE) Study. *American Journal of Preventive Medicine, 14*(4), 245–258.

Fox, M., Entringer, S., Buss, C., De Haene, J., & Wadhwa, D. (2015). Intergenerational transmission of the effects of acculturation on health in Hispanic Americans: A fetal programming perspective. *American Journal of Public Health, 105*, S409–S423. https://doi.org/10.2105/AJPH.2015.302571

Gilbert, L. K., Breiding, M. J., Merrick, M. T., Thompson, W. W., Ford, D. C., Dhingra, S. S., & Parks, S. E. (2015). Childhood adversity and adult chronic disease: An update from ten states and the District of Columbia, 2010. *American Journal of Preventive Medicine, 48*(3), 345–349.

Gonzalez, F. R., Benuto, L. T., & Casas, J. B. (2020). Prevalence of interpersonal violence among Latinas: A systematic review. *Trauma, Violence, & Abuse, 21*(5), 977–990.

Hoggatt, K. J, Flores, M., Solario, R., Wilhelm, M., & Ritz, B. (2012). The "Latina epidemiologic paradox" revisited: The role of birthplace and acculturation in predicting infant low birth weight for Latinas in Los Angeles, CA. *Journal of Immigrant and Minor Health, 14*(5), 875–884. https://doi.org/10.1007/s10903-011-9556-4.

Hughes, K., Bellis, M. A., Hardcastle, K. A., Sethi, D., Butchart, A., Mikton, C., Jones, L., & Dunne, M. P. (2017). The effect of multiple adverse childhood experiences on health: A systematic review and meta-analysis. *The Lancet Public Health, 2*(8), e356–e366. https://doi.org/10.1016/S2468-2667(17)30118-4

Kim, C., Harrall, K. K., Glueck, D. H., Needham, B. L., & Dabelea, D. (2022). Gestational diabetes mellitus, epigenetic age and offspring metabolism. *Diabetic Medicine, 39*(11), Article e14925.

Martin, C. L., Ghastine, L., Lodge, E. K., Dhingra, R., & Ward-Caviness, C. K. (2022). Understanding health inequalities through the lens of social epigenetics. *Annual Review of Public Health, 43*, 235–254.

Ryznar, R. J., Phibbs, L., & Van Winkle, L. J. (2021). Epigenetic modifications at the center of the barker hypothesis and their transgenerational implications. *International Journal of Environmental Research and Public Health, 18*(23), 12728.

REFERENCES

Abraído-Lanza, A. F., Chao, M. T., & Flórez, K. R. (2005). Do healthy behaviors decline with greater acculturation?: Implications for the Latino mortality paradox. *Social Science & Medicine, 61*(6), 1243–1255.

Abraido-Lanza, A. F., Dohrenwend, B. P., Ng-Mak, D. S., & Turner, J. B. (1999). The Latino mortality paradox: A test of the "salmon bias" and healthy migrant hypotheses. *American Journal of Public Health, 89*(10), 1543–1548.

ACE Interface website: https://www.aceinterface.com/

Akinyemiju, T., Do, A. N., Patki, A., Aslibekyan, S., Zhi, D., Hidalgo, B., Tiwari, H. K., Abdsher, D., Geng, X., Arnett, D. K., & Irvin, M. R. (2018). Epigenome-wide association study of metabolic syndrome in African-American adults. *Clinical Epigenetics*, 10, Article 49.

Alegría, M., Canino, G., Shrout, P. E., Woo, M., Duan, N., Vila, D., Torres, M., Chen, C.-N., & Meng, X.-L. (2008). Prevalence of mental illness in immigrant and non-immigrant U.S. Latino groups. *American Journal of Psychiatry, 165*(3), 359–369.

Alegría, M., Mulvaney-Day, N., Torres, M., Polo, A., Cao, Z., & Canino, G. (2007). Prevalence of psychiatric disorders across Latino subgroups in the United States. *American Journal of Public Health, 97*(1), 68–75.

Allen, B., Cisneros, E. M., & Tellez, A. (2015). The children left behind: The impact of parental deportation on mental health. *Journal of Child and Family Studies, 24*, 386–392.

Almeida, J., Biello, K. B., Pedraza, F., Wintner, S., & Viruell-Fuentes, E. (2016). The association between anti-immigrant policies and perceived discrimination among Latinos in the U.S.: A multilevel analysis. *SSM-Population Health, 2*, 897–903.

Anda, R. F., Felitti, V. J., Bremner, J. D., Walker, J. D., Whitfield, C. H., Perry, B. D., Dube, S. R., & Giles, W. H. (2006). The enduring effects of abuse and related adverse experiences in childhood: A convergence of evidence from neurobiology and epidemiology. *European Archives of Psychiatry and Clinical Neuroscience, 256*(3), 174–186.

Bagby, S. P., Martin, D., Chung, S. T., & Rajapakse, N. (2019). From the outside in: Biological mechanisms linking social and environmental exposures to chronic disease and to health disparities. *American Journal of Public Health, 109*(Suppl. 1), S56–S63.

Banaudha, K., Kumar, V., & Verma, M. (2018). Challenges and opportunities in social epigenomics and cancer. *Methods in Molecular Biology, 1856*, 233–243. https://doi.org/10.1007/978-1-4939-8751-1_13

Barker, D. J. (1995). Fetal origins of coronary heart disease. *British Medical Journal, 311*(6998), 171–174.

Barker, D. J. (1998). In utero programming of chronic disease. *Clinical Science, 95*(2), 115–128.

Barker, D. J. (1999a). Fetal origins of cardiovascular disease. *Annals of Medicine, 31*(Suppl. 1), 3–6.

Barker, D. J. (1999b). The fetal origins of type 2 diabetes mellitus. *Annals of Internal Medicine, 130*(4 Part 1), 322–324.

Barker, D. J. (2007). The origins of the developmental origins theory. *Journal of Internal Medicine, 261*(5), 412–417.

Bethel, J. W., & Schenker, M. B. (2005). Acculturation and smoking patterns among Hispanics: A review. *American Journal of Preventive Medicine, 29*(2), 143–148.

Beydoun, H., & Saftlas, A. F. (2008). Physical and mental health outcomes of prenatal maternal stress in human and animal studies: A review of recent evidence. *Paediatric and Perinatal Epidemiology, 290*, 595–596.

Binder, E. B., Bradley, R. G., Liu, W., Epstein, M. P., Deveau, T. C., Mercer, K. B., Tang, Y., Gillespie, C. F., Heim, C. M., Nemeroff, C. B., Schwatz, A. C., Cubells, J. F., & Ressler, K. J. (2008). Association of FKBP5 polymorphisms and childhood abuse with risk of posttraumatic stress disorder symptoms in adults. *JAMA, 299*, 1291–1305

Biswas, S., & Rao, C. M. (2017). Epigenetics in cancer: fundamentals and beyond. *Pharmacology & Therapeutics, 173*, 118–134.

Blasi, G., Lo Bianco, L., Taurisano, P., Gelao, B., Romano, R., Fazio, L., Papzacharias, A., Di Giorgio, A., Caforio, G., Rampino, A, Masellis, R., Papp, A., Ursini, G., Sinibaldi, L., Popolizio, T., Sadee, W., & Bertolino, A. (2009). Functional variation of the dopamine D2 receptor gene is associated with emotional control as well as brain activity and connectivity during emotion processing in humans. *Journal of Neuroscience, 29*, 14812–14819

Bonomi, A. E., Anderson, M. L., Cannon, E. A., Slesnick, N., & Rodriguez, M. A. (2009). Intimate partner violence in Latina and non-Latina women. *American Journal of Preventive Medicine, 36*(1), 43–48.

Bosquet Enlow, M., Devick, K. L., Brunst, K. J., Lipton, L. R., Coull, B. A., & Wright, R. J. (2017). Maternal lifetime trauma exposure, prenatal cortisol, and infant negative affectivity. *Infancy, 22*(4), 492–513.

Boullier, M., & Blair, M. (2018). Adverse childhood experiences. *Paediatrics and Child Health, 28*(3), 132–137.

Bowleg, L., & Landers, S. (2023). Intergenerational trauma and structural racism: New mentorship approaches to HIV and substance use prevention and treatment. *American Journal of Public Health, 113*(Suppl. 2), S92–S92.

Brabeck, K. M., & Xu, Q. (2010). The impact of detention and deportation on Latino immigrant children and families: A quantitative exploration. *Hispanic Journal of Behavioral Sciences, 32*(3) 341–361.

Bradley, R. G., Binder, E. B., Epstein, M. P., Tang, Y., Nair, H. P., Liu, W., Gillespie, C. F., Berg, T., Evces, M., Jeffrey Newport, D., Stowe, Z. N., Heim, C. M., Nemeroff, C B., Schwartz, A., Cubells, J. F., & Ressler, K. J. (2008). Influence of child abuse on adult depression: Moderation by the corticotropin-releasing hormone receptor gene. *Archives of General Psychiatry, 65*, 190–200

Braveman, P., Marchi, K., Egerter, S., Kim, S., Metzler, M., Stancil, T., & Libet, M. (2010). Poverty, near-poverty, and hardship around the time of pregnancy. *Maternal and Child Health Journal, 14*, 20–35.

Breast Cancer Association Consortium, Dorling, L., Carvalho, S., Allen, J., González-Neira, A., Luccarini, C., Wahlström, C., Pooley, K. A., Parsons, M. T., Fortuno, C., Wang, Q., Bolla, M. K., Dennis, J., Keeman, R., Alonso, M. R., Álvarez, N., Herraez, B., Fernandez, V., Núñez-Torres, R., Osorio, A., ... Easton, D. F. (2021). Breast cancer risk genes: Association analysis in more than 113,000 women. *The New England Journal of Medicine, 384*(5), 428–439. https://doi.org/10.1056/NEJMoa1913948

Brockie, T. N., Heinzelmann, M., & Gill, J. (2013). A framework to examine the role of epigenetics in health disparities among Native Americans. *Nursing Research and Practice*, Article 410395.

Brown, D. W., Anda, R. F., Tiemeier, H., Felitti, V. J., Edwards, V. J., Croft, J. B., & Giles, W. H. (2009). Adverse childhood experiences and the risk of premature mortality. *American Journal of Preventive Medicine, 37*(5), 389–396.

Brummett, B. H., Kuhn, C. M., Boyle, S. H., Babyak, M. A., Siegler, I. C., & Williams, R. B. (2012). Cortisol responses to emotional stress in men: Association with a functional polymorphism in the 5HTR2C gene. *Biological Psychology, 89*, 94–98.

Buitelaar, J. K., Huizink, A. C., Mulder, E. J., De Medina, P. G. R., & Visser, G. H. (2003). Prenatal stress and cognitive development and temperament in infants. *Neurobiology of Aging, 24*, S53–S60.

Burris, H. H., & Hacker, M. R. (2017, October). Birth outcome racial disparities: A result of intersecting social and environmental factors. *Seminars in Perinatology, 41*(6), 360–366.

Caballero, T. M., Johnson, S. B., Buchanan, C. R. M., & DeCamp, L. R. (2017). Adverse childhood experiences among Hispanic children in immigrant families versus U.S.-native families. *Pediatrics, 140*(5).

Calkins, K., & Devaskar, S. U. (2011). Fetal origins of adult disease. *Current Problems in Pediatric and Adolescent Health Care, 41*(6), 158–176.

Campbell, R. K., Curtin, P., Bosquet Enlow, M., Brunst, K. J., Wright, R. O., & Wright, R. J. (2020). Disentangling associations among maternal lifetime and prenatal stress, psychological functioning during pregnancy, maternal race/ethnicity, and infant negative affectivity at age 6 months: A mixtures approach. *Health Equity, 4*(1), 489–499.

Cao-Lei, L., Laplante, D. P., & King, S. (2016). Prenatal maternal stress and epigenetics: Review of the human research. *Current Molecular Biology Reports, 2*, 16–25.

Centers for Disease Control and Prevention. (2023, June 29). *Fast facts: Preventing adverse childhood experiences*. https://www.cdc.gov/violenceprevention/aces/fastfact.html

Cerdeña, J. P., Rivera, L. M., & Spak, J. M. (2021). Intergenerational trauma in Latinxs: A scoping review. *Social Science & Medicine, 270*, Article 113662.

Charil, A., Laplante, D. P., Vaillancourt, C., & King, S. (2010). Prenatal stress and brain development. *Brain Research Reviews, 65*(1), 56–79.

Cobb, C. L., Salas-Wright, C. P., John, R., Schwartz, S. J., Vaughn, M., Martínez, C. R., Awad, G., Pinedo, M., & Cano, M. Á. (2021). Discrimination trends and mental health among native-and foreign-born Latinos: Results from national surveys in 2004 and 2013. *Prevention Science, 22*(3), 397–407.

Coker, E. S., Gunier, R., Huen, K., Holland, N., & Eskenazi, B. (2018). DNA methylation and socioeconomic status in a Mexican-American birth cohort. *Clinical Epigenetics, 10*(1), 61.

Conching, A. K. S., & Thayer, Z. (2019). Biological pathways for historical trauma to affect health: A conceptual model focusing on epigenetic modifications. *Social Science & Medicine, 230*, 74–82

Crimmins, E. M., Thyagarajan, B., Levine, M. E., Weir, D. R., & Faul, J. (2021). Associations of age, sex, race/ethnicity, and education with 13 epigenetic clocks in a nationally representative U.S. sample: The Health and Retirement Study. *Journal of Gerontology. Series A, Biological Science and Medical Sciences, 76*(6), 1117–1123.

Crouch, E., Probst, J. C., Radcliff, E., Bennett, K. J., & McKinney, S. H. (2019). Prevalence of adverse childhood experiences (ACEs) among U.S. children. *Child Abuse & Neglect, 92*, 209–218.

Cunliffe, V. T. (2015). Experience-sensitive epigenetic mechanisms, developmental plasticity, and the biological embedding of chronic disease risk. *Wiley Interdisciplinary Reviews: Systems Biology and Medicine, 7*(2), 53–71.

Cunliffe, V. T. (2016).The epigenetic impacts of social stress: How does social adversity become biologically embedded? *Epigenomics, 8*(12), 1653–1669.

De Boo, H. A., & Harding, J. E. (2006). The developmental origins of adult disease (Barker) hypothesis. *Australian and New Zealand Journal of Obstetrics and Gynaecology, 46*(1), 4–14.

De Rooij, S. R., Bleker, L. S., Painter, R. C., Ravelli, A. C., & Roseboom, T. J. (2022). Lessons learned from 25 years of research into long term consequences of prenatal exposure to the Dutch famine 1944–45: The Dutch famine birth cohort. *International Journal of Environmental Health Research, 32*(7), 1432–1446.

DiPietro, J. A. (2004). The role of prenatal maternal stress in child development. *Current Directions in Psychological Science, 13*(2), 71–74.

DiPietro, J. A., Hilton, S. C., Hawkins, M., Costigan, K. A., & Pressman, E. K. (2002). Maternal stress and affect influence fetal neurobehavioral development. *Developmental Psychology, 38*, 659–668.

Donner, J., Sipila, T., Ripatti, S., Kananen, L., Chen, X., Kendler, K. S., Lönnqvist, J., Pirkola, S., Hettema, J. M., & Hovatta, I. (2012). Support for involvement of glutamate decarboxylase 1 and neuropeptide Y in anxiety susceptibility. *American Journal of Medical Genetics Part B: Neuropsychiatric Genetics, 159B*(3), 316–327.

Dreby, J. (2012). The burden of deportation on children in Mexican immigrant families. *Journal of Marriage and Family, 74*(4), 829–845.

Dube, S. R., Felitti, V. J., Dong, M., Giles, W. H., & Anda, R. F. (2003). The impact of adverse childhood experiences on health problems: Evidence from four birth cohorts dating back to 1900. *Preventive Medicine, 37*(3), 268–277. https://doi.org/10.1016/s0091-7435(03)00123-3

Dunkel Schetter, C., & Tanner, L. (2015). Anxiety, depression and stress in pregnancy: Implications for mothers, children, research, and practice. *Current Opinions in Psychiatry, 25*(2), 141–148. https://doi.org/10.1097/YCO.0b013e3283503680.

Esteller, M. (2008). Epigenetics in cancer. *New England Journal of Medicine, 358*, 1148–1159

Estrada, A. L. (2009). Mexican Americans and historical trauma theory: A theoretical perspective. *Journal of Ethnicity in Substance Abuse, 8*(3), 330–340.

Felitti, V. J. (2019). Origins of the ACE Study. *American Journal of Preventive Medicine, 56*(6), 787–789.

Felitti, V. J., & Anda, R. (2003, March 31–April 5). *The relationship of adverse childhood experiences to adult health status: A collaborative effort of Kaiser Permanente and the Centers for Disease Control* [Paper presentation]. 14th National Conference on Child Abuse and Neglect, St. Louis, Missouri, United States. https://www.acf.hhs.gov/sites/default/files/documents/cb/nccan14_opening_plenary.pdf

Felitti, V. J., Anda, R. F., Nordenberg, D., & Williamson, D. F. (1998a). Adverse childhood experiences and health outcomes in adults: The ACE Study. *Journal of Family and Consumer Sciences, 90*(3), 31.

Felitti, V. J., Anda, R. F., Nordenberg, D., Williamson, D. F., Spitz, A. M., Edwards, V., & Marks, J. S. (1998b). Relationship of childhood abuse and household dysfunction to many of the leading causes of death in adults: The Adverse Childhood Experiences (ACE) Study. *American Journal of Preventive Medicine, 14*(4), 245–258.

Flores, M. E., Simonsen, S. E., Manuck, T. A., Dyer, J. M., & Turok, D. K. (2012). The "Latina epidemiologic paradox": Contrasting patterns of adverse birth outcomes in U.S.-born and foreign-born Latinas. *Women's Health Issues, 22*(5), e501–e507.

Foss, S., Petty, C., Howell, C., Mendonca, J., Bosse, A., Waber, D., Wright, R. J., & Bosquet Enlow, M. (2023). Associations among maternal lifetime trauma, psychological symptoms in pregnancy, and infant stress reactivity and regulation. *Development and Psychopathology, 35*(4), 1714–1731. https://doi.org/10.1017/S0954579422000402

Fox, M., Entringer, S., Buss, C., De Haene, J., Wadhwa, D. (2015). Intergenerational transmission of the effects of acculturation on health in Hispanic Americans: A fetal programming perspective. *American Journal of Public Health, 105*, S409–S423. https://doi.org/10.2105/AJPH.2015.302571

Frustaci, A., Pozzi, G., Gianfagna, F., Manzoli, L., & Boccia, S. (2008). Meta-analysis of the brain-derived neurotrophic factor gene (BDNF) Val66Met polymorphism in anxiety disorders and anxiety-related personality traits. *Neuropsychobiology, 58*, 163–170.

Gallo, L. C., & Matthews, K. A. (2003). Understanding the association between socioeconomic status and physical health: Do negative emotions play a role? *Psychological Bulletin, 129*, 10–51.

Gallo, L. C., Penedo, F. J., Espinosa de los Monteros, K., & Arguelles, W. (2009). Resiliency in the face of disadvantage: Do Hispanic cultural characteristics protect health outcomes? *Journal of Personality, 77*(6), 1707–1746.

Gatt, J. M., Burton, K. L., Williams, L. M., & Schofield, P. R. (2015). Specific and common genes implicated across major mental disorders: A review of meta-analysis studies. *Journal of Psychiatric Research, 60*, 1–13.

Gatt, J. M., Nemeroff, C. B., Dobson-Stone, C., Paul, R. H., Bryant, R. A., Schofield, P. R., Gordon, E., Kemp, A. H., & Williams, L. M. (2009). Interactions between BDNF Val66Met polymorphism and early life stress predict brain and arousal pathways to syndromal depression and anxiety. *Molecular Psychiatry, 14*(7), 681–695

Gatt, J. M., Nemeroff, C. B., Schofield, P. R., Paul, R. H., Clark, C. R., Gordon, E., & William, L. M. (2010). Early life stress combined with serotonin 3A receptor and brain-derived neurotrophic factor valine 66 to methionine genotypes impacts emotional brain and arousal correlates of risk for depression. *Biological Psychiatry, 68*(9), 818–824.

Gilbert, L. K., Breiding, M. J., Merrick, M. T., Thompson, W. W., Ford, D. C., Dhingra, S. S., & Parks, S. E. (2015). Childhood adversity and adult chronic disease: An update from ten states and the District of Columbia, 2010. *American Journal of Preventive Medicine, 48*(3), 345–349.

Godoy, L. D., Rossignoli, M. T., Delfino-Pereira, P., Garcia-Cairasco, N., & de Lima Umeoka, E. H. (2018). A comprehensive overview on stress neurobiology: basic concepts and clinical implications. *Frontiers in Behavioral Neuroscience, 12*, 127.

Gonzalez, F. R., Benuto, L. T., & Casas, J. B. (2020). Prevalence of interpersonal violence among Latinas: A systematic review. *Trauma, Violence, & Abuse, 21*(5), 977–990.

Gonzalez-Quintero, V. H., Tolaymat, L., Luke, B., Gonzalez-Garcia, A., Duthely, L., O'Sullivan, M. J., & Martin, D. (2006). Outcome of pregnancies among Hispanics: Revisiting the epidemiologic paradox. *The Journal of Reproductive Medicine, 51*(1), 10–14.

Grant, C. D., Jafari, N., Hou, L., Li, Y., Stewart, J. D., Zhang, G., Lamichhane, A., Manson, J. E., Baccarelli, A. A., Whitsel, E. A., & Conneely, K. N. (2017). A longitudinal study of DNA methylation as a potential mediator of age-related diabetes risk. *Geroscience, 39*(5–6), 475–489.

Gunn, S., Wainberg, M., Song, Z., Andersen, S., Boudreau, R., Feitosa, M. F., Tan, Q., Montasser, M. E., O'Connell, J. R., Stitziel, N., Price, N., Perls, T., Schork, N. J., & Sebastiani, P. (2022). Distribution of 54 polygenic risk scores for common diseases in long lived individuals and their offspring. *Geroscience, 44*(2), 719–729. https://doi.org/10.1007/s11357-022-00518-2

Harper, K. N., Zuckerman, M. K., Harper, M. L., Kingston, J. D., & Armelagos, G. J. (2011). The origin and antiquity of syphilis revisited: An appraisal of Old World pre-Columbian evidence for treponemal infection. *American Journal of Physical Anthropology, 146*(S53), 99–133.

Hazen, A. L., & Soriano, F. I. (2007). Experiences with intimate partner violence among Latina women. *Violence Against Women, 13*(6), 562–582.

Heijmans, B. T., Tobi, E. W., Stein, A. D., Putter, H., Blauw, G. J., Susser, E. S., Slagboom, P. E., & Lumey, L. H. (2008). Persistent epigenetic differences associated with prenatal exposure to famine in humans. *Proceedings of the National Academy of Sciences, 105*(44), 17046–17049.

Heinz, A., & Smolka, M. N. (2006). The effects of catechol O-methyltransferase genotype on brain activation elicited by affective stimuli and cognitive tasks. *Reviews in the Neurosciences, 17*, 359–367.

Herzog, J. I., & Schmahl, C. (2018). Adverse childhood experiences and the consequences on neurobiological, psychosocial, and somatic conditions across the lifespan. *Frontiers in Psychiatry, 9*, 357654.

Hoggatt, K. J, Flores, M., Solario, R., Wilhelm, M., & Ritz, B. (2012). The "Latina epidemiologic paradox" revisited: The role of birthplace and acculturation in predicting infant low birth weight for Latinas in Los Angeles, CA. *Journal of Immigrant and Minority Health, 14*(5), 875–884. https://doi.org/10.1007/s10903-011-9556-4

Horvath, S. (2013). DNA methylation age of human tissues and cell types. *Genome Biology, 14*(10), 1–20.

Hughes, K., Bellis, M. A., Hardcastle, K. A., Sethi, D., Butchart, A., Mikton, C., Jones, L., & Dunne, M. P. (2017). The effect of multiple adverse childhood experiences on health: A systematic review and meta-analysis. *The Lancet Public Health, 2*(8), e356–e366. https://doi.org/10.1016/S2468-2667(17)30118-4

Joassart-Marcelli, P., Rossiter, J. S., & Bosco, F. J. (2017). Ethnic markets and community food security in an urban "food desert." *Environment and Planning, 49*(7), 1642–1663.

Jones, P. A., & Takai, D. (2001). The role of DNA methylation in mammalian epigenetics. *Science, 293*(5532), 1068–1070.

Kapoor, A., Dunn, E., Kostaki, A., Andrews, M. H., & Matthews, S. G. (2006). Fetal programming of hypothalamo-pituitary-adrenal function: Prenatal stress and glucocorticoids. *The Journal of Physiology, 572*(1), 31–44.

Karg, K., Burmeister, M., Shedden, K., & Sen, S. (2011). The serotonin transporter promoter variant (5-HTTLPR), stress, and depression meta-analysis revisited: Evidence of genetic moderation. *Archives of General Psychiatry, 68*, 444–454.

Kelly-Irving, M., Lepage, B., Dedieu, D., Bartley, M., Blane, D., Grosclaude, P., Land, T., & Delpierre, C. (2013). Adverse childhood experiences and premature all-cause mortality. *European Journal of Epidemiology, 28*(9), 721-734.

Kessler, R. C., & Wang, P. S. (2008). The descriptive epidemiology of commonly occurring mental disorders in the United States. *Annual Review of Public Health, 29*, 115–129.

Khashan, A. S., McNamee, R., Abel, K. M., Mortensen, P. B., Kenny, L. C., Pedersen, M. G., Webb, R. T., & Baker, P. N. (2009). Rates of preterm birth following antenatal maternal exposure to severe life events: A population-based cohort study. *Human Reproduction, 24*(2), 429–437.

Khashan, A. S., McNamee, R., Abel, K. M., Pedersen, M. G., Webb, R. T., Kenny, L. C., Bo Mortenson, P., & Baker, P. N. (2008). Reduced infant birthweight consequent upon maternal exposure to severe life events. *Psychosomatic Medicine, 70*(6), 688–694.

Kim, C., Harrall, K. K., Glueck, D. H., Needham, B. L., & Dabelea, D. (2022). Gestational diabetes mellitus, epigenetic age and offspring metabolism. *Diabetic Medicine, 39*(11), Article e14925.

Kim, H. K., Kim, S. J., Lee, Y. J., Lee, H.-J., Kang, S.-G., Choi, J.-E., Yun, K.-W., & Kim, W.-J. (2011). Influence of the interaction between the serotonin 1A receptor C-1019G polymorphism and negative life stressors on the development of depression. *Neuropsychobiology, 64*(1), 1–8.

Kinsella, M. T., & Monk, C. (2009). Impact of maternal stress, depression, and anxiety on fetal neurobehavioral development. *Clinical Obstetrics and Gynecology, 52*, 425–440.

Klevens, J. (2007). An overview of intimate partner violence among Latinos. *Violence Against Women, 13*(2), 111–122.

Kostović, I., Sedmak, G., & Judaš, M. (2019). Neural histology and neurogenesis of the human fetal and infant brain. *Neuroimage, 188*, 743–773.

Kristensen, L. S., Nielsen, H. M., & Hansen, L. L. (2009). Epigenetics and cancer treatment. *European Journal of Pharmacology, 625*(1–3), 131–142.

Kuzawa, C. W., & Sweet, E. (2009). Epigenetics and the embodiment of race: developmental origins of US racial disparities in cardiovascular health. *American Journal of Human Biology: The Official Journal of the Human Biology Association, 21*(1), 2–15.

Kwon, E. J., & Kim, Y. J. (2017). What is fetal programming?: A lifetime health is under the control of in utero health. *Obstetrics & Gynecology Science, 60*(6), 506–519.

Leaune, E., Dealberto, M. J., Luck, D., Grot, S., Zeroug-Vial, H., Poulet, E., & Brunelin, J. (2019). Ethnic minority position and migrant status as risk factors for psychotic symptoms in the general population: A meta-analysis. *Psychological Medicine, 49*(4), 545–558.

Liu, C. H., Giallo, R., Doan, S. N., Seidman, L. J., & Tronick, E. (2016). Racial and ethnic differences in prenatal life stress and postpartum depression symptoms. *Archives of Psychiatric Nursing, 30*(1), 7–12.

Llabre, M. M., Schneiderman, N., Gallo, L. C., Arguelles, W., Daviglus, M. L., Gonzalez, F., II, Isasi, C. r., Perreira, K. M., & Penedo, F. J. (2017). Childhood trauma and adult risk factors and disease in Hispanics/Latinos in the U.S.: Results from the Hispanic Community Health Study/Study of Latinos (HCHS/SOL) Sociocultural Ancillary Study. *Psychosomatic Medicine, 79*(2), 172–180.

Loi, M., Del Savio, L., & Stupka, E. (2013). Social epigenetics and equality of opportunity. *Public Health Ethics, 6*(2), 142–153.

López-León, S., Janssens, A. C. J. W., Gonzalez-Zuloeta Ladd, A. M., Del-Favero, J., Claes, S. J., Oostra, B. A., & Van Duijn, C. M. (2008). Meta-analyses of genetic studies on major depressive disorder. *Molecular Psychiatry, 13*(8), 772–785.

Lu, M. C., & Chen, B. (2004). Racial and ethnic disparities in preterm birth: The role of stressful life events. *American Journal of Obstetrics and Gynecology, 191*, 691–699.

MacDonald, J. L., & Roskams, A. J. (2009). Epigenetic regulation of nervous system development by DNA methylation and histone deacetylation. *Progress in Neurobiology, 88*, 170–183. https://doi.org/10.1016/j.pneurobio.2009.04.002

Mackenbach, J. P. (2005). Genetics and health inequalities: Hypotheses and controversies. *Journal of Epidemiology & Community Health, 59*(4), 268–273.

MacNell, L., Elliott, S., Hardison-Moody, A., & Bowen, S. (2017). Black and Latino urban food desert residents' perceptions of their food environment and factors that influence food shopping decisions. *Journal of Hunger & Environmental Nutrition, 12*(3), 375–393.

Mamtani, M., Kulkarni, H., Dyer, T. D., Göring, H. H., Neary, J. L., Cole, S. A., Kent, J. W., Kumar, S., Glahn, D. C., Mahaney, M. C., Comuzzie, A. G., Almasy, L., Curran, J. E., Duggirala, R., Blangero, J., & Carless, M. A. (2016). Genome-and epigenome-wide association study of hypertriglyceridemic waist in Mexican American families. *Clinical Epigenetics, 8*, 1–14.

Mancilla, V. J., Peeri, N. C., Silzer, T., Basha, R., Felini, M., Jones, H. P., Phillips, N., Tao, M.-H., Thyagarajan, S., & Vishwanatha, J. K. (2020). Understanding the interplay between health disparities and epigenomics. *Frontiers in Genetics, 11*, 903.

Marioni, R. E., Shah, S., McRae, A. F., Chen, B. H., Colicino, E., Harris, S. E., Gibson, J., Henders, A. K., Redmond, P., Cox, S. R., Pattie, A., Corley, J., Murphy, L., Martin, N. G., Montgomery, G. W., Feinberg, A. P., Fallin, M. D., Multhaup, M. L., Jaffe, A. E., ... Deary, I. J. (2015). DNA methylation age of blood predicts all-cause mortality in later life. *Genome Biology, 16*(1), 1–12.

Mars, N., Lindbohm, J. V., Della Briotta Parolo, P., Widén, E., Kaprio, J., Palotie, A., FinnGen, & Ripatti, S. (2022). Systematic comparison of family history and polygenic risk across 24 common diseases. *American Journal of Human Genetics, 109*(12), 2152–2162. https://doi.org/10.1016/j.ajhg.2022.10.009

Martin, C. L., Ghastine, L., Lodge, E. K., Dhingra, R., & Ward-Caviness, C. K. (2022). Understanding health inequalities through the lens of social epigenetics. *Annual Review of Public Health, 43*, 235–254.

McCance-Katz, E. F. (2019). *The National Survey on Drug Use and Health: 2017.* Substance Abuse and Mental Health Services Administration.

McEwen, B. S. (2016). In pursuit of resilience: Stress, epigenetics, and brain plasticity. *Annals of the New York Academy of Sciences, 1373*(1), 56–64.

McKnight-Eily, L. R., Okoro, C. A., Strine, T. W., Verlenden, J., Hollis, N. D., Njai, R., Mitchell, E. W., Board, A., Puddy, R., & Thomas, C. (2021). Racial and ethnic disparities in the prevalence of stress and worry, mental health conditions, and increased substance use among adults during the COVID-19 pandemic—United States, April and May 2020. *Morbidity and Mortality Weekly Report, 70*(5), 162–166.

Menselson, T., Rehkopf, D. H., & Kubzansky, L. D. (2008). Depression among Latinos in the United States: A meta-analytic review. *Journal of Consulting and Clinical Psychology, 76*(3), 355–366.

Mersky, J. P., & Janczewski, C. E. (2018). Racial and ethnic differences in the prevalence of adverse childhood experiences: Findings from a low-income sample of U.S. women. *Child Abuse & Neglect, 76*, 480–487.

Metz, G. A., Ng, J. W., Kovalchuk, I., & Olson, D. M. (2015). Ancestral experience as a game changer in stress vulnerability and disease outcomes. *Bioessays, 37*(6), 602–611.

Miller W. L. (2018). The Hypothalamic-Pituitary-Adrenal Axis: A Brief History. *Hormone Research in Paediatrics, 89*(4), 212–223

Mulligan, C. J., D'Errico, N. C., Stees, J., & Hughes, D. (2012) Methylation changes at NR3C1 in newborns associate with maternal prenatal stress exposure and newborn birth weight. *Epigenetics, 7*(8), 853–857.

Myers, H. F. (2009). Ethnicity-and socio-economic status-related stresses in context: An integrative review and conceptual model. *Journal of Behavioral Medicine, 32*, 9–19.

Oblak, L., van der Zaag, J., Higgins-Chen, A. T., Levine, M. E., & Boks, M. P. (2021). A systematic review of biological, social and environmental factors associated with epigenetic clock acceleration. *Ageing Research Reviews, 69*, 101348.

O'Donnell, K., O'Connor, T. G., & Glover, V. (2009). Prenatal stress and neurodevelopment of the child: Focus on the HPA axis and role of the placenta. *Developmental Neuroscience, 31*, 285–292.

Oyama, S., & Terry, S. F. (2016). Epigenetics and racial health inequities. *Genetic Testing and Molecular Biomarkers, 20*(9), 483–484. https://doi.org/10.1089/gtmb.2016.29021.sj

Phillips-Beck, W., Sinclair, S., Campbell, R., Star, L., Cidro, J., Wicklow, B., Guillemette, L., Morris, M. I., & McGavock, J. M. (2019). Early-life origins of disparities in chronic diseases among Indigenous youth: Pathways to recovering health disparities from intergenerational trauma. *Journal of Developmental Origins of Health and Disease, 10*(1), 115–122.

Powers, R. A., Moule, R. K., & Severson, R. E. (2022). Adverse childhood experiences and offending among Hispanic adults in the U.S.: Examining differences in prevalence and effects across nativity. *Journal of Criminal Justice, 79*, Article 101893.

Ptacek, R., Kuzelova, H., & Stefano, G. B. (2011). Dopamine D4 receptor gene DRD4 and its association with psychiatric disorders. *Medical Science. Monitor, 17*, RA215–RA220.

Roberts, S., Keers, R., Lester, K. J., Coleman, J. R. I., Breen, G., Arendt, K., Blatter-Meunier, J., Cooper, P., Creswell, C., Fjermestad, K., Havik, O. E., Herren, C., Hogendoorn, S. M., Hudson, J. L., Krause, K., Lyneham, H. J., Morris, T., Nauta, M., Rapee, R. M., ... Wong, C. C. Y. (2015). HPA axis related genes and response to psychological therapies: Genetics and epigenetics. *Depression and Anxiety, 32*(12), 861–870.

Rodriguez, M. A., Heilemann. M. V., Fielder, E., Ang, A., Nevarez, F., & Mangione, C. M. (2008). Intimate partner violence, depression, and PTSD among pregnant Latina women. *Annals of Family Medicine, 6*, 44–52.

Roseboom, T., de Rooij, S., & Painter, R. (2006). The Dutch famine and its long-term consequences for adult health. *Early Human Development, 82*(8), 485–491.

Rosenberg, T. J., Raggio, T. P., & Chiasson, M. A. (2005). A further examination of the "epidemiologic paradox": Birth outcomes among Latinas. *Journal of the National Medical Association, 97*(4), 550.

Rutten, B. P., Hammels, C., Geschwind, N., Menne-Lothmann, C., Pishva, E., Schruers, K., van den Hove, D., Kenis, G., van Os, J., & Wichers, M. (2013) Resilience in mental health: Linking psychological and neurobiological perspectives. *Acta Psychiatrica Scandinavica, 128*, 3–20.

Ryan, J., Wrigglesworth, J., Loong, J., Fransquet, P. D., & Woods, R. L. (2020). A systematic review and meta-analysis of environmental, lifestyle, and health factors associated with DNA methylation age. *The Journals of Gerontology: Series A, 75*(3), 481–494.

Ryznar, R. J., Phibbs, L., & Van Winkle, L. J. (2021). Epigenetic modifications at the center of the barker hypothesis and their transgenerational implications. *International Journal of Environmental Research and Public Health, 18*(23), 12728.

Sabina, C., Cuevas, C. A., & Zadnik, E. (2015). Intimate partner violence among Latino women: Rates and cultural correlates. *Journal of Family Violence, 30*(1), 35–47.

Salas, L. A., Peres, L. C., Thayer, Z. M., Smith, R. W., Guo, Y., Chung, W., Si, J., & Liang, L. (2021). A transdisciplinary approach to understand the epigenetic basis of race/ethnicity health disparities. *Epigenomics, 13*(21), 1761–1770.

Sanchez-Vaznaugh, E. V., Braveman, P. A., Egerter, S., Marchi, K. S., Heck, K., & Curtis, M. (2016). Latina birth outcomes in California: Not so paradoxical. *Maternal and Child Health Journal, 20*, 1849–1860.

Sapkota, Y., Qiu, W., Dixon, S. B., Wilson, C. L., Wang, Z., Zhang, J., Leisenring, W., Chow, E. J., Bhatia, S., Armstrong, G. T., Robison, L. L., Hudson, M. M., Delaney, A., & Yasui, Y. (2022). Genetic risk score enhances the risk prediction of severe obesity in adult survivors of childhood cancer. *Nature Medicine, 28*(8), 1590–1598. https://doi.org/10.1038/s41591-022-01902-3

Schultz, M., Timme, U., & Schmidt-Schultz, T. H. (2007). Infancy and childhood in the pre-Columbian North American Southwest: First results of the palaeopathological investigation of the skeletons from the Grasshopper Pueblo, Arizona. *International Journal of Osteoarchaeology, 17*(4), 369–379.

Scott Yoshizawa, R. (2012). The Barker hypothesis and obesity: Connections for transdisciplinarity and social justice. *Social Theory & Health, 10*, 348–367.

Scribner, R. (1996). Paradox as paradigm: The health outcomes of Mexican Americans. *American Journal of Public Health, 86*(3), 303–305. https://doi.org/10.2105/AJPH.86.3.303

Segman, R. H., Cooper-Kazaz, R., Macciardi, F., Goltser, T., Halfon, Y., Dobroborski, T., & Shalev, A. Y. (2002). Association between the dopamine transporter gene and posttraumatic stress disorder. *Molecular Psychiatry, 7*(8), 903–907.

Sheridan, M. A., & McLaughlin, K. A. (2014). Dimensions of early experience and neural development: deprivation and threat. *Trends in Cognitive Sciences, 18*(11), 580–585.

Shevell, M. C., & Denov, M. S. (2021). A multidimensional model of resilience: Family, community, national, global and intergenerational resilience. *Child Abuse & Neglect, 119*, Article 105035.

Skelton, K., Ressler, K. J., Norrholm, S. D., Jovanovic, T., & Bradley-Davino, B. (2012). PTSD and gene variants: New pathways and new thinking. *Neuropharmacology, 62*, 628–637.

Sotero, M. M. (2006). A Conceptual model of historical trauma: Implications for public health practice and research. *Journal Health Disparities Research and Practice, 1*(1), 93–108.

Spry, E., Moreno-Betancur, M., Becker, D., Romaniuk, H., Carlin, J. B., Molyneaux, E., Howard, L. M., Ryan, J., Letcher, P., McIntosh, J., Macdonald, J. A., Greenwood, C. J., Thomson, K. C., McAnally, H., Hancox, R., Hutchinson, D. M., Youssef, G. J., Olsson, C. A., & Patton, G. C. (2020). Maternal mental health and infant emotional reactivity: A 20-year two-cohort study of preconception and perinatal exposures. *Psychological Medicine, 50*(5), 827–837.

Steckel, R. H. (2005). Health and nutrition in pre-Columbian America: The skeletal evidence. *Journal of Interdisciplinary History, 36*(1), 1–32.

Steegers-Theunissen, R. P., Twigt, J., Pestinger, V., & Sinclair, K. D. (2013). The periconceptional period, reproduction and long-term health of offspring: The importance of one-carbon metabolism. *Human Reproduction Update, 19*(6), 640–655.

Storey, R. (1986). Perinatal mortality at pre-Columbian Teotihuacan. *American Journal of Physical Anthropology, 69*(4), 541–548.

Swedo, E. A., Aslam, M. V., Dahlberg, L. L., Niolon, P. H., Guinn, A. S., Simon, T. R., & Mercy, J. A. (2023). Prevalence of adverse childhood experiences among U.S. Adults—Behavioral Risk Factor Surveillance System, 2011–2020. *Morbidity and Mortality Weekly Report, 72*, 707–715. https://doi.org/10.15585/mmwr.mm7226a2

Tampa, M., Sarbu, I., Matei, C., Benea, V., & Georgescu, S. R. (2014). Brief history of syphilis. *Journal of Medicine and Life, 7*(1), 4.

Taouk, L., & Schulkin, J. (2016). Transgenerational transmission of pregestational and prenatal experience: Maternal adversity, enrichment, and underlying epigenetic and environmental mechanisms. *Journal of Developmental Origins of Health and Disease, 7*(6), 588–601.

Thayer, Z. M., & Kuzawa, C. W. (2011). Biological memories of past environments: Epigenetic pathways to health disparities. *Epigenetics, 6*(7), 798–803.

Torres, L., Driscoll, M. W., & Voell, M. (2012). Discrimination, acculturation, acculturative stress, and Latino psychological distress: A moderated mediational model. *Cultural Diversity and Ethnic Minority Psychology, 18*(1), 17.

Tsuang, M. T., Stone, W. S., & Faraone, S. V. (1999). Schizophrenia: A review of genetic studies. *Harvard Review of Psychiatry, 7*(4), 185–207.

Uddin, M., Aiello, A. E., Wildman, D. E., Koenen, K. C., Pawelec, G., de Los Santos, R., Goldmann, E., & Galea, S. (2010). Epigenetic and immune function profiles associated with posttraumatic stress disorder. *Proceedings of the National Academy of Sciences, 107*(20), 9470–9475.

Van den Bergh, B. R. H., Mulder, E. J. H., Mennes, M., & Glover, V. (2005). Antenatal maternal anxiety and stress and the neurobehavioural development of the fetus and child: Links and possible mechanisms. A review. *Neuroscience & Biobehavioral Reviews, 29*, 237–258.

Vargas, E. D., & Ybarra, V. D. (2017). U.S. citizen children of undocumented parents: The link between state immigration policy and the health of Latino children. *Journal of Immigrant and Minority Health, 19*, 913–920.

Vick, A. D., & Burris, H. H. (2017). Epigenetics and health disparities. *Current Epidemiology Reports, 4*, 31–37.

Will, D., & Wang, F. (2021). On the intergenerational transmission of health inequality. *Science Insights, 39*(5), 407–418.

Witt, W. P., Cheng, E. R., Wisk, L. E., Litzelman, K., Chatterjee, D., Mandell, K., & Wakeel, F. (2014). Maternal stressful life events prior to conception and the impact on infant birth weight in the United States. *American Journal of Public Health, 104*(Suppl. 1), S81–S89.

Witt, W. P., Litzelman, K., Cheng, E. R., Wakeel, F., & Barker, E. S. (2014). Measuring stress before and during pregnancy: A review of population-based studies of obstetric outcomes. *Maternal and Child Health Journal, 18*, 52–63.

Wong, C. C., Mill, J., & Fernandes, C. (2011). Drugs and addiction: An introduction to epigenetics. *Addiction, 106*(3), 480–489.

World Health Organization. (2006). *Promoting optimal fetal development: Report of a technical consultation*. https://iris.who.int/bitstream/handle/10665/43409/9241594004_eng.pdf?sequence=1&isAllowed=y

Wu, G., Feder, A., Cohen, H., Kim, J. J., Calderon, S., Charney, D. S., & Mathé, A. A. (2013). Understanding resilience. *Frontiers in Behavioral Neuroscience, 7*, 10.

Zannas, A. S., & West, A. E. (2014). Epigenetics and the regulation of stress vulnerability and resilience. *Neuroscience, 264*, 157–170.

Zemore, S. E. (2007). Acculturation and alcohol among Latino adults in the United States: A comprehensive review. *Alcoholism: Clinical and Experimental Research, 31*(12), 1968–1990.

Zimmermann, P., Bruckl, T., Nocon, A., Pfister, H., Binder, E. B., Uhr, M., Lieb, R., Moffitt, T. E., Caspi, A., Holsboer, F., & Ising, M. (2011). Interaction of FKBP5 gene variants and adverse life events in predicting depression onset: Results from a 10-year prospective community study. *American Journal of Psychiatry, 168*, 1107–1116.

Figure Credits

Fig. 6.2: Heather H. Burris and Michele R. Hacker, "Conceptual Model of Socioenvironmental," Seminars in Perinatology. Copyright © 2017 by Elsevier B.V.

Fig. 6.3: Hector F. Myers, "Myers' Conceptual Model of Cumulative Vulnerability," Journal of Behavioral Medicine, vol. 32. Copyright © 2009 by Springer Nature.

Fig. 6.8: Adapted from ACE Interface, LLC, "Population Attributable Risk, ACEs, and Health," https://pinetreeinstitute.org/aces/. Copyright © by Pinetree Institute.

Fig. 6.10: National Human Genome Research Institute, "A Diagram of DNA Epigenomics," https://www.genome.gov/about-genomics/fact-sheets/Epigenomics-Fact-Sheet.

Fig. 6.11: ACE Interface, LLC, "Pyramidic Influences of Intergenerational Trauma," https://www.dhcs.ca.gov/Documents/AB-340-Workgroup-Terris-Presentation.pdf, p. 3, 2017.

Fig. 6.11a: Copyright © 2023 Depositphotos/Piscine.

Fig. 6.12: Linda C Gallo, Frank J Penedo, Karla Espinosa de los Monteros, and William Arguelles, "The Reserve Capacity Model (RCM)," https://pubmed.ncbi.nlm.nih.gov/19796063/. Copyright © 2009 by John Wiley & Sons, Inc.

CHAPTER 7

Major Communicable Disease Inequalities Among Mexican Americans

LEARNING OBJECTIVES

- Assess vaccine hesitancy and the factors that influence it.
- Describe the negative social influences in naming diseases after a country or population.
- Analyze the extent of vaccination coverage among Mexican Americans compared to non-Latino White Americans and non-Latino Black Americans.
- Illustrate how the social determinants of health influence communicable disease among Latinos of Mexican descent.
- Explain how cultural factors are important to consider in HIV prevention among Latinos.
- Assess some of the factors that led to the reversal of the Latino mortality paradox.
- Evaluate some of the factors that increased the risk for COVID-19 morbidity and mortality among Latinos.
- Explain why Mexican Americans may be more susceptible and vulnerable to communicable diseases than non-Latino White Americans.

Communicable Disease Inequalities

Severe epidemics and pandemics of communicable diseases have occurred in the early 21st century. The revelation of social inequalities in economic stability, access to quality health care, and other social determinants of health has led to a renewed focus on social justice in public health to remediate the current situation (Blacksher & Lovasi, 2012; Marmot, 2017; Noonan et al., 2016; Ruger, 2004). In this chapter we examine several major communicable disease inequalities among Latinos that are fundamentally based on social inequalities. More recently, the COVID-19 pandemic laid bare several inequalities in the social determinants of health among historically marginalized populations, especially non-Latino Black Americans and Latinos (Antequera et al., 2021; Fortuna et al., 2020; McNeely et al., 2020).

Vaccination hesitancy—that is, the reluctance to obtain a vaccine for oneself or family members—is a strong predictor of vaccination coverage (Hudson & Montelpare; 2021; Khosa et al., 2022). It is a common barrier in influenza, COVID-19, and HPV vaccination coverage. Reasons for vaccine hesitancy are framed in three general areas: 1) lack of knowledge regarding the efficacy of the vaccine, 2) misinformation on precautionary countermeasures, unknown ingredients, and rush to make vaccine, and 3) fear of potential side effects (Dhama et al., 2021; Troiano & Nardi, 2021). For example, COVID-19 countermeasures like wearing masks and obtaining a vaccine when available continue to be highly politized in the United States and have led to increased COVID-19 incidence and related morbidity and mortality (Clark et al., 2022; Muric et al., 2021). Dr. Ashish Jha, former COVID-19 response coordinator, was quoted in a Politico article saying, "Hundreds of thousands of Americans have died in this pandemic because of the bad information about vaccines and treatments" (Messerly, 2023, para. 11). The Associated Press-NORC Center for Public Affairs Research (AP-NORC; 2023) analysis of the 2022 General Social Survey (GSS) found that political divisions surrounding confidence in the scientific community and medicine persisted during and after the COVID-19 pandemic. Overall, 39% of U.S. adults said they had "a great deal of confidence" in the scientific community, down from 48% in 2018 and 2021. An additional 48% of adults in the latest survey reported "only some" confidence, while 13% reported "hardly any," according to AP-NORC's analyses.

The unequal distribution of resources within the social determinants of health was discussed in Chapter 3. Latinos of Mexican descent are disproportionately impacted by high poverty rates, lower educational attainment, lack of health insurance coverage, and overall lack of access to health care. Coupled with a high prevalence of chronic disease risk factors, occupational exposure risks contribute to multiple disparities and an increased likelihood of disease burden among Latinos of Mexican descent.

The prevention of communicable disease is a public health priority. Moreover, the distribution or lack thereof of effective and efficacious vaccinations for many communicable diseases makes transmission almost negligible for those who use them. Unfortunately, we have not learned from our mistakes with the H1N1 pandemic of 2009, which provided an inadequate foundation for mounting rigorous public health campaigns to prevent disease transmission, as seen with COVID-19 only a decade later.

Blumenshine et al. (2008) developed a model that included possible sources of inequalities during the influenza pandemic that is useful for other communicable diseases, like COVID-19, HIV/AIDS, and other sexually transmitted infections (STIs). The flow of components presented in Figure 7.1 illustrates the pattern of relationships between these sources of health and social inequalities.

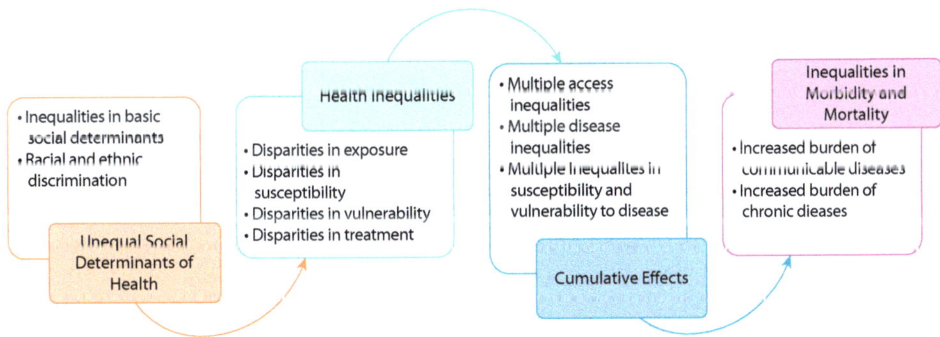

FIGURE 7.1 Sources of Inequalities Associated With Increased Morbidity and Mortality

Adapted from: Blumenshine et al. (2008).

A discussion of inequalities in the social determinants of health and racial/ethnic discrimination provided a foundation for examining health disparities in Chapter 3. The discussion of theories related to ethnic and racial differences encompassed disparities in risk exposure, riskscapes, susceptibility and vulnerability to disease, and chronic disease burden.

Influenza Vaccine Effectiveness and Vaccination Coverage Rates

Influenza vaccine effectiveness in the United States is assessed by Flu Vaccine Effectiveness Network that determines the effectiveness in several demographic subgroups through randomized controlled clinical trials (Gaglani et al., 2016; McLean et al., 2015; Ohmit et al., 2014). For example, Gaglani et al. (2016) found that the overall effectiveness of H1N1 flu vaccine was 54% (95% confidence interval [CI] was 46%-61%). During the 2015-2016 influenza season, Jackson et al. (2017) found that the effectiveness of the influenza vaccine against any influenza illness was 48% (95% confidence interval [CI] was 41%-55%).

According to the Centers for Disease Control and Prevention (CDC, 2009), as of mid-December 2009, only 24.7% of Latino adults had received the seasonal influenza vaccine, compared to 38.6% of non-Latino White adults. No significant differences were seen in cumulative 2009 H1N1 vaccination coverage by race/ethnicity among adults overall. Remarkably—and very disheartening from a prevention perspective—only 11.6% of adults aged 25-64 years with high-risk conditions were vaccinated (CDC, 2010a).

These low vaccination rates are associated with higher 2009 H1N1 hospitalization rates for persons with underlying health conditions (CDC, 2010b). According to the CDC (2010c), the highest hospitalization rates among adults for 2009 H1N1 influenza were for asthma (30%), diabetes (23%), chronic cardiovascular disease (20%), COPD (14%), and pregnancy (9%). Among children, the highest hospitalization rates were for asthma (33%), neuro/developmental conditions (11%), moderate-severe developmental delay (8%), and seizure disorder (6%). In addition, CDC (2010d) reported that Latinos had higher hospitalization rates than non-Latino White Americans and non-Latino Black Americans from September 1, 2009, through January 26, 2010 (30.7/100,00 compared to 16.3/100,000 and 29.7/1000,000, respectively These extremely low vaccination rates, especially among those at increased risk for hospitalization and death from influenza and pneumonia, are sobering and confirm the lack of preparedness among Latinos and others.

Data collected by the CDC (2009) for the 2008-2009 influenza season shows extremely low vaccination coverage among at-risk and high-risk groups (Table 7.1). For example, among youth 5-17 years of age, Latino Americans reported the lowest coverage rates (14.8%) in comparison to non-Latino White Americans (20.8%) and non-Latino Black Americans (16.8%). In addition, among Latino Americans 18-49 years of age who are at high risk due to comorbid conditions, only 27.2% have coverage, compared to 33.5% of non-Latino White Americans and 41.6% of non-Latino Black Americans. Elderly Latino Americans also have lower vaccination coverage than non-Latino White Americans. For every age group, including at-risk and high-risk groups, Latino Americans had lower vaccination coverage rates than non-Latino White Americans and lower than non-Latino Black Americans in several age groups.

TABLE 7.1 Estimated Seasonal Influenza Vaccination Coverage, by Age and Race/Ethnicity, Behavioral Risk Factor Surveillance System (BRFSS), Selected States,* 2008–2009 Season

Age group	Total (%)	Non-Latino White (%)	Non-Latino Black (%)	Latino (%)
All age groups (≥6 mos)	32.6	36.7	24.9	22.0
6 mos–17 yrs	24.0	24.9	20.0	18.4
6–23 mos	40.9	37.2	-	-
2–4 yrs	32.0	39.6	-	16.1
5–17 yrs	20.8	21.0	20.5	16.8
18–49 yrs	22.2	25.3	16.8	14.8
18–49 yrs at high risk**	32.1	33.5	41.6	27.2
50–64 yrs	42.3	43.7	29.8	40.6
≥65 yrs	67.2	69.0	56.3	65.8

* Alaska, California, Connecticut, Delaware, Hawaii, Illinois, Iowa, Kansas, Maine, Michigan, Nevada, New Mexico, Ohio, Texas, Utah, Washington, West Virginia, Wisconsin, and Wyoming.

**Respondents who have diabetes, heart disease, or asthma.

Source: CDC (2009)

Inequalities in Childhood Immunizations for Prevalent Communicable Diseases

Several studies have shown that immunization coverage for Latino children was lower than non-Latino White children (Anandappa et al., 2018; Hill et al., 2017; Niederhauser & Stark, 2005). For example, the gap between non-Latino White children and Latino children widened by an average of 0.5% each year between 1996 and 2001 (Chu et al., 2004). Even though immunization coverage rates have significantly increased, there are still gaps between Latinos and non-Latino White Americans and more so between non-Latino Black Americans and non-Latino White Americans (Hill et al., 2019).

Childhood immunizations can prevent communicable diseases like rubella, whooping cough, and other life-threatening diseases early in life. National data on vaccine coverage for children at least 24 months of age shows that Latino children have slightly lower rates compared to non-Latino White children but higher than non-Latino Black children (National Center for Health Statistics, 2021a; see Figure 7.2).

However, vaccination coverage for children 13–17 years of age shows inequalities for Latinos vis-à-vis non-Latino White Americans (National Center for Health Statistics, 2021b) (Figure 7.3). Latino children have lower vaccination coverage for measles, mumps, and rubella, hepatitis B, varicella, and tetanus-diphtheria than either non-Latino white or non-Latino Black Americans. Only for meningitis vaccine were coverage rates higher for Latinos than non-Latino White Americans. This difference in vaccination coverage places Latino children more at-risk for acquiring these preventable communicable diseases and resulting complications like hospitalization than non-Latino white children.

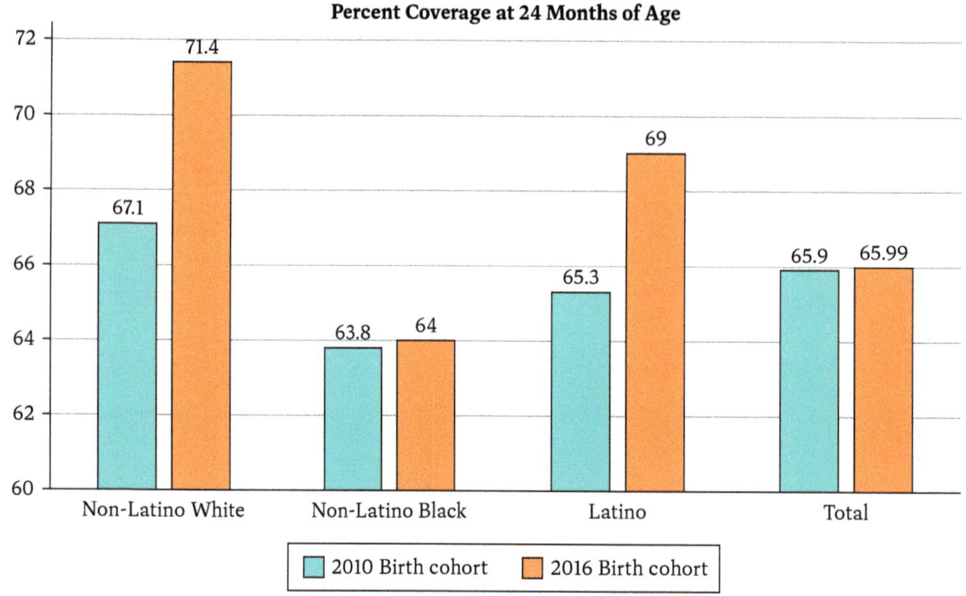

FIGURE 7.2 Vaccine Coverage for Combined Seven-Vaccine Series by Age 24 months, by Race and Latino Origin, United States, Birth Years 2010 and 2016

Source: National Center for Health Statistics (2021a)

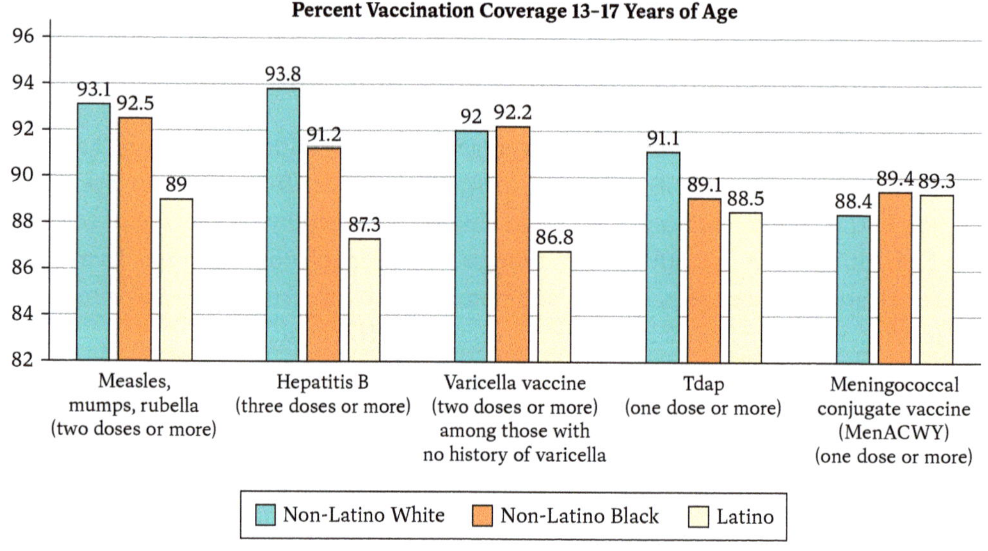

FIGURE 7.3 Vaccination Coverage for Selected Diseases Among Adolescents Aged 13–17 Years, United States, 2008–2019

Source: National Center for Health Statistics (2021b)

2009 H1N1 (Swine Flu) Inequalities Among Latinos

The "swine flu" epidemic originated in Mexico and soon came to be known as the "Mexican flu." While some researchers have indicated that the term is not pejorative or blaming of Mexicans (see de Lamballerie & Gould, 2009) but simply indicates that the first outbreak was in Mexico. However, the stigmatization of Mexicans as a "diseased population" date back to the early 20th century and is very real. Mexicans, especially migrant and seasonal farmworkers, became scapegoats (Schoch-Spana et al., 2010). Vigsø (2010) suggests that naming the epidemic the "Mexican flu" framed the public response and negative perceptions of Mexicans. For example, there was the idea that avoiding Mexicans was one countermeasure to avoid infection. Unfortunately, perceptions of Mexicans as dirty and diseased has a long history in the American Southwest.

National data collected by the CDC (2009, 2010b, 2010c) show systematic influenza inequalities among historically marginalized populations, including those living in poverty and racial/ethnic groups like non-Latino Black Americans, American Indians/Alaska Natives, and Latinos. For example, the CDC reported age-adjusted incidence of influenza-related hospitalizations by census tract poverty level for the years 2010–2012 (Hadler et al., 2016). They found that influenza-related hospitalizations increased with each poverty level (0%–4%, 5%–9%, 10%–19%, >20%) among all racial/ethnic groups, but non-Latino Black Americans and Latinos had higher influenza-related hospitalization rates than non-Latino White Americans across every poverty level. A comparison between those living at the highest poverty level (<5%) with those at the lowest poverty level (≥20%) showed a direct relationship with hospitalizations, with a 96% higher risk of being hospitalized in an intensive care unit, twice as high requiring mechanical ventilation, and 82% higher deaths within 30 days from being hospitalized. Furthermore, there was an inverse relationship between vaccination coverage and hospitalizations, with 35% of those living in the highest poverty census tracts compared with 48% of those living in the lowest poverty tracts having been vaccinated.

The H1N1 pandemic was first detected in the United States in April 2009 and ended in April 2010 (CDC, 2010c). During the spring of 2009, Latinos comprised 30% of all H1N1 influenza cases in the United States from April 15–August 31, 2009, and 15% of people hospitalized with H1N1 in 2009 from 13 metropolitan areas representing 10 states were Latino. The CDC (2010a) notes that in prior influenza seasons, Latinos without underlying medical conditions were overrepresented in hospitalized cases (ranging from 16%–25% of cases without an underlying medical condition). Latino children younger than 18 years of age account for 27% of 210 reported 2009 H1N1 influenza-associated deaths in the United States.

Persons with comorbid conditions were more likely to be hospitalized than those without (CDC, 2010d). Comorbid conditions that increase the risk for hospitalization include asthma, chronic lung diseases like obstructive pulmonary disease and cystic fibrosis, neurological conditions (cerebral palsy), heart disease (e.g., congenital heart disease, congestive heart failure and coronary artery disease), diabetes mellitus, kidney disorders, liver disorders, metabolic disorders (e.g., inherited metabolic disorders and mitochondrial disorders), and a weakened immune system due to disease or medication (such as people with HIV/AIDS, lupus, cancer, or those on chronic steroids).

Age-adjusted hospitalization rates for H1N1 during September 1, 2009, through January 26, 2010 (CDC, 2010b) show that Latino Americans have slightly higher rates than non-Latino Black Americans and almost twice the rate as compared to non-Latino White Americans (30.7/100,000 compared to

16.3/100,000) during the flu season beginning in September 2009 and ending in January 2010 (Figure 7.4). Data shows that off-season influenza hospitalizations were 2.7 times higher for Latino Americans compared to non-Latino White Americans (CDC, 2010b). According to the CDC (2010a), there is no epidemiological or clinical evidence that suggests that Latinos are more susceptible to either 2009 H1N1 or seasonal influenza or to poorer health outcomes by virtue of their ethnicity alone. Data confirms that differences in socioeconomic status, regular source of health care, and lack of health insurance coverage coupled with closer living conditions exacerbated the H1N1 infection and hospitalization rates for Latinos.

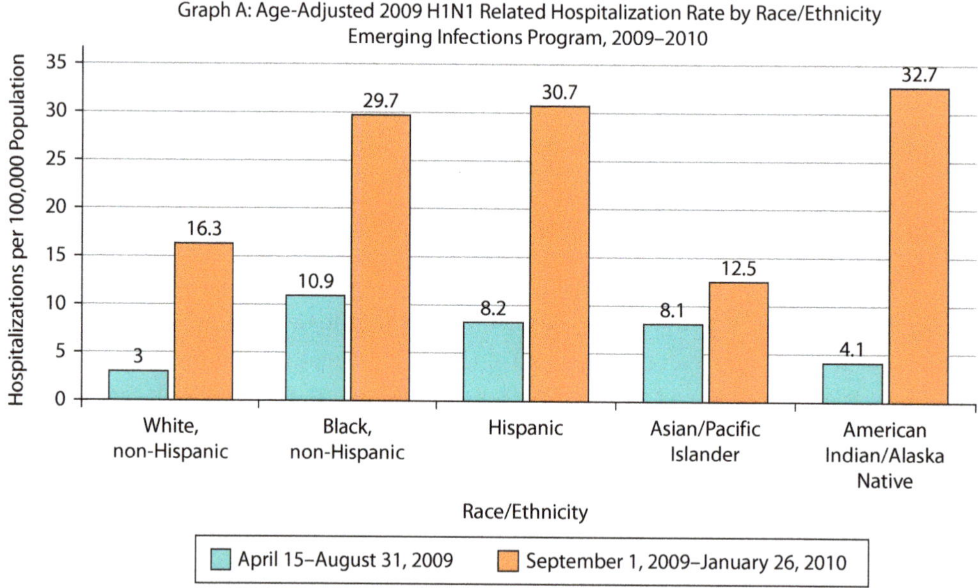

FIGURE 7.4 H1N1 Hospitalization Rates by Race/Ethnicity, 2009–2010

Mortality associated with H1N1 reveal that the highest rates were among American Indians/ Alaska Natives (3.7/100,000), Latinos (1.4/100,000), non-Latino White Americans (0.8/100,000), and non-Latino Black Americans (0.7/100,000) (CDC, 2009). Mortality was higher among those with comorbid conditions like asthma and diabetes mellitus (CDC, 2010d). Influenza-associated pediatric deaths have been nationally notifiable since October 2004. As of August 8, 2009, CDC had received 477 deaths associated with the 2009 pandemic influenza A (H1N1) in the United States, including 36 deaths among children aged <18 years. Among these 36 deaths, 28 (78%) had an underlying high-risk medical condition.

Overall, for 2009 H1N1 influenza Latinos had higher hospitalization rates than non-Latino White Americans and non-Latino Black Americans (CDC, 2009) and some of the lowest vaccination coverage rates, especially for at-risk and high-risk population groups (Ayers et al., 2021). Research shows that Latinos face several barriers associated with vaccination coverage, like time taken from work, childcare responsibilities, transportation, fear of deportation for those who are undocumented, and general mistrust of providers (Anderson et al., 1997; Galbraith et al., 2016; Morales-Campos et al., 2022; Wilson et al., 2018).

As noted previously, historically marginalized population groups like Latinos, American Indians, and non-Latino Black Americans have lower influenza vaccination rates, resulting in higher complications requiring hospitalization, especially for those at-risk and high-risk groups. O'Halloran et al. (2021) showed that age-specific hospitalization rates were highest for Latino Americans compared to non-Latino White Americans for every age group except those ≥ 75 years of age.

Age-specific rate ratios show this inequality gap more directly. O'Halloran et al. (2021) reported that during the 2009 influenza A H1N1 pandemic season, age-adjusted hospitalization rates compared with non-Latino White Americans were higher among American Indian/Alaska Natives (RR, 1.82; 95% CI, 1.48–2.22) and Latino Americans (RR, 1.89; 95% CI, 1.77–2.02), and ICU admission rates were higher among Latinos (RR, 1.77; 95% CI, 1.53–2.04). During that same season, rates of in-hospital deaths were higher among Latinos (RR, 1.87; 95% CI, 1.28–2.74) compared to non-Latino White Americans (O'Halloran et al., 2021). According to O'Halloran et al., in 2019 Latino hospitalization rates were 87% higher than non-Latino White Americans for persons ≤ 4 years of age, 96% higher for ICU admissions, and almost 3 times higher for in-hospital deaths (Table 7.2). Non-Latino Black Americans had the highest rates in all three categories for each age group.

TABLE 7.2 Age-Specific Rate Ratios and Confidence Intervals of Hospitalization, ICU Admission, and In-Hospital Death by Race and Ethnicity, Influenza, 2019

Outcome	Non-Latino White	Latino OR and CI	Non-Latino Black OR and CI
Hospitalization, age group			
≤4	1 (Reference)	1.87 (1.77–1.97)	2.21 (2.10–2.33)
5–17	1 (Reference)	1.28 (1.19–1.36)	1.99 (1.88–2.11)
18–49	1 (Reference)	1.29 (1.24–1.34)	2.52 (2.44–2.59)
50–64	1 (Reference)	1.25 (1.20–1.31)	2.50 (2.43–2.57)
65–74	1 (Reference)	1.18 (1.12–1.25)	1.74 (1.68–1.81)
≥75	1 (Reference)	0.93 (0.89–0.98)	1.05 (1.02–1.09)
ICU admission, age group			
≤4	1 (Reference)	1.96 (1.73–2.23)	2.74 (2.43–3.09)
5–17	1 (Reference)	1.16 (1.00–1.34)	2.00 (1.77–2.26)
18–49	1 (Reference)	1.14 (1.04–1.24)	1.85 (1.72–1.99)
50–64	1 (Reference)	1.04 (0.93–1.15)	2.09 (1.96–2.23)

(continued)

TABLE 7.2 ***(continued)***

Outcome	Non-Latino White	Latino OR and CI	Non-Latino Black OR and CI
65–74	1 (Reference)	1.11 (0.98–1.27)	1.50 (1.37–1.64)
≥75	1 (Reference)	0.88 (0.77–1.00)	1.26 (1.15–1.37)
In-hospital death, age group			
≤4	1 (Reference)	2.98 (1.23–7.19)	3.39 (1.40–8.18)
5–17	1 (Reference)	0.80 (0.38–1.69)	1.19 (0.62–2.28)
18–49	1 (Reference)	1.07 (0.81–1.41)	1.22 (0.94–1.57)
50–64	1 (Reference)	1.08 (0.83–1.40)	1.53 (1.28–1.83)
65–74	1 (Reference)	1.07 (0.77–1.48)	1.19 (0.94–1.51)
≥75	1 (Reference)	0.71 (0.56–0.91)	0.93 (0.79–1.10)

Source: O'Halloran et al. (2021)

Overall, stark inequalities in influenza vaccination coverage are associated with increased influenza-related hospitalizations and increased mortality from influenza, especially among young children and elderly. Moreover, there is a higher risk for hospitalizations and mortality for persons with underlying health conditions like asthma and other upper respiratory conditions and diabetes mellitus. Latinos, non-Latino Black Americans, and American Indians/Alaska Natives are at greater risk than non-Latino White Americans because of these comorbid conditions, lower vaccination coverage, crowded housing conditions, higher poverty rates, and lack of access to health care.

Several scholars have proposed several vaccination barriers that may preclude Latinos from obtaining a needed vaccine (Kim et al., 2015; Quinn et al., 2011; Rubin et al., 2009). Cultural factors like familism and fatalism, health beliefs such as perceptions of risk linked to perceived vulnerability and susceptibility to H1N1, and lack of knowledge regarding the efficacy of the vaccination have all been associated with vaccine hesitancy. For example, Rubin et al. (2009) found that perceptions of increased risk of acquiring H1N1 and that it would lead to severe health consequences were associated with preventive behaviors. Additionally, perceiving that the H1N1 pandemic would continue for a lengthy period was a predictor of whether people engaged in recommended preventive behaviors like washing hands frequently or avoiding crowded venues, probably because of the perceived associated higher level of risk over the longer term.

Kim et al. (2015) identified concerns regarding family exposure and perceptions of risk and severity among Latinos in Arizona. They found that Latinos perceived a higher likelihood of getting infected than non-Latino respondents, and those with children younger than 18 years old in the household perceived a higher likelihood of becoming infected than those without children. Additionally, Latinos reported a higher level of perceived concern than the non-Latinos, and those with children younger than 18 years old in the household perceived a higher concern of becoming infected with H1N1. However, in terms of perceived susceptibility and vulnerability to H1N1, Quinn et al. (2011) found that Mexican Americans reported less susceptibility and vulnerability than non-Latino White Americans and non-Latino Black Americans.

Inequalities in Human Papilloma Virus (HPV) Initiation and Completion Rates

HPV has been identified as a leading causal agent in cervical, esophageal, and other oral cancers (Saraiya et al., 2015). For example, Saraiya et al. (2015) found that HPV DNA was detected in 70% of oropharyngeal cancers (back of the throat, including the base of the tongue and tonsils), 90.6% of cervical cancers, and 91.1% of anal cancers in the United States. Like other STIs, it is conflated with negative perceptions of sexual behaviors and those who engage in such behaviors. Again, social, and cultural determinants like poverty, low educational attainment, and sexual silence play pivotal roles in determining whether one obtains the HPV vaccination. Moreover, during the COVID-19 pandemic, vaccination coverage decreased for almost all vaccinations, including HPV (Chao et al., 2022).

There are over 200 HPV types, but only 14 are determined to be high-risk cancers by the National Cancer Institute (NCI, 2023). Of these, two are responsible for most HPV-related cancers: HPV16 and HPV18. Cancers that are highly associated with HPV infection are presented in Table 7.3.

Latino inequalities in HPV vaccination coverage had been noted prior to widespread availability of the vaccine, with Spanish-speaking Latinos possessing less knowledge regarding vaccine effectiveness but willing to have their daughters vaccinated due to the possibility of developing cancers (Aragones et al.,

TABLE 7.3 HPV-Related Cancers

HPV-related cancers	Description
Cervical cancer	Virtually all cervical cancers are caused by HPV. Routine screening can prevent most cervical cancers by allowing health care providers to find and remove precancerous cells before they develop into cancer. As a result, cervical cancer incidence rates in the United States are decreasing.
Oropharyngeal cancers	Most of these cancers, which develop in the throat (usually the tonsils or the back of the tongue), are caused by HPV (70% of those in the United States). The number of new cases is increasing each year, and oropharyngeal cancers are now the most common HPV-related cancer in the United States.
Anal cancers	Over 90% of anal cancers are caused by HPV. The number of new cases and deaths from anal cancer are increasing each year. Anal cancer is nearly twice as common in women as in men.
Penile cancer	Most penile cancers (over 60%) are caused by HPV.
Vaginal cancer	Most vaginal cancers (75%) are caused by HPV.
Vulvar cancer	Most vulvar cancers (70%) are caused by HPV.

Source: National Cancer Institute (2023)

2016; Bodson et al., 2016; Chando et al., 2013; Galbraith et al., 2016; Glenn et al., 2015; Reiter et al., 2014). National, regional, and state-level data show that Latinos have some of the highest rates of HPV vaccine coverage (Walker et al., 2019). Lack of coverage may be due to provider hesitancy in discussing the value of obtaining an HPV vaccine. For example, rates of physician-recommended HPV vaccinations for children were found to be 52% for Mexicans, 58% for Cubans, and 62.4% for Puerto Ricans (Reiter et al., 2020). Reiter et al. (2020) also found that Spanish-speaking Latinos across all Latino subgroups had higher rates of HPV vaccine coverage than English-speaking Latinos, especially among Spanish-speaking Mexican women.

The data presented by Reiter et al. (2020) (Figure 7.5) shows low percentages of HPV vaccine initiation (≤ 1 dose), and completion (≥3 doses) rates among Latino adolescent males. The lowest HPV initiation rate for adolescent males was found among South Americans (50.6 %), and the highest HPV initiation rate was found among Puerto Rican females (71.2%). The lowest HPV vaccine completion rate was found among Puerto Ricans males (22.8%) and the highest HPV vaccine completion rate was found for South American females (48.7%). From a public health and cancer prevention perspective, an HPV vaccine initiation rate of 50% is cause for major concern. Moreover, the fact that HPV completion rates hover around one quarter for Latino adolescent males means more culturally tailored prevention messages should target this group given the higher transmission dynamics in the spread of STIs from men to women.

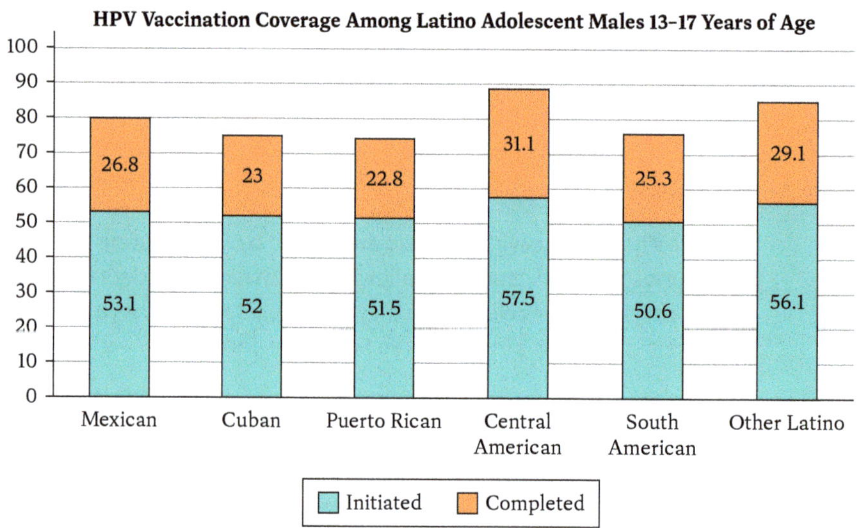

FIGURE 7.5 HPV Vaccination Coverage Among Latino Adolescent Males 13–17 Years of Age, United States, 2012–2016

Adapted from: Reiter et al. (2020).

Among Latinas in the Reiter et al. (2020) study, the lowest HPV vaccine initiation rate was found among Cuban women (63.4%), and the lowest HPV vaccine completion rate was found for "other" Latina descent women (33.6%; see Figure 7.6). The highest HPV vaccine initiation rates are found among Puerto Rican women (71.2%), and the highest HPV vaccine completion rates were found among other Latina descent women (68.5%). It is worth noting that the HPV vaccine initiation and completion rates for adolescent women are higher than like rates for adolescent men. Undoubtedly, this difference can be attributed to a more aggressive and comprehensive targeting approach directed toward women than men (Daley et al., 2017; Dykens et al., 2023).

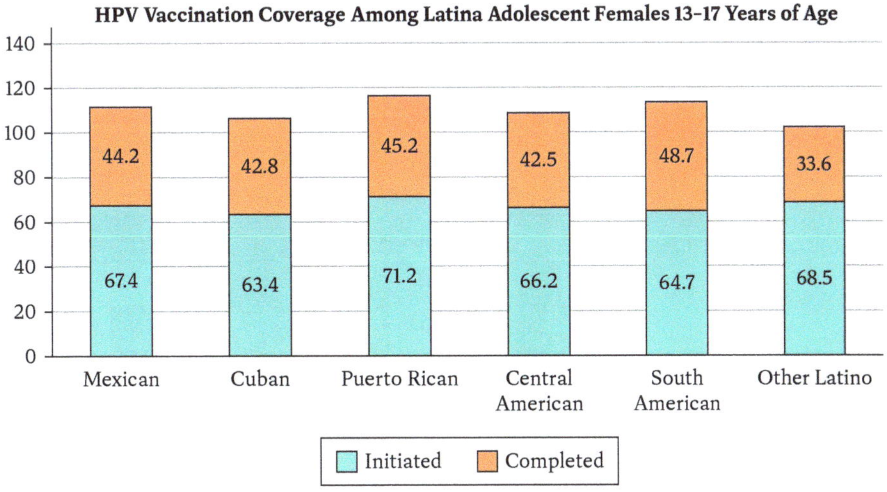

FIGURE 7.6 HPV Vaccination Coverage Among Latina Adolescent Females 13–17 Years of Age, United States, 2012–2016

Adapted from: Reiter et al. (2020).

Sexually Transmitted Infections and HIV/AIDS

Sexually transmitted infections (STIs) are often referred to as "hidden epidemics" due to several factors: the reluctance to discuss sexual issues, symptoms that are present in private body parts, and negative perceptions of having multiple sexual partners. Rooted in human sexual behaviors that are fundamentally influenced by the social and cultural determinants of health, STIs (including HIV) present a social and cultural challenge.

Sexually Transmitted Infection (STI) Inequalities Among Latinos

According to the CDC (2022), there were more than 2.5 million cases of chlamydia, gonorrhea, and syphilis reported in 2021. The age-adjusted prevalence of primary and secondary syphilis was 16.2/100,000, for gonorrhea 214/100,000, and for chlamydia 494.5/100,000. Men who have sex with men (MSM) comprise almost one third of the primary and secondary syphilis infections across all racial and ethnic groups.

Non-Latino White Americans have significantly lower STI rates than non-Latino Black Americans and Latino Americans. The underlying inequalities in the social determinants of health and sexual risk-taking behaviors have been well researched (Harling et al., 2013). Sexual networks and gender imbalance have been recognized as primary drivers of the continuing STI epidemic among historically disadvantaged populations (Adimora & Schoenbach, 2005; Aral et al., 2008; Laumann & Youm, 1999).

Data collected by the CDC (2022) shows several STI inequalities by race and gender. Non-Latino Black Americans show the highest STI infection rates for chlamydia (Figure 7.7). Latino males and females have almost twice the rate for chlamydia as their non-Latino White counterparts. Chlamydia is the only STI examined that has a higher incidence among women than men across all racial/ethnic groups.

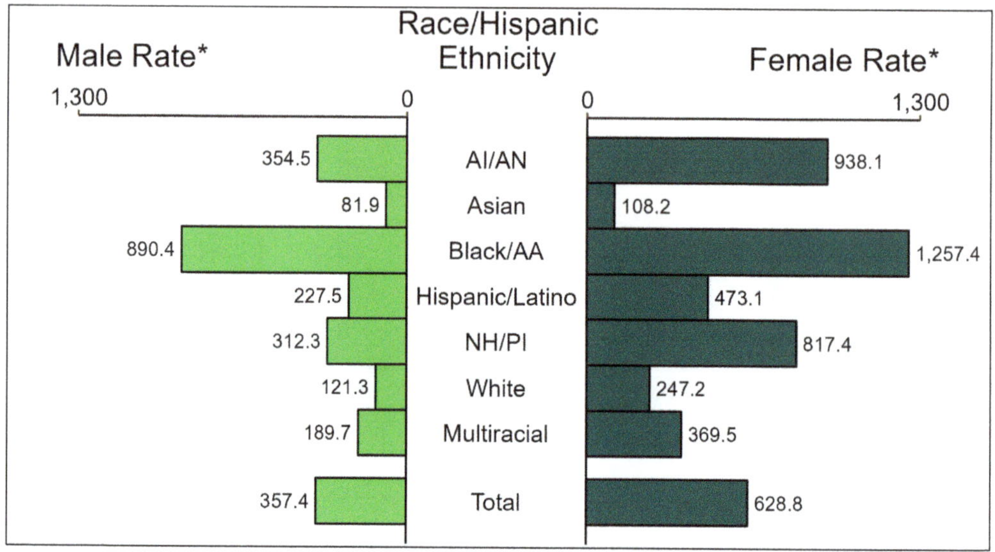

FIGURE 7.7 Chlamydia Rates of Reported Cases per 100,000 by Race/Hispanic Ethnicity and Sex, United States, 2021

The rates of reported gonorrhea cases are shown in Figure 7.8. Non-Latino Black men and women have higher incidence rates than Latino Americans and non-Latino White Americans. Latino men have an incidence rate 1.96 times higher than non-Latino White men, and Latina Americans have a rate that is

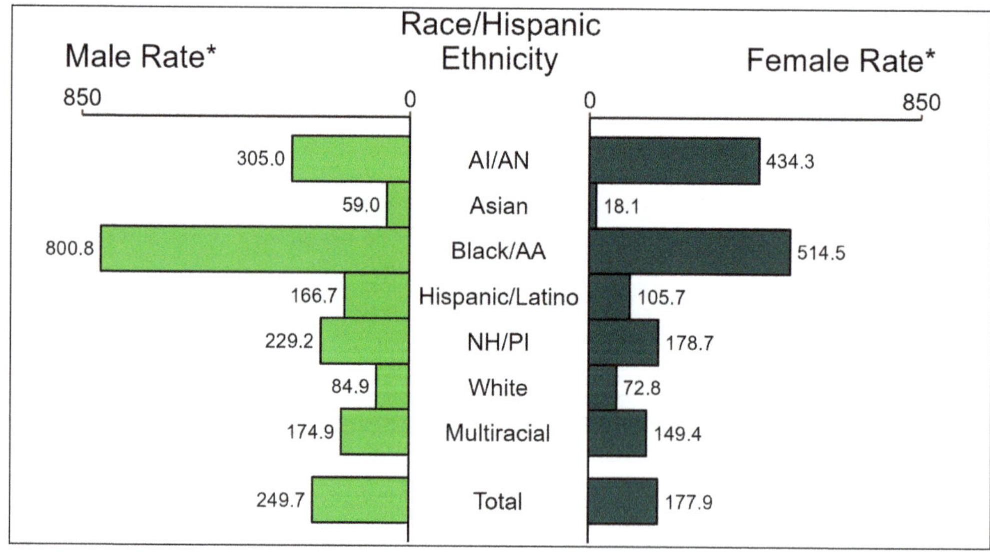

FIGURE 7.8 Gonorrhea Rate of Reported Cases per 100,000 by Race/Hispanic Ethnicity and Sex, United States, 2021

1.45 times higher than non-Latina White women. Overall, men have substantially higher rates of gonorrhea than women (CDC, 2022).

For reported cases of primary or secondary syphilis, Latinos, men have almost 5 times the infection rate for primary or secondary syphilis as women (27.8/100,000 compared to 6.1/100,000, respectively) (CDC, 2022). Additionally, Latino men have twice the rate as non-Latino White men, and Latina women have a 1.27 or 27% higher rate than non-Latina White women. Having an ulcerative STI, like syphilis, increases the risk for HIV transmission due to direct contact of infected fluids with an open entry point to the blood stream (Figure 7.9).

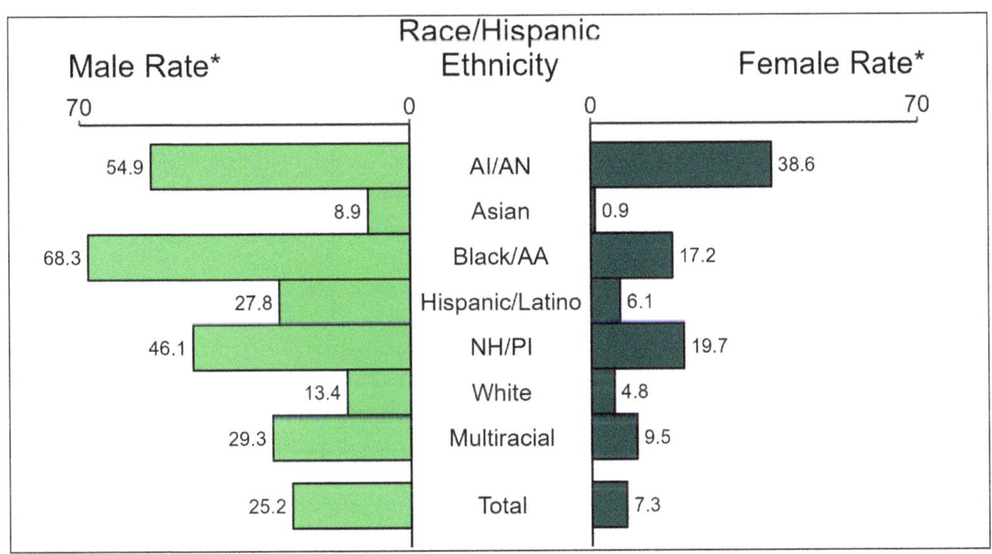

FIGURE 7.9 Primary and Secondary Syphilis Rates of Reported Cases per 100,000 by Race/Hispanic Ethnicity and Sex, United States, 2021

HIV/AIDS Inequalities Among Latinos

The HIV/AIDS epidemic entered its 4th decade in the United States in 2021 with approximately 1.2 million living with HIV disease (CDC, 2023b). There were 36,136 new HIV diagnoses (incidence) in the United States and dependent areas in 2021. The "Ending the HIV Epidemic" national goal is to reduce this number down to 9,588 new diagnoses by 2025 and 3,000 by 2030. Unfortunately, these goals will not be realized with the large number of new HIV infections detected. It is worth noting that the CDC (2023c) estimates that about 40% of incident (new) HIV infections are transmitted by people who do not know their HIV serostatus (estimated to be about 13% of HIV infections) and about 33% of those who do know their HIV serostatus (87% of those diagnosed with HIV infection). Currently, there is not an effective vaccine for HIV, though clinical trials continue.

HIV and AIDS are staged depending on the level of CD4+ cells and whether there is an AIDS-defining condition (e.g., opportunistic infections) (CDC, 2023b). Beginning in 2014 case definition was used to classify cases diagnosed in 2014 and later. It is like the 2008 case definition except for the inclusion of criteria for Stage 0. The stages of HIV infection in the 2014 case definition are based on age-specific CD4+ counts or percentages of total lymphocytes and are defined as follows: HIV infection, Stages 1, 2, and 3. Documentation of an AIDS-defining condition is Stage 3. Otherwise, the stage is determined by the lowest CD4+ test result. For HIV infection, stage unknown there is no information on AIDS-defining conditions and no information available on CD4+ count or percentage. The 2008 stages of HIV infection are presented in Table 7.4.

TABLE 7.4 HIV and AIDS Infection Stages

Stage of infection	Definition (2008)
HIV infection, Stage 0	First positive HIV test result within 6 months after a negative HIV test result. The stage remains stage 0 until 6 months after the first positive test result. After 6 months, the stage may be reclassified as 1, 2, 3, or unknown if based on a CD4 test result or the diagnosis of an opportunistic illness. The diagnosis of an AIDS-defining condition or a low CD4 test result before the 6 months have elapsed does not change the stage from Stage 0 to Stage 3.
HIV infection, Stage 1	No AIDS-defining condition and either a CD4 count of ≥500 cells/µL or a CD4 percentage of total lymphocytes of ≥29.
HIV infection, Stage 2	No AIDS-defining condition and either a CD4 count of 200–499 cells/µL or a CD4 percentage of total lymphocytes of 14–28.
HIV infection, Stage 3 (AIDS)	Documentation of an AIDS-defining condition or either a CD4 count of <200 cells/µL or a CD4 percentage of total lymphocytes of <14. Documentation of an AIDS-defining condition supersedes a CD4 count or percentage that would not, by itself, be the basis for a Stage 3 (AIDS) classification.
HIV infection, stage unknown	No reported information on AIDS-defining conditions and no information available on CD4 count or percentage.

Source: CDC (2019)

The transmission of HIV is dependent on two major interconnected factors: (a) the sociocultural context of risk factors, attitudes, and beliefs and (b) engagement in behavioral risk practices that increase the potential for HIV transmission (Sattenspiel & Castro-Chavez, 1990). Additionally, several intertwined factors enhance the probability of HIV transmission:

- The local HIV seroprevalence rate (sexual/injection network viral load, HIV infection rate, undetected HIV infections)
- Individual risk practices (sexually related risk behaviors, injection-mediated risk behaviors); biological factors than enhance transmission (HIV viral load, CD4+ percentage, CD8+ cells, presence, or history of sexually transmitted infections)

- Socioeconomic and sociocultural conditions (e.g., economic inequalities, HIV-related sigma, homophobia and transphobia, homelessness, serious mental illness, substance abuse, and access to care)
- Perceptions of vulnerability and susceptibility, self-efficacy, and behavioral intentions to reduce risk practices; important epidemiological terminology related to HIV includes *seroprevalence*, or the HIV prevalence in the population or community, and *serostatus*, or whether a person is HIV positive or HIV negative

Social determinants of HIV influence the context of population and individual vulnerability that contributes to increased risk of exposure or compromises the ability to enact preventive behaviors. Social determinants like HIV-related stigma, poverty, and homelessness can also impede access to and receipt of antiretroviral therapy (De Jesus & Williams, 2018; CDC, 2019). For example, in 2018 the CDC (2019) reported higher rates of diagnoses of HIV infection among individuals living below the 18% poverty level. HIV infection rates among those living at the lowest poverty level show dramatic inequalities. HIV-related stigma from the lay public and health professionals profoundly influences HIV-testing rates, disclosure of HIV status, and continuation in HIV care (De Jesus & Williams, 2018).

The CDC *HIV Surveillance Report* provided important information on the social determinants of health among adults diagnosed with HIV infection in 2017 (CDC, 2019). The report analyzed census tract-level data on social determinants using the following definitions:

- Federal poverty status: the proportion of residents in the census tract who were living below the U.S. poverty level (i.e., below a specified threshold) at any time during the 12 months before the survey response (individuals aged 18 years and older)
- Education level: the proportion of residents in the census tract with less than a high school diploma (individuals aged 18 years and older)
- Median household income: median income for a household within the census tract during the 12 months before the survey response
- Health insurance coverage: the proportion of residents in the census tract without health insurance or health coverage plan (individuals aged 18 years and older)

Results are presented in Figures 7.10 and Figures 7.11 for males and females, respectively.

As shown in the CDC (2019) data in Figure 7.10, among male adults 18 years of age and over, HIV-infected non-Latino Black Americans have the highest percentages for those living at or below 19% federal poverty, less than a high school diploma, median household income less than $40,000, and not having health insurance (Figure 7.10). Latino Americans are three times more likely than non-Latino White Americans to live at or below 19% federal poverty, over two times less likely to have a high school diploma, three times more likely to have household incomes less than $40,000 annually, and almost 4 times more likely not to have health insurance coverage. These results clearly demonstrate that non-Latino Black Americans and Latino Americans are significantly more socioeconomically disadvantaged than non-Latino White Americans as measured by these four social determinants.

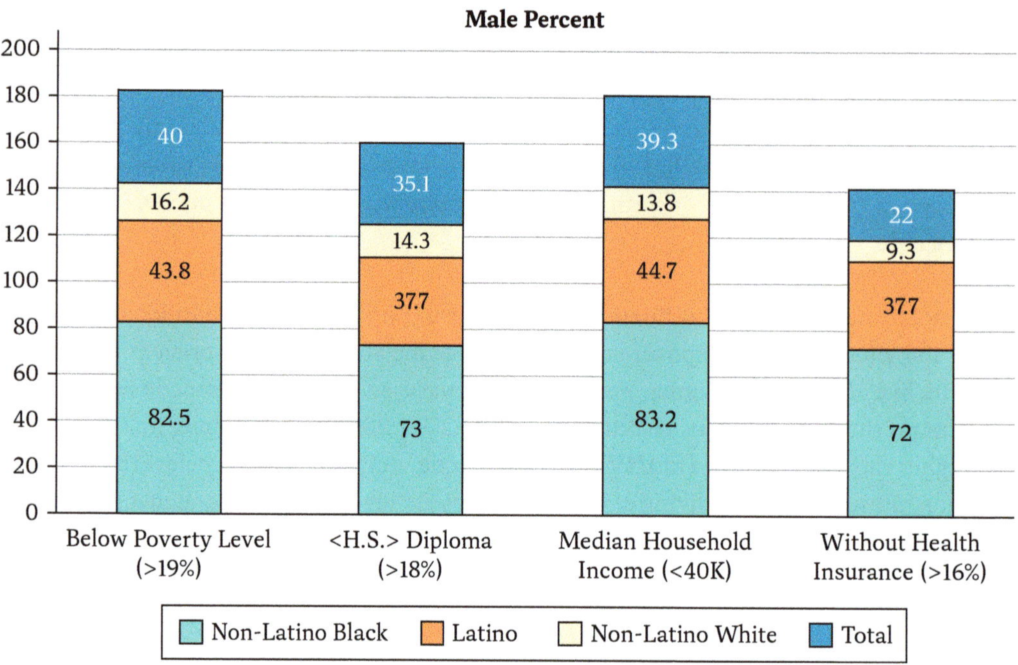

FIGURE 7.10 Diagnoses of HIV Infection Among Adults, by Race/Ethnicity, Sex, and Selected Social Determinants of Health, 2017—Census Tract Level, United States and Puerto Rico

Source: CDC (2019)

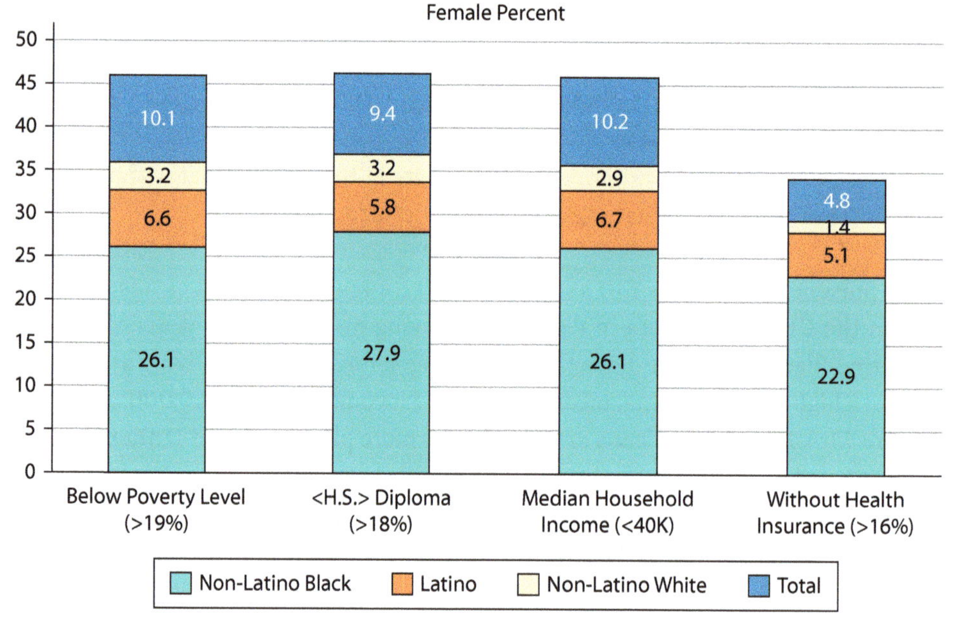

FIGURE 7.11 Diagnoses of HIV Infection Among Adults, by Race/Ethnicity, Sex, and Selected Social Determinants of Health, 2017—Census Tract Level, United States and Puerto Rico

Source: CDC (2019)

The large gaps between non-Latino Black Americans, Latino Americans, and non-Latino White Americans are also present among women (CDC, 2019; Figure 7.11). Still, non-Latina Black Americans have the highest rates in percentages living below 19% federal poverty, not having a high school diploma, median household incomes less than $40,000 annually, and not having health insurance. Among HIV-infected Latinas, a ratio of 2:1 exists for percentage living below 19% poverty, having less than a high school diploma, and median household income less than $40,000 annually. However, lack of health insurance was almost 5:1 among Latina Americans compared to non-Latina White Americans. The persistence of detrimental social determinants among HIV-infected persons reduces the effectiveness for medical linkages to HIV specialty care and viral suppression.

Historically marginalized and disadvantaged populations, especially non-Latino Black Americans and Latino Americans are overrepresented in HIV diagnoses, persons living with HIV/AIDS, and HIV mortality compared to non-Latino White Americans. In the early 1980s, most people perceived that HIV/AIDS was a disease mainly of White, gay men and perceived little or no risk to themselves. Nothing could be further from the truth then or now. For example, in 2018, 39.5% of diagnoses were among non-Latino Black Americans, 28.1% were among Latino Americans, and 26.8% were among non-Latino White Americans (CDC, 2019). Moreover, the proportion of HIV diagnoses that were among Latino adult and adolescent males was greater than the proportion of diagnoses that were among non-Latino White adult and adolescent males.

According to the CDC (2023a), the rate of diagnosed HIV infection in 2021 was higher among non-Latino Black Americans than among Latino Americans and non-Latino White Americans (Table 7.5). Non-Latino Black men have about 7.5 times the rate of non-Latino White men, and Latino men have 4 times the rate as non-Latino White men. Among women, non-Latina Black Americans have almost 11 times the rate of diagnoses of HIV infection than non-Latina White Americans, and Latina Americans have 2.6 times the rate as non-Latina White Americans.

TABLE 7.5 Diagnoses of HIV Infection Among Persons Aged ≥ 13 Years by Race/Ethnicity and Sex at Birth, 2021—United States

Race/ethnicity	No.	Rate/100,000
Non-Latino Black		
• **Men**	10,978	66.5
• **Women**	3,544	19.5
Latino		
• **Men**	8,895	35.7
• **Women**	1,164	4.8
Non-Latino White		
• **Men**	7,536	8.9
• **Women**	1,522	1.8

Source: CDC (2023a)

In 2021, the prevalence rate of persons living with an HIV diagnosis among non-Latino Black men was 5.6-times higher than non-Latino White men, and among Latino men it was almost 3-times higher than non-Latino White men. Non-Latina Black women had a rate of HIV infection 17-times higher than non-Latina White women, and Latinas' HIV infection rate was 4-times higher than non-Latina White women (Table 7.6).

TABLE 7.6 Persons Aged >13 Years Living With Diagnosed HIV infection by Race/Ethnicity and Sex assigned at Birth, 2021, United States

Race/Ethnicity	No.	Rate/100,000
Non-Latino Black		
• **Men**	289,847	1,756.8
• **Women**	142,380	781.6
Latino		
• **Men**	209,118	839.6
• **Women**	45,983	188.6
Non-Latino White		
• **Men**	265,798	313.6
• **Women**	40,630	46.8

Source: CDC (2023a)

The most affected subpopulations in 2021, as reported by the CDC (2023a), are non-Latino Black and Latino MSM, followed by non-Latino White MSM, heterosexual non-Latina Black women, heterosexual non-Latino Black men, heterosexual Latinas, and heterosexual non-Latina White women. Significant gender differences by race/ethnicity are also apparent, with Latina adult and adolescent HIV infection rates lower than Latino males (17% compared to 28%, respectively; Figure 7.12). The highest rates of HIV infection among Latinos were among those born in the United States (32% men, 31% women). Mexico-born males had higher HIV infection rates than Puerto Rico-born males (11% vs. 6%, respectively), while Mexico-born women had lower HIV infection rates than Puerto Rican-born women (7% vs. 10%, respectively).

Transmission categories varied as well, with 85% of Latino males contracting HIV through male-male sex and 88% of Latinas contracting HIV through heterosexual contact (CDC, 2023a). A notable racial/ethnic and gender difference is identified with injection drug use as a transmission category, with non-Latina White women having the highest percentage (34%), in comparison to non-Latina Black women (8%) and Latinas (12%).

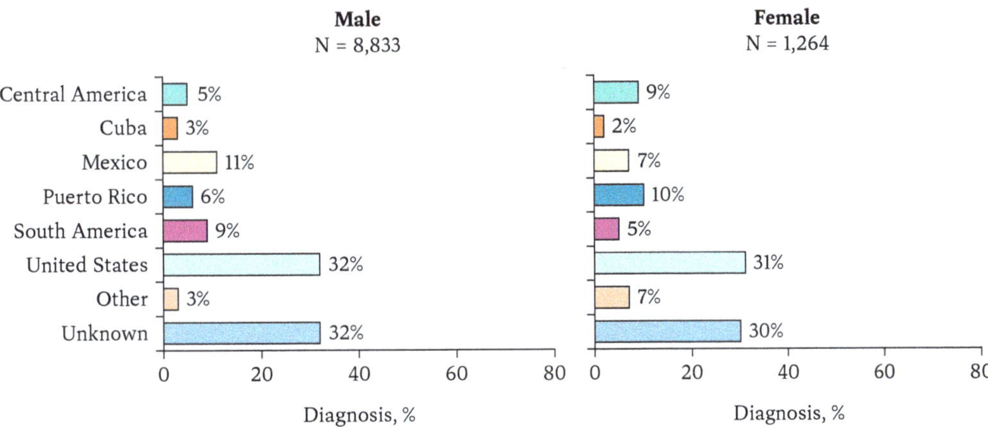

FIGURE 7.12 Diagnoses of HIV Infection Among Hispanic/Latino/a Adults and Adolescents, by Sex and Place of Birth, 2018—United States and Six Dependent Areas

Employing the CDC WONDER Online Database (AIDS Public Use Data; CDC, n.d.-a), the top-10 states with the largest Latino populations were identified. A wide variation in rate-ratio differences in HIV infection between Latinos and non-Latino White Americans was found (Table 7.7). The lowest rate-ratio difference is in New Mexico (4.4), and the largest rate-ratio difference is in New York (25.8). In all states listed, Latinos have higher rates of HIV infection per 100,000 than non-Latino White Americans.

TABLE 7.7 Rates of Diagnoses of HIV Infection Among Latinx Adults and Adolescents, 2018, 10 Largest Latino-Origin States, per 100,000

State	Latino	Non-Latino White	Excess morbidity (rate ratio)
New Mexico	7.7	3.3	2.3
California	17.5	8.4	2.1
Texas	20.6	8.8	2.3
Arizona	18.8	8	2.4
Nevada	22.9	12.1	1.9
Florida	35	11	3.2
Colorado	16.1	5.3	3.0
New Jersey	26.4	4.6	5.7
New York	29.6	3.8	7.8
Illinois	18.5	4.5	4.1

Source: CDC (n.d.-c)

Stage 3 AIDS infection is the most severe in terms of decreased immunological response and increased mortality (CDC, 2023b). According to the CDC (n.d.-b), in 2021, among adults and adolescents living with diagnosed HIV infection that was ever classified as Stage 3 (AIDS), non-Latino Black Americans accounted for 40%, non-Latino White Americans accounted for 37.9%, and Latinos accounted for 18.6% of all cases (Table 7.8). However, the rate per 100,000 was 7.2 times higher for non-Latino Black Americans compared to non-Latino White Americans. The 35–39 age group had the highest percentage of deaths (17.3% of deaths), followed by those 40–44 years of age (16.7% of deaths) at the end of 2021.

TABLE 7.8 Stage 3 (AIDS) Classifications and Deaths of Persons With Stage 3 (AIDS) by Race/Ethnicity, Cumulative as of Year-End 2021, United States and Six Dependent Areas

	Classifications		Deaths	
Race/ethnicity	No.	%	No.	%
Non-Latino Black	532,799	39.9	318,284	40.0
Latino	284,524	21.3	147,695	18.6
Non-Latino White	450,066	33.7	301,474	37.9

Source: CDC (n.d.-b.)

Using the AIDS Public Use Data accessed through CDC WONDER (CDC, n.d.-a), in the 10-largest Latino population states, the rates of diagnosed HIV infections ever classified as Stage 3 (AIDS) are higher for Latino Americans than non-Latino White Americans (Table 7.9). The highest differential between Latino Americans and non-Latino White Americans is in New York (9.3 times the rate) and New Jersey (6.4 times the rate). The lowest rate ratios for Latino Americans are Nevada (60% higher than non-Latino White Americans), California, and Arizona where the rates are twice as high as non-Latino White Americans.

TABLE 7.9 Rates of Diagnosed HIV Infections Classified as Stage 3 (AIDS) per 100,000 Among Latinx Adults and Adolescents, 2018 in the 10 Largest Latino-Origin States

State	Latino	Non-Latino White	Excess morbidity (rate ratio)
New Mexico	3.7	1.6	2.3
California	6.6	3.3	2.0
Texas	8.5	3.3	2.6
Arizona	6.6	3.2	2.0
Nevada	8.6	5.5	1.6

State	Latino	Non-Latino White	Excess morbidity (rate ratio)
Florida	10.9	4.8	2.3
Colorado	7.8	2.1	3.7
New Jersey	11.5	1.8	6.4
New York	15.8	1.7	9.3
Illinois	6.7	1.9	3.5

Source: CDC (n.d.-b)

Data for adults and adolescents diagnosed with HIV infection in 2018 and residing in the 10-largest Latino population states are presented in Table 7.10 (CDC, n.d.-a). All the rate ratios shown in the Table 7.11 indicate that Latinos have an excess morbidity associated with diagnosed HIV infection when compared to non-Latino White Americans. The highest differentials are in New Jersey (4.6 times higher) and New York (6.3 times higher), and the lowest are in California (10% higher than non-Latino White Americans) and New Mexico (20% higher than non-Latino White Americans).

TABLE 7.10 Adults and Adolescents Living With Diagnosed HIV Infection, 2018

State	Latino	Non-Latino White	Excess morbidity (rate ratio)
New Mexico	209.9	176.9	1.2
California	410.5	374.4	1.1
Texas	360.7	213.8	1.7
Arizona	298.1	224.3	1.3
Nevada	398.8	316.5	1.3
Florida	596.4	298.9	2.1
Colorado	313.3	215.1	1.5
New Jersey	711.3	154.2	4.6
New York	1511.2	239.0	6.3
Illinois	422.1	142.5	3.0

Source: CDC (n.d.-b)

Inequalities in HIV-Related Mortality Among Latinos

AIDS mortality has been declining since the introduction of highly active antiretroviral medications (HAART) in 1985. Non-Latino Black Americans have the highest age-adjusted mortality rates when compared to other racial/ethnic groups in the United States. The lifespan for those living with HIV/AIDS has increased from an average of 36 years in 1987 to an average of 54 years in 2018 (CDC, n.d.-d). Mortality in HIV-infected persons depends on several factors: the duration of the infection, the age at the time of seroconversion, and the effectiveness of antiretroviral treatment. These factors in turn depend on when treatment was initiated, whether previous treatment responses were suboptimal, and the presence of opportunistic infections. For those HIV-infected people not receiving HAART, the survival rates are very low, with 48% surviving 2 years, 26% surviving 4 years, and 18% surviving after 6 years of an AIDS diagnosis. Most AIDS patients who receive HAART will survive for >10 years after the onset of AIDS, whereas most of the patients who do not receive HAART die within 2 years of the onset of AIDS (Stage 3). Latinos with AIDS have survival rates that are higher than non-Latino White Americans and non-Latino Black Americans (CDC, n.d.-d).

In 2021, non-Latino Black men had the highest mortality rate (34.5 deaths per 100,000 population), which was about 6 times higher than non-Latino white men (Table 7.11). Latino males had 1.86 times the mortality rate as non-Latino White Americans. Among women, non-Latina Black Americans had the highest rates, followed by Latinas, and non-Latina White Americans. Mortality rates for non-Latina Black Americans were 14 times higher than non-Latina White Americans, and almost 5 times higher than Latina Americans, whereas Latina American mortality rates were about 3 times that of non-Latina White Americans.

TABLE 7.11 Deaths of Persons With Diagnosed HIV Infection by Race/Ethnicity and Assigned Sex at Birth, 2021—United States

Race/ethnicity	Number	Rate/100,000
Non-Latino Black		
• **Men**	5,698	34.5
• **Women**	2,704	14.8
Latino		
• **Men**	2,778	11.2
• **Women**	720	3.0
Non-Latino White		
• **Men**	5,102	6.0
• **Women**	923	1.1

Source: CDC (n.d.-c)

Mortality differentials are presented in Table 7.12 for the 10-largest Latino population states. Latinos have an HIV morality advantage in California and Arizona where the rates are higher for non-Latino White Americans than for Latinos. However, New Jersey and New York continue to show the consequences of delayed HIV treatment with Latino-non-Latino White differentials almost 4 times and 8 times higher, respectively.

TABLE 7.12 Age-Adjusted Mortality Rates Among Persons Diagnosed With HIV by 10 Largest Latino States, 2021, United States

State	Latino	Non-Latino White	Excess Mortality (Rate Ratio)
New Mexico	3.3	2.7	1.22
California	4.1	6.2	0.66
Texas	4.3	4.3	1.00
Arizona	2.5	3.9	0.64
Nevada	4.6	5.5	0.84
Florida	7.2	6.5	1.10
Colorado	2.2	1.6	1.38
New Jersey	9.2	2.5	3.68
New York	21.9	2.7	8.11
Illinois	4.3	2.2	1.95

Source: CDC (n.d.-d)

In 2021, the annual mortality rate among Latinos with HIV disease as the underlying cause versus the five leading causes of death among persons aged 25–44 were unintentional injuries (60.5/100,000), COVID-19 (36.9/100,000), cancer (14.3/100,000), suicide (12.3/100,000), homicide (11.9/100,000), and HIV (1.4/100,000).

Inequalities in the HIV Care Continuum

Once an individual is diagnosed with HIV infection, it is extremely important that they be linked to care within 1 month after diagnosis, receive antiretroviral therapy as warranted, be retained in care for ongoing monitoring, and achieve viral suppression to undetectable levels within 6 months of HIV diagnosis. The national goals outlined in "Ending the HIV Epidemic" (EHE) (CDC, n.d.-e) coordinated by the U.S. Department of Health and Human Services are to increase the percentage of people with diagnosed HIV who are virally suppressed to at least 95% by 2025 and remain there through 2030 (CDC, n.d.-e). Currently, according to the CDC (2023d), for every 100 Latinos with diagnosed HIV, 72% received some form of HIV-related care, 51% were retained in care, and only 64% were virally suppressed (based on the most recent viral load test).

According to the CDC (2023d), only 80.2% of persons > 13 years of age who were diagnosed with HIV were linked to care within 1 month of their diagnosis. Analysis by race and ethnicity shows that non-Latino White Americans have the highest percentage of persons linked to care (82.6%) and non-Latino Black Americans the lowest percentage of persons linked to care (77.1%), with Latino Americans about the same as non-Latino White Americans (82.4%). Viral suppression within 6 months of HIV diagnosis was very low, only 66.8%. Viral suppression was highest among Latino Americans (71%), then non-Latino White Americans (68.3%), with non-Latino Black Americans having the lowest viral suppression among

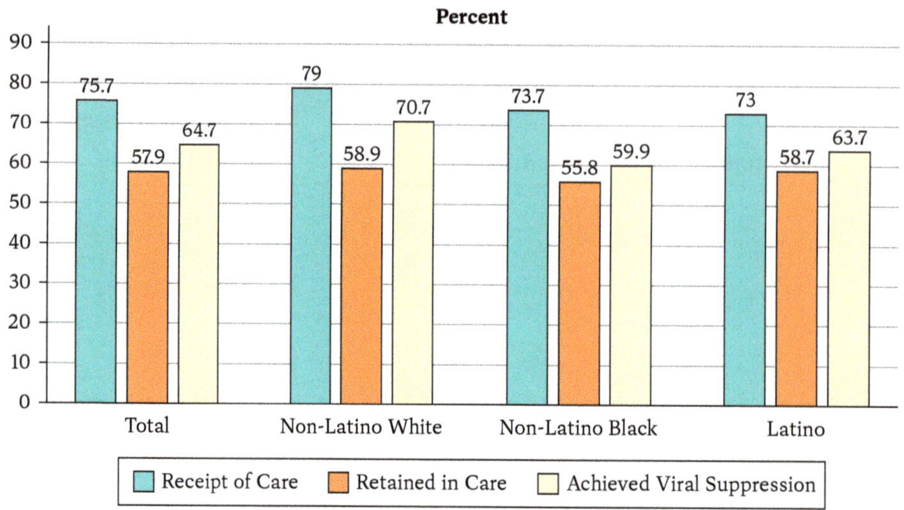

FIGURE 7.13 Receipt of HIV Medical Care, Retention in Care, and Viral Suppression Among Persons Aged ≥13 Years Living With Diagnosed HIV Infection, by Race/Ethnicity 2018—41 States and the District of Columbia

the three groups (62.6%). Among those diagnosed and living with HIV among persons aged ≥ 13 years, receipt of medical care, retention in care, and viral suppression varied significantly, with 75.7% receiving HIV medical care, 57.9% being retained in care, and 64.7% achieving viral suppression. Racial and ethnic inequalities are particularly noteworthy (Figure 7.13).

In 2018, among persons living with diagnosed or undiagnosed HIV infection, the HIV care continuum outcomes show that, overall, 86% were diagnosed with HIV infection, and of these, 65% received HIV medical care, 50% were retained in care, and 56% achieved viral suppression (CDC, 2023d). This is not a great trend for those diagnosed with HIV infection. Would this be acceptable if the disease were cancer or diabetes mellitus? There are also racial and ethnic inequalities related to the HIV care continuum outcomes (Figure 7.14).

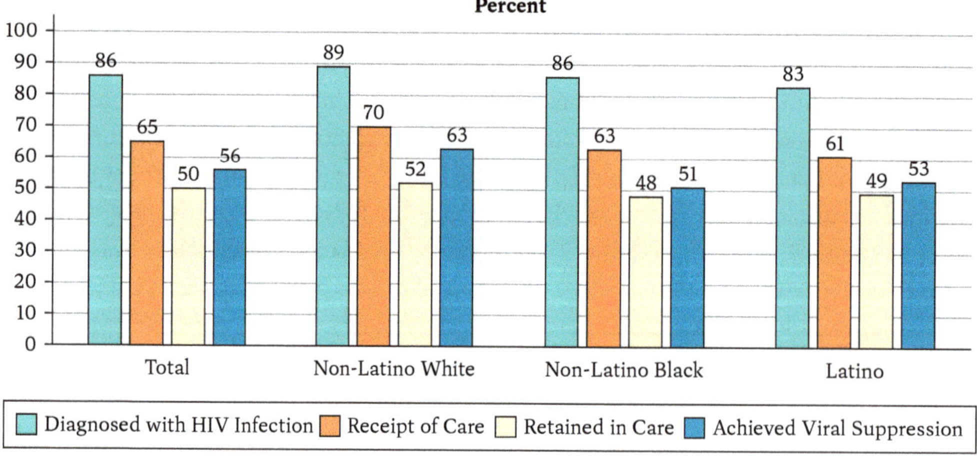

FIGURE 7.14 Persons Living With Diagnosed or Undiagnosed HIV Infection HIV Care Continuum Outcomes, by Race/Ethnicity, 2018—United States

Latinos have the lowest percentage of persons diagnosed with HIV, which translates into a significant percentage (about 17%) who do not know they are infected and can transmit the virus to others through high-risk behaviors (CDC, 2023d). The HIV care continuum outcomes are lower for Latino Americans compared to non-Latino White Americans, with 61% receiving medical care and only 53% achieving viral suppression, compared to 70% of non-Latino White Americans receiving HIV medical care and 63% achieving viral suppression. Viral suppression is lowest for non-Latino Black Americans.

As noted previously, social determinants associated with HIV exert a powerful influence on all aspects of the HIV care continuum, from low HIV testing rates to suboptimal viral suppression (CDC, 2023e). Latinos are disproportionately represented in HIV incidence, have low percentages of receiving HIV medical care, less than 50% are retained in care, and they have very low viral suppression rates.

Cultural and Social Influences on Sexual Risk Behaviors

Consistent condom use with casual sexual partners and the sterilization of injection-related paraphernalia are the two primary prevention practices for HIV and other sexually transmitted and blood-borne infections (Bertozzi et al., 2006; Stine, 2014). Also, reducing the number of sexual partners and decreasing the amount of time syringes are circulating creates an initiative-taking context for HIV prevention (Strathdee & Vlahov, 2001; Vlahov et al., 2001).

The probability of becoming infected with HIV depends on several factors: transmission efficiency, number of sexual partners, and HIV seroprevalence (Stine, 2014). Typically, multiple sexual exposures are necessary for someone to become infected with HIV. The greatest risk for transmission occurs soon after seroconversion when viremia (viral load) is highest. HIV has another important secondary means of spread through blood or blood products: Direct exposure to blood and blood products is the most highly efficient method of HIV transmission—from 67% to over 90% per encounter. The primary risk group for HIV transmission via blood exposure are those who inject drugs, sharing infected needles and other injection paraphernalia. A compilation of HIV risk behaviors available in the literature is presented in Table 7.13. The frequency of syringe-mediated and sexual risk behaviors, coupled with the HIV seroprevalence, increases the risk of HIV transmission.

TABLE 7.13 HIV Syringe-Mediated and Sexual Risks

Syringe-mediated risk behaviors	Sexual risk behaviors
Frequency of injection	Sexual relations under the influence of drugs/alcohol
Injecting last	Exchanging sex for money or drugs
Type of drug injected (cocaine, meth, heroin)	Sexual bingeing with anonymous sexual partners
Common drug purchases (pooling money to buy drugs)	Unprotected sex with an HIV-positive person without using pre-exposure prophylaxis

(continued)

TABLE 7.13 *(continued)*

Syringe-mediated risk behaviors	Sexual risk behaviors
Multiperson reuse of needle/syringe	Unprotected sex with an HIV-positive persons who inject drugs without using pre-exposure prophylaxis
Lack of appropriate bleaching of needle/ syringe	Increased risk of unprotected sexual transmission, low–high risk: • Oral • Vaginal • Insertive anal • Receptive anal
Sharing the cooker, cotton, rinse water	Presence of a sexually transmitted infection, especially syphilis and gonorrhea
Syringe-mediated drug dispersal: • **Front-loading and back-loading**	Inconsistent disclosure of HIV serostatus to casual or main sexual partners

Most Latinos do not perceive themselves to be at risk for HIV infection (Campbell et al., 2008, Herbst et al., 2007). Because of this, many do not take safety precautions like using condoms or disinfecting their syringes and other injection paraphernalia. Studies have shown that condoms are inconsistently used among Latino heterosexuals, men who have sex with men (MSM), and people who inject drugs (PWID; Deardorff et al., 2010; Sibthorpe, 1992; Teitelman et al., 2008). For example, in a multisite sample of PWID, Estrada (1998) found Latino PWID (Mexican American and Puerto Rican) injected more frequently and shared syringes more often than African American PWID, thus increasing their risk for HIV exposure. Non-Latino Black PWID used bleach to disinfect their syringes a higher proportion of time (49%) compared to Puerto Rican PWID (46%) and Mexican American PWID (35%). In addition, Mexican American PWID shared a higher proportion of the time (25%). There are several cultural factors and influences among Latinos that must be taken into consideration for effective, culturally tailored HIV prevention planning (Table 7.14).

TABLE 7.14 **Cultural and Social Influences and HIV Among Latinos**

Cultural and social factors	Implications
Sexual silence	Not discussing sex or sexuality with family or peers.
Conservative attitudes toward sex and sexuality	Unlikely to carry condoms or discuss sexual behaviors.
Beliefs about virginity	Influences sexual risks: oral and/or anal sex rather than vaginal sex.

Cultural and social factors	Implications
Double standards for sexual behavior	Men can and are expected to engage in multiple sexual relationships with women; women are not allowed the same.
Behaviorally bisexual males	Can serve as a bridge to heterosexual women; Mexican men are defined by the sexual role performed—passive or receptive.
Homophobia	"Coming out" issues and homophobia in the Latino community.
Addictophobia	Stigmatization of people who use drugs in the Latino community.
Lack of awareness of IDU partner	Leads to increased risk for non-using partners and uneven exposure.
Denial of HIV risk	Negatively impacts HIV testing rates and timely access to HIV medical treatment.

Regarding sexuality, studies have shown that higher acculturation level among Latino youth, adolescents, and young adults is associated with negative attitudes about and use of condoms (Marin et al., 1993). Among Latino college students, Gurman and Borzekowski (2004) found inconsistent and low rates of condom use, with fewer than half of recently sexually active Latino students reporting condom use during their last oral (4.9%), vaginal (41.3%), or anal (27.8%) sexual encounter. Other issues and challenges to prevention for Latinos include:

- Relationship power dynamics: *machismo* beliefs
- Acculturation, gender, and cultural expectations
- Intimate partner violence
- Sexual and reproductive health decisions
- Parenting and caregiving responsibilities
- Lack of access to specialty HIV medical care
- Low medication adherence and retention in HIV medical care
- Low rates of disclosure of both HIV status and sexual orientation to intimate or casual sexual or injection partners

Social and cultural determinants of health, along with biological and behavioral factors in HIV transmission, are inherently associated with HIV disease at every level, from initial HIV testing, linkage to care, retention in care, viral suppression, and death.

COVID-19 Inequalities Among Latinos

Although there were other recent epidemics, the COVID-19 pandemic was the worst pandemic the world has experienced since the worldwide flu pandemic of 1918. At the beginning of the COVID-19 pandemic when appropriate preventive precautions could be initiated, as was done for the 2009 H1N1 pandemic, failure of U.S. government leadership, a politically compromised CDC, and political hysteria and disinformation over precautionary measures, like wearing masks when in public, the effectiveness of social distancing protocols, and frequency of handwashing, lead to unnecessary COVID-19 mortality and morbidity (Cuan-Baltazar et al., 2020; Enders et al., 2020; Filkuková et al., 2021). This was especially true for historically marginalized and disadvantaged populations like non-Latino Black Americans, Latinos, and American Indians and Alaska Natives (Lopez et al., 2021).

The COVID-19 pandemic not only compromised existing comorbidities among vulnerable populations but also delayed needed treatment for cancer, STIs, and heart disease due to the acute and long-term characteristics of COVID-19 and precautionary safeguards in hospitals. Unlike previous respiratory disease pandemics, there was no existing or immediate vaccine available for COVID-19, and due to its characteristics as a retrovirus, it was prone to rapid mutation, like HIV (Simula et al., 2022; Stine, 2014).

According to CDC (n.d.-f) data, as of September 2023, the COVID-19 pandemic has resulted in 1.14 million deaths and 6.3 million hospitalizations in the United States, with approximately 75% of deaths occurring among adults aged ≥65 years. In 2020 COVID-19 became the third leading cause of death nationally and has led to a 1.8-year decrease in lifespan (CDC, n.d.-f).

According to Tenforde et al., (2022) vaccine effectiveness (VE) against invasive mechanical ventilation (IMV) and in-hospital death was 90% for mRNA COVID-19 vaccines with similar results found by Lauring et al. (2022). Lauring et al. (2022) provided three periods within which various COVID-19 variants were identified—alpha (March 11 to July 3, 2021), Delta (July 4 to December 25, 2021), and Omicron (December 26, 2021, to January 14, 2022). Lauring et al. (2022) found that VE for two doses of mRNA vaccine to prevent hospitalization was 85% in the alpha period, 85% in the delta period, and 65% in the omicron period. They suggest that three doses rather than two would achieve the same level of VE of Omicron as the other two variants.

COVID-19 Vaccination Coverage Among Latinos

In August 2020, Latino Americans had 2.8 times the number of COVID-19 cases, 4.6 times higher rates of hospitalization, and 1.1 times higher mortality compared to non-Latino White Americans (CDC, n.d.-g). COVID-19 vaccination coverage shows inequalities by racial and ethnic group (Kriss et al., 2022). For instance, Kriss et al. (2022) found that while non-Latino White Americans had 59% vaccination coverage, non-Latino Black Americans had 46% and Latinos had 47% coverage by the end of April 2021. By the end of November 2021, however, national ≥1-dose COVID-19 vaccination coverage was similar for non-Latino Black adults (78.2%), Latino American adults (81.3%), and non-Latino White adults (78.7%). There was wide variation among Latino subgroups who had one or more doses, with South Americans having the highest vaccination rates (90.6%) and Mexicans the lowest vaccination rates (79.3%). However, the percentage of persons who had received a booster dose among those who completed their primary dose (s) was higher for non-Latino White Americans than non-Latino Black Americans, and lowest for Latino Americans (Figure 7.15).

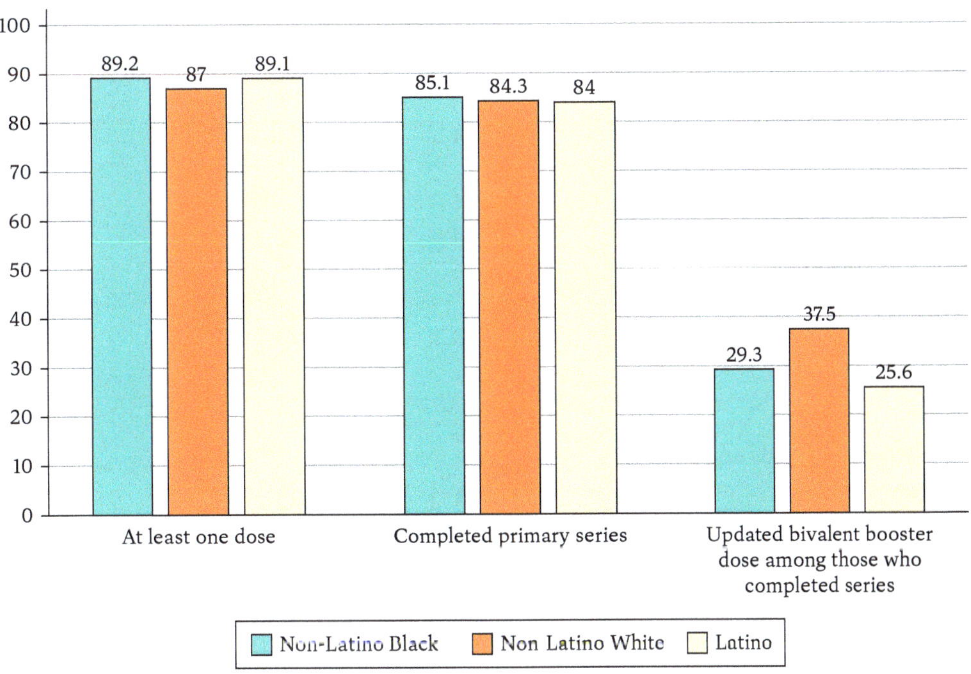

FIGURE 7.15 Estimated Percentage of People 18 Years and Older by Race/Ethnicity Reporting COVID-19 Vaccination, April 2021–March 2023.

In 2022–2023, among adults aged 18 years and older, COVID-19 unvaccinated rates were highest among non-Latino Black Americans (32.3%), followed by non-Latino White Americans (23.1%) and Latino Americans (16.8%; Link-Gelles et al., 2023).

According to several behavioral theories of health behavior, perceptions of vulnerability and susceptibility to a disease and behavioral intentions to prevent disease are valid predictors of whether one engages in preventive health behaviors. For example, Ajzen (1980) theorizes that behavioral intentions and attitudes are related to whether one engages in preventive health behaviors (theory of reasoned action and planned behavior), and Becker's (1974) health belief model that includes behavioral self-efficacy.

Kriss et al (2021) found that Latino Americans have the lowest confidence in COVID 19 vaccine safety (53.0 %), and lower percentages of a health provider recommending a COVID-19 vaccine (30.4 %) than non-Latino Black Americans and White Americans. However, Latino Americans have higher percentages of confidence that COVID-19 is important for protection and that almost all their family and friends have been vaccinated (75.7 and 74.3 %, respectively) than non-Latino White Americans, and that work, or school requires a COVID-19 vaccination (28.2 %). About 16 % of Latinos indicated that they had trouble in getting vaccinated (Table 7.15).

TABLE 7.15 Behavioral Intentions, Concerns, and Confidence in COVID-19 Vaccination

Items	Non-Latino Black % and CI	Non-Latino White % and CI	Latino % and CI
Concerned about COVID-19 disease.	39.7 (35.0–44.5)	27.7 (25.7–29.4)	27.8 (22.9–32.7)
Confidence in COVID-19 vaccine safety.	59.7 (54.8–64.6)	60.3 (58.3–62.3)	53.0 (47.56–58.7)
Confidence that COVID-19 vaccine is important to protect me (somewhat or very important responses).	85.4 (82.5–88.3)	69.6 (67.8–71.4)	75.7 (70.9–80.4)
Many or almost all of friends and family are vaccinated.	70.4 (66.0–74.7)	72.7 (71.0–74.4)	74.2 (69.4–79.0)
Health provider recommended I get COVID-19 vaccine.	52.4 (47.7–57.2)	53.7 (51.8–55.7)	49.2 (43.8–54.6)
Health provider recommended I get COVID-19 vaccine booster.	33.6 (29.1–38.1)	35.1 (33.2–36.9)	30.4 (25.6–35.3)
Work or school requires COVID-19 vaccination.	30.6 (26.0–35.3)	17.0 (15.5–18.5)	28.2 (23.5–32.9)
Not at all or little difficulty in getting vaccinated.	91.0 (88.6–93.5)	83.1 (81.6–84.6)	83.6 (79.5–87.7)
Had difficulty getting vaccinated.	9.0 (6.5–11.4)	16.9 (15.4–18.4)	16.4 (12.3–20.5)

Source: CDC (2021)

COVID-19 Infection and Risk for Hospitalization Among Latinos

The risk for COVID-19 infection varies within populations based on exposure levels, especially among essential and/or frontline workers (Chen et al., 2021; Cummings et al., 2022). For example, poultry and meat production plants were hardest hit initially where most workers were Latino or non-Latino Black (Klein & Shiro, 2020; Olayo-Méndez et al., 2021). After adjusting for covariates like health system, age, sex, body mass index, and smoking status, Shortreed et al. (2023) found lower relative risk for Latinos compared to non-Latino White Americans in the general population, and risk of severe COVID-19 infection 10% higher (Figure 7.16). The authors conclude that their results indicate increased incidence of severe COVID-19 among non-Latino Black Americans and Latino Americans is due to higher COVID-19 infection rates, not increased susceptibility to disease progression, and that social rather than biological factors are involved in COVID-19 inequalities observed among historically disadvantaged and marginalized population groups (Mackey et al., 2021; Tai et al., 2021).

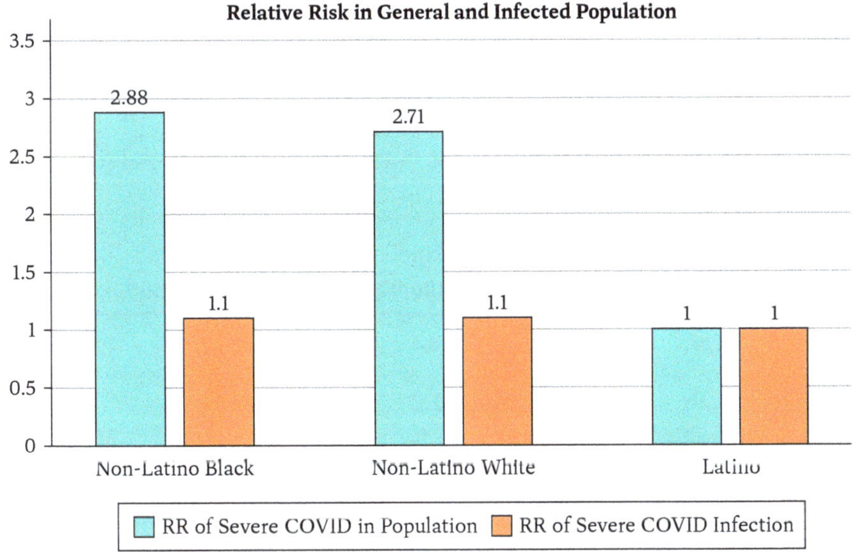

FIGURE 7.16 Relative Risk in the General and COVID-19–Infected population

Rodriguez-Diaz et al. (2020) examined COVID-19 infection and mortality rates in counties with at least a 17% Latino population. They found that COVID-19 cases were greater in Northeastern and Midwestern Latino counties (42% and 70%, respectively) and that COVID-19 deaths were greater in Midwestern Latino counties (≥17% Latino population). Additionally, COVID-19 diagnoses were associated with counties with greater monolingual Spanish speakers, higher employment rates, higher heart disease deaths, less social distancing, and number of days since the first reported case. The authors also note the heterogeneity of COVID-19 diagnoses and deaths among Latinos in various geographic regions, including the U.S.–Mexico border.

COVID-19 Mortality Inequalities Among Latinos

Among COVID-19 patients, Gross et al. (2020), found the relative risk (RR) of death for non-Latino Black Americans compared to non-Latino White Americans was 3.57, or 3.5 times the risk. For Latinos, findings showed that they experienced an 88% higher risk of death than non-Latino White patients (RR for Latinx vs. White was 1.88). Also, Rodriguez-Diaz et al. (2020) found that COVID-19 deaths were associated with household occupancy density, air pollution, employment, days since the first reported case, and age (fewer <35 years of age), and rates were higher among Latino Midwestern counties. Others have found similar results, with Latino Americans and non-Latino Black Americans disproportionately represented in the mortality data (Gold et al., 2020).

Further examining the heterogeneity of COVID-19 mortality rates among Latinos in the 10 largest states of the Latino population shows remarkable variation like that reported by Rodriguez-Diaz et al. (2020). Mortality due to COVID-19 was higher among Latino Americans compared to non-Latino White Americans, from a low of 36% higher mortality in Florida, to 278% higher mortality in California (CDC, n.d.-a) (Table 7.16). Across all 10 Latino population states, there was no state where the COVID-19 mortality rate was lower for non-Latino White Americans than Latino Americans. There is no Latino epidemiological paradox with respect to COVID-19 mortality.

TABLE 7.16 COVID-19 Age-Adjusted Mortality Rates in 10 Largest Latino Population States, 2018–2021

State	Primary Latino origin	Latino rate/100,000	Non-Latino rate/100,000	Mortality rate-ratio differences
New Mexico	Mexican	74.4	54.1	1.38
California	Mexican	81.3	29.2	2.78
Texas	Mexican	103.5	50.6	2.05
Arizona	Mexican	104.4	47.7	2.19
Nevada	Mexican	86.6	53.4	1.62
Florida	Cuban	54.5	40.1	1.36
Colorado	Mexican	81.1	32.9	2.47
New Jersey	Puerto Rican	89.3	48.3	1.85
New York	Puerto Rican	91.3	49.5	1.84
Illinois	Mexican	75.1	39.8	1.89

Source: CDC (n.d.-b)

For another regional focus, looking at the U.S.-Mexico border region shows higher COVID-19 mortality rates (crude rates) among Latinos residing in the U.S.-Mexico border region compared to non-border regions (CDC, n.d.-a) (Figure 7.17). Interestingly, COVID-19 mortality rates are lower for non-Latino White Americans and non-Latino Black Americans in the U.S.-Mexico border regions than in non-border regions, perhaps an indicator of systemic migration back to their original states.

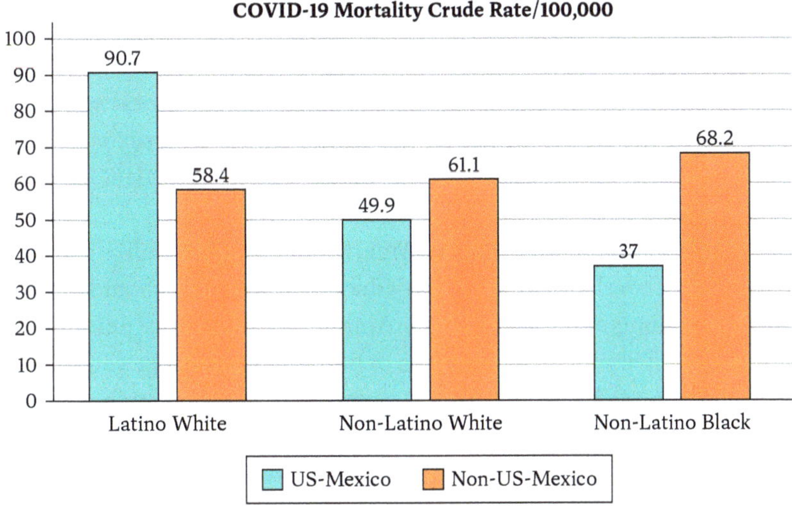

FIGURE 7.17 U.S.–Mexico Border Region COVID-19 Mortality Crude Rates

CHAPTER SUMMARY

Communicable diseases remain a public health priority and highlight the foundational inequalities in the social determinants of health. The intersection of poverty, gender, education, lack of access to health care, and race/ethnicity compounds the socioeconomic disadvantages experienced by Latino Americans and non-Latino Black Americans, which translates to increased morbidity and mortality from preventable diseases. HIV/AIDS and COVID-19 are prime examples.

Vaccine hesitancy is the result of many factors, including lack of knowledge regarding vaccine effectiveness, fear of unknown or new mRNA treatments, potential adverse side effects, and political indoctrination. In addition, deliberate misinformation fueled resistance to effective precautionary measures like wearing masks and social distancing in the case of COVID-19.

Sources of inequalities associated with increased morbidity and mortality among historically marginalized and disadvantaged populations are anchored in the unequal distribution of resources and racial/ethnic discrimination. Health inequalities are the result of the differential exposure, susceptibility, vulnerability, and treatment of Latinos within their social and built environments. The cumulative effect leads to increased burden of chronic and communicable diseases (Blumenshine et al., 2008).

Latino Americans of all ages have lower influenza vaccination coverage than non-Latino White Americans and non-Latino Black Americans and are therefore at higher risk for becoming infected and transmitting influenza to others. Latino children also have lower vaccination coverage for measles, mumps, and rubella; hepatitis B; varicella; and tetanus-diphtheria than either non-Latino White or non-Latino Black Americans.

The H1N1 or "Mexican flu" pandemic of 2009–2010 stigmatized Latinos of Mexican descent as a diseased population, rhetoric harking back to the early 20th century. H1N1 hospitalizations were higher for Mexican Americans than non-Latino White Americans and Black Americans. Moreover, H1N1 mortality among Latinos was higher than non-Latino White Americans.

HPV is known to cause several types of cancers, yet vaccination rates among Latino men and women are suboptimal, even though women have higher vaccination rates, with the highest rate among Puerto Rican women at 71%. In association with sexual practices and especially oral sex to preserve a women's virginity, increases in oral cancers have been observed. Additionally, other sexually transmitted infections like chlamydia, gonorrhea, and syphilis are more substantially more prevalent among Latino Americans than non-Latino White Americans.

Diagnoses of HIV infection among Mexican Americans are appreciably higher for those living in areas where there are higher levels of poverty, less education, less household income, and lower health insurance coverage than among non-Latino White Americans, especially among Latino men. Overall, the HIV epidemic has negatively impacted Latinos, with higher incidence rates, prevalence rates, and mortality rates than non-Latino White Americans. Among the 10-largest Latino population states, Latinos had excess HIV morbidity, with Latinos of Mexican descent and Puerto Rican descent having more than twice the excess HIV morbidity. Latinos of Mexican descent have lower HIV mortality compared to non-Latino White Americans, while Latinos of Puerto Rican descent have higher HIV mortality compared to non-Latino White Americans and Latinos of Mexican descent. Stark inequalities in the receipt of HIV medical care, retention in care and especially viral suppression suggest inadequate screening and linkage to HIV care among Latinos. Only 64% of Latinos with HIV infection achieved viral suppression, which is far lower than the national goal of 95% set for 2025–2030.

There are several important cultural influences that influence the context of risk among Latinos. Of primary importance is sexual silence, virginity beliefs that can influence risky sexual practices, behavioral double standards for men and women, *machismo*, and acculturation level, which is also involved in risk-taking behaviors.

The persistence of social inequalities among Latinos and other historically marginalized populations were revealed during the COVID-19 pandemic. Among Latinos, especially frontline workers, close working conditions and lack of prophylaxis led to increased infection, hospitalization, and death. Research has shown that Latinos have the lowest confidence in vaccine safety and lower percentages of having a physician recommend getting a COVID-19 vaccine.

Prior to COVID-19, Latino Americans were defined by their exceptional mortality differential, which was better than non-Latino White Americans and non-Latino Black Americans. However, COVID-19 reversed the epidemiological mortality paradox. Latinos had higher mortality from COVID-19 than non-Latino White Americans in the 10-largest Latino population states.

Taken together, Latinos and Latinos of Mexican descent show increased morbidity and mortality from several major communicable diseases compared to non-Latino White Americans. These health inequalities are the direct result of foundational inequalities among the various social determinants of health.

QUESTIONS TO CONSIDER

1. What are the differences in the preventive approaches to the H1N1 virus and COVID-19?
2. How does the politization of a disease make it more difficult to muster public health prevention and intervention programs?

3. Does the social determinants of health paradigm adequately explain the risk and vulnerability of historically marginalized populations to communicable disease?
4. What are several cultural factors that exert an influence on HIV risk reduction among Latinos?
5. How can the synthesis of social and cultural determinants better explain reasons for vaccine hesitancy?

SUGGESTED READINGS

Adimora, A. A., & Schoenbach, V. J. (2005). Social context, sexual networks, and racial disparities in rates of sexually transmitted infections. *The Journal of Infectious Diseases, 191*(Suppl. 1), S115–S122.

Blumenshine, P., Reingold, A., Egerter, S., Mockenhaupt, R., Braveman, P., & Marks, J. (2008). Pandemic influenza planning in the United States from a health disparities perspective. *Emerging Infectious Diseases, 14*(5), 709.

Cuan-Baltazar, J. Y., Muñoz-Perez, M. J., Robledo-Vega, C., Pérez-Zepeda, M. F., & Soto-Vega, E. (2020). Misinformation of COVID-19 on the internet: Infodemiology study. *JMIR Public Health and Surveillance*, 6(2), Article e18444.

De Jesus, M., & Williams, D. R. (2018). The care and prevention in the United States demonstration project: A call for more focus on the social determinants of HIV/AIDS. *Public Health Reports, 133*(Suppl. 2), 28S–33S.

Elam-Evans, L. D., Yankey, D., Singleton, J. A., Sterrett, N., Markowitz, L. E., Williams, C. L., Fredua, B., McNamara, L., & Stokley, S. (2020). National, regional, state, and selected local area vaccination coverage among adolescents aged 13–17 years—United States, 2019. *Morbidity and Mortality Weekly Report*, 69(33), 1109–1116.

Fortuna, L. R., Tolou-Shams, M., Robles-Ramamurthy, B., & Porche, M. V. (2020). Inequity and the disproportionate impact of COVID-19 on communities of color in the United States: The need for a trauma-informed social justice response. *Psychological Trauma: Theory, Research, Practice, and Policy, 12*(5), 443.

Galbraith, K. V., Lechuga, J., Jenerette, C. M., Moore, L. A. D., Palmer, M. H., & Hamilton, J. B. (2016). Parental acceptance and uptake of the HPV vaccine among African-Americans and Latinos in the United States: A literature review. *Social Science & Medicine, 159*, 116–126.

Marmot, M. (2017). Social justice, epidemiology and health inequalities. *European Journal of Epidemiology, 32*, 537–546.

O'Halloran, A. C., Holstein, R., Cummings, C., Kirley, P. D., Alden, N. B., Yousey-Hindes, K., Anderson, E. J., Ryan, P., Kim, S., Lynfield, R., McMullen, C., Bennett, N. M., Spina, N., Billing, L. M., Sutton, M., Schaffner, W., Keipp Talbot, H., Price, A., Fry, A., ... Garg, S. (2021). Rates of influenza-associated hospitalization, intensive care unit admission, and in-hospital death by race and ethnicity in the United States from 2009 to 2019. *JAMA Network Open*, 4(8), e2121880–e2121880.

Reiter, P. L., Pennell, M. L., Martinez, G. A., Perkins, R. B., & Katz, M. L. (2020). HPV vaccine coverage across Hispanic/Latinx subgroups in the United States. *Cancer Causes & Control, 31*, 905–914.

Rodriguez-Diaz, C. E., Guilamo-Ramos, V., Mena, L., Hall, E., Honermann, B., Crowley, J. S., Baral, S., Prado, G. J., Marzan-Rodriguez, M., Beyrer, C., Sullivan, P. S., & Millett, G. A. (2020). Risk for COVID 19 infection and death among Latinos in the United States: Examining heterogeneity in transmission dynamics. *Annals of Epidemiology, 52*, 46–53.

Schoch-Spana, M., Bouri, N., Rambhia, K. J., & Norwood, A. (2010). Stigma, health disparities, and the 2009 H1N1 influenza pandemic: How to protect Latino farmworkers in future health emergencies. *Biosecurity and Bioterrorism: Biodefense Strategy, Practice, and Science*, 8(3), 243–254.

REFERENCES

Adimora, A. A., & Schoenbach, V. J. (2005). Social context, sexual networks, and racial disparities in rates of sexually transmitted infections. *The Journal of Infectious Diseases, 191*(Suppl. 1), S115–S122.

Ajzen, I. (1980). *Understanding attitudes and predicting social behavior.* Englewood Cliffs.

Anandappa, M., Boakye, E. A., Li, W., Zeng, W., Rebmann, T., & Chang, J. J. (2018). Racial disparities in vaccination for seasonal influenza in early childhood. *Public Health, 158*, 1–8.

Anderson, L. M., Wood, D. L., & Sherbourne, C. D. (1997). Maternal acculturation and childhood immunization levels among children in Latino families in Los Angeles. *American Journal of Public Health, 87*(12), 2018–2021.

Antequera, A., Lawson, D. O., Noorduyn, S. G., Dewidar, O., Avey, M., Bhutta, Z. A., Chamberlain, C., Ellingwood, H., Francis, D., Funnell, S., Ghogomu, E., Greer-Smith, R., Horsley, T., Juando-Prat, C., Jull, J., Kristjansson, E., Little, J., Nicholls, S. G., Nkangu, M., ... Welch, V. (2021). Improving social justice in COVID-19 health research: Interim guidelines for reporting health equity in observational studies. *International Journal of Environmental Research and Public Health, 18*(17), 9357.

Aragones, A., Genoff, M., Gonzalez, C., Shuk, E., & Gany F. (2016). HPV vaccine and Latino immigrant parents: If they offer it, we will get it. *Journal of Immigrant and Minority Health, 18*, 1060–1065.

Aral, S. O., Adimora, A. A., & Fenton, K. A. (2008). Understanding and responding to disparities in HIV and other sexually transmitted infections in African Americans. *The Lancet, 372*(9635), 337–340.

Associated Press-NORC Center for Public Affairs Research. (2023, June 15). *Major declines in the public's confidence in science in the wake of the pandemic.* https://apnorc.org/projects/major-declines-in-the-publics-confidence-in-science-in-the-wake-of-the-pandemic/

Ayers, C. K., Kondo, K. K., Williams, B. E., Kansagara, D., Advani, S. M., Smith, M., ... & Saha, S. (2021). Disparities in H1N1 vaccination rates: a systematic review and evidence synthesis to inform COVID-19 vaccination efforts. *Journal of General Internal Medicine, 36*, 1734–1745.

Becker, M. H. (1974). The health belief model and sick role behavior. *Health Education Monographs, 2*(4), 409–419.

Bertozzi, S., Padian, N. S., Wegbreit, J., DeMaria, L. M., Feldman, B., Gayle, H., Gold, J., Grant, R., & Isbell, M. T. (2006). HIV/AIDS prevention and treatment. In D. T. Jamison, Joel, G. Breman, et al. (Eds.), *Disease control priorities in developing countries* (2nd ed., pp. 331–370). The World Bank.

Blacksher, E., & Lovasi, G. S. (2012). Place-focused physical activity research, human agency, and social justice in public health: Taking agency seriously in studies of the built environment. *Health & Place, 18*(2), 172–179.

Blumenshine, P., Reingold, A., Egerter, S., Mockenhaupt, R., Braveman, P., & Marks, J. (2008). Pandemic influenza planning in the United States from a health disparities perspective. *Emerging Infectious Diseases, 14*(5), 709–715.

Bodson, J., Warner, E. L., & Kepka, D. (2016). Moderate awareness and limited knowledge relating to cervical cancer, HPV, and the HPV vaccine among Hispanics/Latinos in Utah. *Health Promotion Practice, 17*(4), 548–556.

Burakoff, M. (2023, June 15). *Confidence in science fell in 2022 while political divides persisted, poll shows.* AP News. https://apnews.com/article/trust-science-medicine-social-survey-725ab3401f27900be6cc957eec52e45e

Campbell, J. C., Baty, M. L., Ghandour, R. M., Stockman, J. K., Francisco, L., & Wagman, J. (2008). The intersection of intimate partner violence against women and HIV/AIDS: A review. *International Journal of Injury Control and Safety Promotion, 15*(4), 221–231.

Centers for Disease Control and Prevention. (2009, October 9). Influenza vaccination coverage among children and adults—United States, 2008–2009 influenza season. *Morbidity and Mortality Weekly Report, 58*(39), 1091–1095. https://www.cdc.gov/mmwr/preview/mmwrhtml/mm5839a1.htm

Centers for Disease Control and Prevention. (2010a, January 22). Interim results: Influenza A (H1N1) 2009 monovalent vaccination coverage—United States, October–December 2009, 2010. *Morbidity and Mortal Weekly Report, 59*(2), 44–48.

Centers for Disease Control and Prevention. (2010b, February 16). *2009 H1N1 and seasonal influenza and Hispanic communities: Questions and answers.* https://www.cdc.gov/H1N1flu/qa_hispanic.

Centers for Disease Control and Prevention. (2010c, February 24). 2009 H1N1 Flu: Underlying health conditions among hospitalized adults and children. https://www.cdc.gov/H1N1flu/eip_underlying_conditions.htm

Centers for Disease Control and Prevention. (2010d, February 24). *Information on 2009 H1N1 impact by race and ethnicity.* https://www.cdc.gov/h1n1flu/race_ethnicity_qa.htm

Centers for Disease Control and Prevention. (2019). Social determinants of health among adults with diagnosed HIV infection, 2017. Part A: Census-tract level social determinants of health and diagnosed HIV infection—United States and Puerto Rico. Part B: County-level social determinants of health, selected care outcomes, and diagnosed HIV infection—41 states and the District of Columbia. *HIV Surveillance Supplemental Report, 24*(4). https://www.cdc.gov/hiv/pdf/library/reports/surveillance/cdc-hiv-surveillance-supplemental-report-vol-24-4.pdf

Centers for Disease Control and Prevention. (2022). *Sexually transmitted infections surveillance 2022.* Retrieved September 15, 2023, from https://www.cdc.gov/std/statistics/default.htm

Centers for Disease Control and Prevention. (2023a). Diagnoses of HIV infection in the United States and dependent areas, 2021. *HIV Surveillance Report, 34.* http://www.cdc.gov/hiv/library/reports/hiv-surveillance.html .

Centers for Disease Control and Prevention. (2023b). Behavioral and clinical characteristics of persons with diagnosed HIV infection—Medical Monitoring Project, United States, 2021 Cycle (June 2021–May 2022). *HIV Surveillance Special Report, 32.* https://www.cdc.gov/hiv/library/reports/hiv-surveillance.html

Centers for Disease Control and Prevention. (2023c). Estimated HIV incidence and prevalence in the United States, 2017–2021. *HIV Surveillance Supplemental Report, 28*(3). http://www.cdc.gov/hiv/library/reports/hiv-surveillance.html

Centers for Disease Control and Prevention. (2023d). Monitoring selected national HIV prevention and care objectives by using HIV surveillance data—United States and 6 dependent areas, 2021. *HIV Surveillance Supplemental Report, 28*(4). https://www.cdc.gov/hiv/library/reports/hiv-surveillance/vol-28-no-4/index.html

Centers for Disease Control and Prevention. (2023e). Social determinants of health among adults with diagnosed HIV infection in the United States and Puerto Rico, 2020. *HIV Surveillance Supplemental Report, 28*(2). http://www.cdc.gov/hiv/library/reports/hiv-surveillance.html

Centers for Disease Control and Prevention. (n.d.-a). CDC WONDER. Retrieved September 19, 2023 from https://wonder.cdc.gov/

Centers for Disease Control and Prevention. (n.d.-b). *National Center for Health Statistics. National Vital Statistics System, Mortality 2018–2021 on CDC WONDER Online Database, released in 2021. Data are from the Multiple Cause of Death Files, 2018–2021, as compiled from data provided by the 57 vital statistics jurisdictions through the Vital Statistics Cooperative Program.* Accessed at http://wonder.cdc.gov/ucd-icd10-expanded.html on Sep 6, 2023 5:04:25 PM

Centers for Disease Control and Prevention (n.d.-c). *HIV Mortality - 2021.* Retrieved September 20, 2023, from https://www.cdc.gov/hiv/library/slideSets/index.html

Centers for Disease Control and Prevention. (n.d.-d). HIV, Hepatitis, STD, TB, Social Determinants of Health Data. Accessed on September 21, 2023, from ttps://www.cdc.gov/nchhstp/Atlas/

Centers for Disease Control and Prevention. (n.d.-e). *About EHE.* Retrieved September 20, 2023, from https://www.cdc.gov/endhiv/about-ehe/index.html

Centers for Disease Control and Prevention. (n.d.-f). *COVID Data Tracker: Trends in demographic characteristics of people receiving COVID-19 Vaccinations in the United States.* Retrieved September 21, 2023, from https://covid.cdc.gov/covid-data-tracker/#vaccination-demographics-trends

Centers for Disease Control and Prevention. (n.d.-g). *COVID data tracker: Demographic trends of COVID-19 cases and deaths in the U.S. reported to CDC.* U.S. Department of Health and Human Services. Retrieved September 6, 2023, from https://covid.cdc.gov/covid-data-tracker/#demographics

Centers for Disease Control and Prevention. (n.d.-h). *HIV Infection Stage 3 (AIDS) - 2021.* Retrieved September 20, 2023, from https://www.cdc.gov/hiv/library/slideSets/index.html

Centers for Disease Control and Prevention. (2021, September 23). *For immunization managers: Adults.* https://www.cdc.gov/vaccines/imz-managers/coverage/covidvaxview/interactive/adults.html

Chando, S., Tiro, J. A., Harris, T. R., Kobrin, S., & Breen, N. (2013). Effects of socioeconomic status and health care access on low levels of human papillomavirus vaccination among Spanish-speaking Hispanics in California. *American Journal of Public Health, 103*(2), 270–272.

Chao, C. R., Xu, L., Cannizzaro, N., Bronstein, D., Choi, Y., Riewerts, R., Mittman, B., Zimmerman, R. K., Gilkey, M., Glenn, B., Shen, E., Hsu, C., & Hahn, E. E. (2022). Trends in HPV vaccine administration and HPV vaccine coverage in children by race/ethnicity and socioeconomic status during the COVID 19 pandemic in an integrated health care system in California. *Vaccine, 40*(46), 6575–6580. https://doi.org/10.1016/j.vaccine.2022.09.073

Chen, Y. H., Glymour, M., Riley, A., Balmes, J., Duchowny, K., Harrison, R., Matthay, E., & Bibbins-Domingo, K. (2021). Excess mortality associated with the COVID-19 pandemic among Californians 18–65 years of age, by occupational sector and occupation: March through November 2020. *PloS One, 16*(6), Article e0252454.

Chu, S. Y., Barker, L. E., & Smith, P. J. (2004). Racial/ethnic disparities in preschool immunizations: United States, 1996–2001. *American Journal of Public Health, 94*(6), 973–977.

Clark, S. E., Bledsoe, M. C., & Harrison, C. J. (2022). The role of social media in promoting vaccine hesitancy. *Current Opinion in Pediatrics, 34*(2), 156–162.

Cuan-Baltazar, J. Y., Muñoz-Perez, M. J., Robledo-Vega, C., Pérez-Zepeda, M. F., & Soto-Vega, E. (2020). Misinformation of COVID-19 on the internet: Infodemiology study. *JMIR Public Health and Surveillance, 6*(2), Article e18444.

Cummings, K. J., Beckman, J., Frederick, M., Harrison, R., Nguyen, A., Snyder, R., Chan, E., Gibb, K., Rodriguez, A., Wong, J., Murray, E. L., Jain, s., & Vergara, X. (2022). Disparities in COVID-19 fatalities among working Californians. *PLoS One, 17*(3), Article e0266058.

Daley, E. M., Vamos, C. A., Thompson, E. L., Zimet, G. D., Rosberger, Z., Merrell, L., & Kline, N. S. (2017). The feminization of HPV: How science, politics, economics and gender norms shaped U.S. HPV vaccine implementation. *Papillomavirus Research, 3*, 142–148.

De Jesus, M., & Williams, D. R. (2018). The care and prevention in the United States demonstration project: A call for more focus on the social determinants of HIV/AIDS. *Public Health Reports, 133*(Suppl. 2), 28S–33S.

de Lamballerie, X., & Gould, E.A. (2009). With reference to Mexican flu. *Influenza and Other Respiratory Viruses, 3*(5), 203. https://doi.org/10.1111/j.1750-2659.2009.00097.x

Deardorff, J., Tschann, J. M., Flores, E., & Ozer, E. J. (2010). Sexual values and risky sexual behaviors among Latino youths. *Perspectives on Sexual and Reproductive Health, 42*(1), 23–32.

DeCuir, J. (2023). Effectiveness of monovalent mRNA COVID-19 vaccination in preventing COVID-19-associated invasive mechanical ventilation and death among immunocompetent adults during the Omicron variant period—IVY Network, 19 U.S. States, February 1, 2022–January 31, 2023. *Morbidity and Mortality Weekly Report, 72*(17), 463–468.

Dhama, K., Sharun, K., Tiwari, R., Dhawan, M., Emran, T. B., Rabaan, A. A., & Alhumaid, S. (2021). COVID-19 vaccine hesitancy–reasons and solutions to achieve a successful global vaccination campaign to tackle the ongoing pandemic. *Human Vaccines & Immunotherapeutics, 17*(10), 3495–3499.

Dykens, J. A., Peterson, C. E., Holt, H. K., & Harper, D. M. (2023). Gender neutral HPV vaccination programs: Reconsidering policies to expand cancer prevention globally. *Frontiers in Public Health, 11*, Article 1067299.

Elam-Evans, L. D., Yankey, D., Singleton, J. A., Sterrett, N., Markowitz, L. E., Williams, C. L., Fredua, B., McNamara, L. A., Stokley, S., & Singleton, J. A. (2021). National, regional, state, and selected local area vaccination coverage among adolescents aged 13–17 years—United States, 2019. *Morbidity and Mortality Weekly Report, 69*(33), 1109–1116.

Enders, A. M., Uscinski, J. E., Klofstad, C., & Stoler, J. (2020). *The different forms of COVID-19 misinformation and their consequences.* The Harvard Kennedy School Misinformation Review.

Estrada, A. L. (1998). Drug use and HIV risks among African American, Mexican American, and Puerto Rican drug injectors. *Journal of Psychoactive Drugs, 30*(3), 247–253.

Filkuková, P., Ayton, P., Rand, K., & Langguth, J. (2021). What should I trust? Individual differences in attitudes to conflicting information and misinformation on COVID-19. *Frontiers in Psychology, 12*, Article 588478.

Fortuna, L. R., Tolou-Shams, M., Robles-Ramamurthy, B., & Porche, M. V. (2020). Inequity and the disproportionate impact of COVID-19 on communities of color in the United States: The need for a trauma-informed social justice response. *Psychological Trauma: Theory, Research, Practice, and Policy, 12*(5), 443.

Gaglani, M., Pruszynski, J., Murthy, K., Clipper, L., Robertson, A., Reis, M., Chung, J. R., Piedra, P. A., Avadhanula, V., Nowalk, M. P., Zimmerman, R. K., Jackson, M. L., Jackson, L. A., Petrie, J. G., Ohmit, S. E., Monto, A. S., McLean, H. Q., Belongia, E. A., Fry, A. M., & Flannery, B. (2016). Influenza vaccine effectiveness against 2009 pandemic influenza A (H1N1) virus differed by vaccine type during 2013–2014 in the United States. *The Journal of Infectious Diseases, 213*(10), 1546–1556.

Galbraith, K. V., Lechuga, J., Jenerette, C. M., Moore, L. A. D., Palmer, M. H., & Hamilton, J. B. (2016). Parental acceptance and uptake of the HPV vaccine among African-Americans and Latinos in the United States: A literature review. *Social Science & Medicine, 159*, 116–126.

Glenn, B. A., Tsui, J., Coronado, G. D., Fernandez, M. E., Savas, L. S., Taylor, V. M., & Bastani, R. (2015). Understanding HPV vaccination among Latino adolescent girls in three U.S. regions. *Journal of Immigrant and Minority Health, 17*, 96–103.

Gold, J. A., Rossen, L. M., Ahmad, F. B., Sutton, P., Li, Z., Salvatore, P. P., Coyle, J. P., DeCuir, J., Baack, B. N., Durant, T. M., Dominguez, K. L., Henley, S. J., Annor, F. B., Fuld, J., Dee, D. L., Bhattaria, A., & Jackson, B. R. (2020). Race, ethnicity, and age trends in persons who died from COVID-19—United States, May–August 2020. *Morbidity and Mortality Weekly Report, 69*(42), 1517–1521.

Gross, C. P., Essien, U. R., Pasha, S., Gross, J. R., Wang, S. Y., & Nunez-Smith, M. (2020). Racial and ethnic disparities in population-level COVID-19 mortality. *Journal of General Internal Medicine, 35*, 3097–3099.

Gurman, T., & Borzekowski, D. L. (2004). Condom use among Latino college students. *Journal of American College Health, 52*(4), 169–178.

Hadler, J. L., Yousey-Hindes, K., Perez, A., Anderson, E. J. Bargsten, M., Bohm, S. R., Hill, M., Hogan, B., Laidler, M., Lindergren, M. L., Lung, K. L., Mermel, E., Miller, L., Morin, C., Parker, H., Zansky, S. M., & Chaves, S. C. (2016, February 12). Influenza-related hospitalization and poverty levels—United States, 2020. *Morbidity and Mortality Weekly Report, 65*(5), 101–105.

Harling, G., Subramanian, S. V., Bärnighausen, T., & Kawachi, I. (2013). Socioeconomic disparities in sexually transmitted infections among young adults in the United States: Examining the interaction between income and race/ethnicity. *Sexually Transmitted Diseases, 40*(7), 575.

Hatton, C. R., Barry, C. L., Levine, A. S., McGinty, E. E., & Han, H. (2022). American trust in science & institutions in the time of COVID-19. *Daedalus, 151*(4), 83–97.

Herbst, J. H., Kay, L. S., Passin, W. F., Lyles, C. M., Crepaz, N., & Marín, B. V. (2007). A Systematic review and meta-analysis of behavioral interventions to reduce HIV risk behaviors of Hispanics in the United States and Puerto Rico. *AIDS and Behavior, 11*, 25–47. https://doi.org/10.1007/s10461-006-9151-1

Hill, H. A., Elam-Evans, L. D., Yankey, D., Singleton, J. A., & Kang, Y. (2017). Vaccination coverage among children aged 19–35 months—United States, 2016. *Morbidity and Mortality Weekly Report, 66*(43), 1171.

Hill, H. A., Singleton, J. A., Yankey, D., Elam-Evans, L. D., Pingali, S. C., & Kang Y. (2019). Vaccination coverage by age 24 months among children born in 2015 and 2016—National Immunization Survey-child, United States, 2016, 2018. *Morbidity and Mortality Weekly Report, 68*(41), 913–918.

Hudson, A., & Montelpare, W. J. (2021). Predictors of vaccine hesitancy: Implications for COVID-19 public health messaging. *International Journal of Environmental Research and Public Health, 18*(15), 8054.

Jackson, M. L., Chung, J. R., Jackson, L. A., Phillips, C. H., Benoit, J., Monto, A. S., Martin, E. T., Belongia, E. A., McLean, H. Q., Gaglani, M., Murthy, K., Zimmerman, R., Nowalk, M. P., Fry, A. M., & Flannery, B. (2017). Influenza vaccine effectiveness in the United States during the 2015–2016 season. *New England Journal of Medicine, 377*(6), 534–543.

Khosa, L. A., Meyer, J. C., Motshwane, F. M., Dochez, C., & Burnett, R. J. (2022). Vaccine hesitancy drives low human papillomavirus vaccination coverage in girls attending public schools in South Africa. *Frontiers in Public Health, 10*, 860809.

Kim, Y., Zhong, W., Jehn, M., & Walsh, L. (2015). Public risk perceptions and preventive behaviors during the 2009 H1N1 influenza pandemic. Disaster medicine and public health preparedness, 9(2), 145–154.

Klein, A., & Shiro, A. G. (2020, October 1). *The COVID-19 recession hit Latino workers hard. Here's what we need to do.* Brookings Institute. https://www.brookings.edu/articles/the-covid-19-recession-hit-latino-workers-hard-heres-what-we-need-to-do/

Kriss, J. L., Hung, M. C., Srivastav, A., Black, C. L., Lindley, M. C., Lee, J. T., Koppaka, R., Tsai, Y., Lu, P.-J., Yankey, D., Elam-Evans, L. D., & Singleton, J. A. (2022). COVID-19 vaccination coverage, by race and ethnicity—national immunization survey adult COVID module, United States, December 2020–November 2021. *Morbidity and Mortality Weekly Report, 71*(23), 757–763.

Kriss, J.L, Hung, M.C., Srivastav, A., Black, C.L., Lu, P.J., Yankey, D., Elam-Evans, L.D., & Singleton, J.A. (2021). *Intent to receive COVID-19 vaccine and behavioral and social drivers of vaccination by race and ethnicity, National Immunization Survey Adult COVID Module — United States, October 31–December 31, 2021.* Retrieved on October 1, 2023, from: https://www.cdc.gov/vaccines/imz-managers/coverage/covidvaxview/pubs-resources/intent-receive-covid19-vaccine-behavioral-social-drivers.html

Laumann, E. O., & Youm, Y. (1999). Racial/ethnic group differences in the prevalence of sexually transmitted diseases in the United States: A network explanation. *Sexually Transmitted Diseases, 25*(5), 250–261.

Lauring, A. S., Tenforde, M. W., Chappell, J. D., Gaglani, M., Ginde, A. A., Mcneal, T., Ghamande, S., Douin, D. J., Talbot, H. K., Casey, J. D., Mohr, N. M., Zepeski, A., Shapiro, N. I., Gibbs, K. W., Files, D. C., Hager, D. N., Sheju, A., Prekker, M. E., Erickson, H. L., Exline, M. C., ... Peltan, I. D. (2022). Clinical severity of, and effectiveness of mRNA vaccines against, COVID-19 from omicron, delta, and alpha SARS-CoV-2 variants in the United States: Prospective observational study. *BMJ, 376*, Article e069761. https://doi.org/10.1136/bmj-2021-069761

Link-Gelles, R., Weber, Z. A., Reese, S. E., Payne, A. B., Gaglani, M., Adams, K., Kharbanda, A. B., Natarajan, K., DeSilva, M. B., Dascomb, K., Irving, S. A., Klein, N. P., Grannis, S. J., Ong, T. C., Embi, P. J., Dunne, M. M., Dickerson, M., McEvoy, C., Andorfer, J., ... Tenforde, M. W. (2023). Estimates of bivalent mRNA vaccine durability in preventing COVID-19–associated hospitalization and critical illness among adults with and without immunocompromising conditions—VISION Network, September 2022–April 2023. *Morbidity and Mortality Weekly Report, 72*(21), 579–588.

Lopez, L., Hart, L. H., & Katz, M. H. (2021). Racial and ethnic health disparities related to COVID-19. *JAMA, 325*(8), 719–720.

Mackey, K., Ayers, C. K., Kondo, K. K., Saha, S., Advani, S. M., Young, S., Spencer, H., Rusek, M., Anderson, J., Veazie, S., Smith, M., & Kansagara, D. (2021). Racial and ethnic disparities in COVID-19–related infections, hospitalizations, and deaths: A systematic review. *Annals of Internal Medicine, 174*(3), 362–373.

Marin, B. V., Gomez, C. A., & Tschann, J. M. (1993). Condom use among Hispanic men with secondary female sexual partners. *Public Health Reports, 108*(6), 742.

Marmot, M. (2017). Social justice, epidemiology and health inequalities. *European Journal of Epidemiology, 32*, 537–546.

Martinez, M. L., & Coles, S. (2020). Addressing immunization health disparities. *Primary Care: Clinics in Office Practice, 47*(3), 483–495.

McLean, H. Q., Thompson, M. G., Sundaram, M. E., Kieke, B. A., Gaglani, M., Murthy, K., Piedra, P. A., Zimmerman, R. K., Nowalk, M. P., Raviotta, J. M., Jackson, M. L., Jackson, L., Ohmit, S. E., Petrie, J. G., Monto, A. S., Meece, J. K., Thaker, S. N., clippard, J. R., Spencer, S. M., ... Belongia, E. A. (2015). Influenza vaccine effectiveness in the United States during 2012–2013: Bariable protection by age and virus type. *The Journal of Infectious Diseases, 211*(10), 1529–1540.

McNeely, C. L., Schintler, L. A., & Stabile, B. (2020). Social determinants and COVID-19 disparities: Differential pandemic effects and dynamics. *World Medical & Health Policy, 12*(3), 206–217.

Messerly, M. (2023, September 21). *"I can't believe we're talking about polio": Health experts are sounding the alarm over the anti-vaccine movement's rise.* Politico. https://www.politico.com/news/2023/09/21/covid-vaccines-science-2024-election-00116520

Morales-Campos, D. Y., Flores, B. E., Donovan, E., Burdick, S., Parra-Medina, D., & Kahn, J. A. (2022). A qualitative descriptive study of providers' perspectives on human papillomavirus vaccine administration among Latino/a adolescents in South Texas clinics: Barriers and facilitators. *BMC Public Health, 22*(1), 1–11.

Muric, G., Wu, Y., & Ferrara, E. (2021). COVID-19 vaccine hesitancy on social media: Building a public Twitter data set of antivaccine content, vaccine misinformation, and conspiracies. *JMIR Public Health and Surveillance*, 7(11), Article e30642.

National Cancer Institute. (2023, October 18). *HPV and cancer.* Retrieved November 5, 2023, from https://www.cancer.gov/about-cancer/causes-prevention/risk/infectious-agents/hpv-and-cancer

National Center for Health Statistics (2021a). *Health, United States, (2020–2021): Table (VaxTn).* Hyattsville, MD. Available from: https://www.cdc.gov/nchs/hus/data-finder.htm

National Center for Health Statistics (2021b). *Health, United States, (2020–2021): Table (VaxCh).* Hyattsville, MD. Available from: https://www.cdc.gov/nchs/hus/data-finder.htm

Niederhauser, V. P., & Stark, M. (2005). Narrowing the gap in childhood immunization disparities. *Pediatric Nursing, 31*(5).

Noonan, A. S., Velasco-Mondragon, H. E., & Wagner, F. A. (2016). Improving the health of African Americans in the USA: An overdue opportunity for social justice. *Public Health Reviews, 37*, 1–20.

O'Halloran, A. C., Holstein, R., Cummings, C., Kirley, P. D., Alden, N. B., Yousey-Hindes, K., Anderson, E. J., Ryan, P., Kim, S., Lynfield, R., McMullen, C., Bennett, N. M., Spina, N., Billing, L. M., Sutton, M., Schaffner, W., Talbot, H. K., Price, A., Fry, A. M., ... Garg, S. (2021). Rates of influenza-associated hospitalization, intensive care unit admission, and in-hospital death by race and ethnicity in the United States from 2009 to 2019. *JAMA Network Open, 4*(8), e2121880–e2121880.

Ohmit, S. E., Thompson, M. G., Petrie, J. G., Thaker, S. N., Jackson, M. L., Belongia, E. A., Zimmerman, R. K., Gaglani, M., Lamerato, L., Spencer, S. M., Jackson, L., Meece, J. K., Nowalk, M. P., Song, J., Zervos, M., Cheng, P.-Y., Rinaldo, C. R., Clipper, L., ... Monto, A. S. (2014). Influenza vaccine effectiveness in the 2011–2012 season: Protection against each circulating virus and the effect of prior vaccination on estimates. *Clinical Infectious Diseases, 58*(3), 319–327.

Olayo-Méndez, A., Vidal De Haymes, M., García, M., & Cornelius, L. J. (2021). Essential, disposable, and excluded: The experience of Latino immigrant workers in the U.S. during COVID-19. *Journal of Poverty, 25*(7), 612–628.

Quinn, S. C., Kumar, S., Freimuth, V. S., Musa, D., Casteneda-Angarita, N., & Kidwell, K. (2011). Racial disparities in exposure, susceptibility, and access to health care in the U.S. H1N1 influenza pandemic. *American Journal of Public Health, 101*(2), 285–293.

Reiter, P. L., Brewer, N. T., Gilkey, M. B., Katz, M. L., Paskett, E. D., & Smith, J. S. (2014). Early adoption of the human papillomavirus vaccine among Hispanic adolescent males in the United States. *Cancer, 120*, 3200–3207

Reiter, P. L., Pennell, M. L., Martinez, G. A., Perkins, R. B., & Katz, M. L. (2020). HPV vaccine coverage across Hispanic/Latinx subgroups in the United States. *Cancer Causes & Control, 31*, 905–914.

Robinson, C. L., Bernstein, H., Poehling, K., Romero, J. R., & Szilagyi, P. (2020). Advisory Committee on Immunization Practices recommended immunization schedule for children and adolescents aged 18 years or younger—United States, 2020. *Morbidity and Mortality Weekly Report, 69*(5), 130–132.

Rodriguez-Diaz, C. E., Guilamo-Ramos, V., Mena, L., Hall, E., Honermann, B., Crowley, J. S., Baral, S., Prado, G. J., Marzan-Rodriguez, M., Beyrer, C., Sullivan, P. S., & Millett, G. A. (2020). Risk for COVID 19 infection and death among Latinos in the United States: Examining heterogeneity in transmission dynamics. *Annals of Epidemiology, 52*, 46–53.

Rubin, G. J., Amlôt, R., Page, L., & Wessely, S. (2009). Public perceptions, anxiety, and behaviour change in relation to the swine flu outbreak: Cross sectional telephone survey. *BMJ, 339*. https://doi.org/10.1136/bmj.b2651

Ruger, J. P. (2004). Health and social justice. *The Lancet, 364*(9439), 1075–1080.

Saraiya, M., Unger, E. R., Thompson, T. D., Lynch, C. F., Hernandez, B. Y., Lyu, C. W., Steinau, M., Watson, M., Wilkinson, E. J., Hopenhayn, C., Copeland, G., Cozen, W., Peters, E. S., Huang, Y., Saber, M. S., Altekruse, S., & Goodman, M. T. (2015). HPV Typing of Cancers Workgroup. U.S. assessment of HPV types in cancers: Implications for current and 9-valent HPV vaccines. *Journal of the National Cancer Institute, 107*(6), Article djv086. https://doi.org/10.1093/jnci/djv086

Sattenspiel, L., & Castillo-Chavez, C. (1990). Environmental context, social interactions, and the spread of HIV. *American Journal of Human Biology, 2*(4), 397–417.

Schoch-Spana, M., Bouri, N., Rambhia, K. J., & Norwood, A. (2010). Stigma, health disparities, and the 2009 H1N1 influenza pandemic: How to protect Latino farmworkers in future health emergencies. *Biosecurity and Bioterrorism: Biodefense Strategy, Practice, and Science, 8*(3), 243–254.

Shortreed, S. M., Gray, R., Akosile, M. A., Walker, R. L., Fuller, S., Temposky, L., Fortmann, s. P., Albertson-Junkans, L., Floyd, J. S., Bayliss, E. A., Harrington, L. B., Lee, M. H., & Dublin, S. (2023). Increased COVID-19 infection risk drives racial and ethnic disparities in severe COVID-19 outcomes. *Journal of Racial and Ethnic Health Disparities, 10*(1), 149–159.

Sibthorpe, B. (1992). The social construction of sexual relationships as a determinant of HIV risk perception and condom use among injection drug users. *Medical Anthropology Quarterly*, 6(3), 255–270.

Simula, E. R., Manca, M. A., Noli, M., Jasemi, S., Ruberto, S., Uzzau, S., Rubino, S., Manca, P., Sechi, L. A., & Sechi, L. A. (2022). Increased presence of antibodies against type I interferons and human endogenous retrovirus W in intensive care unit COVID-19 patients. *Microbiology Spectrum*, *10*(4), Article e0128022.

Stine, G. J. (2014). *AIDS Update 2014: An annual survey of acquired immune deficiency syndrome*. McGraw-Hill Education.

Strathdee, S. A., & Vlahov, D. (2001). The effectiveness of needle exchange programs: A review of the science and policy. *AIDScience*, *1*(16), 1–33.

Tai, D. B. G., Shah, A., Doubeni, C. A., Sia, I. G., & Wieland, M. L. (2021). The disproportionate impact of COVID-19 on racial and ethnic minorities in the United States. *Clinical Infectious Diseases*, *72*(4), 703–706.

Teitelman, A. M., Ratcliffe, S. J., Morales-Aleman, M. M., & Sullivan, C. M. (2008). Sexual relationship power, intimate partner violence, and condom use among minority urban girls. *Journal of Interpersonal Violence*, *23*(12), 1694–1712.

Tenforde, M. W., Self, W. H., Gaglani, M., Ginde, A. A., Douin, D. J., Talbot, H. K., Casey, J. D., Mohr, N. M., Zepeski, A., McNeal, T., Ghamande, S., Gibbs, K. W., Files, D. C., Hager, D., Sheju, A., Prekker, M. E., Frosch, A. E., Gong, M. N., Monhamed, A., ... Johnson, N. J. (2022). IVY Network. Effectiveness of mRNA vaccination in preventing COVID-19–associated invasive mechanical ventilation and death—United States, March 2021–January 2022. *Morbidity and Mortality Weekly Report*, *71*, 459–465. https://doi.org/10.15585/mmwr.mm7112e1

Troiano, G., & Nardi, A. (2021). Vaccine hesitancy in the era of COVID-19. *Public Health*, *194*, 245–251.

Vigsø, O. (2010). Naming is framing: Swine flu, new flu, and A (H1N1). *Observatorio*, *4*(3).

Vlahov, D., Des Jarlais, D. C., Goosby, E., Hollinger, P. C., Lurie, P. G., Shriver, M. D., & Strathdee, S. A. (2001). Needle exchange programs for the prevention of human immunodeficiency virus infection: Epidemiology and policy. *American Journal of Epidemiology*, *154*(12), S70–S77.

Walker, T. Y., Elam-Evans, L. D., Yankey, D. Markowitz, L. E., Williams, C. L., Fredua, B., Singleton, J. A., & Stokley, S. (2019). National, regional, state, and selected local area vaccination coverage among adolescents aged 13–17 years—United States, 2018. *Morbidity and Mortality Weekly Report*, *68*, 718–723

Wilson, L., Rubens-Augustson, T., Murphy, M., Jardine, C., Crowcroft, N., Hui, C., & Wilson, K. (2018). Barriers to immunization among newcomers: A systematic review. *Vaccine*, *36*(8), 1055–1062.

Figure Credits

Fig. 7.1: Adapted from Philip Blumenshine, Arthur Reingold, Susan Egerter, Robin Mockenhaupt, Paula Braveman, and James Marks, "Sources of Inequalities associated with Increased Morbidity and Mortality," Pandemic influenza planning in the United States from a health disparities perspective, 2008.

Fig. 7.4: Centers for Disease Control and Prevention, "H1N1 Hospitalization Rates by Race/Ethnicity, 2009-2010," https://www.cdc.gov/H1N1flu/race_ethnicity_qa.htm, 2010.

Fig. 7.7: Centers for Disease Control and Prevention, "Chlamydia Rates of Reported Cases per 100,000 by Race/Hispanic Ethnicity and Sex, United States, 2021," https://www.cdc.gov/std/statistics/2021/, 2021.

Fig. 7.8: Centers for Disease Control and Prevention, "Gonorrhea Rate of Reported Cases per 100,000 by Race/Hispanic Ethnicity and Sex," https://www.cdc.gov/std/statistics/2021/, 2021.

Fig. 7.9: Centers for Disease Control and Prevention, "Primary & Secondary Syphilis Rates of Reported Cases per 100,000 by Race/Hispanic Ethnicity and Sex," https://www.cdc.gov/std/statistics/2021/, 2021.

Fig. 7.12: CDC, "Diagnoses of HIV Infection among Hispanic/Latino/a Adults and Adolescents, by Sex and Place of Birth, 2018—United States and 6 Dependent Areas," HIV Surveillance Report, 2020.

CHAPTER 8

Health Status and Major Chronic Disease Inequalities Among Mexican Americans

LEARNING OBJECTIVES

- What are some health care inequalities that Mexican Americans encounter?
- Describe the general health status of Mexican Americans compared to non-Latino Black Americans and non-Latino White Americans.
- What are some mental health inequalities found among Mexican Americans?
- What are three cancer inequalities found among Mexican Americans?
- What are some factors in persons not obtaining a vaccination for HPV?
- Compare and contrast the prevalence of STIs among Mexican Americans, non-Latino Black Americans, and non-Latino White Americans. What are some factors that may contribute to observed differences?
- Describe the HIV continuum of care. How do Mexican Americans compare to non-Latino White Americans and non-Latino Black Americans in each of the areas?
- What is the overarching national goal of the "Ending the HIV Epidemic in the United States" initiative?
- How did COVID-19 exacerbate the social determinants of health?
- Why were Mexican Americans more at risk than non-Latino White Americans for COVID-19 infection and mortality?

Past research has clearly demonstrated that (a) the Latino mortality paradox exists for all-cause mortality, (b) the Latino mortality paradox is driven primarily by Latinos of Mexican descent, and (c) selective migration is the hypothesis best supported by available data.

Latinos of Mexican descent exhibit lower all-cause mortality rates than other Latino subgroups, non-Latino White Americans, and non-Latino Black Americans (see Chapter 5). Does the paradox also apply to specific morbidity characteristics among Latinos? For example, are there observed Latino inequalities relative to non-Latino White Americans for specific chronic diseases like diabetes mellitus, gallbladder disease, and liver disease? Are certain types of cancers more prevalent among Mexican Americans than non-Latino White Americans? Additionally, does acculturation level influence important chronic disease risk factors? In this chapter, several important modifiable risk factors are examined in comparison to non-Latino White Americans and non-Latino Black Americans. Further, an examination of incidence, prevalence, morbidity, and mortality differences for noncommunicable and communicable diseases may assist in discerning patterns or trends that may or may not support a Latino morbidity paradox.

The conflation of poor health status with poverty, educational attainment, gender, and race/ethnicity is at the core of health inequities in the United States, especially among non-Latino Black Americans and some Latino subgroups, like Puerto Ricans. However, the health status of Latinos of Mexican descent continues to present a paradox. Intersectionality analyses show how socioeconomically disadvantaged groups within the larger Latino population suffer from poorer health status than their healthier Latino counterparts.

Health Status Characteristics Among Latinos

In general, morbidity and mortality characteristics of Mexican Americans are better than non-Latino White Americans and show lower rates of morbidity and mortality than non-Latino Black Americans who have similar socioeconomic status. More than 2 decades ago, Vega and Amaro (2002) described the health prognosis of Latinos as "uncertain" given changes in public health policy that limit health care access of undocumented Latino immigrants, the number of second- and third-generation Latino youth engaging in behaviors that place them at risk for adverse health consequences, and the overall influence of acculturation and lived experiences on health and psychological well-being of Latinos. There is an overall mortality paradox among Latinos, especially among those of Mexican descent (Abraido-Lanza et al., 1999). Nevertheless, Latinos do have higher mortality rates than non-Latino White Americans for a host of obesity-related diseases (Hales et al., 2020). There is also greater morbidity for diseases like COVID-19, HIV/AIDS, diabetes mellitus, end-stage renal disease (ESRD), and cancer of the cervix, stomach, and gallbladder (Macias Gil et al., 2020; Velasco-Mondragon et al., 2016). In addition, Latinos tend to have lower vaccination rates for preventable communicable diseases, like measles, pertussis, influenza, and COVID-19 (Adorador et al., 2011; Herrera et al., 2001; Khubchandani et al., 2021; Lu et al., 2015). Moreover, Latino children have higher rates of infectious respiratory diseases than non-Latino White children and higher rates of asthma and obesity in the U.S.–Mexico border region, which increases their vulnerability to chronic diseases (De Cosio & Boadella, 1999; Jones et al., 2023; Shen et al., 2016; Sumaya, 1991).

Inequalities in Health Care Access

Numerous studies have shown that Latinos, especially Latinos of Mexican descent, have inequalities in health care access (Parchman & Byrd, 2001; Vega & Amaro, 2002; Velasco-Mondragon et al., 2016). Historically, Latinos of Mexican descent have been disadvantaged relative to non-Latino White Americans in access to quality health care (Bruhn & Fuentes, 1977; Roberts & Lee, 1980). This social determinant is enhanced by having health insurance coverage, having a regular source of health care, and utilization of health providers. However, Latino health care barriers include (a) cost of care and prescriptions, (b) institutional barriers, like hours of available service and lack of cultural competency, and (c) provider-related barriers, like the inability to speak Spanish (as discussed in Chapter 4).

Enabling factors predictive of health care utilization include health insurance coverage, having a regular source of health care, and cost of care (Phillips et al., 1998). It is well-established that economic stability influences health care utilization in predicted directions, with those living in poverty and having lower educational attainment and being unemployed lacking a usual source of health care, health insurance coverage, and financial means to pay for prescription medications. For example, Rodríguez et al. (2009) found that undocumented Latino immigrants had significantly lower percentages of health insurance coverage (37% vs. 77% for U.S.-born) and usual source of care (58% vs. 79% U.S.-born).

Health Insurance Coverage

Of course, one of the major determinants of health care utilization is whether a person has health insurance coverage and a regular source of health care. Historically, Latino Americans have been found to have lower rates of health insurance coverage than non-Latino White Americans and non-Latino Black Americans (Alcalá et al., 2016; Estrada et al., 1990; NCHS, n.d-a; Perez-Escamilla, 2010), and especially Latinos of Mexican descent (Trevino et al., 1991).

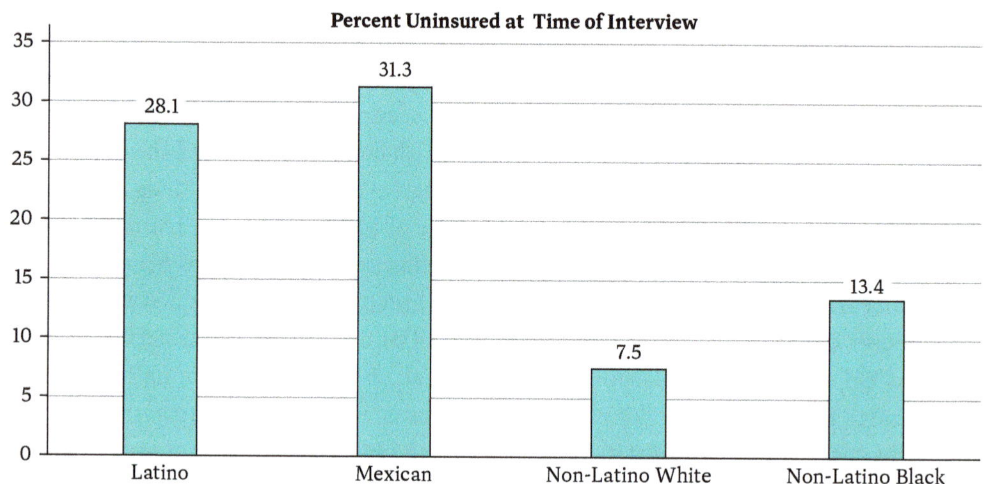

FIGURE 8.1 Percentage of Being Uninsured at the Time of Interview for Adults Aged 18–64, Race and Latino Origin, United States, 2022

Cohen and Cha (2023), reporting data from the 2022 National Health Interview Survey, show that in 2022 the Latino American uninsured rate was 4 times higher than non-Latino White Americans and 2 times higher than non-Latino Black Americans (Figure 8.1). Among Latinos of Mexican descent, almost one third were uninsured at the time of their interview for the survey.

Usual Source of Health Care

Having a usual source of health care is an important access-related factor and is correlated with increased health care utilization (Alcalá et al., 2016; Burgos et al., 2005). National data collected in 2012–2013 as part of the National Health Interview Survey showed that about one third of Latinos and over one third (34.5%) of Latinos of Mexican descent did not have a regular source of health care (González et al., 2009). According to 2022 data retrieved from the National Center for Health Statistics (NCHS, n.d.-b) 20% of Latinos of Mexican descent did not have a regular source of care, a dramatic reduction since the implementation of the Affordable Care Act (ACA) but still lower than non-Latino White Americans and non-Latino Black Americans (Figure 8.2). Additionally, having a regular source of health care among Latinos of Mexican descent did not differ substantially during the COVID-19 pandemic (2020–2022).

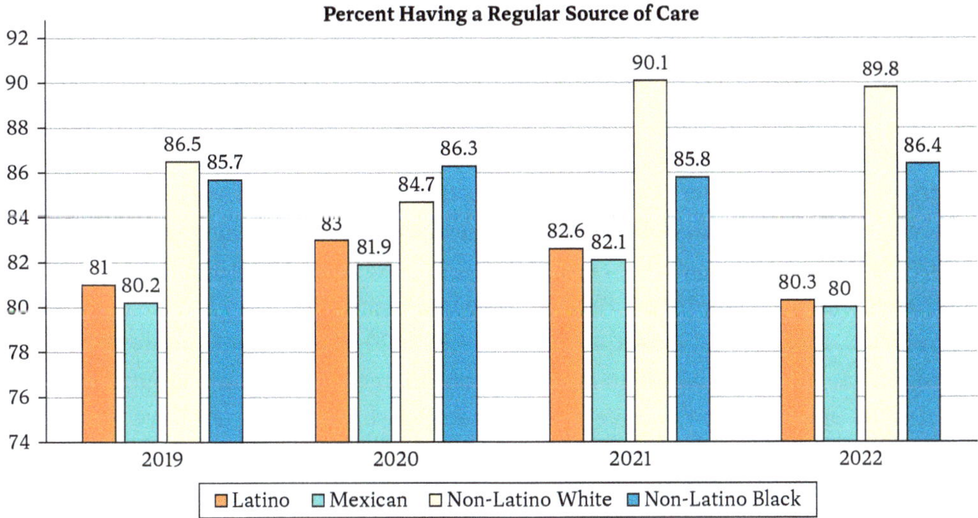

FIGURE 8.2 Percentage of Having a Usual Place of Health Care for Adults Aged 18 and Over, United States, 2019–2022, by Race and Latino Origin

Physician Visits in the Past Year

Data collected as part of the National Health Interview Survey (NCHS, n.d.-b.) on health care utilization among Latino Americans continues to show lower rates of physician visits than non-Latino White Americans and non-Latino Black Americans. (Figure 8.3). Several factors have been suggested to account for underutilization of health care among Latinos of Mexican descent, including use of folk remedies and curanderos (Bruhn & Fuentes, 1977; Higgenbotham et al., 1990), lack of knowledge about the system of health care in the United States, lack of education and health literacy, and mixed-status families (undocumented parents with U.S.-born children) fearing possible deportation (Cabral & Cuevas, 2020; Vargas Bustamante et al., 2012).

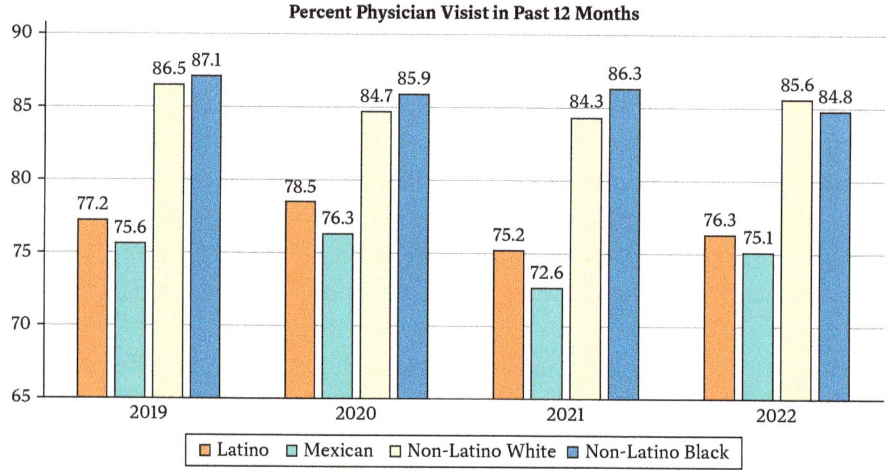

FIGURE 8.3 Percentage Having a Doctor Visit for Any Reason in the Past 12 Months for Adults Aged 18 and Over, United States, 2019–2022, by Race and Latino Origin

Health Care Cost-Related Barriers

The most important types of health care barriers are related to the cost of care and prescription medications (Compton et al., 2010; Estrada et al., 1990). Research has consistently shown that Latinos Americans, especially those who are undocumented, experience more cost-related barriers to health care than non-Latino White Americans and non-Latino Black Americans (Figure 8.4).

Overall, regional, and national data (Cabral & Cuevas, 2020; Vargas Bustamante et al., 2012, Estrada et al., 1990) show that Latinos of Mexican descent carry an unequal burden related to access to quality health care. Almost one third do not have health insurance, one fifth do not have a regular source of health care, they have lower rates of physician visits, and they have a higher percentage of cost-related barriers to health care. Coupled with cultural barriers discussed in previous chapters, Latinos of Mexican descent should experience higher rates of morbidity in comparison to non-Latino White Americans.

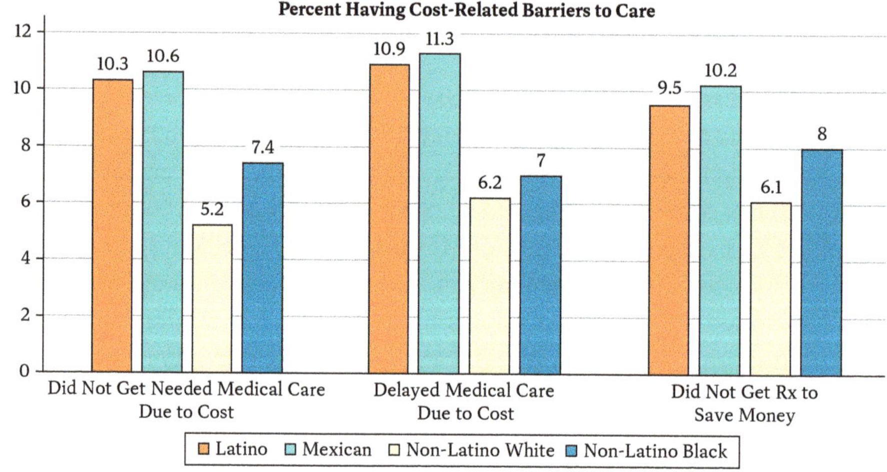

FIGURE 8.4 Percentage of Adults Aged 18 and Over Who Experienced Cost-Related Barriers in the Past 12 Months, by Race and Latino Origin, United States, 2022

General Health Status

A common question in national health surveys is whether the health of the individual is better or worse compared to others. This type of question is referred to as *subjective health status* because the individual is assessing, subjectively, their own health. For example, in the National Health and Nutrition Examination Survey (NHANES), the subjective health status question asked is "Would you say your health in general is excellent, very good, good, fair, or poor?" with the respondent choosing a response (Martinez & Clarke, 2021).

Data obtained from the 2019 National Health Interview Survey and reported by Martinez and Clarke (2021) show that for every age group, Latinos report the highest percentages in "fair or poor" health, with over 40% of Latinos 65 years of age and over reporting "fair or poor" health (Figure 8.5).

The social determinants of health (SDOH) are strongly associated with self-ratings of health in predictable patterns as noted with age. In 2019 the percentage of respondents who rated their health status as fair or poor substantially increased with poverty level, with 24.6% of those 100% below the federal poverty level rating their health as fair or poor, compared to 5.3% among those at 400% or more of the federal poverty level (NCHS, n.d.-c). There is an upward trend observed for fair or poor health ratings among all

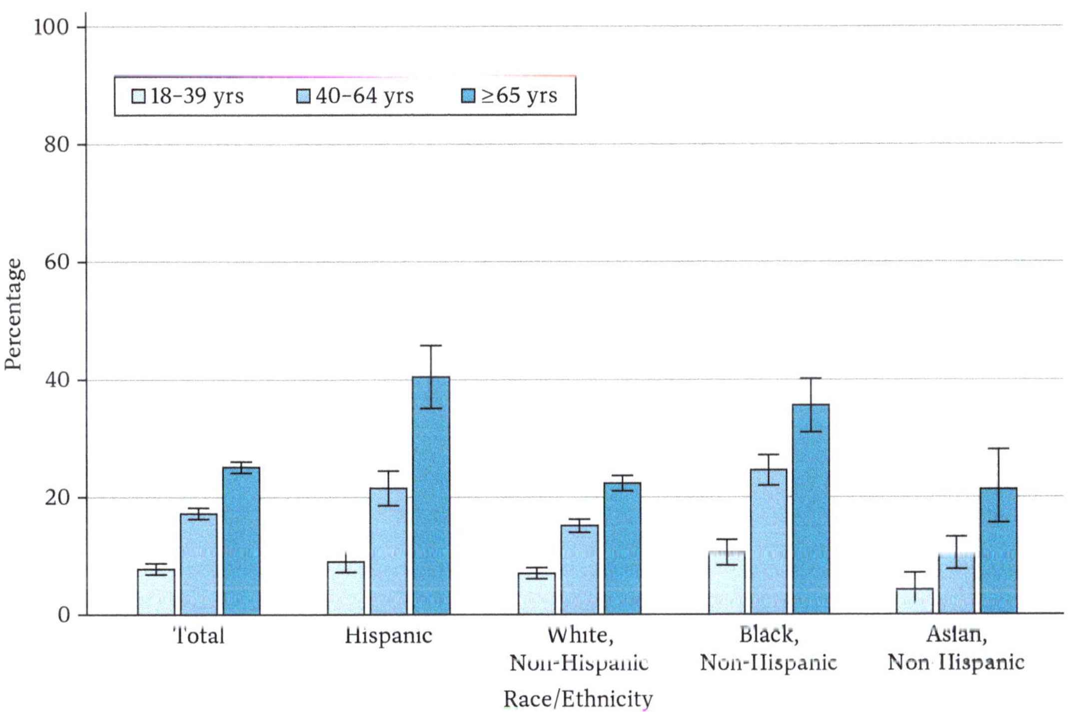

FIGURE 8.5 Percentage of Adults in Fair or Poor Health by Age Group and Race and Ethnicity—National Health Interview Survey, United States, 2019

racial/ethnic groups in Table 8.1. African Americans had higher rates of fair or poor health ratings from 2015–2019. Latino Americans and non-Latino White Americans have identical ratings in 2018 and 2019.

According to NCHS (n.d.-c) data, among those at 400% or more of the federal poverty level, African Americans again have the highest self-ratings of their health as fair or poor in comparison to Latino Americans and non-Latino White Americans (Table 8.2). Additionally, from 2015–2019, Latino Americans have higher self-ratings of fair of poor health than non-Latino White Americans. The data displayed in Table 8.2 shows a racial and ethnic paradox at these higher levels of income, with Latino Americans and non-Latino Black Americans reporting higher self-ratings of fair or poor health. Overall, however, those living at 400% or above the federal poverty threshold have significantly lower self-ratings of fair or poor health in comparison to those living at 100% below poverty: about 3 times the rate for non-Latino Black Americans, 5 times the rate for non-Latino White Americans, and 3 times the rate for Latino Americans. There is an apparent paradox among Latino Americans and non-Latino Black Americans compared to non-Latino White Americans among those living above 400% poverty with higher ratings of fair or poor health than non-Latino White Americans.

TABLE 8.1 Fair or Poor Health Rating by Race/Ethnicity and 100% Below Poverty

Race/Ethnicity	2015	2017	2018	2019
Latino	21.3	20.0	20.5	24.3
Non-Latino White	20.7	21.8	20.5	24.3
Non-Latino Black	23.3	24.0	23.8	28.2

Source: NCHS (n.d.-c)

TABLE 8.2 Fair or Poor Health Rating by Race/Ethnicity and 400% Above Poverty

Race/ethnicity	2015	2017	2018	2019
Latino	5.7	5.7	5.7	6.8
Non-Latino White	3.7	3.9	3.7	5.0
Non-Latino Black	6.3	6.0	6.3	7.5

NCHS (n.d.-c)

Health status self-rating comparisons obtained from the National Center for Health Statistics (NCHS, n.d.-c) for the years 2015–2019 are shown in Figure 8.6. Increases in subjective health status self-rating among all groups can be seen in 2019, prior to the first full year of the COVID-19 pandemic. Non-Latino White Americans have the lowest self-ratings of fair or poor health (9.6%). Mexicans and non-Latino Black Americans have similar self-ratings of fair or poor health of 15.8 and 15.6%, respectively. Additionally, Mexicans have slightly higher percentages than other Latinos in for the years 2017, 2018, and 2019. Overall, the data shows that a slightly higher percentage of Latinos rate their health as fair or poor in comparison to non-Latino Black Americans, with Latinos of Mexican descent reporting higher percentages of fair or poor health status.

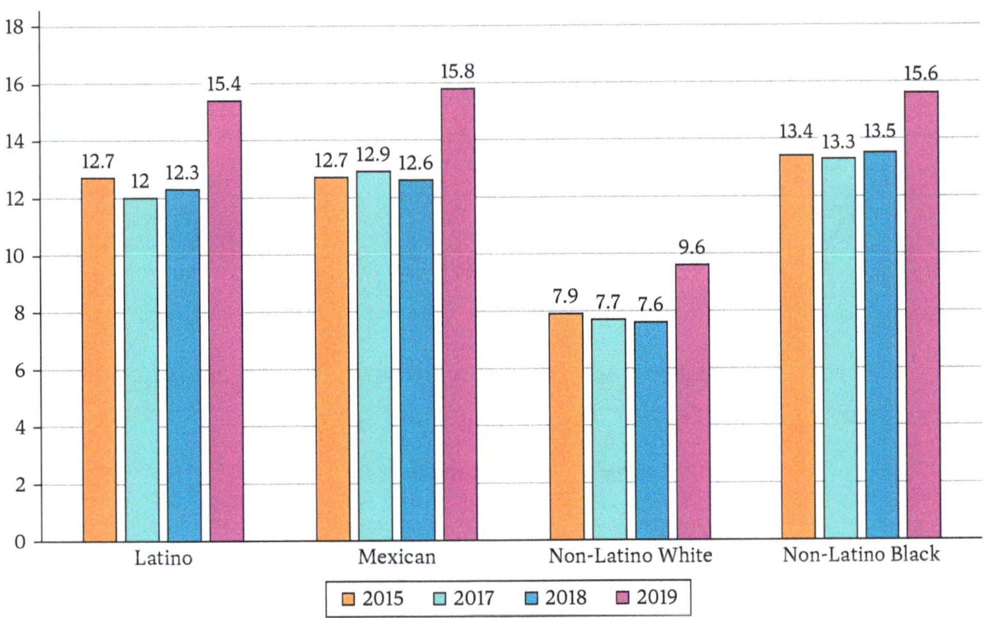

FIGURE 8.6 Respondent-Assessed Fair or Poor Health Status (Percent) by Race/Ethnicity, 2015–2019

Functional Limitations

Functional limitations are an important health assessment that can inform us about the relative lack of access to health care, work-related injuries, and age-related limitations. In general, functional limitations increase with age and are influenced by occupation (Garcia et al., 2020). Research examining functional limitations among Mexican Americans have shown differences with non-Latino White Americans (Melvin et al., 2014). For example, Melvin et al. (2014) examined functional limitations, limitations in activities of daily living (ADL), and limitations in instrumental activities of daily living (IADL) among foreign-born and U.S.-born Latinos. Their data show that among all age groups (50–64, 65–74, 75–84, and 85+) Latinas born in Mexico and Latinas born on Puerto Rico have significantly more functional limitations than non-Latina White women. Additionally, among U.S.-born Latinas, those of Mexican descent had significantly higher rates of functional limitations than non-Latina White women in the 50–64 and 65–74 age categories in ADL and IADL. Elderly Latinas (75+) had higher functional limitations overall and in ADL and IADL. Among Latino men born in Mexico or Puerto Rico, all age groups reported higher levels of overall functional limitations than non-Latino White men. Among U.S.-born Latinos of Mexican descent, all age groups also reported higher levels of functional limitations than non-Latino White men born in the United States.

The percentages reported by Melvin et al. (2014) are similar to national data collected in 2019, as shown in Figures 8.7 and 8.8 (NCHS, n.d.-d). Similar age-related trends are noted, with those older than age 65 reporting more functional limitations than those 18–64 years of age.

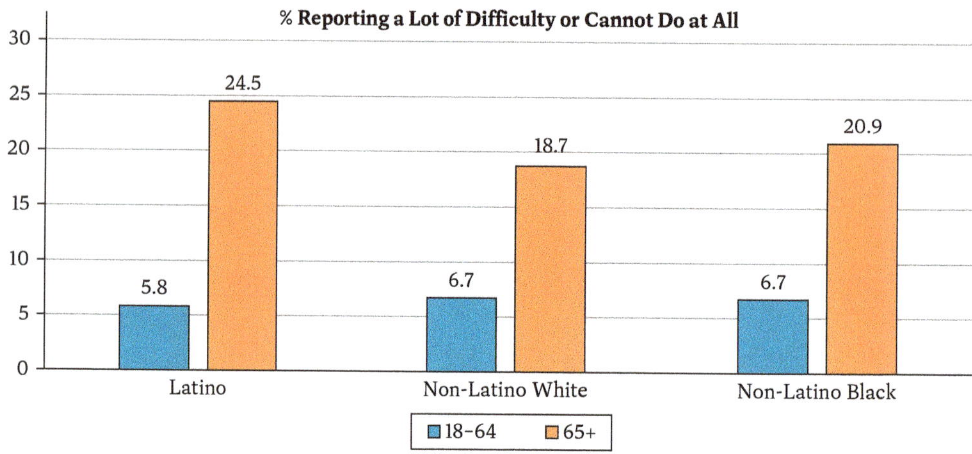

FIGURE 8.7 Functional Limitation in Adults Aged 18 and Over by Race/Ethnicity, 2019

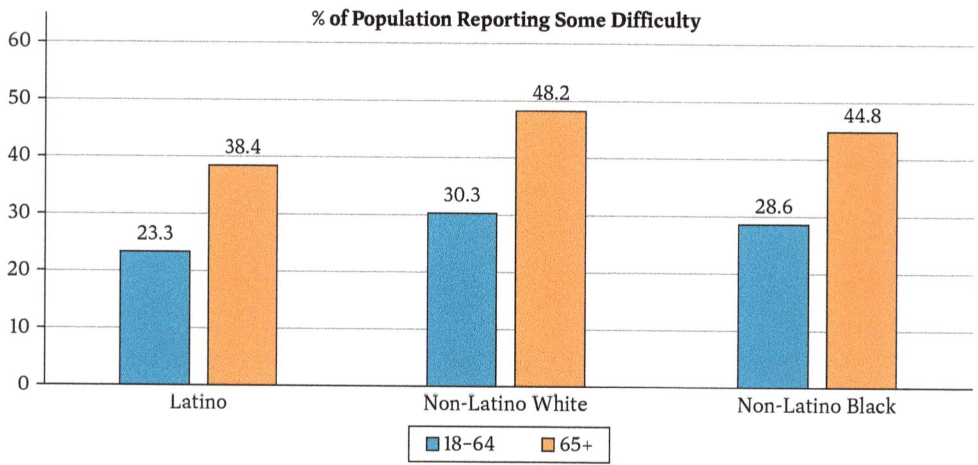

FIGURE 8.8 Functional Limitations in Adults by Race/Ethnicity, 2019

The percentage reporting "a lot of difficulty or cannot do things" for themselves among Latino Americans aged 65 and over is substantially higher than non-Latino White Americans and non-Latino Black Americans. This observation is like those studies noted above with elderly Latinos reporting more functional limitations than others. Conversely, Latinos aged 18–64 have reported lower rates than non-Latinos.

As seen in Figure 8.8, the percentage of adults reporting "some difficulty" in doing things for themselves was higher among non-Latino White Americans and non-Latino Black Americans than Latino Americans for those aged 18–4 and 65 years and over (NCHS, n.d.-d).

Garcia et al. (2020) using data from the 1999–2015 Health Interview Survey among adults 50 to 85 years of age, found that among women, U.S.-born Mexicans, foreign-born Mexicans, and foreign-born Cubans spent less years without functional limitations, while Puerto Rican women had more years with functional limitations. For men, Garcia et al. (2020) found that among the Latino subgroups, Puerto Rican men experienced more years living with functional limitations than others.

Prescription Drug Use (Prescribed by Physician)

Use of prescription drugs that are legitimately prescribed by a physician is another indicator of health status, albeit for those who have utilized health care. It is generally assumed that persons who are prescribed medications by their physicians have some type of health condition. Nationally, data shows that prescription drug use increases with age and is more prevalent among women than men across all racial and ethnic groups (NCHS, n.d.-i). Prescription drug use in the past 30 days is shown in Figure 8.9, with percentages for at least one prescription drug, three or more prescription drugs, and five or more prescription drugs (available from https://www.cdc.gov/nchs/data/hus/2017/079.pdf).

Substantial inequalities are identified in Figure 8.9. Prescription drug use is lower among Latino males and females compared to their non-Latino White and non-Latino Black counterparts. Latinas of Mexican descent also have lower rates of prescription drug use than their non-Latina White and non-Latina Black counterparts for each category of prescription drug use. Barriers to prescription drug use have been documented in the literature and primarily include the cost of prescriptions, not having a regular source of health care, and lack of health insurance coverage (Carroll & Hill, 2019; Compton et al., 2010; Estrada et al., 1990).

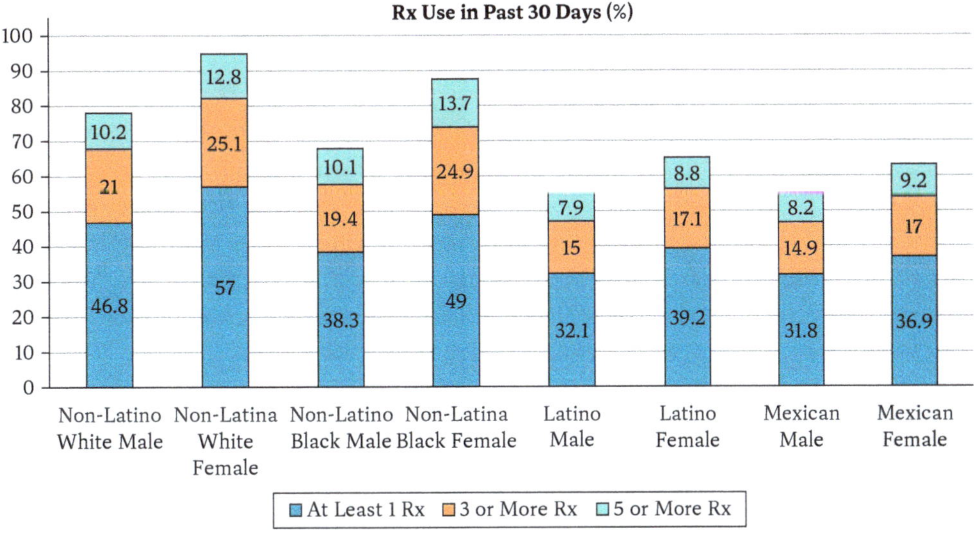

FIGURE 8.9 Prescription Drug Use in the Past 30 Days by Race and Latino Origin, 2011–2014

Psychological Well-Being

Psychological well-being is an important component that contributes to overall health status. Research in the field of Latino mental health has demonstrated how psychological distress is manifested in somatic complaints and symptoms (Bagayogo et al., 2013; Bucay-Harari et al., 2020; Escovar et al., 2018; Letamendi et al., 2013). Lara-Cinisomo et al. (2020), for instance, conducted a systematic review of the literature on somatic symptoms and found a trend for Latinas with depression or depressive symptoms to be more likely to report somatic symptoms compared with non-Latino White women. A study by Escovar et al. (2018) showed that Latina patients had higher levels of somatization than non-Latina White women patients.

An examination of psychological well-being among Latinos may reveal an underlying association with physical health status. National epidemiological studies on the prevalence of serious mental illness among adults 18 years of age and older show that Latino Americans have lower rates than non-Latino White Americans and higher rates than non-Latino Black Americans (4.9% vs. 4%, respectively; Substance Abuse and Mental Health Services Administration (SAMHSA, 2020). Historically, data trends show that Latino Americans underutilize mental health services compared to non-Latino White Americans, even if there is a higher need for services (Alegria et al., 2002; López, 2002). In 2019, data reported by SAMHSA (2020) shows that Latino Americans with a mental illness underutilized mental health services relative to non-Latino White Americans in the past year (33.9 % compared to 50.3 %, respectively). Moreover, among those diagnosed with a serious mental illness, 52.8% of Latinos compared to 57.9% of non-Latino Black Americans and 70.5% of non-Latino White Americans received mental health services in the past year. Inequalities clearly exist in utilization of mental health services based on need among Latinos, which places Latinos at higher risk for more severe forms of mental disorders.

Serious Psychological Distress

The prevalence of serious psychological distress, depression, and anxiety have been shown to be associated with health self-ratings and overall physical health status (SAMHSA, 2020). The prevalence of serious psychological distress in the past 3 -days (serious psychological distress is measured by a six-question scale that asks respondents how often they experienced each of the six symptoms of psychological distress in the past 30 days) was higher among other Latino Americans than non-Latino White Americans and non-Latino Black Americans for the years 1999–2011 (Figure 8.10). However, Latinos of Mexican descent compared to other Latinos reported lower rates of serious psychological distress during this same period. Nevertheless, Latinos of Mexican descent reported higher rates than non-Latino White Americans from 1999–2011. It is interesting to note how the rates of all racial/ethnic groups converge from 2015–2016, with very slight differences in prevalence of serious psychological distress.

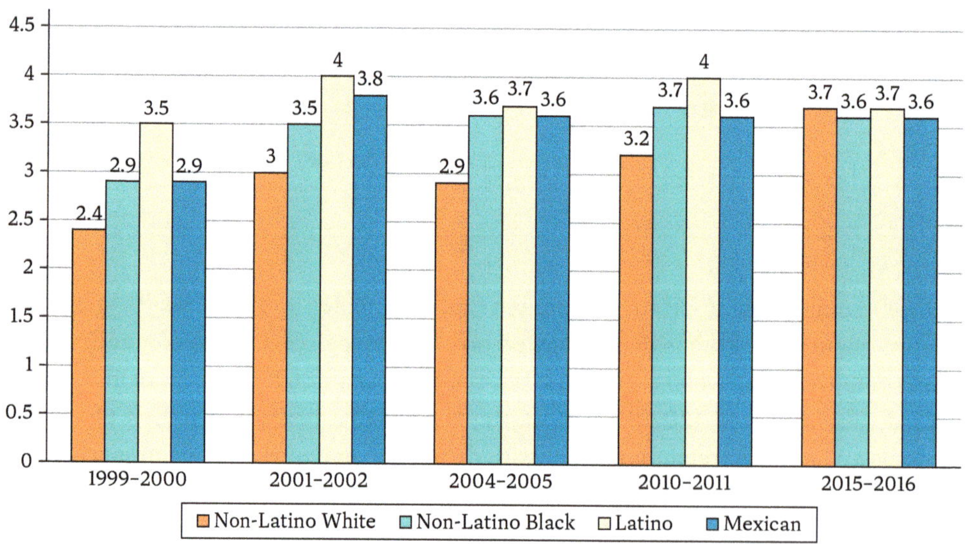

FIGURE 8.10 Percentage of Adults With Serious Psychological Distress, 1999–2016

Poverty level is inextricably associated with psychological well-being. National data shows that people living below the federal poverty level have higher rates of depression and anxiety than those living above the federal poverty level (Pratt & Brody, 2014).

Data collected by the National Center for Health Statistics (NCHS, n.d.-e) clearly shows a linear association among non-Latino White Americans, non-Latino Black Americans, and Latinos with those living at less than the federal poverty level having substantially higher rates of serious psychological distress (Figure 8.11). The difference is most pronounced among non-Latino White Americans, with those living below 100% poverty having almost 11 times the rate as non-Latino White Americans living at 400% above poverty. However, Latino Americans living above 400% poverty had 2 times the rate of serious psychological distress compared to non-Latino Black Americans and non-Latino White Americans. Higher income Latino Americans are more distressed than higher income White Americans and Black Americans, which is a paradoxical finding similar to that reported for non-Latino Black Americans. That is, high-income non-Latino Black Americans have poorer health outcomes compared to their high-income non-Latino White counterparts, known as the *weathering hypothesis* (Braveman, 2023; Forde et al., 2019; Simons et al., 2021). Perhaps a similar process is occurring for Latinos.

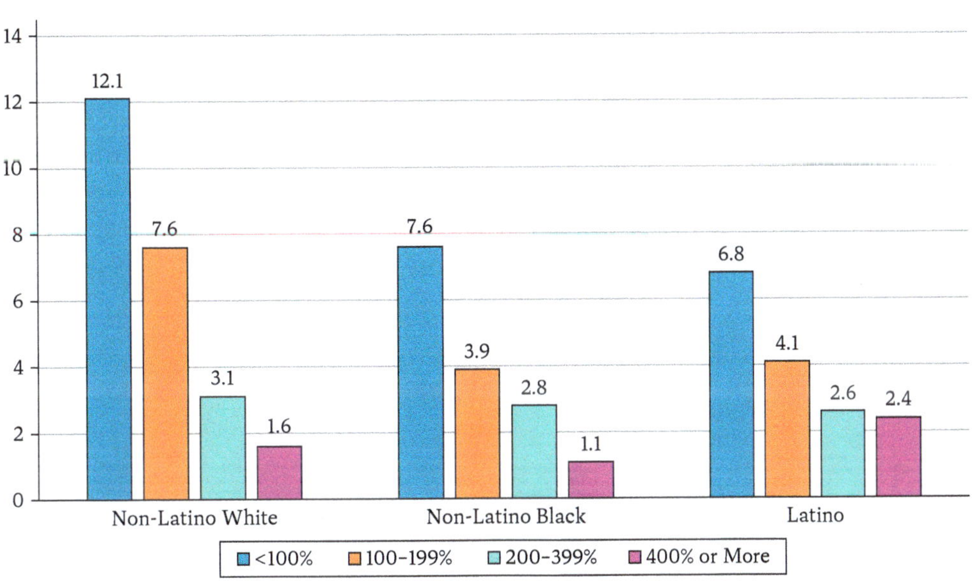

FIGURE 8.11 Percentage of Adults With Serious Psychological Distress by % Federal Poverty Level

Prevalence of Depression

As noted in Chapter 5, the prevalence of depression is lower among Latino Americans in comparison to non-Latino White Americans and lower among foreign-born Latinos than U.S.-born Latinos. National data (Brody et al., 2018) shows that women have higher prevalence rates of depression than men (Figure 8.12). Latino men have a higher prevalence of depression than non-Latino White men, but Latinas have identical rates as non-Latina White women. In 2013–2016, non-Latino Black men and women had the highest prevalence rates of depression (7.1% and 11.0%, respectively).

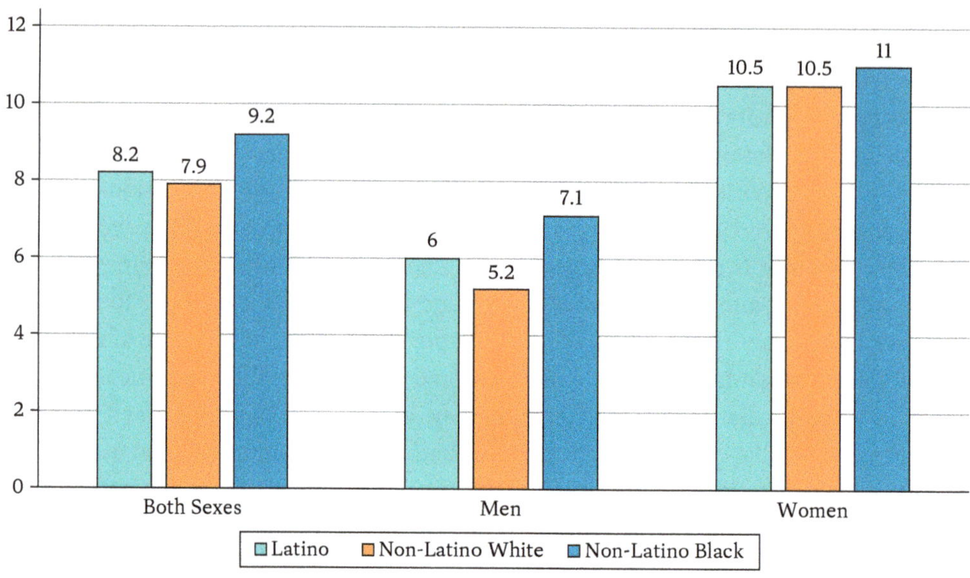

FIGURE 8.12 Percentage of Persons Aged 20 and Over With Depression, by Race and Latino Origin and Sex: United States, 2013–2016

Prevalence of Worry, Nervousness, or Anxiety

In 2019, 2020, and 2022, data from the NCHS (n.d.-f) showed that Latinos reported the lowest rate of feelings of worry, nervousness, or anxiety (Figure 8.13). All racial/ethnic groups shown reported the highest prevalence in 2022, especially among non-Latino White Americans (14.1%) compared to non-Latino Black Americans (10.8%) and Latino Americans (10%). From 2019–2022, Latinos of Mexican descent reported

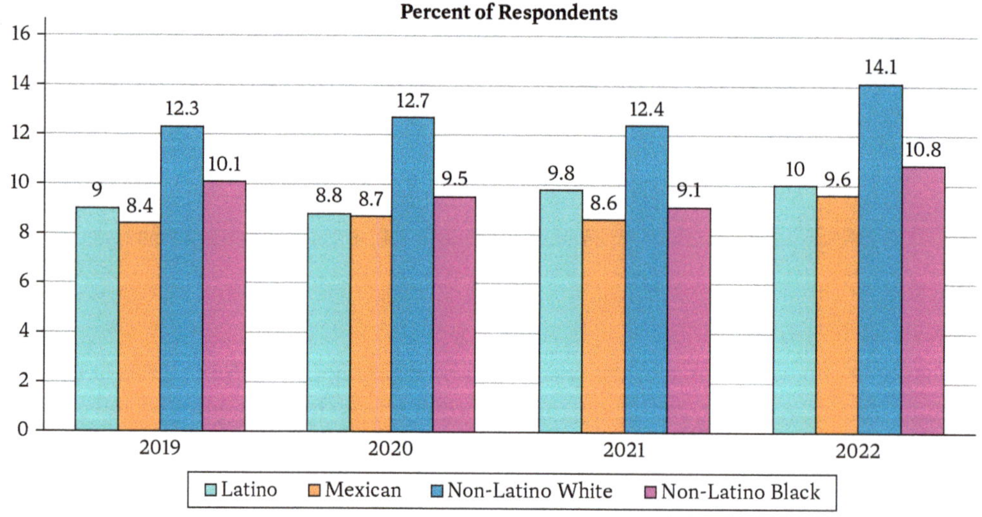

FIGURE 8.13 Percentage of Persons Who Regularly Had Feelings of Worry, Nervousness, or Anxiety for Adults Aged 18 and Over, United States, 2019–2022

the lowest prevalence rates of worry, nervousness, or anxiety than other Latino Americans, non-Latino White Americans, and non-Latino Black Americans.

The examination of Latino subgroups, activities of daily living and rating of fair or poor heath shows some notable differences. For example, Gallo et al. (2014) found that Latinos of Mexican descent had higher self-reported rates of fair or poor health status and a higher percentage reporting that they are unable to do things for themselves, especially among the elderly. However, Latinos of Mexican descent report lower ratings of worry, anxiety, and nervousness than non-Latino White Americans and non-Latino Black Americans. Latino Americans overall report higher rates of depression and serious psychological distress than non-Latino White Americans and non-Latino Black Americans, which adds to their burden of disease.

Major Chronic Disease Risk Factors Among Latinos

Chronic disease risk factors include biobehavioral and socioenvironmental risks (Table 8.3). These known risk factors contribute to disease causation through their underlying biological, physiological, and psychosocial processes (Balfour et al., 2016; Daviglus et al., 2012; Gomez et al., 2022). Chronic diseases are the major killers of the U.S. population. In previous chapters we have discussed several of the socioenvironmental risk factors identified in Table 8.3. In the current chapter, biobehavioral risk factors will be evaluated.

TABLE 8.3 Risk Factors for Chronic Disease

Biobehavioral risk factors	Socioenvironmental risk factors
• Current cigarette smoking	• Stress and stressful life events
• Alcohol consumption	• Poverty
• Hypertension	• Discrimination
• Physical inactivity	• Institutional racism
• Hypercholesterolemia	• Epigenetics
• Overweight and obesity	
• Lack of fruit and vegetable intake	
• Increased fat intake	

Risk factors can also be discussed in terms of modifiable and nonmodifiable risks. *Modifiable risk factors* can be reduced or eliminated through intervention. *Nonmodifiable risk factors*, by definition, cannot be reduced or eliminated by interventions, or can they? We have discussed how epigenetic modifications can enhance or minimize disease vulnerability, and treatments for certain types of cancers are based on modifications of methylated genes (Oyama & Terry, 2016). Among the nonmodifiable risk factors, DNA-encoded hereditary risk is the most common. For example, Native Americans and Latinos of Mexican descent are at higher risk than other groups for gallbladder disease (Hanis et al., 1985; Maurer et al., 1989; Samet et al., 1988).

The interrelationships between selected chronic diseases and modifiable risk factors are shown in Table 8.4. It is also important to recognize that several chronic diseases are considered comorbid conditions and causes of other chronic diseases. For example, type 2 diabetes is strongly associated with cardiovascular disease, and people with type 2 diabetes are likely to have heart disease as well (Kaplan et al., 2014). Moreover, nonalcoholic fatty liver disease (NAFLD) is more prevalent among Latinos and is associated with chronic liver disease (Rector & Thyfault, 2011; Saab et al., 2016). NAFLD severity includes the co-occurrence of nonalcoholic steatohepatitis (NASH), with significant fibrosis of the liver, and the development of cirrhosis complications and increased mortality (Rich et al., 2018).

TABLE 8.4 Interrelationships Between Various Chronic Diseases and Modifiable Risk Factors Among Latinos, United States

	Cardiovascular disease	Cancer	Chronic lung diseases	Type 2 diabetes	Nonalcohol fatty liver disease (NAFLD)	Gallbladder disease (GBD)
Cigarette smoking	+	+	+	+	?	+
Alcohol consumption	+	+	?	+	?	+
Illicit drug use	+	+	+	+	+	?
High cholesterol	+	+	+	+	+	+
High blood pressure	+	?	+	+	+	+
Poor dietary practices	+	+	?	+	+	+
Overweight & obesity	+	+	+	+	+	+
Physical inactivity	+	+	+	+	+	+
Psychosocial stress	+	+	+	+	+	?
Environmental pollution	+	+	+	?	?	?
Socioeconomic status	+	+	+	+	+	+
Adverse childhood experiences (ACES)	+	+	+	+	?	?

Legend: + indicates a positive association; ? indicates more research is needed to clarify association.

Adapted from: Allen et al. (2013)

Acculturation level has been shown to be an important cultural determinant among Latinos. Research has shown that acculturation level is associated with an increase in risk behaviors like tobacco use, alcohol use, illicit drug use, and poor dietary practices. For example, several studies have documented increases in alcohol, tobacco, and other drug use among Latinos who are highly acculturated compared to lower acculturated Latinos (Caetano & Clark, 2003; Bethel & Schenker, 2005). While acculturation in and of itself is not a risk factor for disease, it does influence risk engagement and disease susceptibility.

Current Cigarette Smoking

Early studies of acculturation and current cigarette smoking among Latinos clearly show that more acculturated Latinos smoke more cigarettes than less acculturated Latinos independent of gender (Marin et al., 1989). However, in the Marin et al. (1989) study and others, lower acculturated Latino males tend to smoke more than higher acculturated Latino males, and higher acculturated Latina's smoke more than lower acculturated Latinas (Bethel & Schenker, 2005), and those born in the United States have higher rates of smoking than Mexican-born Latinos (Wilkinson et al., 2005) (see Figure 8.14).

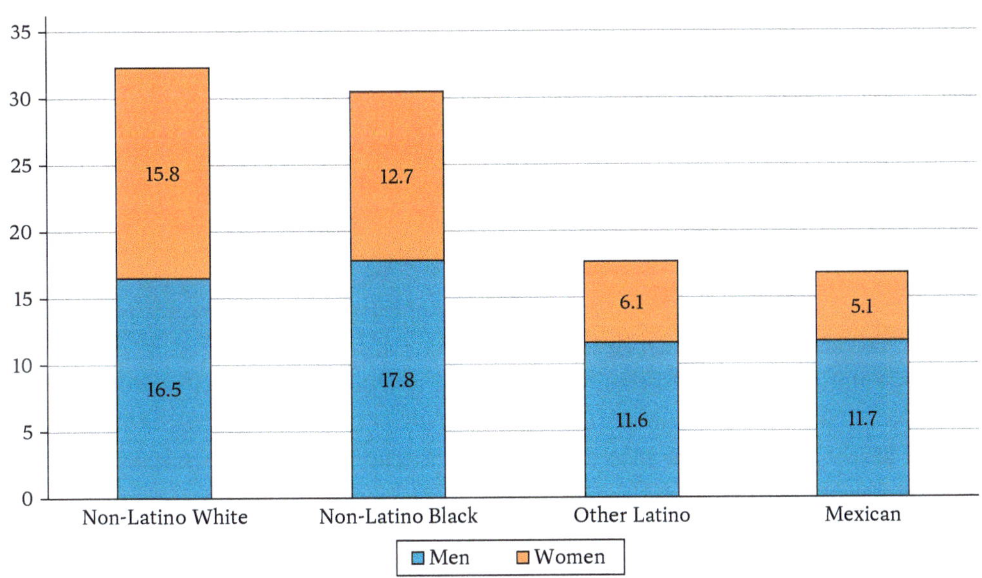

FIGURE 8.14 Current Cigarette Smoking Among Adults Aged 18 and Over by Race/Ethnicity and Gener, Age-Adjusted, 2019

Current cigarette smoking has declined substantially since 1997, but e-cigarette vaping has increased (Goldenson et al., 2017). National data collected by the National Health Interview Survey (NCHS, n.d.-g) shows that age-adjusted rates for men aged 18 and over in 1997 was 27.1% and declined to 15.5% in 2019, a reduction of over half. Among women 18 aged and over, 22.2% were current cigarette smokers in 1997 compared to 13% in 2019. Similarly, among Latinos rates declined from 25.4% in 1997 to 6.1% in

2019, a substantial reduction in current cigarette smoking. Again, current cigarette smoking rates vary significantly by federal poverty level, with higher rates among those persons living in poverty than those who are not across all racial/ethnic groups. Additionally, in 2019, Latinas of Mexican descent have 3 times lower rates of current cigarette smoking than non-Latina White Americans, and 2 times lower rates than non-Latina Black Americans (Figure 8.14). The prevalence rate difference between men is much less, with about 12 % of Latinos of Mexican descent compared to 18 % of non-Latino Black Americans and 17 % of non-Latino White Americans reporting current cigarette smoking in 2019.

Alcohol and Drug Use

Significant acculturation differences have been found for Latinos associated with alcohol and drug use. Much of the extant research clearly shows that higher acculturated Latinos compared to lower acculturated Latinos consume more alcohol and drugs and are more likely to have an alcohol or drug use disorder (Caetano & Clark, 2003; Gil et al., 2000; Zemore, 2007).

National data from the Monitoring the Future Study (Johnson et al., 2020; Miech et al., 2020) show that Latino youth (8th, 10th, and 12th graders) had higher rates for any illicit drug use than non-Latino White youth, and non-Latino Black youth had the lowest rates. For example, among Latino 12th graders, 39.7% reported any illicit drug use compared to 38.5% among non-Latino White 12th graders and 35.6% among non-Latino Black 12th graders. Additionally, Latino 12th graders had the highest reported rate of lifetime marijuana use and use in the past 12 months at 50.3% compared to 43.6% among non-Latino White 12th graders and 41.8% among non-Latino Black 12th graders. Past month use of marijuana was also higher among Latinos than non-Latino White and non-Latino Black 12th graders. Other illicit drugs that had a higher prevalence of use among Latinos 12th graders than non-Latino White and non-Latino Black students were inhalants, hallucinogens, cocaine, and over-the-counter cold/cough medicines.

Alcohol consumption data for non-Latino White Americans, Black Americans and Latino Americans from the National Survey on Drug Use and Health (NSDUH) conducted by SAMHSA is shown in Figure 8.15 (Center for Behavioral Health Statistics and Quality, National Survey on Drug Use and Health, 2016). Non-Latino White Americans have the highest prevalence of alcohol use, binge alcohol use, and heavy alcohol use than the other groups. Latino and non-Latino Black Americans have very similar rates for alcohol use.

Binge alcohol use for men is defined as drinking five or more drinks on the same occasion on at least 1 day in the past 30 days. Starting in 2015, *binge alcohol use for women* is defined as drinking four or more drinks on the same occasion on at least 1 day in the past 30 days. *Occasion* is defined as at the same time or within a couple of hours of each other (CDC, n.d.-h). *Heavy alcohol use* is defined as drinking five or more drinks on the same occasion on each of 5 or more days in the past 30 days. According to the CDC definition, all heavy alcohol users are also binge alcohol users.

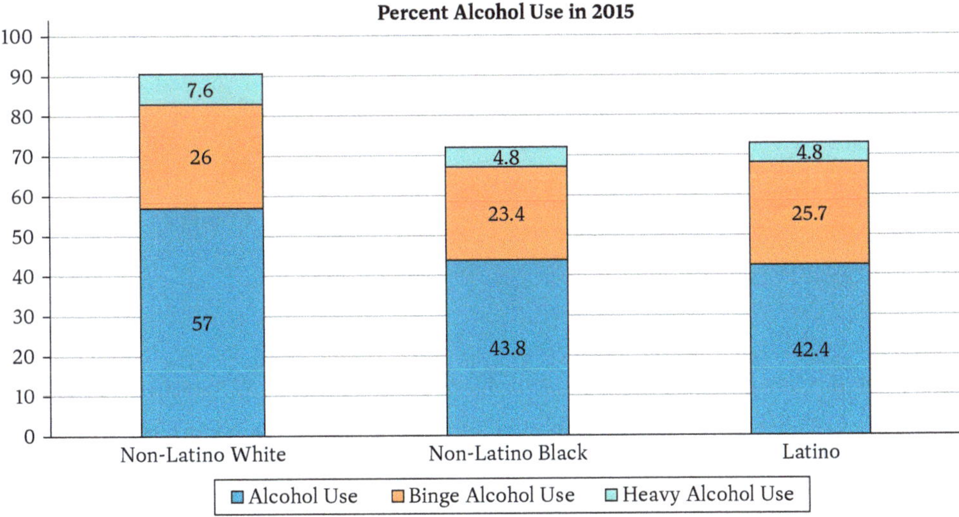

FIGURE 8.15 Use of Alcohol in the Past Month Among Persons Aged 12 and Over by Race/Ethnicity, 2015

Source: Substance Abuse and Mental Health Services Administration, Center for Behavioral Health Statistics and Quality, National Survey on Drug Use & Health. Available from: http://www.samhsa.gov/data/population-data-nsduh

Unlike the Monitoring the Future Study, data obtained from NSDUH shows lower rates for marijuana use among Latino Americans aged 12 and over in comparison to non-Latino White Americans and non-Latino Black Americans (Figure 8.16). Latino Americans show higher rates of prescription drug misuse than non-Latino Black Americans, but lower than non-Latino White Americans.

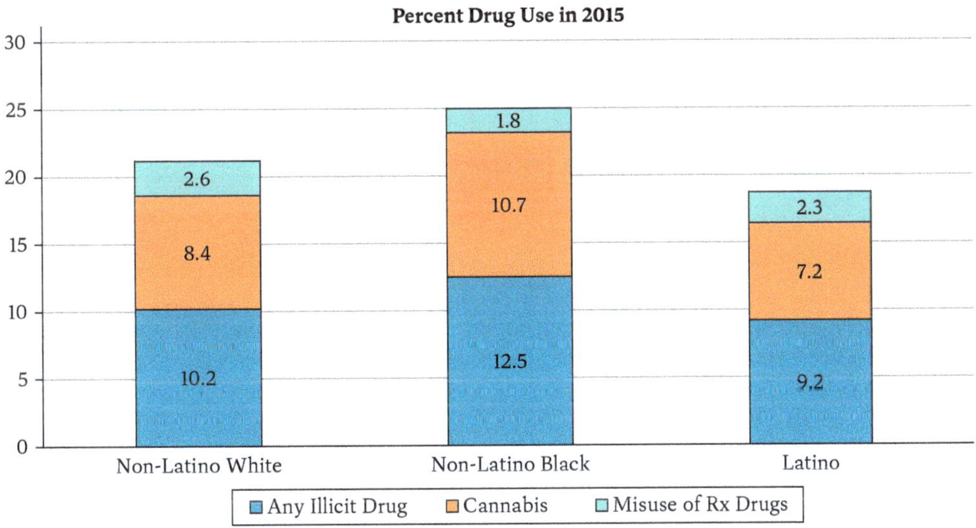

FIGURE 8.16 Use of Selected Drugs in the Past Month Among Persons Aged 12 and Over by Race/Ethnicity, 2015

Source: Substance Abuse and Mental Health Services Administration, Center for Behavioral Health Statistics and Quality, National Survey on Drug Use & Health. Available from: http://www.samhsa.gov/data/population-data-nsduh . See Appendix I, National Survey on Drug Use & Health (NSDUH).

Any illicit drug includes marijuana, cocaine (including crack), heroin, hallucinogens (including LSD, PCP, peyote, mescaline, psilocybin mushrooms, MDMA/"ecstasy," ketamine, DMT/AMT/"Foxy," and *Salvia divinorum*), inhalants, methamphetamine, or the misuse of prescription pain relievers, tranquilizers, stimulants, and sedatives (Center for Behavioral Health Statistics and Quality, NSDUH, 2016). *Misuse of prescription psychotherapeutic drugs* is defined as use in any way not directed by a doctor, including use without a prescription of one's own; use in greater amounts, more often, or longer than told to take a drug; or use in any other way not directed by a doctor.

Hypertension or High Blood Pressure (HBP)

Hypertension or high blood pressure (HBP) is significantly associated with increased morbidity and mortality in the United States (Cushman, 2003). Moreover, if not controlled, hypertension can lead to stroke and increase functional limitations. National data (Ostchega et al., 2020) show that women of Mexican descent have higher rates of hypertension than non-Latino White women and the same as other Latinas (Figure 8.17). Likewise, Mexican men have almost identical rates as non-Latino White men and other Latino men. Non-Latino Black men and women have the highest prevalence rate of hypertension.

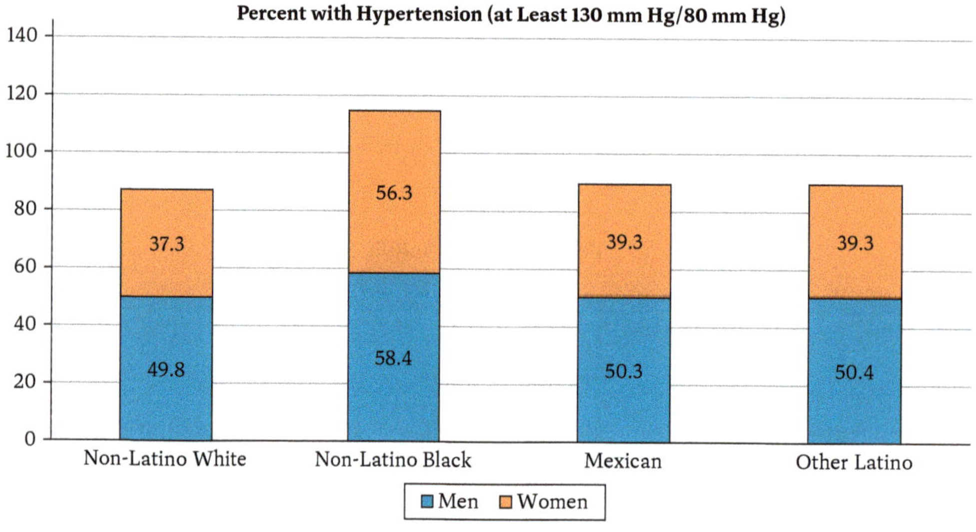

FIGURE 8.17 Hypertension Prevalence Among Adults Aged 18 and Over by Race/Ethnicity and Gender, 2017–2018

Early detection and treatment of hypertension can prevent heart failure, kidney failure, and death and disability from stroke. In fact, hypertension is the single most important risk factor for stroke, so its control is essential for reducing death and disability. Typically, hypertension does not manifest in symptoms, so screening is essential for proper control of the condition. Unfortunately, studies show that Latino Americans are less likely to receive a blood pressure screening compared to non-Latino White Americans. Further,

Latinos 18–44 years of age are less likely to receive a blood pressure screening compared to Latinos 65 and over (Campos & Rodriguez, 2019).

Among those with hypertension, evidence shows that a significant proportion do not have it controlled (Ostchega et al., 2020), with variation by race and Latino origin (Figure 8.18). Among men, almost 70% of Mexican men do not have their hypertension under control compared to about 57% of non-Latino White men. Similarly, Mexican women have higher rates of uncontrolled hypertension than non-Latina White women, 45% compared to 37%, respectively. There is an increased risk for stroke and disability among Latinos of Mexican descent compared to non-Latino White women.

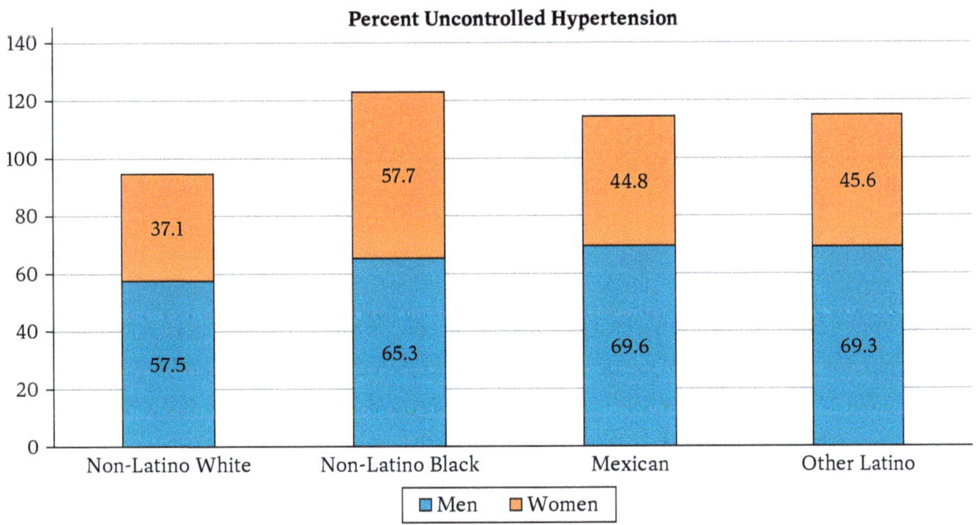

FIGURE 8.18 Uncontrolled Hypertension Among Adults Aged 18 and Over by Race/Ethnicity and Gender, 2013–2016

Physical Inactivity

Physical inactivity is a risk factor for obesity, heart disease, NAFLD, and diabetes mellitus (Rector & Thyfault, 2011; Keating et al., 2012). NCHS data (NCHS, n.d.-h) shows that the percentages of the U.S. population engaged in aerobic activity or muscle strengthening guidelines vary significantly by income, gender, race/ethnicity, and age (Figure 8.19).

Physical inactivity significantly varies by poverty status (NCHS, n.d.-f). Twice as many people living below 100% poverty compared to people living at 400% or more were physically inactive (18.7% compared to 35.1%, respectively). Likewise, among Latino Americans, non-Latino White Americans, and non-Latino Black Americans, those living below 100% poverty had almost twice the rate of physical inactivity than people living at 400% or more of the federal poverty level.

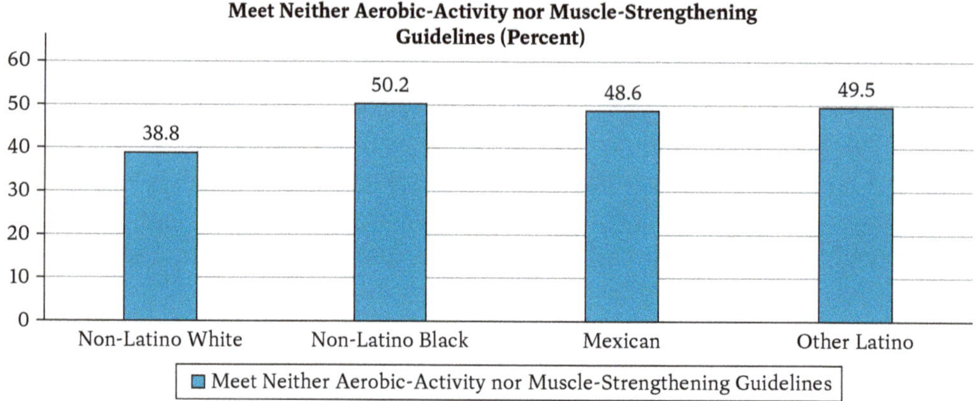

FIGURE 8.19 Physical Inactivity Among Racial/Ethnic Groups, 2018

Source: NCHS, National Health Interview Survey, Family Core and Sample Adult questionnaires. Data for level of difficulty are from the 2010 Quality of Life, 2011–2017 Functioning and Disability, and 2018 Sample Adult questionnaires. See Appendix I, National Health Interview Survey (NHIS)

Hypercholesterolemia (High Cholesterol)

Risk for heart disease is associated with high levels of cholesterol, known as *hypercholesterolemia* (Wilkins et al., 2014). Mexican men have higher rates of high cholesterol than non-Latino Black men but lower than non-Latino White men (Figure 8.20). Alternatively, Mexican women have lower rates than non-Latina White and non-Latina Black women.

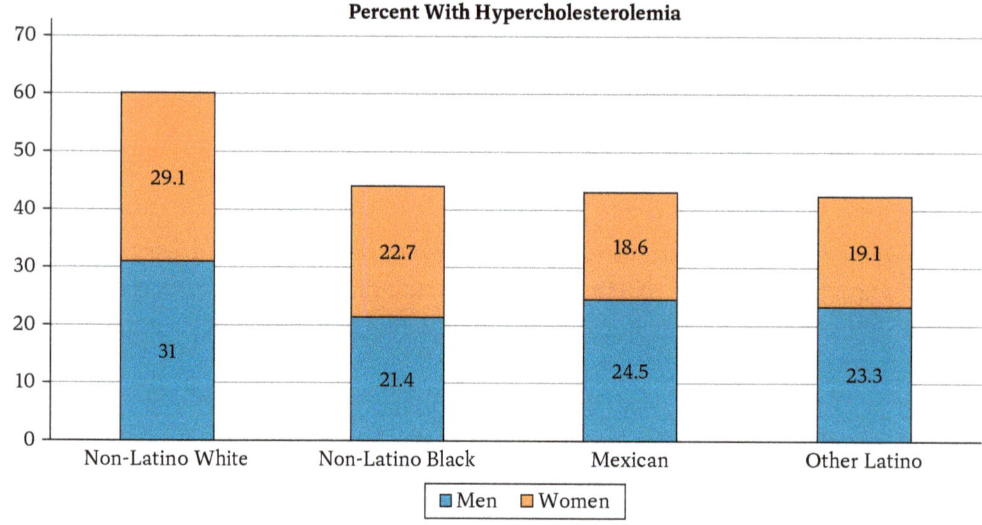

FIGURE 8.20 Percentage with Hypercholesterolemia (Serum Total Cholesterol Greater Than or Equal to 240 mg/dL or Taking Cholesterol-Lowering Medications) by Race/Ethnicity, 2015–2018

Dietary Practices

The Dietary Guidelines for the United States are jointly issued every 5 years by the U.S. Department of Health and Human Services (DHHS) and the U.S. Department of Agriculture (USDA; Figure 8.21). Dietary Guidelines identify daily amounts of foods, in nutrient-dense forms, to be consumed from five major food groups and their subgroups. The primary aim of these Dietary Guidelines is disease prevention (USDA & DHHS, 2020). Nevertheless, Dietary Guidelines are ideal and poorly understood by most people. Moreover, persons living at or below the federal poverty threshold cannot follow the guidelines due to the cost of many of the food groups.

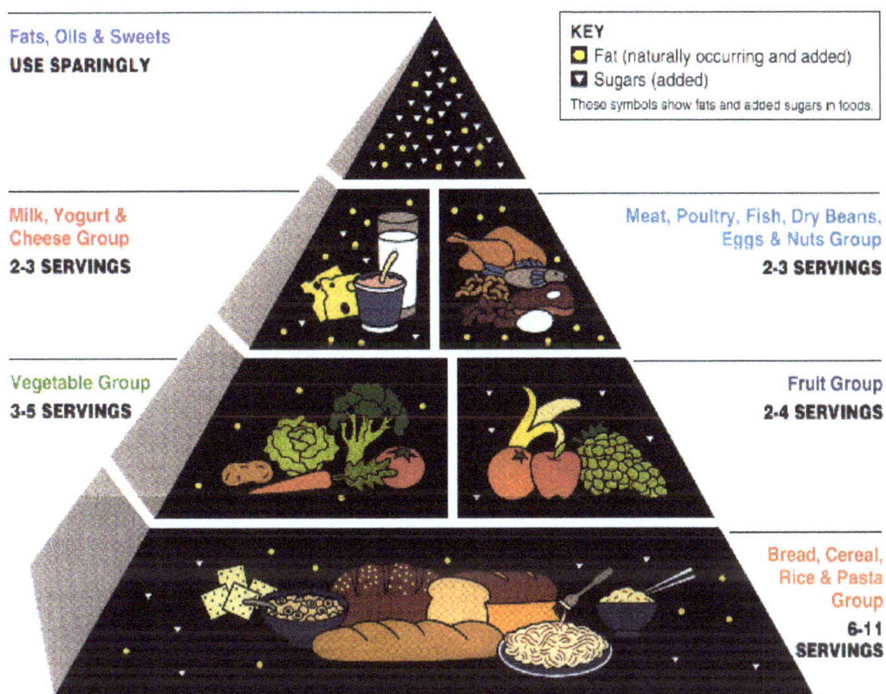

FIGURE 8.21 USDA Dietary Guidelines

Food insecurity is one of the major problems facing historically marginalized populations, as seen in Chapter 5. In 2018, about one fifth of non-Latino Black Americans and 16.2% of Latinos compared to 8.1% of non-Latino White Americans were *food insecure*, defined by the USDA and DHHS (2020) as occurring "when access to nutritionally adequate and safe food is limited or uncertain" (p. 50). Poor nutrition undermines many attempts at improving individual and population level health, especially for historically marginalized population groups. Studies have shown how poor nutrition negatively impacts one's immune system.

National data shows little variation in the recommended fruit and vegetable consumption by race and ethnicity (Lee et al., 2022). All the percentages for recommended intake of fruit and vegetable consumption are low, with Latinos reporting higher percentages for both fruit and vegetable consumption than non-Latino White Americans and Black Americans (Table 8.5). Overall, however, adherence to dietary guidelines was less than 60% for all Americans in 2015–2016 (USDA & DHHS, 2020).

TABLE 8.5 Percentage of Respondents Meeting Federal Fruit Intake Recommendations by Race and Ethnicity, BRFSS, 2019

	Non-Latino White	Latino	Non-Latino Black
Federal fruit recommendation	11.1	16.4	12.9
Federal vegetable recommendation	10.1	11.0	6.9

Source: Lee et al. (2022).

One of the most comprehensive studies to date on the Latino population residing in the United States was conducted by Siega-Riz et al. (2014) who examined food group and nutrient-density intakes among Latinos using the Hispanic Community Health Study/Study of Latinos. They found that Cubans had higher intakes of total energy, macronutrients (including all subtypes of fat), and alcohol than those of other Latino subgroups, which may reflect their overall better access to healthy foods and higher incomes. Mexicans had higher intakes of vitamin C, calcium, and fiber. Puerto Ricans had lowest intakes of vitamin C and fiber. Dominicans reported the lowest intakes of total energy, macronutrients, folate, iron, and calcium.

Siega-Riz et al. (2014) also found that food-group servings reflected nutrient intakes, with Cubans reporting higher intakes of refined grains, vegetables, red meat, and fats; Dominicans having higher intakes of fruit and poultry; and Puerto Ricans reporting the lowest intakes of fruit and vegetables. Central and South Americans were second in their reported intakes of fruit and poultry and were the highest in fish consumption in comparison with other Latino subgroups.

Overall, recommended dietary consumption patterns among U.S. residents are very low, with Latino Americans having higher consumption of fruits and vegetables than non-Latino White Americans and non-Latino Black Americans. Latino subgroup differences in fruit and vegetable consumption are also found, with Latinos of Cuban descent having higher consumption rates than other Latino subgroups, as noted by Siega-Riz et al. (2014). There is much room for improvement among all groups residing in the United States.

Research clearly demonstrates that Latinos have an excess of modifiable risk factors for the major chronic diseases like cardiovascular disease (Daviglus et al., 2012) and diabetes mellitus (Marquez et al., 2019), for which they have a higher prevalence and mortality rate than non-Latino White Americans (Figure 8.22).

Nevertheless, this excess in risk factors does not translate into higher morbidity or mortality associated with heart disease, congestive heart failure, or stroke. Unhealthy behaviors, including physical inactivity, poor dietary practices, excessive alcohol consumption, elevated cholesterol, increasing obesity, and uncontrolled hypertension and diabetes, account for upwards of 50% of heart disease and stroke mortality in the United States. Yet national data do not show an elevated mortality rate for Latino Americans over

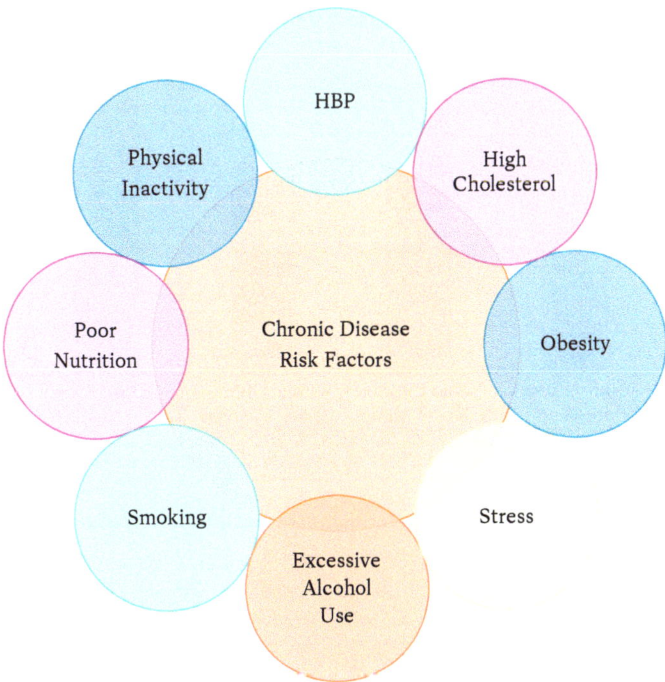

FIGURE 8.22 Modifiable Risk Factors for Chronic Disease

non-Latino White Americans, though diseases of the heart is the second leading cause of death among Latino Americans and cerebrovascular disease is the fourth leading cause of death.

Major Chronic Disease Inequalities Among Latinos

There are several major chronic disease inequalities identified among Latinos vis-à-vis non-Latino White Americans. These inequalities include certain types of cancers, obesity and obesity-related diseases, metabolic syndrome, diabetes mellitus, and gallbladder disease as we shall see below.

Cancer Inequalities

Many factors are related to cancer incidence among Latinos (Pinheiro et al., 2009; Espinosa de Los Monteros & Gallo, 2011). These include inadequate screening facilities, access and financial issues, delayed presentation, and cultural factors (e.g., fatalism). Cultural factors can also include talking about "private parts," touching private parts, someone else touching or looking at private parts, embarrassment, modesty, fatalism, and *machismo*, especially in relation to undergoing a digital rectal exam to check for prostate cancer.

According to the American Cancer Society (2023, Table 9) compared to non-Latino White Americans and Black Americans, Latinos have lower cancer incidence rates for all cancer sites (352.2/100,000 compared to 466.6/100,000 and 453.7/100,000, respectively). There are noted exceptions. For example, Latinas have a higher incidence than non-Latino White women for cancer of the kidney and renal pelvis (13.1/100,000 compared to 11.9/100,000). Cancer inequalities among Latinos compared to non-Latino White

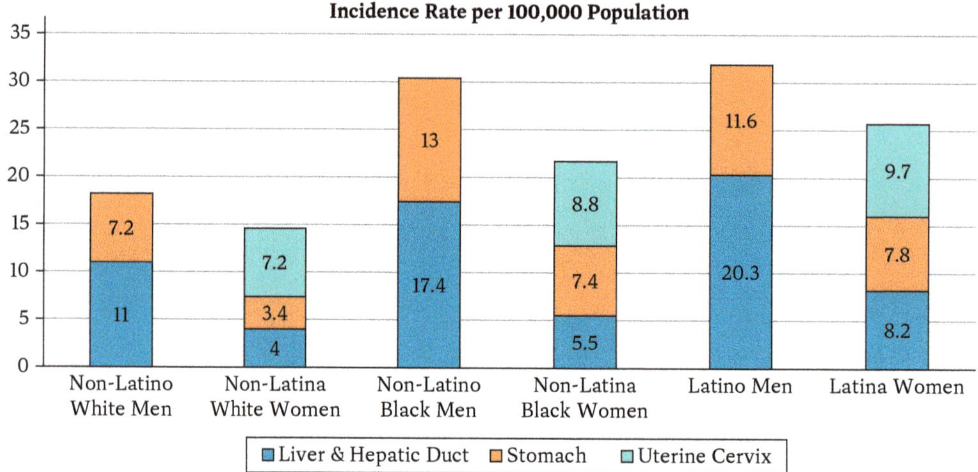

FIGURE 8.23 Incidence of Selected Cancer Inequalities by Race/Ethnicity and Gender, United States, 2015–2019

Rates are per 100,000 population, age adjusted to the 2000 U.S. standard population, and exclude data from Puerto Rico

Source: American Cancer Society, Table 9, 2023. https://www.cancer.org/content/dam/cancer-org/research/cancer-facts-and-statistics/annual-cancer-facts-and-figures/2023/mr8-race-and-ethnicity-2023-cff.pdf

Americans are found for cancer incidence (Figure 8.23) and mortality (Figure 8.24) associated with the liver and intrahepatic bile duct, the stomach, and uterine cervix in women.

One method to quantify the health burden of a population is using the Population Attributable Fraction (PAF), which shows the relative contribution of risk factors to a specific disease (Flegal et al., 2015). For example, Makarova-Rusher et al., (2016) shows that Latinos have higher population attributable risk (PAF) for liver and hepatic duct cancer (hepatocellular carcinoma) with metabolic disorders contributing 39.3% to this risk, followed by hepatitis C (21.1% contribution), alcohol (20% contribution), smoking and hepatitis B (contributing 1.1% each), and genetic disorders (0.3% contribution) for a total PAF of 63.1%, which is higher than non-Latino White Americans and non-Latino Black Americans indicating a higher disease burden for Latino Americans.

Cancer mortality rates are associated with several factors, including access and financial issues (Singh, 2003), later stage of cancer presentation (Ward et al., 2004), lack of awareness regarding efficacious cancer treatment options (Costas-Muniz et al., 2013), as well as cultural factors like fatalism (Yanez et al., 2016).

Prior to the COVID-19 pandemic, cancer was the leading cause of death among Latinos. National mortality data shows that compared to non-Latino White Americans, Latino Americans have lower overall rates for the most common cancers (e.g., female breast, colorectum, lung, and prostate) but have the highest rates for cancers associated with infectious agents like the human papilloma virus (HPV) and perhaps *H. pylori* (Huerta-Franco et al., 2018; Kumar et al., 2020; Tsang et al., 2022). For instance, data from the American Cancer Society (2023) indicates that cervical cancer incidence is more than 30% higher in Latinas than in non-Latina White women, and liver and stomach cancer rates in Latino Americans are double those in non-Latino White Americans (see Figure 8.23). Cancer incidence rates, however, vary substantially by country of origin, generation, birthplace, and length of residence in the United States due to acculturation and other factors. For example, prostate cancer incidence is about 16% lower in Latino men than in non-Latino

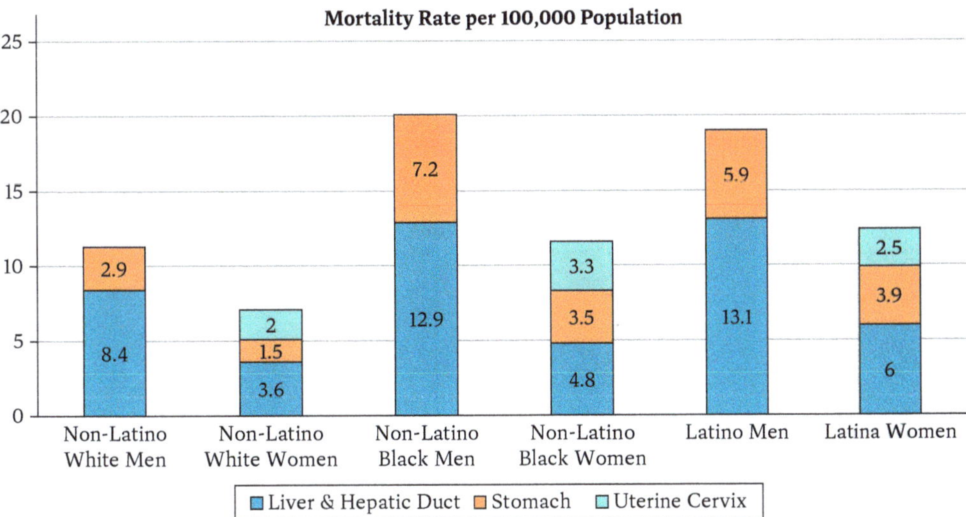

FIGURE 8.24 Mortality Rates for Selected Cancer Inequalities by Race/Ethnicity and Gender, United States, 2015–2019

Rates are per 100,000 population, age adjusted to the 2000 U.S. standard population, and exclude data from Puerto Rico

Source: American Cancer Society, Table 9, 2023. https://www.cancer.org/content/dam/cancer-org/research/cancer-facts-and-statistics/annual-cancer-facts-and-figures/2023/mr8-race-and-ethnicity-2023-cff.pdf

White men but 44% higher in men residing in Puerto Rico, which is 99% comprised of Latinos of Puerto Rican descent (American Cancer Society, 2023).

Overweight and Obesity

There are clear health inequalities among Latinos associated with obesity and severe obesity. Certain types of cancers, like gallbladder and stomach cancers, and liver disease and cirrhosis are etiologically linked to severe obesity (BMI > 40) among Latinos of Mexican descent. Overweight and obesity are defined internationally by the calculation of body mass index (BMI; Kaplan et al., 2014). BMI is calculated by using one's weight divided by height (in meters) squared (Pietrzak et al., 2019, p. 3, Table 8.6).

TABLE 8.6 **Body Mass Index and Overweight and Obesity**

Body mass index (BMI) (Kg/m^2)	Grade
25.0–29.9	Overweight
30.0–34.9	Grade 1 obesity: Obese
35.0–39.9	Grade 2 obesity: Severe obesity
>40	Grade 3 obesity: Morbid obesity

Source: Adapted from Pietrzak et al., 2019, p.3

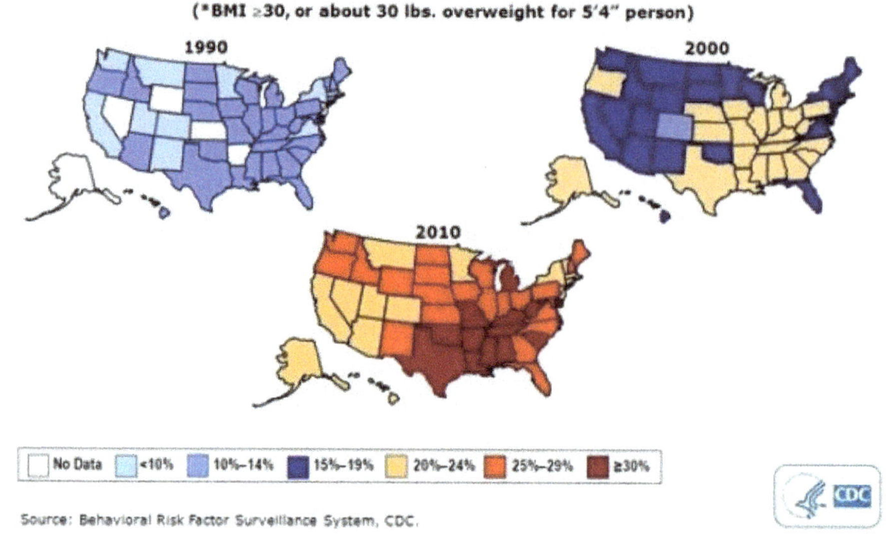

FIGURE 8.25 Obesity Trends Among U.S. Adults, 1990–2010

Obesity trends in the United States have increased dramatically over the past 2 decades (CDC, n.d.-c). In 1990, among states participating in the Behavioral Risk Factor Surveillance System (BRFSS), 10 states had a prevalence of obesity less than 10% and no state had prevalence greater than or equal to 15%. In 2000, no state had a prevalence of obesity less than 10%, 23 states had a prevalence between 20% and 24%, and no state had prevalence greater than or equal to 25%. By 2010, no state had a prevalence of obesity less than 20%, 36 states had a prevalence equal to or greater than 25%, and 12 of these states (Alabama, Arkansas, Kentucky, Louisiana, Michigan, Mississippi, Missouri, Oklahoma, South Carolina, Tennessee, Texas, and West Virginia) had a prevalence equal to or greater than 30% (see Figure 8.25).

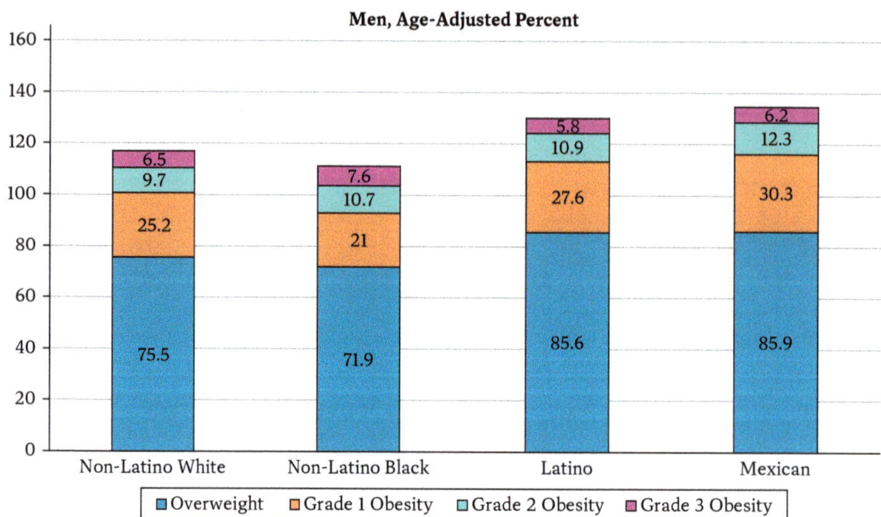

FIGURE 8.26 Overweight and Graded Obesity Prevalence Among Men by Race/Ethnicity, 2013–2015

Trend maps used by the CDC (n.d.-c) show racial and ethnic differences among men and women regarding overweight and obesity classes, and are shown in Figures 8.26 and 8.27, respectively, for the years 2013–2015. The highest overweight prevalence is observed for Mexican men and other Latino men in comparison to non-Latino Black men and White men. Mexican men also have the highest prevalence rates of Grade 1 and Grade 2 obesity at 30.3% and 12.3%, respectively. However, non-Latino White men and Black men have higher prevalence rates of Grade 3 obesity than Mexicans and other Latinos.

Overweight and obesity differences among women are also observed in the trend maps from the CDC (n.d.-c). Almost 84% of Mexican women are overweight, the highest among the racial and ethnic groups considered. Non-Latina White women have the lowest prevalence rates of overweight and obesity compared to the other groups. Non-Latina Black women have the highest prevalence rates of Grades 1, 2, and 3 of obesity compared to others.

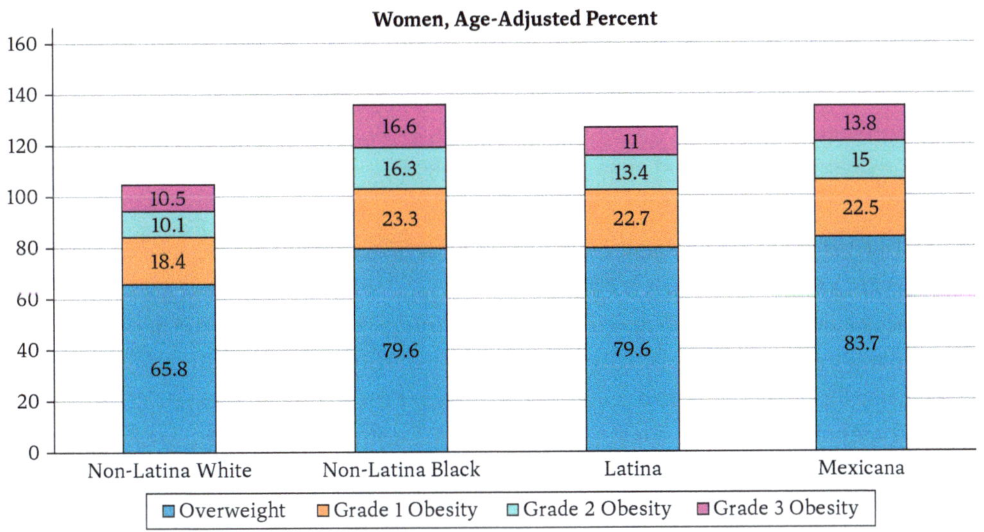

FIGURE 8.27 Overweight and Graded Obesity Prevalence Among Women by Race/Ethnicity, 2013–2015

According to the CDC obesity trend maps (CDC, n.d.-c), in 2015–2017 among Latino adults, ≥ 35% obesity rates were found in Arizona, Texas, Oklahoma, North Dakota, South Dakota, Illinois, and Michigan (Figure 8.28).

According to Hales et al. (2020), during 2017–2018, increases in overweight and obesity continued, though not significantly so. Among Latinos, 45.7% of men and 43.7% of women over 20 years of age were obese, which was higher than the national average of 42.4%. Hales et al. found that non-Latina White women had the lower obesity rates than Latina or African American women.

According to Mokdad et al. (2003), persons with severe obesity are likely to have significant comorbidities like diabetes mellitus (26%), asthma (23%), arthritis (44%), hypertension (51%), and cancer (52%). Other studies have shown that the percentages of cancer attributed to obesity were 11% for colon

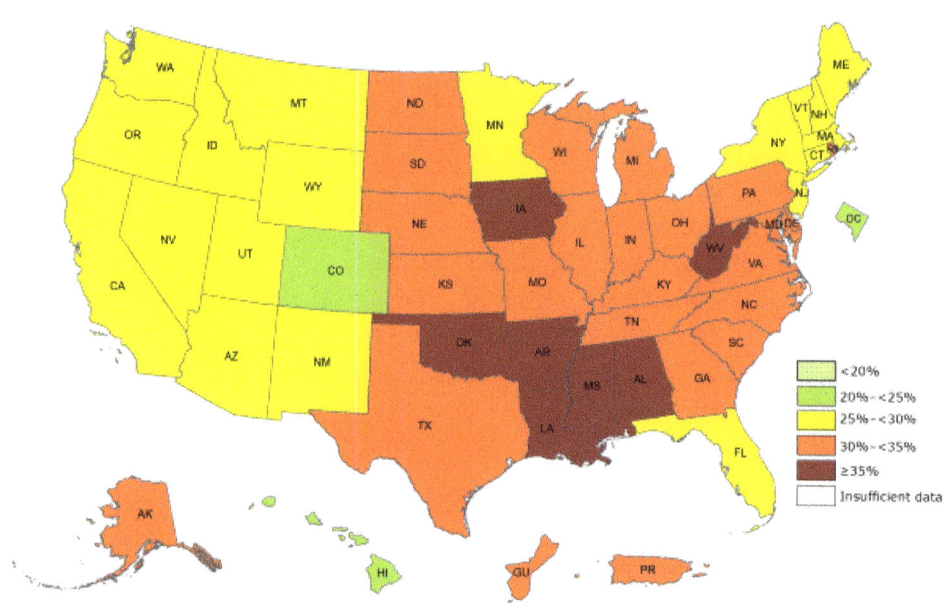

FIGURE 8.28 Obesity Rates Among Latinos, 2015–2017, BRFSS

cancer, 9% for postmenopausal breast cancer, 39% for endometrial cancer, 25% for kidney cancer, and 37% for esophageal cancer (Vainio & Bianchini, 2002).

Similarly, Calle et al. (2003) found a dose-response relationship between increased obesity and certain types of cancers. For overweight and obese women, relative to those women with a BMI < 25, the risk of developing cancer was 8% higher for a BMI 25.0–29.9; 18% higher for a BMI 30 .0–34.9; 32% higher for a BMI 35.0–39.9; and 62% higher for a BMI ≥ 40. For men, only BMI ≥ 30 was associated with increased cancer risk; a BMI of 30.0–34.9 elevated risk by 9%; 35.0–39.9 by 20%; and ≥ 40 by 52%. Calle et al. also estimated the population attributable fraction (PAF) in 2000 to be 14% for men and 20% for women, meaning that 14% of all cancers in men and 20% of all cancers in women are attributable to obesity, especially Grade 3 obesity and above (BM ≥ 35; Table 8.7).

TABLE 8.7 Obesity-Associated Cancer Mortality

Cancer type and BMI	Men (RR)	Women (RR)
Liver (≥35)	4.52	1.68
Pancreas (≥35)	2.61	2.76
Stomach (≥35)	1.94	-
Colorectal (≥35)	1.84	1.46
Gallbladder (≥30)	1.76	2.13
Multiple myeloma (≥35)	1.71	1.44
Kidney (≥35)	1.70	4.75

Cancer type and BMI	Men (RR)	Women (RR)
All other cancers (≥40)	1.68	2.51
Non-Hodgkin's lymphoma (≥35)	1.49	1.95
Prostate (≥35)	1.34	-
Ovarian (≥35)	-	1.51
Breast (≥40)	-	2.12
Cervical (≥35)	-	3.20
Uterus (≥40)	-	6.25

Source: Calle and Thun (2004)

The observed dose-response relationship and relative risk profiles for each of the cancers shown in Table 8.7 hints at the higher rates seen for stomach, gallbladder, and liver cancers found among obese Latinos of Mexican descent (Stern et al., 2016).

Metabolic Syndrome (MeS)

Metabolic syndrome is also known as *insulin resistance syndrome*. It represents a cluster of risk factors that are responsible for excess cardiovascular disease mortality among overweight and obese people and those who have diabetes mellitus (type 2 diabetes). The major characteristics of metabolic syndrome include insulin resistance, central fat or abdominal obesity, elevated blood pressure, and lipid abnormalities such as elevated levels of triglycerides and low levels of high-density lipoprotein cholesterol (HDL).

Latino men and women have a higher prevalence of metabolic syndrome (MeS) than either non-Latino White Americans or Black Americans. Ford et al. (2002), using national data from the National Health and Nutrition Examination Survey III (1988–1994), found that the age-adjusted prevalence of metabolic syndrome was 23.7% among U.S. adults 20 years or older. Moreover, they found Mexican Americans had the highest age-adjusted prevalence of metabolic syndrome (31.9%). The age-adjusted prevalence was similar for men (24.0%) and women (23.4%). However, among African Americans, women had about a 57% higher prevalence than men did, and among Mexican Americans women had about a 26% higher prevalence than men. According to Heiss et al. (2014), the prevalence of MeS varies from a low of 27.3% among South Americans to a high of 37.1% for Puerto Ricans, with about 35% of Latino men and women 18–74 years of age having MeS.

The age-adjusted prevalence of metabolic abnormalities associated with metabolic syndrome are shown in Figure 8.29. Mexican Americans have higher rates of metabolic abnormalities than non-Latino White Americans and Black Americans. Studies have shown a positive association between metabolic syndrome and liver/liver duct cancer, with a risk estimate of 1.5–2.5 (50% to 2.5 times the risk!) with a population attributable fraction (PAF) between 30% and 40% (El-Serag & Kanwal, 2014).

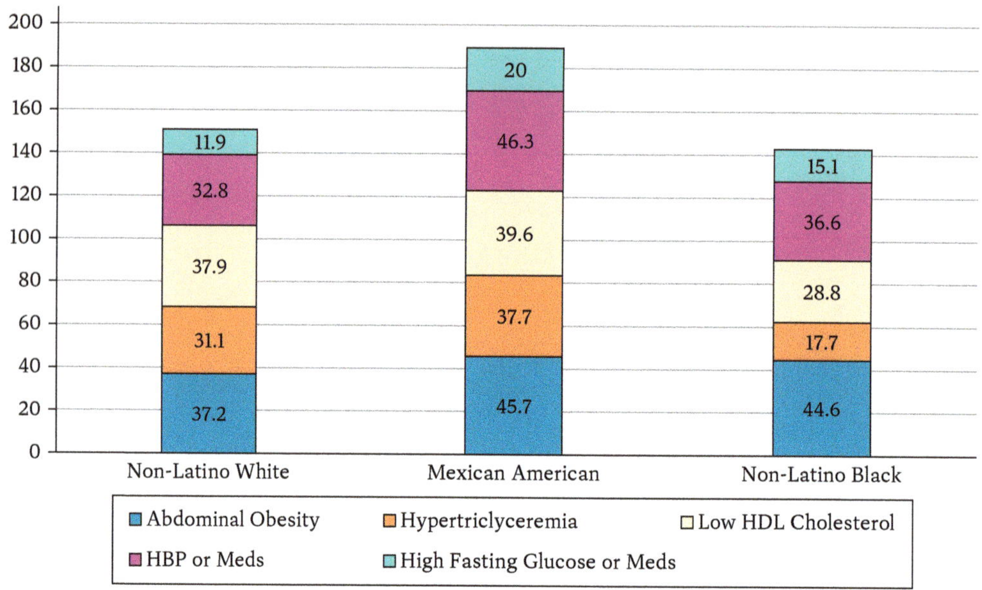

FIGURE 8.29 Age-Adjusted Prevalence (%) of Metabolic Abnormalities of Metabolic Syndrome Among Adults Aged 20 and Older by Race and Ethnicity, United States, NHANES III

Ford et al. (2002) found wide variations by race/ethnicity and gender as well (Figure 8.30). Mexican American women have higher rates of abdominal obesity and low HDL cholesterol than Mexican American men. However, Mexican American men have higher rates of hypertriglyceridemia, HBP or medication use, and high fasting glucose or medication use. The overall prevalence of metabolic syndrome among Mexican American men compared to Mexican American women was 28% and 36%, respectively. The probability of developing comorbid diseases like heart disease, liver and bile duct cancer, female breast cancer, endometrial cancer, and colorectal cancer increases with higher prevalence of metabolic syndrome and obesity. For example, a study of Medicare patients by Makarova-Rusher et al. (2016) found that metabolic disorders had the largest population attributable fraction (PAF) among Latinos (39.3%) and non-Latino

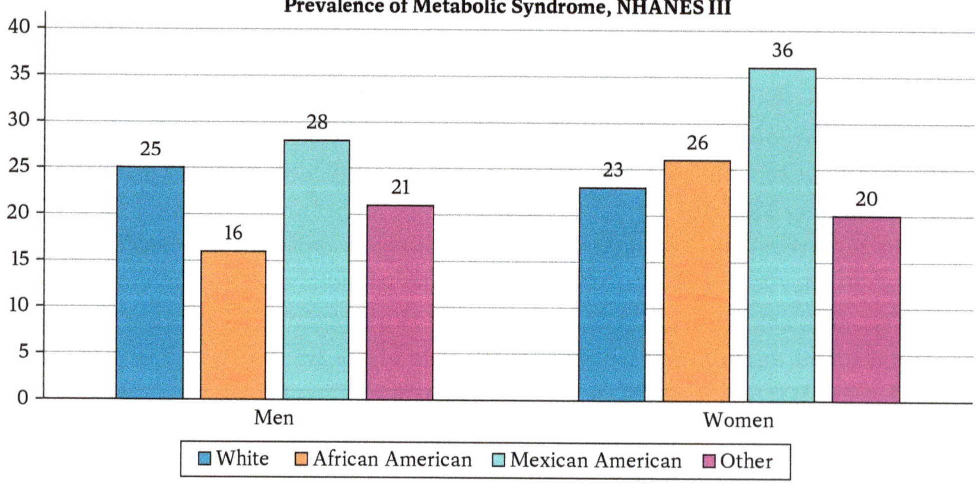

FIGURE 8.30 Prevalence of Metabolic Syndrome, NHANES III

White Americans (34.8%) and that they contribute more to the burden of liver cancer than any other risk factor they examined, including hepatitis b, hepatitis c, smoking, alcohol, and genetics.

Type 2 Diabetes

Diabetes mellitus is also known as *type 2 diabetes* and *non-insulin dependent diabetes mellitus* (*NIDDM*). Type 2 diabetes is a metabolic disorder characterized by abnormal glucose metabolism. People with type 2 diabetes have a relative rather than an absolute deficiency in insulin production. This is caused by the body's resistance to the action of insulin and to impaired insulin secretion. Low insulin sensitivity is referred to as *insulin resistance*. Insulin resistance is linked to overeating, being overweight, physical inactivity, aging, medication use, hyperglycemia, and elevated free fatty acids (FFAs). FFAs have been shown to be associated with inhibiting insulin-stimulated glucose uptake and glycogen synthesis (Delarue & Magnan, 2007).

Insulin sensitivity describes how sensitive the body is to the effects of insulin and its uptake. It is influenced by lifestyle and dietary practices as well as heredity. Insulin resistance is associated with abnormal beta-cell function in the pancreas, which in turn influences relative insulin deficiency leading to hyperglycemia and type 2 diabetes. High insulin sensitivity means the body is having difficulty metabolizing glucose in the blood stream. A person who has high insulin sensitivity will require smaller amounts of insulin to lower blood glucose levels than someone who has low insulin sensitivity. People with low insulin sensitivity will require larger amounts of insulin either from their own pancreas or from injections to keep blood glucose stable. Most people, including 90%–95% of Latino diabetics have type 2 diabetes. Chiu et al. (2000) showed that Mexican Americans in their study had significantly lower rates of low insulin sensitivity (i.e., higher levels of insulin resistance) than non-Latino White Americans.

Insulin resistance is associated with cardiomyopathy, urinary frequency, light-headedness, bloating, heartburn, constipation, erectile dysfunction, abdominal fat, elevated blood sugar, hypertension, elevated triglycerides, inflammation of the liver and cirrhosis, sleep apnea, polycystic ovarian disease, atherosclerosis which contributes to heart attacks, strokes, ad peripheral vascular disease, increased blood clots, and low levels of HDL (Azziz, 2007; Castro et al., 2014; Ormazabal et al., 2018; Polsky & Ellis, 2015).

Prediabetes is a serious health condition where blood glucose level is higher than normal but not high enough for a diagnosis of type 2 diabetes. Prediabetes increases the risk of developing type 2 diabetes, heart disease, and stroke. The National Diabetes Statistics Report (CDC, n.d.-b) estimates the prevalence of prediabetes among Latinos between 2017–2020 at 34.5%, which was lower than non-Latino White Americans (38.7 %) and non-Latino Black Americans (39.2%). About 90% of people with prediabetes are unaware that they have the condition. For example, the prevalence of prediabetes awareness in 2019 was lower among Latinos (20.9%) than non-Latino White Americans (17.3%) but not non-Latino Black Americans (21.9%). According to the CDC (n.d.-c) Risk factors for prediabetes include:

- Being overweight
- Being 45 years or older
- Having a parent, brother, or sister with type 2 diabetes
- Being physically active less than three times/week
- Ever having gestational diabetes (diabetes during pregnancy) or giving birth to a baby who weighed more than 9 pounds
- Having polycystic ovarian syndrome

Type 2 Diabetes Incidence

According to the CDC (n.d.-a), in 2018–2019, an estimated 1.4 million new cases of diabetes (5.9 per 1,000 persons) were diagnosed among U.S. adults aged 18 years or older. Compared to adults aged 18–44 years, incidence rates of diagnosed diabetes were higher among adults aged 45–64 years and those aged 65 years and older. Incidence rates did not vary significantly by racial/ethnic group, but Latinos had the highest incidence rate of 7.0/1,000 compared to non-Latino Black Americans (6.5/1,000) and non-Latino White Americans (6/1,000).

Type 2 Diabetes Prevalence

According to the CDC (n.d.-a), about 38.4 million adults over the age of 18 years, or 11.6% of all U.S. adults, have type 2 diabetes, and of these, about 23% were undiagnosed. Type 2 diabetes prevalence is correlated with increases in overweight and obesity. There are significant variations in type 2 diabetes prevalence by age, education level, and race/ethnicity. For example, 29.2% of adults aged 65 and older have type 2 diabetes (CDC, n.d.-a; Narayan et al., 2003). Additionally, 12.6% of adults with less than a high school education compared to 7.2% of those with more than a high school education were diagnosed with type 2 diabetes. In 2018, Latinos had higher type 2 diabetes prevalence rates than non-Latino White Americans and non-Latino Black Americans (12.5% compared to 7.5% and 11.7%, respectively). Among the Latino subgroups, Latinos of Mexican descent had the highest type 2 diabetes prevalence (14.4%), followed by Puerto Ricans (12.4%), Central and South Americans (8.3%), and Cubans (6.5%). Among U.S. adults aged 18 years or older, age-adjusted data for 2017–2018 showed that among Latino subgroups, Mexicans (14.4%) and Puerto Ricans (12.4%) had the highest prevalence rates for diagnosed type 2 diabetes, followed by Central/South Americans (8.3%) and Cubans (6.5%). Data from 2017–2020, however, shows that non-Latino Black Americans have higher rates than Latino Americans, and Latino Americans and non-Latino White Americans have similar rates (Table 8.8).

Type 2 Diabetes Complications

Miller et al. (2013) discuss several major complications of type 2 diabetes that include:

- Heart disease
- Eye disease (blindness, retinopathy)
- Kidney disease (renal failure)
- Nerve disease (diabetic neuropathy)
- Peripheral vascular disease
- Inadequate circulation leading to infection, injury, and lower limb amputations
- Higher incidence of myocardial infarction
- Higher incidence of congestive heart failure
- Higher incidence of stroke

Higher rates of complications related to type 2 diabetes have been documented in studies of Mexican Americans (Haw et al., 2021). End-stage renal disease (ESRD) and lower limb amputation are the most common type 2 diabetes complications among Latinos (Ricardo et al., 2015). For example, Ricardo et al.

(2015, p. 1757) reported that the age-adjusted incidence of ESRD due to type 2 diabetes among Latinos was "50% greater" than non-Latinos.

TABLE 8.8 Estimated Crude Prevalence of Diagnosed Diabetes, Undiagnosed Diabetes, and Total Diabetes Among Adults Aged 18 Years or Older, United States, 2017–2020

	% Diagnosed (95% CI)	% Undiagnosed (95%CI)	% Total (95% CI)
Non-Latino White	11.0 (9.4–12.8)	2.7 (1.7–4.2)	13.6 (11.4–16.2)
Non-Latino Black	12.7 (10.7–15.0)	4.7 (3.3–6.5)	17.4 (15.2–19.8)
Latino	11.1 (9.5–13.0)	4.4 (3.3–5.8)	15.5 (13.8–17.3)

Source: CDC (n.d.-a)

A recently updated definition of Stages 1–4 of chronic kidney disease shows that non-Latino Black Americans have the highest crude rate (46.6%), followed by Latino Americans (38.5 %), and non-Latino White Americans (38.2%; CDC, n.d.-b). Only about 30% of all groups were aware of their condition, with lower rates of awareness among Latinos.

TABLE 8.9 Association Between Type 2 Diabetes Complications and Modifiable Risk Factors

Modifiable risk factors	Stroke	Coronary heart disease (CHD)	Peripheral vascular disease (PVD)	Retinopathy	End stage renal disease (ESRD)	Lower limb amputation
Obesity	+	+	+	+	+	+
Lack of self-management skills and access to care	+	+	+	+	+	+
Hypertension	+	+	+	+	+	+
Cigarette smoking	+	+	+	+	+	+
Hyperlipidemia	+	+	+	?	?	+
Hyperglycemia	+	+	+	?	?	+

Adapted from Miller et al. (2013).

Type 2 Diabetes Mortality

Between 2019 and 2020, the mortality rates for type 2 diabetes increased by almost 15% (Murphy et al., 2021). However, Kochanek et al. (2023) reported that from 2021 to 2022 the age-adjusted mortality rate for type 2 diabetes decreased from 25.4/100,000 in 2021 to 24.1/100,000 in 2022. Overall, in 2022, type 2 diabetes was the eighth leading cause of mortality in the United States (Kochanek, et al., 2023).

According to data from the CDC (n.d.-b), type 2 diabetes is the sixth leading cause of mortality among Latinos in 2020. A study by Lv et al. (2022), found that type 2 diabetes mortality increased by more than 30% during the COVID-19 pandemic, with adults 25–44 years of age having the greatest increase in mortality. Moreover, Latino Americans were found to have the highest excess of deaths, which were three times higher than non-Latino White Americans.

However, because many people die of complications related to type 2 diabetes rather than the disease itself, type 2 diabetes tends to be underreported as the underlying or even the contributing cause of death (Chukwueke & Cordero-MacIntyre, 2010; Gu et al., 1998). Nevertheless, according to data released by the Kaiser Family Foundation (Nambi-Ndugga & Artiga, 2023) type 2 diabetes mortality rates are substantially higher among Latino Americans in comparison to non-Latino White Americans (29.4/100,000 vs. 22.4/100,000).

Gallbladder Disease (GBD)

Gallbladder disease (GBD) has a 15% prevalence rate among adults in the United States (Stinton et al., 2010). GBD includes gallstones, the surgical removal of the gallbladder (cholecystectomy), and cholecystitis. The incidence of GBD is associated with genetics, lifestyle behaviors related to abdominal obesity, and dietary practices (Hanis et al., 1985; Maurer et al., 1989; Samet et al., 1988).

One of the early hypotheses advanced to account for the higher observed prevalence of GBD among Latinos of Mexican descent is that the proportion of American Indian admixture in their genetic profile contributes to these higher rates (Hanis et al., 1985; Samet et al., 1988). Scholars note the similar epidemiology between Mexican Americans residing in the Southwest and American Indians, who also have very high rates of comorbid conditions like hypertension, type 2 diabetes, and obesity.

The Hispanic Health and Nutrition Examination Survey (HHANES) conducted between 1982 and 1984, was the first nationally representative sample of Latino health in the United States that provided a baseline for studying GBD among Puerto Ricans, Cubans, and Mexican Americans (Maurer et al., 1989). Maurer et al. (1989) found that the age-adjusted prevalence of GBD (gallstones + cholecystectomy) was higher among Mexican American men (7.2%), which was 1.7 times higher than Cuban men and 1.8 times higher than Puerto Rican men. The prevalence of GBD for Mexican American women (23.2%) was 1.5 times higher than Cuban women and 1.7 times higher than Puerto Rican women. Women had 3 times higher rates than men, with increasing rates with age, except for older Puerto Rican women. A very high rate of GBD (44.1%) was found among Mexican American women aged 60–74 years. When compared to other Latino subgroups, evidence shows that Latinos of Mexican descent have higher rates of GBD than others, again suggesting a genetic association with American Indian ancestry.

Figueiredo et al. (2017) examined the incidence and prevalence of gallbladder disease among a longitudinal cohort of Latinos born in the United States and Mexico/South America. The prevalence of GBD was lower among Latinos (17.9% among U.S.-born and 17.3% among Mexico/South America–born) than

African Americans (18.4%) and highest among non-Latino White Americans (19.4%). Higher rates were found for women than men. Among U.S.-born Latinos significant risk factors for GBD included obesity, type 2 diabetes, and smoking. Additionally, consumption of dietary fiber, vegetables, red meat, percentage of calories from saturated fat, and cholesterol were significantly associated with GBD incidence among U.S.-born Latinos. The study authors concluded that "the overall body of evidence supports the hypothesis that a diet characterized by high caloric intake, refined carbohydrates, animal protein and cholesterol and low in vegetables and dietary fiber increase risk of GBD" (Figueiredo et al., 2017, Discussion section).

Chronic Liver Disease

Chronic liver disease (CLD) is a major cause of morbidity and mortality in the United States, resulting in approximately 66,000 deaths each year, with the major underlying causes being alcohol-related liver disease, hepatitis C, and nonalcoholic fatty liver disease (NAFLD), with many patients having a high prevalence of NAFLD. Overall, Latino Americans are 50% more likely to die from CLD than non-Latino White Americans and it is the sixth leading cause of mortality (CDC, 2015).

Browning et al. (2004) found an overall NAFLD prevalence of 31% in their large sample (n = 2287). They also found that the frequency of NAFLD varied significantly by race and ethnicity, with 45% of Latino Americans, 33% of non-Latino White Americans, and 24% of non-Latino Black Americans being diagnosed with NAFLD, with higher rates among men than women. The authors suggest that the higher prevalence of NAFLD in Latinos was due to their higher prevalence of obesity and insulin resistance and not due to increased alcohol consumption. Setiawan et al. (2016) used the multiethnic cohort prospective design of more than 215,000 men and women, aged 45–75 years, enrolled between 1993 and 2012, and found the prevalence of CLD ranged from a low of 3.9% in African Americans, to 4.1% in non-Latino White Americans, and 6.7% in Latino Americans. NAFLD was the most common cause of CLD in all ethnic groups combined (52%), followed by alcoholic liver disease (21%). NAFLD was the most common cause of cirrhosis in the entire cohort, with Latino Americans having the highest comorbidity prevalence (45.6%), followed by non-Latino White Americans (40.7%) and Black Americans (39.2%).

Carrion et al. (2011) conducted a meta-analysis on CLD and NAFLD and found that the prevalence was almost 2 times higher in Latinos than in Black Americans and 1.4 times higher than in non-Latino White Americans. Latinos with NAFLD were found to have more advanced fibrosis than other ethnic groups, and Latinos had the highest prevalence of alcoholic liver disease. Moreover, the incidence of hepatic cancer in Latino Americans is 2.7 times higher than in non-Latino White Americans; mortality from hepatic cancer is 9% higher than in non-Latino White Americans.

Burden of Disease: Examining Heart Disease, Cancer, Diabetes, and Stroke Inequalities Among Latinos

Social inequalities in cardiovascular disease (CVD) risk factors, incidence, and mortality are well-documented in the research literature (Havranek et al., 2015). Researchers have also documented the high prevalence of CVD risk factors found among Latinos (Crespo et al., 1996; Mitchell et al., 1990; Sundquist & Winkleby, 1999) but without finding a corresponding increase in CVD mortality in comparison to non-Latino White Americans and non-Latino Black Americans (Daviglus et al., 2012). However, studies among older Latino participants show that the combination of depression and type 2 diabetes increases the risk of CVD mortality (Inoue et al., 2021). Although there is no evidence to support a finding that Latino Americans experience higher CVD mortality than non-Latino White Americans, the prevalence of several CVD risk factors is cause for concern.

Prior to COVID-19, the five leading causes of death in the United States in 2019 were heart disease, cancer, unintentional injuries, chronic lower respiratory diseases, and stroke. Together, these five leading causes of death accounted for 61% of all deaths. Heart disease and cancer are the major contributors of mortality in the United States, accounting for about 44% of all deaths in 2019 (Heron, 2021).

In comparison to other historically disadvantaged populations, Latinos of Mexican descent tend to have better all-cause mortality rates even in the face of economic hardship and *a lack* of health-enhancing social determinants like access to quality education, access to quality medical care, residing in segregated neighborhoods, and living in built environments that emit hazardous emissions. Discussion of potential factors for better mortality outcomes include the Latino mortality paradox, social support networks, and cultural values that mitigate against engagement in high-risk behaviors. However, there are known cultural values that increase risk behaviors, namely *machismo* and *marianismo*, one by commission and the other by omission. Additionally, assimilation into the non-Latino White mainstream culture increases risk behaviors for many chronic and communicable diseases like obesity, diabetes, and HIV.

Using data from NCHS (n.d.-k) an examination of the *chronic disease burden*, defined as the prevalence of heart disease, cancer, diabetes mellitus, and stroke, showed that non-Latino Black Americans had the highest additive chronic disease burden than any other group from 2017–2018 (Figure 8.31). Latinos of Mexican descent have the lowest prevalence of heart disease, cancer, and stroke but the highest prevalence for diabetes mellitus, as shown in Figure 8.30. Other Latinos also report lower prevalence rates of heart disease, cancer, and stroke than non-Latino White Americans and non-Latino Black

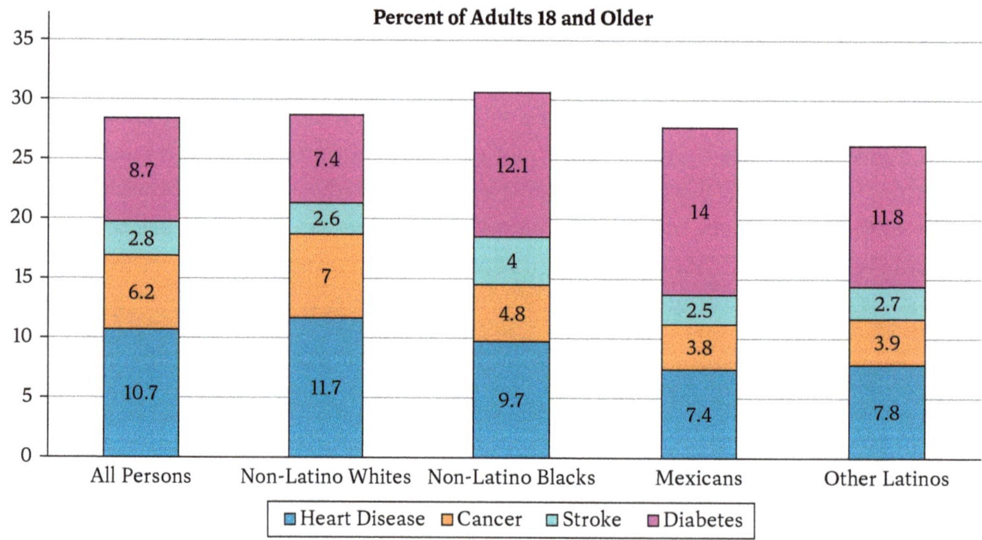

FIGURE 8.31 Respondent-Reported Prevalence of Heart Disease, Cancer, Diabetes, and Stroke Among Adults Aged 18 and Over by Race/Ethnicity, 2017–2018, Age-Adjusted

Source: NCHS, Health, United States, 2019

Americans. Diabetes mellitus prevalence is higher in Latinos, as many studies have documented. If untreated or not detected early, it can lead to severe complications requiring increased medical expenses and premature death.

Latino Health Inequalities in the U.S.–Mexico Border Region

Within the social determinants of health framework, place is important. As noted in Chapter 4, the U.S.-Mexico border region is a unique place and very different from non-border regions, in part due to high levels of socioeconomic poverty, younger ages, shared border infrastructures, and lack of access to medical care. Though on a national level there appears to be a Latino mortality paradox, this is primarily in the U.S.-Mexico border region, where predominantly Latinos of Mexican descent reside. Recall that some of the research related to the Latino mortality paradox suggests that Latinos of Mexican descent are the primary drivers of mortality differences (Abraido-Lanza et al., 1999).

The following data and associated figures were derived from CDC WONDER (n.d.) online database comparing U.S.-Mexico border regions to non-border regions. Latinos were compared to non-Latino White Americans and non-Latino Black Americans for "diseases of the digestive system," "endocrine, nutritional, and metabolic diseases," and "certain infectious and parasitic diseases."

According to CDC WONDER (n.d.) data, age-adjusted mortality rates from diseases of the digestive system are higher among Latinos living in the U.S.-Mexico border region compared to Latinos living in non- border regions and higher than non-Latino White Americans and Black Americans living in the U.S.-Mexico border region (Figure 8.32).

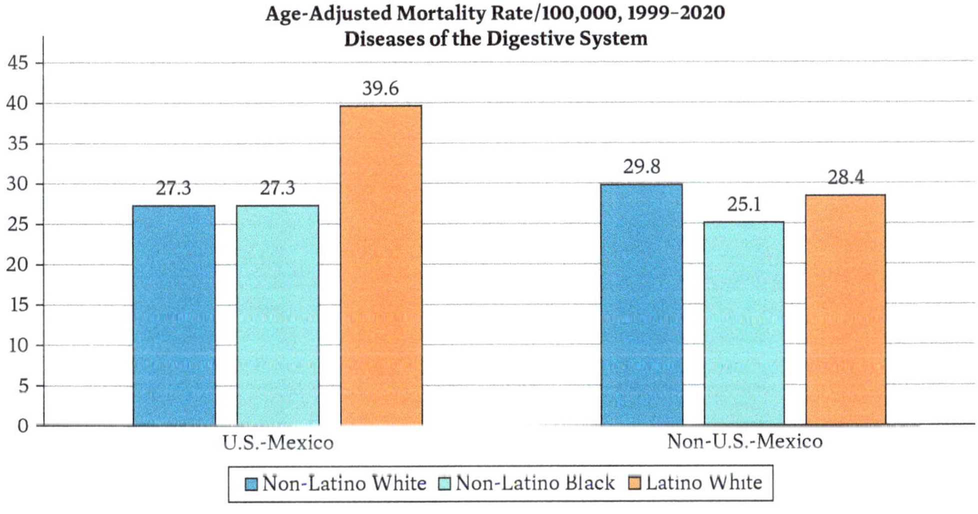

FIGURE 8.32 Age-Adjusted Mortality Rate for Diseases of the Digestive System

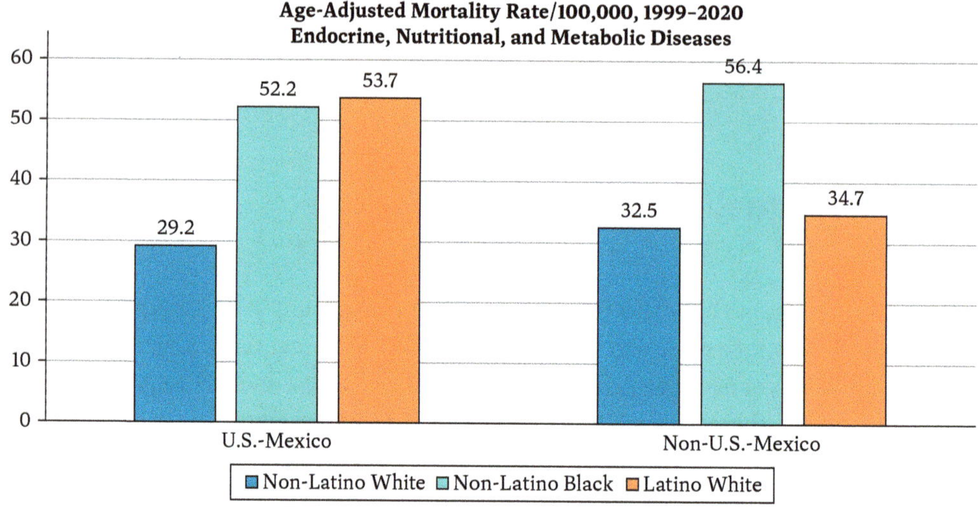

FIGURE 8.33 Age-Adjusted Mortality Rate for Endocrine, Nutritional, and Metabolic Diseases

Latino living in the U.S.-Mexico border region have substantially higher mortality rates than non-Latino White Americans and Latinos living in non-border regions of endocrine, nutritional, and metabolic diseases (CDC WONDER, n.d.; Figure 8.33).

Diabetes mellitus mortality rates are substantially higher among Latinos than non-Latinos residing in the U.S.-Mexico border states of Arizona, California, New Mexico, and Texas (CDC WONDER, n.d.; Table 8.10). The highest diabetes mellitus mortality rate relative to non-Latinos is in Arizona.

TABLE 8.10 Age-Adjusted Diabetes Mortality Rates, 2021

State	Primary Latino origin	Percentage Latino	Latino rate/100,000	Non-Latino rate/100,000
New Mexico	Mexican	47.7	34.5	24.5
California	Mexican	39.4	33.2	20.7
Texas	Mexican	39.3	34.6	21.7
Arizona	Mexican	30.7	38.8	22.5

Source: CDC WONDER (n.d.)

Similar to national data showing Latinos have higher rates of liver and intrahepatic duct cancers, Latinos residing in the U.S.-Mexico border states have significantly higher rates than non-Latinos, reaching almost twice the mortality rate in New Mexico and Ariona (CDC WONDER, n.d.; Table 8.11).

TABLE 8.11 **Age-Adjusted Liver and Intrahepatic Duct Cancer, 2021**

State	Primary Latino origin	Percentage Latino	Latino rate/100,000	Non-Latino rate/100,000
New Mexico	Mexican	47.7	12.5	6.5
California	Mexican	39.4	10	6.8
Texas	Mexican	39.3	11.4	7.3
Arizona	Mexican	30.7	9	5.7

Source: CDC WONDER (n.d.)

Certain infectious and parasitic disease mortality is also higher among Latinos compared to non-Latino White Americans (almost twice the rate) and non-Latino Black Americans living in the U.S.-Mexico border region (CDC WONDER, n.d.; Figure 8.34). Their rates are also higher than Latinos not living in the U.S.-Mexico border region. The rate for non-Latino Black Americans living in non-border regions is almost 2 times the rate for non-Latino White Americans and Latino Americans.

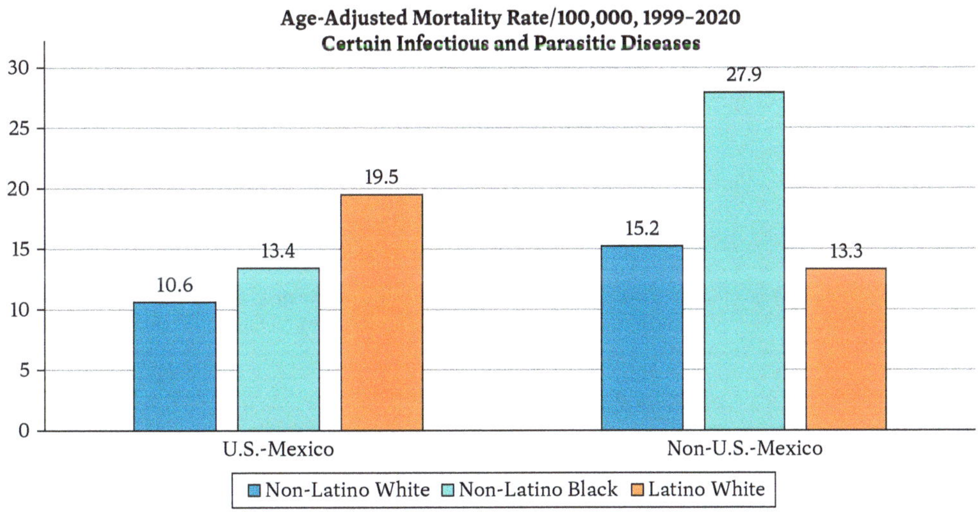

FIGURE 8.34 Age-Adjusted Mortality Rate for Certain Infectious and Parasitic Diseases

Compared to non-Latino White Americans, Latinos living in the U.S.-Mexico border region have significant mortality inequalities with reference to diseases of the digestive system, endocrine, nutritional, and metabolic diseases, and for certain infectious and parasitic diseases, as noted above. Latinos living in the U.S.-Mexico border region are unique and have tremendous socioeconomic inequalities and poorer health status Latinos living in non-border regions. National comparisons between Latinos and other racial and ethnic groups should take these differences into consideration, as well as the paradoxical relationship between health and socioeconomic status and other social determinants of health. These differences along the U.S.-Mexico border provide a stark difference in relation to Latinos and non-Latinos not living in the region.

Modifying Disease Risk Factors Among Latinos

Prevention of health inequalities among Latinos should focus on macro and micro factors that are amenable to change. Among the macro factors, a concerted effort to eliminate inequalities in the basic social determinants of health requires social justice and a reallocation of resources to reduce poverty, enhance access to quality education and health care, and provide prevention services in the Latino community.

Attention to the public health tenets of primary, secondary, and tertiary prevention can facilitate a reduction in risk factors Moreover, using Latino cultural strengths and values can assist in modifying behaviors and attitudes. The basic public health model includes prevention strategies that are targeted to the population's disease status and desired outcomes (Figure 8.35).

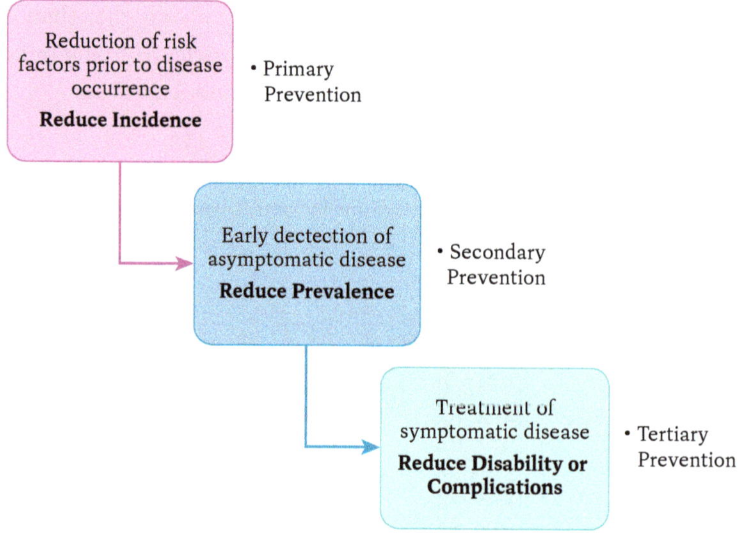

FIGURE 8.35 Public Health Model of Prevention

Increasing screening rates, access to health care, remaining in care, following prescriptive recommendations, and achieving positive health outcomes are the goals of chronic disease prevention. An integration of educational communications and cultural values can effectively reach Latino populations, as several studies have demonstrated (Caballero, 2005; Larkey & Gonzalez, 2007; Rivera, 2018).

Incidence and prevalence rates are associated with inadequate screening facilities, lack of access to health care and financial burden, delayed presentation of asymptomatic and symptomatic disease, lack of knowledge and awareness of efficacious treatments and treatment side effects, and several cultural factors that can enhance or hinder prevention among Latinos (Buki & Selem, 2009). For example, fatalism can prevent screening and engagement in health maintenance. *Machismo* can prevent Latino men from obtaining prostate cancer prevention screening, like digital rectal exams. It can also act as a deterrent for women to obtain mammograms and pelvic exams because their Latino partners may not want others to see their body (Getrich et al., 2012). *Marianismo* among Latinas can prevent them from obtaining timely medical care because they are placing their families' needs first and their own needs last (D'Orazio et al., 2014).

Fear and anxiety associated with heart disease and cancer treatments can be paralyzing for many people, Latinos included. Lack of knowledge regarding specific treatments can be alleviated through education by persons who have survived the procedure and create positive social networks (Alligood-Percoco & Kesterson, 2016; Dean et al., 2018; Elder et al., 2009; Fairley et al., 2009). Connecting familism, the value and importance of the family, to survivorship is another means for enhancing treatment and rehabilitation among Latinos. Identifying and acknowledging cultural barriers and then using cultural values to work through these barriers can facilitate increased preventive screening and survivorship (Table 8.12).

TABLE 8.12 Prevention Strategy and Areas of Communication for Latinos

Prevention strategy	Areas of communication
Primary: focus on susceptible population	• Increase knowledge regarding symptom recognition. • Use age-appropriate screening recommendations. • Engage in nutritional guidelines. • Reduce fear and anxiety regarding disease and treatment. • Increase preventive behaviors. • Identify and acknowledge cultural challenges to engaging in preventive behaviors depending on disease. • Connect early screening to survivorship.
Secondary: focus on asymptomatic population	• Increase knowledge regarding efficacious treatment options and use of biopsies. • Focus on changing modifiable risk factors. • Maintain preventive behaviors, including blood pressure checks, blood-glucose level monitoring, breast self-exams, clinical breast exams, Pap smears, prostate exams and PSA screening, and colonoscopy. • Identify and acknowledge any cultural challenges in engaging in treatment, preventive behaviors, and changing risk behaviors, such as *machismo* and *marianismo*. • Connect treatment to increased survivorship (using familism), and challenge *fatalismo* beliefs and attitudes. • Decrease anxiety and fear regarding treatment options.

(*continued*)

TABLE 8.12 ***(continued)***

Prevention strategy	Areas of communication
Tertiary: focus on treatment of symptomatic population, rehabilitation, recovery and maintenance	• Increase knowledge regarding survivorship (e.g., 5-year survival rates for cancer). • Provide social support and use familism and respeto to enhance adherence to medications and medical regimens. • Maintain preventive behaviors and blood assessments. • Identify and acknowledge any cultural challenges in maintaining treatment and preventive behaviors. • Provide rehabilitation services, including spirituality and religion. • Provide examples of others who have achieved success.

Source: Adapted from Buki and Selem (2009)

CHAPTER SUMMARY

Questions remain unresolved regarding the tenacity of the hypothetical explanations accounting for the Latino mortality paradox. To date, the selective immigration hypothesis appears to be the leading empirically supported proposition. Latino Americans exhibit a mortality advantage relative to non-Latino White Americans and non-Latino Black Americans in the United States as a whole and in the U.S.-Mexico border region. Nevertheless, there are mortality and morbidity inequalities among Latinos compared to non-Latino White Americans.

A substantial proportion of Latinos of Mexican descent (about a quarter) do not have health insurance coverage, which means that out-of-pocket expenses for medical visits and prescription drugs can exceed what they can afford. General health status characteristics of Latino Americans show much higher self-ratings of "fair or poor" health in comparison to non-Latino White Americans across all age-groups and are especially high among elderly Latinos (≥ 65 years of age). Poverty is associated with fair or poor health ratings among all racial and ethnic groups examined. However, a paradoxical finding with Latino Americans and non-Latino Black Americans are higher rates of self-reported fair or poor health than non-Latino White Americans even with those living at 400% poverty or above.

Latino Americans also have a higher percentage of functional limitations (percentage reporting a lot of difficulty or cannot do things at all) than non-Latino White Americans, especially among older adults. Prescribed drug use is also lower among male and female Latinos of Mexican descent than their non-Latino White and non-Latino Black counterparts.

Psychological well-being is intrinsically linked to overall physical health status. Latinos of Mexican descent report higher rates of serious psychological distress in comparison to non-Latino White Americans from 1999–2011. But their rates are lower than other Latinos during the same timeframe. As expected, there is a linear association between poverty level and serious psychological distress across all racial and ethnic groups examined, with those living at less than 100% of the federal poverty showing significantly higher rates of serious psychological distress than those living at 400% or more of the federal poverty level. Again, paradoxically, Latinos living at 400% or more of the federal poverty level have higher rates than non-Latino White Americans and non-Latino Black Americans at almost 2:1. Latinos also report slightly higher rates of depression than non-Latino White Americans. Latinos of Mexican descent reported lower rates of feelings of worry, nervousness, or anxiety than other Latinos, non-Latino White Americans, and non-Latino Black Americans. Overall, Latinos of Mexican descent tend to show better levels of psychological well-being as measured by the reported levels of serious psychological distress, and feelings of worry, nervousness, or anxiety. Higher levels of depression remain a concern given its association with ratings of fair or poor health.

Latinos exhibit several chronic disease risk factors. Of most concern is the increasing prevalence of obesity, metabolic syndrome, and diabetes mellitus, which are all linked and a precursor to cardiovascular disease, cerebrovascular disease, and cancer. Studies have shown that acculturation level among Latinos is significantly associated with the prevalence of risk behaviors and risk factors. Cigarette smoking, alcohol and drug use, physical inactivity, and poor dietary practices are all associated with increased acculturation.

Hypertension rates are higher among Latinos of Mexican descent compared to non-Latino White Americans. Uncontrolled hypertension, however, can be deadly, and results show that Latinos and Latinos of Mexican descent have higher rates of uncontrolled hypertension than non-Latino White men and non-Latino Black men.

There are evident chronic disease inequalities among Latinos in comparison to non-Latino White Americans. The incidence of cancers of the stomach, uterine cervix, and liver and intrahepatic duct are much higher among Latinos and Latinas than non-Latino White men and women. Mortality inequalities are also observed for these same cancers, with higher rates among Latinos.

Rates of being overweight and obesity have dramatically increased in the United States since the 1990s. More U.S. residents are classified into the obesity and severe obesity grades than ever before. This is equally true and perhaps more so for Latinos in general and Latinos of Mexican descent specifically. Latino men of Mexican descent have higher prevalence rates of overweight, Grade 1 obesity, and Grade 2 obesity than other Latino Amerericans, non-Latino Black Americans, and non-Latino White Americans. Latinas of Mexican descent have higher rates of Grade 1 and Grade 2 obesity than non-Latina White women. Grade 2 obesity is significantly correlated with many cancer types, especially the liver, stomach, and gallbladder, all cancers that have a higher incidence and mortality among Latinos.

Metabolic abnormalities of metabolic syndrome are much higher among Mexican Americans than non-Latino White Americans. Moreover, the metabolic profile is worse for Mexican Americans than for non-Latino Black Americans. Research shows that the prevalence of metabolic syndrome is higher among both Mexican American men and women than non-Latino White Americans, non-Latino Black Americans, and other groups. Consequently, morbidity and mortality associated with type 2 diabetes is generally higher among Latinos than non-Latino White Americans.

Other chronic disease inequalities that are more prevalent among Latinos include gallbladder disease and chronic liver disease and cirrhosis. However, other than type 2 diabetes mortality, the burden of chronic disease is lower for Mexican Americans and other Latino Americans than non-Latino White Americans and non-Latino Black Americans.

The U.S.–Mexico border region is a unique place that differs from non-border regions in relation to several social and cultural determinants of health. Higher mortality rates for Latinos are observed for diseases of the digestive system, endocrine, nutritional, and metabolic diseases, type 2 diabetes, certain infectious and parasitic diseases, and liver and intrahepatic duct.

Reducing risk for chronic and infectious diseases is a high priority for public health entering the 21st century (Office of Disease Prevention and Health Promotion, n.d.). The utilization of a public health model for prevention can provide comprehensive prevention from populations who are susceptible to those who need treatment and rehabilitation. Incorporating Latino cultural values and strengths and acknowledging socioeconomic and cultural challenges can effectively reduce risk behaviors.

QUESTIONS TO CONSIDER

1. In examining health differences between Latinos and non-Latino White Americans, is there evidence for a Latino morbidity paradox?
2. Could the higher prevalence of obesity among Latinos of Mexican descent be a primary reason for gallbladder and other obesity-associated cancers?
3. What are the social determinants of HIV disease?
4. What factors might account for lower viral suppression among those infected with HIV?
5. What factors might account for the better health status of Latinos of Mexican descent compared to non-Latino Black Americans?

SUGGESTED READINGS

Abraido-Lanza, A. F., Dohrenwend, B. P., Ng-Mak, D. S., & Turner, J. B. (1999). The Latino mortality paradox: A test of the "salmon bias" and healthy migrant hypotheses. *American Journal of Public Health, 89*(10), 1543–1548.

Alegria, M., Canino, G., Ríos, R., Vera, M., Calderón, J., Rusch, D., & Ortega, A. N. (2002). Mental health care for Latinos: Inequalities in use of specialty mental health services among Latinos, African Americans, and non-Latino Whites. *Psychiatric Services, 53*(12), 1547–1555.

Calle, E. E., Rodriguez, C., Walker-Thurmond, K., & Thun, M. J. (2003). Overweight, obesity, and mortality from cancer in a prospectively studied cohort of U.S. adults. *New England Journal of Medicine, 348*, 1625–1638.

Daviglus, M. L., Talavera, G. A., Avilés-Santa, M. L., Allison, M., Cai, J., Criqui, M. H., Gellman, M., Giachello, A. L., Gouskova, N., Kaplan, R. C., LaVange, L., Penedo, F., Perreira, K., Pirzada, A., Scheniederman, N., Wassertheil-Smoller, S., Sorlie, P. D., & Stamler, J. (2012). Prevalence of major cardiovascular risk factors and cardiovascular diseases among Hispanic/Latino individuals of diverse backgrounds in the United States. *JAMA, 308*(17), 1775–1784.

Estrada, A. L., Trevino, F. M., & Ray, L. A. (1990). Health care utilization barriers among Mexican Americans: Evidence from HHANES 1982–84. *American Journal of Public Health, 80*(Suppl.), 27–31.

Forde, A. T., Crookes, D. M., Suglia, S. F., & Demmer, R. T. (2019). The weathering hypothesis as an explanation for racial disparities in health: A systematic review. *Annals of Epidemiology, 33*, 1–18.

Gomez, S., Blumer, V., & Rodriguez, F. (2022). Unique cardiovascular disease risk factors in Hispanic individuals. Current *Cardiovascular Risk Reports, 16*(7), 53–61.

Jones, E. A., Mitra, A. K., & Malone, S. (2023). Racial disparities and common respiratory infectious diseases in children of the United States: A systematic review and meta-analysis. *Diseases, 11*(1), 23.

Lu, P. J., O'Halloran, A., Williams, W. W., Lindley, M. C., Farrall, S., & Bridges, C. B. (2015). Racial and ethnic disparities in vaccination coverage among adult populations in the US. *Vaccine, 33*, D83–D91.

Miller, K. D., Ortiz, A. P., Pinheiro, P. S., Bandi, P., Minihan, A., Fuchs, H. E., Tyson, D. M., Tortolero-Luna, G., Fedewa, S. A., Jemal, A. M., & Siegel, R. L. (2021). Cancer statistics for the U.S. Hispanic/Latino population, 2021. *CA: A Cancer Journal for Clinicians, 71*(6), 466–487.

Pérez-Escamilla, R., & Putnik, P. (2007). The role of acculturation in nutrition, lifestyle, and incidence of type 2 diabetes among Latinos. *The Journal of Nutrition*, *137*(4), 860–870. https://doi.org/10.1093/jn/137.4.860

Saab, S., Manne, V., Nieto, J., Schwimmer, J. B., & Chalasani, N. P. (2016). Nonalcoholic fatty liver disease in Latinos. *Clinical Gastroenterology and Hepatology*, *14*(1), 5–12.

Vega, W. A., & Amaro, H. (2002). Latino outlook: Good health, uncertain prognosis. In T. A. LaVeist (Ed.), *Race, ethnicity, and health: A public health reader* (pp. 47–75). Jossey-Bass.

Wilkinson, A. V., Spitz, M. R., Strom, S. S., Prokhorov, A. V., Barcenas, C. H., Cao, Y., Saunder, K. C., & Bondy, M. L. (2005). Effects of nativity, age at migration, and acculturation on smoking among adult Houston residents of Mexican descent. *American Journal of Public Health*, *95*(6), 1043–1049.

REFERENCES

Abraido-Lanza, A. F., Dohrenwend, B. P., Ng-Mak, D. S., & Turner, J. B. (1999). The Latino mortality paradox: A test of the "salmon bias" and healthy migrant hypotheses. *American Journal of Public Health*, *89*(10), 1543–1548.

Adorador, A., McNulty, R., Hart, D., & Fitzpatrick, J. J. (2011). Perceived barriers to immunizations as identified by Latino mothers. *Journal of the American Academy of Nurse Practitioners*, *23*(9), 501–508.

Alcalá, H. E., Albert, S. L., Trabanino, S. K., Garcia, R. E., Glik, D. C., Prelip, M. L., & Ortega, A. N. (2016). Access to and use of health care services among Latinos in East Los Angeles and Boyle Heights. *Family & Community Health*, *39*(1), 62.

Alegria, M., Canino, G., Ríos, R., Vera, M., Calderón, J., Rusch, D., & Ortega, A. N. (2002). Mental health care for Latinos: Inequalities in use of specialty mental health services among Latinos, African Americans, and non-Latino Whites. *Psychiatric Services*, *53*(12), 1547–1555.

Allen, P., Sequeira, S., Jacob, R. R., Hino, A. A. F., Stamatakis, K. A., Harris, J. K., Elliott, L., Kerner, J. F., Jones, E., Dobbins, M., Baker, E. A., & Brownson, R. C. (2013). Promoting state health department evidence-based cancer and chronic disease prevention: A multi-phase dissemination study with a cluster randomized trial component. *Implementation Science*, *8*, 1–14.

Alligood-Percoco, N., & Kesterson, J. P. (2016). Addressing the barriers to cervical cancer prevention among Hispanic women. *Journal of Racial and Ethnic Health Disparities*, *3*, 489–495.

American Cancer Society. (n.d.). *The state of cancer disparities in the United States*. Retrieved September 6, 2023, from https://www.cancer.org/research/acs-research-highlights/cancer-health-disparities-research/state-of-cancer-disparities-in-the-united-states.html

American Cancer Society. (2023). Cancer Facts & Figures 2024. Atlanta: American Cancer Society; 2024. Retrieved April 17, 2024 from: https://www.cancer.org/content/dam/cancer-org/research/cancer-facts-and-statistics/annual-cancer-facts-and-figures/2024/2024-cancer-facts-and-figures-acs.pdf.

Asrani, S. K., Larson, J. J., Yawn, B., Therneau, T. M., & Kim, W. R. (2013). Underestimation of liver-related mortality in the United States. *Gastroenterology*, *145*(2), 375–382.

Azziz, R. (2007). Evaluation for insulin resistance and comorbidities related to insulin resistance in polycystic ovary syndrome. In E. Diamanti-Kandarakis, J. E. Nestler, et al. (Eds.), *Insulin resistance and polycystic ovarian syndrome: Pathogenesis, evaluation, and treatment* (pp. 1–13). Springer.

Bagayogo, I. P., Interian, A., & Escobar, J. I. (2013). Transcultural aspects of somatic symptoms in the context of depressive disorders. *Cultural Psychiatry*, *33*, 64–74.

Balfour, P. C., Jr., Ruiz, J. M., Talavera, G. A., Allison, M. A., & Rodriguez, C. J. (2016). Cardiovascular disease in Hispanics/Latinos in the United States. *Journal of Latina/o Psychology*, *4*(2), 98.

Bethel, J. W., & Schenker, M. B. (2005). Acculturation and smoking patterns among Hispanics: A review. *American Journal of Preventive Medicine*, *29*(2), 143–148.

Braveman, P. (2023). The Black-White disparity in preterm birth: Race or racism? *The Milbank Quarterly*, *101*(Suppl. 1), 356–378. https://doi.org/10.1111/1468-0009.12625

Brody, D.J., Pratt, L.A., & Hughes, J. (2018). Prevalence of depression among adults aged 20 and over: United States, 2013–2016. NCHS Data Brief, no. 303. Hyattsville, MD: National Center for Health Statistics.

Browning, J. D., Szczepaniak, L. S., Dobbins, R., Nuremberg, P., Horton, J. D., Cohen, J. C., Grundy, S. M., & Hobbs, H. H. (2004). Prevalence of hepatic steatosis in an urban population in the United States: Impact of ethnicity. *Hepatology*, *40*(6), 1387–1395.

Bruhn, J. G., & Fuentes, R. G. (1977). Cultural factors affecting utilization of services by Mexican Americans. *Psychiatric Annals*, 7(12), 20–29.

Bucay-Harari, L., Page, K. R., Krawczyk, N., Robles, Y. P., & Castillo-Salgado, C. (2020). Mental health needs of an emerging Latino community. *The Journal of Behavioral Health Services & Research, 47*, 388–398.

Buki, L. P., & Selem, M. (2009). Cancer screening and survivorship in Latino populations. In F. A. Villarruel, G. Carlo, et al. (Eds.0, *Handbook of U.S. Latino psychology: Developmental and community-based perspectives* (pp. 363–378). SAGE.

Burgos, A. E., Schetzina, K. E., Dixon, L. B., & Mendoza, F. S. (2005). Importance of generational status in examining access to and utilization of health care services by Mexican American children. *Pediatrics, 115*(3), e322–e330.

Caballero, A. E. (2005). Diabetes in the Hispanic or Latino population: Genes, environment, culture, and more. *Current Diabetes Reports, 5*(3), 217–225.

Cabral, J., & Cuevas, A. G. (2020). Health inequities among Latinos/Hispanics: Documentation status as a determinant of health. *Journal of Racial and Ethnic Health Disparities, 7*, 874–879.

Caetano, R., & Clark, C. L. (2003). Acculturation, alcohol consumption, smoking, and drug use among Hispanics. In K. M. Chun, P. Balls Organista, & G. Marín (Eds.), *Acculturation: Advances in theory, measurement, and applied research* (pp. 223–239). American Psychological Association. https://doi.org/10.1037/10472-014

Calle, E. E,, Rodriguez, C., Walker-Thurmond, K., & Thun, M. J. (2003). Overweight, obesity, and mortality from cancer in a prospectively studied cohort of U.S. adults. *New England Journal of Medicine, 348*, 1625–1638.

Calle, E. E., & Thun, M. J. (2004). Obesity and cancer. *Oncogene, 23*(38), 6365–6378.

Campos, C. L., & Rodriguez, C. J. (2019). High blood pressure in Hispanics in the United States: A review. *Current Opinion in Cardiology, 34*(4), 350–358.

Carrion, A. F., Ghanta, R., Carrasquillo, O., & Martin, P. (2011). Chronic liver disease in the Hispanic population of the United States. *Clinical Gastroenterology and Hepatology, 9*(10), 834–841.

Carroll, W. A., & Hill, S. C. (2019). *Trends in prescribed medication expenditures by age and prescription drug coverage, 2009 to 2016 MEPS-HC*. Agency for Healthcare Research and Quality. https://meps.ahrq.gov/data_files/publications/st522/stat522.pdf

Castro, A. V. B., Kolka, C. M., Kim, S. P., & Bergman, R. N. (2014). Obesity, insulin resistance and comorbidities–Mechanisms of association. *Arquivos Brasileiros de Endocrinologia & Metabologia, 58*, 600–609.

CDC WONDER. (n.d.) *Multiple cause of death with U.S.-Mexico border regions, 1999–2020*. Retrieved September 1, 2023, from http://wonder.cdc.gov/ucd-border.html

Center for Behavioral Health Statistics and Quality. (2016). 2015 National Survey on Drug Use and Health: Detailed Tables. Substance Abuse and Mental Health Services Administration. Available from http://www.samhsa.gov/data/population-data-nsduh

Centers for Disease Control and Prevention. (2015, May). Hispanic health. *Vital Signs*. https://www.cdc.gov/vitalsigns/pdf/2015-05-vitalsigns.pdf

Centers for Disease Control and Prevention. (n.d.-a). *National Diabetes Statistics Report: estimates of diabetes and its burden in the United States*. Retrieved August 22, 2023, from https://www.cdc.gov/diabetes/data/statistics-report/index.html

Centers for Disease Control and Prevention. (n.d.-b). *Diabetes: Appendix Table 11. Crude prevalence of chronic kidney disease among adults aged 18 years or older, overall and by race/ethnicity, United States, 2017–2020*. https://www.cdc.gov/diabetes/data/statistics-report/appendix.html#tabs-1-11

Centers for Disease Control and Prevention. (n.d.-c). *Adult obesity prevalence maps*. Retrieved August 24, 2023, from https://www.cdc.gov/obesity/data/prevalence-maps.html.

Centers for Disease Control and Prevention. (n.d.-d). What is prediabetes? https://www.cdc.gov/diabetes/basics/prediabetes.html

Centers for Disease Control and Prevention. (n.d.-e). What is excessive alcohol use? https://www.cdc.gov/alcohol/onlinemedia/infographics/excessive-alcohol-use.html

Chiu, K. C., Chuang, L. M., & Yoon, C. (2001). Comparison of measured and estimated indices of insulin sensitivity and β cell function: Impact of ethnicity on insulin sensitivity and β cell function in glucose-tolerant and normotensive subjects. *The Journal of Clinical Endocrinology & Metabolism, 86*(4), 1620–1625.

Chukwueke, I., & Cordero-MacIntyre, Z. (2010). Overview of type 2 diabetes in Hispanic Americans. *International Journal of Body Composition Research, 8*(Suppl.), 77.

Cohen, R. A., & Cha, A. E. (2023, May). *Health insurance coverage: Early release of estimates form the National Health Interview Survey, 2022*. National Center for Health Statistics, Centers for Disease Control and Prevention, U.S. Department of Health and Human Services. https://www.cdc.gov/nchs/data/nhis/earlyrelease/insur202305_1.pdf

Compton, S., Haack, S., & Phillips, C. R. (2010). Identification of barriers to medication adherence in a Latino population. *Research in Social and Administrative Pharmacy*, *6*(4), 365–371.

Costas-Muniz, R., Sen, R., Leng, J., Aragones, A., Ramirez, J., & Gany, F. (2013). Cancer stage knowledge and desire for information: mismatch in Latino cancer patients?. *Journal of Cancer Education*, *28*, 458–465.

Crespo, C. J., Loria, C. M., & Burt, V. L. (1996). Hypertension and other cardiovascular disease risk factors among Mexican Americans, Cuban Americans, and Puerto Ricans from the Hispanic Health and Nutrition Examination Survey. *Public Health Reports*, *111*(Suppl. 2), 7.

Cushman, W. C. (2003). The burden of uncontrolled hypertension: morbidity and mortality associated with disease progression. *The Journal of Clinical Hypertension*, *5*(3), 14–22.

Davids, A. H., Sommese, K. J., Roach, M. V., Lee, S. J., Crose, C. E., Khan, S. B., & Leader, A. P. (2020). Clínica Comunitaria Esperanza: Strategy for health promotion and engagement with Hispanic communities. *Health Promotion Practice*, *21*(1), 91–96.

Daviglus, M. L., Talavera, G. A., Avilés-Santa, M. L., Allison, M., Cai, J., Criqui, M. H., Gellman, M., Giachello, A. L., Gouskova, N., Kaplan, R. C., LaVange, L., Penedo, F., Perreira, K., Pirzada, A., Scheniederman, N., Wassertheil-Smoller, S., Sorlie, P. D., & Stamler, J. (2012). Prevalence of major cardiovascular risk factors and cardiovascular diseases among Hispanic/Latino individuals of diverse backgrounds in the United States. *JAMA*, *308*(17), 1775–1784.

De Cosio, F. G., & Boadella, A. (1999). Demographic factors affecting the U.S.-Mexico border health status. In M. O. Loustaunau & M. Sanchez-Bane (Eds.), *Life, death and in-between on the U.S.-Mexico border* (pp. 1–22). Bergin & Garvey.

Dean, L. T., Gehlert, S., Neuhouser, M. L., Oh, A., Zanetti, K., Goodman, M., Thompson, B., Visvanathan, K., & Schmitz, K. H. (2018). Social factors matter in cancer risk and survivorship. *Cancer Causes & Control*, *29*, 611–618.

Delarue, J., & Magnan, C. (2007). Free fatty acids and insulin resistance. *Current Opinion in Clinical Nutrition & Metabolic Care*, *10*(2), 142–148.

D'Orazio, L. M., Taylor-Ford, M., & Meyerowitz, B. E. (2014). Cervical cancer prevention among Latinas in a post-HPV vaccine world: Considering the sociocultural context. *Women & Therapy*, *37*(3–4), 261–281.

Elder, J. P., Ayala, G. X., Parra-Medina, D., & Talavera, G. A. (2009). Health communication in the Latino community: Issues and approaches. *Annual Review of Public Health*, *30*, 227–251.

El-Serag, H. B., & Kanwal, F. (2014). Epidemiology of hepatocellular carcinoma in the United States: Where are we? Where do we go? *Hepatology*, *60*(5), 1767.

Escovar, E. L., Craske, M., Roy-Byrne, P., Stein, M. B., Sullivan, G., Sherbourne, C. D., Bystritsky, A., & Chavira, D. A. (2018). Cultural influences on mental health symptoms in a primary care sample of Latinx patients. *Journal of Anxiety Disorders*, *55*, 39–47.

Espinosa de Los Monteros, K., & Gallo, L. C. (2011). The relevance of fatalism in the study of Latinas' cancer screening behavior: A systematic review of the literature. *International Journal of Behavioral Medicine*, *18*, 310–318.

Estrada, A. L., Trevino, F. M., & Ray, L. A. (1990). Health care utilization barriers among Mexican Americans: Evidence from HHANES 1982–84. *American Journal of Public Health*, *80*(Suppl.), 27–31.

Fairley, T. L., Pollack, L. A., Moore, A. R., & Smith, J. L. (2009). Addressing cancer survivorship through public health: An update from the Centers for Disease Control and Prevention. *Journal of Women's Health*, *18*(10), 1525–1531.

Figueiredo, J. C., Haiman, C., Porcel, J., Buxbaum, J., Stram, D., Tambe, N., Cozen, W., Wilkens, L., Marchand, L. L., & Setiswan, V. W. (2017) . Sex and ethnic/racial-specific risk factors for gallbladder disease. *BMC Gastroenterology*, *17*, Article 153. https://doi.org/10.1186/s12876-017-0678-6

Ford, E. S., Giles, W. H., & Dietz, W. H. (2002). Prevalence of the metabolic syndrome among U.S. adults: Findings from the third National Health and Nutrition Examination Survey. *JAMA*, *287*(3), 356–359.

Forde, A. T., Crookes, D. M., Suglia, S. F., & Demmer, R. T. (2019). The weathering hypothesis as an explanation for racial disparities in health: A systematic review. *Annals of Epidemiology*, *33*, 1–18.

Gallo, L. C., Roesch, S. C., Fortmann, A. L., Carnethon, M. R., Penedo, F. J., Perreira, K., Birnbaum-Weitzman, O., Wassertheil-Smoller, S., Castañeda, S. F., Talavera, G. A., Sotres-Alvarez, D., Daviglus, M., Schneiderman, N. & Isasi, C. R. (2014). Associations of chronic stress burden, perceived stress, and traumatic stress with cardiovascular disease prevalence and risk factors in the HCHS/SOL Sociocultural Ancillary Study. *Psychosomatic Medicine*, *76*(6), 468–475.

Garcia, M. A., Reyes, A. M., García, C., Chiu, C. T., & Macias, G. (2020). Nativity and country of origin variations in life expectancy with functional limitations among older Hispanics in the United States. *Research on Aging*, *42*(7–8), 199–207.

Getrich, C. M., Sussman, A. L., Helitzer, D. L., Hoffman, R. M., Warner, T. D., Sánchez, V., Solares, A., Rhyne, R. L., & Rios Net Clinicians. (2012). Expressions of machismo in colorectal cancer screening among New Mexico Hispanic subpopulations. *Qualitative Health Research*, *22*(4), 546–559.

Gil, A. G., Wagner, E. F., & Vega, W. A. (2000). Acculturation, familism, and alcohol use among Latino adolescent males: Longitudinal relations. *Journal of Community Psychology, 28*(4), 443–458.

Goldenson, N. I., Leventhal, A. M., Stone, M. D., McConnell, R. S., & Barrington-Trimis, J. L. (2017). Associations of electronic cigarette nicotine concentration with subsequent cigarette smoking and vaping levels in adolescents. *JAMA Pediatrics, 171*(12), 1192–1199.

Gomez, S., Blumer, V., & Rodriguez, F. (2022). Unique cardiovascular disease risk factors in Hispanic individuals. *Current Cardiovascular Risk Reports, 16*(7), 53–61.

González, H. M., Vega, W. A., Rodríguez, M. A., Tarraf, W., & Sribney, W. M. (2009). Diabetes awareness and knowledge among Latinos: Does a usual source of healthcare matter? *Journal of General Internal Medicine, 24*, 528–533.

Gu, K., Cowie, C. C., & Harris, M. I. (1998). Mortality in adults with and without diabetes in a national cohort of the U.S. population, 1971–1993. *Diabetes Care, 21*(7), 1138–1145.

Hales, C. M., Carroll, M. D., Fryar, C. D., & Ogden, C. L. (2020). *Prevalence of obesity and severe obesity among adults: United States, 2017–2018*. National Center for Health Statistics.

Hanis, C. L., Ferrell, R. E., Tulloch, B. R., & Schull, W. J. (1985). Gallbladder disease epidemiology in Mexican Americans in Starr county, Texas. *American Journal of Epidemiology, 122*(5), 820–829.

Havranek, E. P., Mujahid, M. S., Barr, D. A., Blair, I. V., Cohen, M. S., Cruz-Flores, S., Davey-Smith, G., Dennison-Himmelfarb, C. R., Lauer, M. S., Lockwood, D. W., Rosal, M., & Yancy, C. W. (2015). Social determinants of risk and outcomes for cardiovascular disease: A scientific statement from the American Heart Association. *Circulation, 132*(9), 873–898.

Haw, J. S., Shah, M., Turbow, S., Egeolu, M., & Umpierrez, G. (2021). Diabetes complications in racial and ethnic minority populations in the USA. *Current Diabetes Reports, 21*, 1–8.

Heiss, G., Snyder, M. L., Teng, Y., Schneiderman, N., Llabre, M. M., Cowie, C., ... & Avilés-Santa, L. (2014). Prevalence of metabolic syndrome among Hispanics/Latinos of diverse background: the Hispanic Community Health Study/Study of Latinos. *Diabetes Care, 37*(8), 2391–2399.

Heron, M. (2021). Deaths: Leading causes for 2019. *National Vital Statistics Reports, 70*(9). https://doi.org/10.15620/cdc:107021

Herrera, G. A., Zhao, Z., & Klevens, R. M. (2001). Variation in vaccination coverage among children of Hispanic ancestry. *American Journal of Preventive Medicine, 20*(4), 69–74.

Higginbotham, J. C., Trevino, F. M., & Ray, L. A. (1990). Utilization of curanderos by Mexican Americans: Prevalence and predictors. Findings from HHANES 1982–84. *American Journal of Public Health, 80*(Suppl.), 32–35.

Huerta-Franco, M. R., Banderas, J. W., & Allsworth, J. E. (2018). Ethnic/racial differences in gastrointestinal symptoms and diagnosis associated with the risk of Helicobacter pylori infection in the US. *Clinical and Experimental Gastroenterology, 11*, 39–49.

Inoue, K., Mayeda, E. R., Nianogo, R., Paul, K., Yu, Y., Haan, M., & Ritz, B. (2021). Estimating the joint effect of diabetes and subsequent depressive symptoms on mortality among older Latinos. *Annals of Epidemiology, 64*, 120–126.

Johnston, L., Miech, R., O'Malley, P., Bachman, J., Schulenberg, J., & Patrick, M. (2020). *Monitoring the Future national survey results on drug use, 1975–2019: Overview, key findings on adolescent drug use*. Institute for Social Research. https://eric.ed.gov/?id=ED604018

Jones, E. A., Mitra, A. K., & Malone, S. (2023). Racial disparities and common respiratory infectious diseases in children of the United States: A systematic review and meta-analysis. *Diseases, 11*(1), 23.

Kaplan, R. C., Avilés-Santa, M. L., Parrinello, C. M., Hanna, D. B., Jung, M., Castañeda, S. F., Hankinson, A. L., Isasi, C. R., Birnbaum-Weitzman, O., Kim, R. S., Daviglus, M. L., Talavera, G. A., Schneiderman, N., & Cai, J. (2014). Body mass index, sex, and cardiovascular disease risk factors among Hispanic/Latino adults: Hispanic Community Health Study/Study of Latinos. *Journal of the American Heart Association, 3*(4), Article e000923.

Keating, S. E., Hackett, D. A., George, J., & Johnson, N. A. (2012). Exercise and non-alcoholic fatty liver disease: A systematic review and meta-analysis. *Journal of Hepatology, 57*(1), 157–166.

Khubchandani, J., Sharma, S., Price, J. H., Wiblishauser, M. J., Sharma, M., & Webb, F. J. (2021). COVID-19 vaccination hesitancy in the United States: A rapid national assessment. *Journal of Community Health, 46*, 270–277.

Kochanek, K.D., Murphy, S.L., Xu, J.Q., & Arias, E. (2023). *Mortality in the United States, 2022. NCHS Data Brief, no 492*. Retrieved on April 18, 2024, from NCHS Data Brief, Number 492, December 2023 (cdc.gov)

Kumar, S., Metz, D. C., Ellenberg, S., Kaplan, D. E., & Goldberg, D. S. (2020). Risk factors and incidence of gastric cancer after detection of Helicobacter pylori infection: A large cohort study. *Gastroenterology, 158*(3), 527–536.

Lara-Cinisomo, S., Akinbode, T. D., & Wood, J. (2020). A systematic review of somatic symptoms in women with depression or depressive symptoms: do race or ethnicity matter? *Journal of Women's Health, 29*(10), 1273–1282.

Larkey, L. K., & Gonzalez, J. (2007). Storytelling for promoting colorectal cancer prevention and early detection among Latinos. *Patient Education and Counseling*, *67*(3), 272–278.

Lee, S. H., Moore, L. V., Park, S., Harris, D. M., & Blanck, H. M. (2022). Adults meeting fruit and vegetable intake recommendations—United States, 2019. *Morbidity and Mortality Weekly Report*, *71*(1), 1.

Letamendi, A. M., Ayers, C. R., Ruberg, J. L., Singley, D. B., Wilson, J., Chavira, D., Palinkas, L., & Wetherell, J. L. (2013). Illness conceptualizations among older rural Mexican-Americans with anxiety and depression. *Journal of Cross-Cultural Gerontology*, *28*(4), 421–433.

López, S. R. (2002). Mental health care for Latinos: A research agenda to improve the accessibility and quality of mental health care for Latinos. *Psychiatric Services*, *53*(12), 1569–1573.

Lu, P. J., O'Halloran, A., Williams, W. W., Lindley, M. C., Farrall, S., & Bridges, C. B. (2015). Racial and ethnic disparities in vaccination coverage among adult populations in the U.S. *Vaccine*, *33*, D83–D91.

Lv, F., Gao, X., Huang, A. H., Zu, J., He, X., Sun, X., ... & Ji, F. (2022). Excess diabetes mellitus-related deaths during the COVID-19 pandemic in the United States. *EClinicalMedicine*, *54*.

Macias Gil, R., Marcelin, J. R., Zuniga-Blanco, B., Marquez, C., Mathew, T., & Piggott, D. A. (2020). COVID 19 pandemic: Disparate health impact on the Hispanic/Latinx population in the United States. *The Journal of Infectious Diseases*, *222*(10), 1592–1595.

Makarova-Rusher, O. V., Altekruse, S. F., McNeel, T. S., Ulahannan, S., Duffy, A. G., Graubard, B. I., Greten, T. F., & McGlynn, K. A. (2016). Population attributable fractions of risk factors for hepatocellular carcinoma in the United States. *Cancer, 122*(11), 1757–1765.

Marin, G., Perez-Stable, E. J., & Marin, B. V. (1989). Cigarette smoking among San Francisco Hispanics: The role of acculturation and gender. *American Journal of Public Health*, *79*(2), 196–198.

Marquez, I., Calman, N., & Crump, C. (2019). A framework for addressing diabetes-related disparities in US Latino populations. *Journal of Community Health*, *44*, 412–422.

Martinez, M. E., & Clarke, T. C. (2021, March 5). QuickStats: Percentage of adults in fair or poor health, by age group and race and ethnicity—National Health Interview Survey, United States, 2019. *Morbidity and Mortality Weekly Report*, *70*, 333. http://doi.org/10.15585/mmwr.mm7009a5

Maurer, K. R., Everhart, J. E., Ezzati, T. M., Johannes, R. S., Knowler, W. C., Larson, D. L., Sanders, R., Shawker, T. H., & Roth, H. P. (1989). Prevalence of gallstone disease in Hispanic populations in the United States. *Gastroenterology*, *96*(2), 487–492.

McPherson, S., & Anstee, Q. M. (2016). Changing epidemiology of chronic liver disease among ethnic groups in the United States. *Hepatology*, *64*(6), 1843–1846.

Melvin, J., Hummer, R., Elo, I., & Mehta, N. (2014). Age patterns of racial/ethnic/nativity differences in disability and physical functioning in the United States. *Demographic Research*, *31*, 497–510.

Miech, R. A., Johnston, L. D., O'Malley, P. M., Bachman, J. G., Schulenberg, J. E., & Patrick, M. E. (2020). *Monitoring the Future National Survey Results on Drug Use, 1975–2019: Vol. 1. Secondary school students.* Institute for Social Research.

Miller, K. D., Ortiz, A. P., Pinheiro, P. S., Bandi, P., Minihan, A., Fuchs, H. E., Tyson, D. M., Tortolero-Luna, G., Fedewa, S. A., Jemal, A. M., & Siegel, R. L. (2021). Cancer statistics for the U.S. Hispanic/Latino population, 2021. *CA: A Cancer Journal for Clinicians*, *71*(6), 466–487.

Miller, R. G., Secrest, A. M., Ellis, D., Becker, D. J., & Orchard, T. J. (2013). Changing impact of modifiable risk factors on the incidence of major outcomes of type 1 diabetes: The Pittsburgh Epidemiology of Diabetes Complications Study. *Diabetes Care*, *36*(12), 3999–4006.

Mitchell, B. D., Stern, M. P., Haffner, S. M., Hazuda, H. P., & Patterson, J. K. (1990). Risk factors for cardiovascular mortality in Mexican Americans and non-Hispanic White Americans: The San Antonio Heart Study. *American Journal of Epidemiology*, *131*(3), 423–433.

Mokdad, A. H., Ford, E. S., Bowman, B. A., Dietz, W. H., Vinicor, F., Bales, V. S., & Marks, J. S. (2003). Prevalence of obesity, diabetes, and obesity-related health risk factors, 2001. *JAMA*, *289*(1), 76–79.

Murphy, S. L., Kochanek, K. D., Xu, J. Q., & Arias, E. (2021). *Mortality in the United States, 2020.* National Center for Health Statistics. https://doi.org/10.15620/cdc:112079.

Nambi Ndugga, L. & Artiga, S. (2023, March 15). Key data on health and health care by race and ethnicity. Retrieved on April 18, 2024 from https://www.kff.org/racial-equity-and-health-policy/report/key-data-on-health-and-health-care-by-race-and-ethnicity/#HealthStatus

Narayan, K. V., Boyle, J. P., Thompson, T. J., Sorensen, S. W., & Williamson, D. F. (2003). Lifetime risk for diabetes mellitus in the United States. *JAMA*, *290*(14), 1884–1890.

National Center for Health Statistics. (n.d.-a). *Percentage of being uninsured at the time of interview for adults aged 18–64, United States, 2019—2022. National Health Interview Survey.* Generated interactively: Sep 12, 2023, from https://wwwn.cdc.gov/NHISDataQueryTool/SHS_adult/index.html

National Center for Health Statistics. (n.d.-b). *Percentage of having a usual place of health care for adults aged 18 and over, United States, 2019—2022. National Health Interview Survey.* Generated interactively: Sep 12, 2023, from https://wwwn.cdc.gov/NHISDataQueryTool/SHS_adult/index.html

National Center for Health Statistics. (n.d.-c). *Health, United States, 2020–2021: Respondent assessed fair or poor health. Table HStat.* Centers for Disease Control and Prevention. https://www.cdc.gov/nchs/data/hus/2020-2021/HStat.pdf

National Center for Health Statistics. (n.d.-d). *Health, United States, (2020–2021) functional limitations: Table (FxLimit).* Hyattsville, MD. Available from: https://www.cdc.gov/nchs/data/hus/2020-2021/FxLimit.pdf

National Center for Health Statistics. (n.d.-e). *Health, United States, (2017): Serious psychological distress, Table (46).* Hyattsville, MD. Available from: https://www.cdc.gov/nchs/hus/contents2017.htm#046

National Center for Health Statistics. (n.d.-f) *Percentage of regularly had feelings of worry, nervousness, or anxiety for adults aged 18 and over, United States, 2019—2022.* National Health Interview Survey. Generated interactively: August 12, 2023, from https://wwwn.cdc.gov/NHISDataQueryTool/SHS_adult/index.html

National Center for Health Statistics. (n.d.-g). *Health, United States, (2020–2021): Table (SmokeSex).* Hyattsville, MD. Available from: https://www.cdc.gov/nchs/hus/contents2020-2021.htm#Table-SmokSex

National Center for Health Statistics. (n.d.-h). *Health, United States, (2018): Participation in leisure-time aerobic and muscle-strengthening activities that meet the federal 2008 Physical Activity Guidelines for Americans among adults aged 18 and over, by selected characteristics: United States, selected years 1998–2017 Table (25).* Available from https://www.cdc.gov/nchs/data/hus/2018/025.pdf

National Center for Health Statistics. (n.d.-i). *Health, United States, (2019): Prescription drug use in the past 30 days, by sex, race and Hispanic origin, and age: United States, selected years 1988–1994 through 2011–2014Table (79).* Hyattsville, MD. Available from: https://www.cdc.gov/nchs/hus/contents2016.htm#079

National Center for Health Statistics. (n.d.-j). *Health, United States, (2018): Hypertension among adults aged 20 and over, by selected characteristics: United States, selected years 1988–1994 through 2013–2016Table (22).* Available from: https://www.cdc.gov/nchs/hus/contents2016.htm#079

National Center for Health Statistics. (n.d.-k). *Health, United States, (2019): Respondent-reported prevalence of heart disease, cancer, and stroke among adults aged 18 and over, by selected characteristics: United States, average annual, selected years 1997–1998 through 2017–2018, Table (13).* Hyattsville, MD. Available from: https://www.cdc.gov/nchs/hus/contents2019.htm#Table-013

Office of Disease Prevention and Health Promotion. (n.d.). *Healthy People 2030.* U.S. Department of Health and Human Services. Retrieved April 17, 2024, from https://health.gov/healthypeople

Olvera Alvarez, H. A., Appleton, A. A., Fuller, C. H. Belcourt, A., & Kubzansky, L. D. (2018). An integrated socio-environmental model of health and well-being: A conceptual framework exploring the joint contribution of environmental and social exposures to health and disease over the life span. *Current Environmental Health Reports, 5*, 233–243. https://doi.org/10.1007/s40572-018-0191-2

Ormazabal, V., Nair, S., Elfeky, O., Aguayo, C., Salomon, C., & Zuñiga, F. A. (2018). Association between insulin resistance and the development of cardiovascular disease. *Cardiovascular Diabetology, 17*, 1–14.

Ostchega, Y., Fryar, C.D., Nwankwo, T., & Nguyen, D.T. (2020). *Hypertension prevalence among adults aged 18 and over: United States, 2017–2018.* NCHS Data Brief, no 364. Hyattsville, MD: National Center for Health Statistics. 2020.

Oyama, S., & Terry, S. F. (2016). Epigenetics and racial health inequities. *Genetic Testing and Molecular Biomarkers, 20*(9), 483–484. https://doi.org/10.1089/gtmb.2016.29021.sj

Parchman, M., & Byrd, T. (2001). Access to and use of ambulatory health care by a vulnerable Mexican American population on the U.S.-Mexico border. *Journal of Health Care for the Poor and Underserved, 12*(4), 404–414.

Pérez-Escamilla, R. (2010). Health care access among Latinos: Implications for social and health care reforms. *Journal of Hispanic Higher Education, 9*(1), 43–60.

Pérez-Escamilla, R. (2011). Acculturation, nutrition, and health disparities in Latinos. *American Journal of Clinical Nutrition, 93*(5), 1163S–1167S. https://doi.org/10.3945/ajcn.110.003467

Pérez-Escamilla, R., & Putnik, P. (2007). The role of acculturation in nutrition, lifestyle, and incidence of type 2 diabetes among Latinos. *The Journal of Nutrition, 137*(4), 860–870. https://doi.org/10.1093/jn/137.4.860

Phillips, K. A., Morrison, K. R., Andersen, R., & Aday, L. A. (1998). Understanding the context of healthcare utilization: Assessing environmental and provider-related variables in the behavioral model of utilization. *Health Services Research, 33*(3 Pt. 1), 571.

Pietrzak, J. R. T., Maharaj, Z., & Mokete, L., Sikhauli, N., & van der Jagt, D. (2019). Total hip arthroplasty in obesity: Separating "fat" from fiction. *British Journal of Hospital Medicine, 80*(6), 325–330. https://doi.org/10.12968/hmed.2019.80.6.325

Pinheiro, P. S., Sherman, R. L., Trapido, E. J., Fleming, L. E., Huang, Y., Gomez-Marin, O., & Lee, D. (2009). Cancer incidence in first generation US Hispanics: cubans, Mexicans, Puerto Ricans, and new Latinos. *Cancer Epidemiology, Biomarkers & Prevention, 18*(8), 2162–2169.

Polsky, S., & Ellis, S. L. (2015). Obesity, insulin resistance, and type 1 diabetes mellitus. *Current Opinion in Endocrinology, Diabetes and Obesity, 22*(4), 277–282.

Pratt, L. A., & Brody, D. J. (2014). Depression and obesity in the U.S. adult household population, 2005–2010. *NCHS Data Briefs, 167*, 1–8.

Rector, R. S., & Thyfault, J. P. (2011). Does physical inactivity cause nonalcoholic fatty liver disease? *Journal of Applied Physiology, 111*(6), 1828–1835.

Ricardo, A. C., Flessner, M. F., Eckfeldt, J. H., Eggers, P. W., Franceschini, N., Go, A. S., Gotman, N. M., Dramer, H. J., Kusek, J. W., Loehr, L. R., Melamed, M. L., Peralta, C. A., Raij, L., Rosas, S. E., Talavera, G. A., & Lash, J. P. (2015). Prevalence and correlates of CKD in Hispanics/Latinos in the United States. *Clinical Journal of the American Society of Nephrology, 10*(10), 1757.

Rich, N. E., Oji, S., Mufti, A. R., Browning, J. D., Parikh, N. D., Odewole, M., Mayo, H., & Singal, A. G. (2018). Racial and ethnic disparities in nonalcoholic fatty liver disease prevalence, severity, and outcomes in the United States: A systematic review and meta-analysis. *Clinical Gastroenterology and Hepatology, 16*(2), 198–210.

Rivera, Y. M. (2018). Reducing cancer health disparities among U.S. Latinos: A Freireian approach. *International Journal of Human Rights in Healthcare, 11*(5), 368–379.

Roberts, R. E., & Lee, E. S. (1980). Medical care use by Mexican-Americans: Evidence from the human population laboratory studies. *Medical Care*, 266–281.

Rodríguez, M. A., Vargas Bustamante, A., & Ang, A. (2009). Perceived quality of care, receipt of preventive care, and usual source of health care among undocumented and other Latinos. *Journal of General Internal Medicine, 24*, 508–513.

Saab, S., Manne, V., Nieto, J., Schwimmer, J. B., & Chalasani, N. P. (2016). Nonalcoholic fatty liver disease in Latinos. *Clinical Gastroenterology and Hepatology, 14*(1), 5–12.

Samet, J. M., Coultas, D. B., Howard, C. A., Skipper, B. J., & Hanis, C. L. (1988). Diabetes, gallbladder disease, obesity, and hypertension among Hispanics in New Mexico. *American Journal of Epidemiology, 128*(6), 1302–1311.

Setiawan, V. W., Wei, P. C., Hernandez, B. Y., Lu, S. C., Monroe, K. R., Le Marchand, L., & Yuan, J. M. (2016). Disparity in liver cancer incidence and chronic liver disease mortality by nativity in Hispanics: The multiethnic cohort. *Cancer, 122*(9), 1444–1452.

Shen, M., Gai, Y., & Feng, L. (2016). Limited access to healthcare among Hispanics in the U.S.-Mexico border region. *American Journal of Health Behavior, 40*(5), 624–633.

Siega-Riz, A. M., Sotres-Alvarez, D., Ayala, G. X., Ginsberg, M., Himes, J. H., Liu, K., Loria, C. M., Mossavar-Rahmani, Y., Rock, C. L., Rodriguez, B., Gellman, M. D., Van Horn, L. (2014). Food-group and nutrient-density intakes by Hispanic and Latino backgrounds in the Hispanic Community Health Study/Study of Latinos. *American Journal of Clinical Nutrition, 99*(6), 1487–1498. https://doi.org/10.3945/ajcn.113.082685.

Simons, R. L., Lei, M. K., Klopack, E., Beach, S. R., Gibbons, F. X., & Philibert, R. A. (2021). The effects of social adversity, discrimination, and health risk behaviors on the accelerated aging of African Americans: Further support for the weathering hypothesis. *Social Science & Medicine, 282*, 113169.

Singh, G. K. (2003). *Area socioeconomic variations in US cancer incidence, mortality, stage, treatment, and survival, 1975–1999* (No. 4). US Department of Health and Human Services, National Institutes of Health, National Cancer Institute.

Stern, M. C., Fejerman, L., Das, R., Setiawan, V. W., Cruz-Correa, M. R., Perez-Stable, E. J., & Figueiredo, J. C. (2016). Variability in cancer risk and outcomes within U.S. Latinos by national origin and genetic ancestry. *Current Epidemiology Reports, 3*, 181–190.

Stinton, L. M., Myers, R. P., & Shaffer, E. A. (2010). Epidemiology of gallstones. *Gastroenterology Clinics, 39*(2), 157–169.

Substance Abuse and Mental Health Services Administration (SAMHSA). (2020). *National Survey on Drug Use and Health (NSDUH)*. https://www.samhsa.gov/data/data-we-collect/nsduh-national-survey-drug-use-and-health

Sumaya, C. V. (1991). Major infectious diseases causing excess morbidity in the Hispanic population. *Archives of Internal Medicine, 151*(8), 1513–1520.

Sundquist, J., & Winkleby, M. A. (1999). Cardiovascular risk factors in Mexican American adults: A transcultural analysis of NHANES III, 1988–1994. *American Journal of Public Health, 89*(5), 723–730.

Trevino, F. M., Moyer, M. E., Valdez, R. B., & Stroup-Benham, C. A. (1991). Health insurance coverage and utilization of health services by Mexican Americans, mainland Puerto Ricans, and Cuban Americans. *JAMA, 265*(2), 233–237.

Tsang, S. H., Avilés-Santa, M. L., Abnet, C. C., Brito, M. O., Daviglus, M. L., Wassertheil-Smoller, S., Castañeda, S. F., Minnerath, S., Talavera, G. A., Graubard, B. I., Thyagarajan, B., & Camargo, M. C. (2022). Seroprevalence and determinants of Helicobacter pylori infection in the Hispanic Community Health Study/Study of Latinos. *Clinical Gastroenterology and Hepatology, 20*(3), e438–e451.

U.S. Department of Agriculture & U.S. Department of Health and Human Services. (2020, December). *Dietary Guidelines for Americans, 2020–2025* (9th ed.). https://www.dietaryguidelines.gov/sites/default/files/2020-12/Dietary_Guidelines_for_Americans_2020-2025.pdf

Vainio, H., & Bianchini, F. (Eds.). (2002). *IARC handbooks of cancer prevention, weight control and physical activity.* IARC Press.

Vargas Bustamante, A., Fang, H., Garza, J., Carter-Pokras, O., Wallace, S. P., Rizzo, J. A., & Ortega, A. N. (2012). Variations in healthcare access and utilization among Mexican immigrants: The role of documentation status. *Journal of Immigrant and Minority Health, 14*, 146–155.

Vega, W. A., & Amaro, H. (2002). Latino outlook: Good health, uncertain prognosis. In T. A. LaVeist (Ed.), *Race, ethnicity, and health: A public health reader* (pp. 47–75). Jossey-Bass.

Velasco-Mondragon, E., Jimenez, A., Palladino-Davis, A. G., Davis, D., & Escamilla-Cejudo, J. A. (2016). Hispanic health in the USA: A scoping review of the literature. *Public Health Reviews, 37*, 1–27.

Ward, E., Jemal, A., Cokkinides, V., Singh, G. K., Cardinez, C., Ghafoor, A., & Thun, M. (2004). Cancer disparities by race/ethnicity and socioeconomic status. *CA: a cancer journal for clinicians, 54*(2), 78–93.

Wilkins, J. T., Ning, H., Stone, N. J., Criqui, M. H., Zhao, L., Greenland, P., & Lloyd-Jones, D. M. (2014). Coronary heart disease risks associated with high levels of HDL cholesterol. *Journal of the American Heart Association, 3*(2), e000519.

Wilkinson, A. V., Spitz, M. R., Strom, S. S., Prokhorov, A. V., Barcenas, C. H., Cao, Y., Saunders, K. C., & Bondy, M. L. (2005). Effects of nativity, age at migration, and acculturation on smoking among adult Houston residents of Mexican descent. *American Journal of Public Health, 95*(6), 1043–1049.

Yanez, B., McGinty, H. L., Buitrago, D., Ramirez, A. G., & Penedo, F. J. (2016). Cancer outcomes in Hispanics/Latinos in the United States: An integrative review and conceptual model of determinants of health. *Journal of Latina/o Psychology, 4*(2), 114.

Zemore, S. E. (2007). Acculturation and alcohol among Latino adults in the United States: A comprehensive review. *Alcoholism: Clinical and Experimental Research, 31*(12), 1968–1990.

Figure Credits

Fig. 8.5: Centers for Disease Control and Prevention, "Percentage of Adults in Fair or Poor Health by Age Group and Race and Ethnicity – National Health Interview Survey, United States, 2019," https://www.cdc.gov/mmwr/volumes/70/wr/mm7009a5.htm?s_cid=mm7009a5_w, 2021.

Fig. 8.21: United States Department of Agriculture, "USDA Dietary Guidelines," https://commons.wikimedia.org/wiki/File:USDA_Food_Pyramid.gif, 1992.

Fig. 8.25: Centers for Disease Control and Prevention, "Obesity Trends Among US Adults, 1990-2010," https://www.hsph.harvard.edu/obesity-prevention-source/us-obesity-trends-map/, 2010.

Fig. 8.28: Centers for Disease Control and Prevention, "Obesity Rates among Latinos, 2015-2017, BRFSS," https://www.cdc.gov/pcd/issues/2019/18_0579.htm, 2019.

CHAPTER 9

Eliminating Mexican American Health Inequalities

LEARNING OBJECTIVES

- Discuss how the U.S. Public Health Service has negatively affected health promotion among Mexican Americans.
- Describe the components that comprise Mexican American community empowerment.
- Describe how social justice applications can be used to improve Mexican American health.
- Evaluate Pennucci's framework for improving the design and implementation of health promotion interventions. How could it be more culturally inclusive?
- Differentiate between culturally sensitive, culturally appropriate, culturally innovative, and socioculturally congruent approaches to Mexican American health. Which one uses cultural values to promote health promotion and reduce health inequalities among Mexican Americans?
- Critically assess Bernal's framework for including culture in research with Mexican Americans.
- Compare and contrast social ecological models with social-cognitive models to reduce health inequalities among Mexican Americans. Which ones could empower Mexican American communities to effect change in the social determinants of health?
- Describe the differences between cultural competency and cultural humility in Mexican American health.
- Discuss the rationale for moving away from assessing acculturation level to examining cognitive referents of acculturation in behavior change with Mexican Americans.
- Discuss several strategies that could potentially be employed to eliminate health inequalities among Mexican Americans.
- Formulate a Mexican American health promotion intervention using concepts derived from Mexican American historical trauma theory and social ecological models.

In the previous chapters, several important Mexican American communicable and chronic disease inequalities were identified. Most of these inequalities are derived from the complex interplay of historical, social, and geopolitical factors that have delimited and undermined important social and cultural determinants of health. Ample empirical evidence suggests that the social determinants of health (SDOH) are fundamentally influenced by historical and geopolitical factors embedded in U.S. society. Several of the life-enhancing qualities of the SDOH have been undermined by these factors, especially for Latinos of Mexican descent, non-Latino Black Americans, and Native Americans.

To improve the health status of Mexican American and eliminate health inequalities, we must examine how past public health initiatives contributed to mistrust and alienation among Mexican Americans and develop new public health approaches that empower rather than disempower them.

U.S. Public Health Service and Development of Latino Mistrust and Resistance

Historically, Latinos of Mexican descent have encountered negative perceptions by non-Latino White Americans as being dirty, diseased, and not fit for U.S. citizenship (Molina, 2006). For example, following a typhus outbreak among Mexican railroad workers, Mexicans were henceforth stigmatized as disease carriers. According to Molina (2006), the public health response was a "campaign against filth and personal hygiene" (pp. 61–62), which would become largely associated with Mexicans and Mexican Americans. The public health response to the "Mexican problem" in the early 20th century was to stigmatize Mexican culture as being unsanitary (Molina, 2006) and attempt to marginalize the population to certain areas and exclude them from interacting with non-Latino White Americans. Common and unfortunately lasting stereotypes of Mexicans as dirty, unsanitary, lacking in hygiene, and disease-ridden were used to socially separate them from "clean" White Americans.

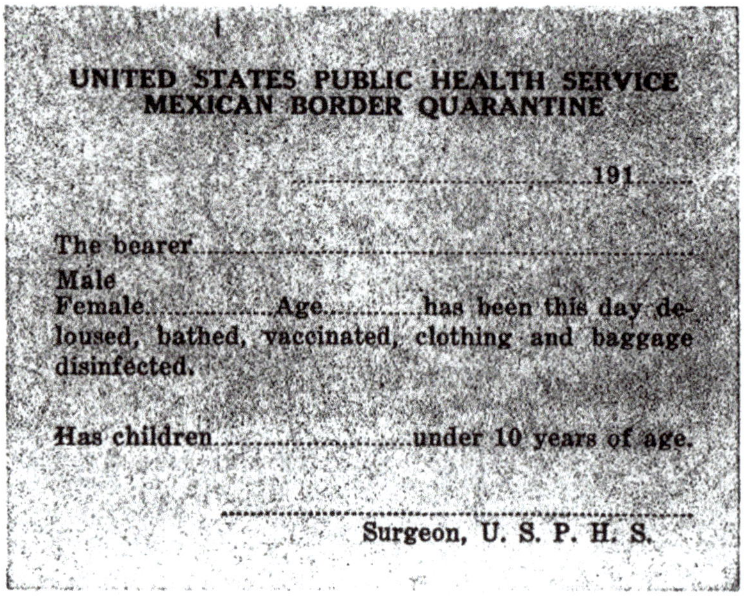

UNITED STATES PUBLIC HEALTH SERVICE
MEXICAN BORDER QUARANTINE

..................................191......

The bearer..
Male
Female..............Age..............has been this day deloused, bathed, vaccinated, clothing and baggage disinfected.

Has children..............................under 10 years of age.

....
Surgeon, U. S. P. H. S.

FIGURE 9.1 Border Quarantine Certification Card

Mexican men and women were segregated and then forced to strip naked and have their clothes washed while they were being deloused. They then were given their clothes back. Subjected to this process of humiliation, Mexican community resistance ensued resulting in the "Bath Riots" of 1917, which lasted for about a week (Romo, 2014). About 200 Mexican women in Ciudad Juarez (the sister city of El Paso) protested the quarantine regulations imposed by the U.S. Public Health Service (USPHS), with little resolution. Those who forcibly participated in the delousing process were provided official certification from the USPHS (Figure 9.1).

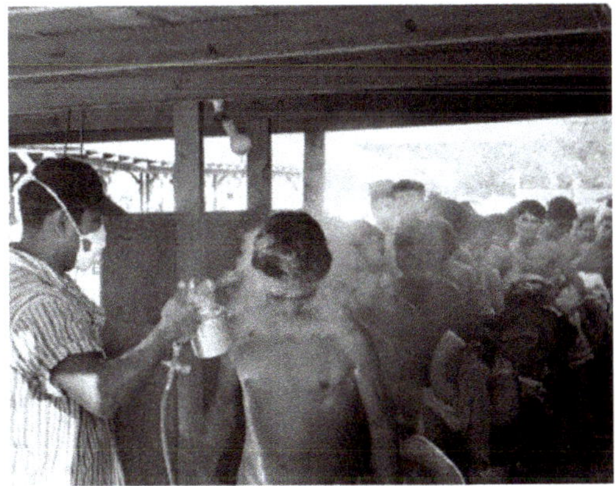

FIGURE 9.2 A Masked Worker Fumigating a Bracero at the Hidalgo Processing Center in Texas

Additionally, Thomas Calloway Jr., the mayor of El Paso at the time, sent a telegram to the US Surgeon General advocating for disinfection by impugning Mexicans as "dirty lousey (sic) destitute Mexicans" (Delgado, 2022, first paragraph) that would spread diseases like typhus. Beginning in 1916, El Paso began a public health program of disinfection targeting Mexican migrants entering the city through the border (Figure 9.2). Disinfectants used included vinegar, kerosene, gasoline, and DDT, a known carcinogen. Mexican migrants, including children, were required to take kerosene and vinegar baths as part of their processing into the United States. Disinfection and fumigation of Mexican migrants were practiced as late as 1963 and were in place during the Bracero Program from 1942–1964 (Walker, 2023).

These negative interactions between the USPHS, community clinics, culturally incompetent physicians, and Latinos of Mexican descent has laid a foundation of mistrust. Social justice for Latinos must first acknowledge the demeaning practices that Mexicans were subjected to, apart from other immigrants to the United States who were not subjected to public nudity and racial medicalization. According to Stern (1999):

> At Ellis Island immigrants underwent a complete medical inspection, and when suspected of disease were required to strip. Delousing was seldom part of detention or extended observation of immigrants. Disinfection and vaccination were almost wholly carried out by the steamship companies. ... On the Mexican border where immigrants entered by foot not ship, medicalization was incorporated directly into the process of entry. (p. 49)

Incorporating an intersectionality and critical race perspective allows for an in-depth understanding of accrued social disadvantage (Bauer, 2014). Recall from Chapter 1 (Table 1.3) that critical race theory and intersectionality theory hypothesize that social identities intersect at the macro (e.g., institutions) and micro (e.g., race, gender) levels to produce social and health inequalities among historically marginalized populations. Both focus on applied social justice as a solution to alleviate these inequalities. Marmot (2007) articulates the vision of the Commission on Social Determinants of Health (Geneva) in discussing collective action and empowerment:

> At the heart of the concern with social determinants of health, and health inequity, is concern for people without the freedom to lead flourishing lives. ... We see empowerment operating along three interconnected dimensions: material, psychosocial, and political. People need the basic material requisites for a decent life, they need to have control over their lives, and they need political voice and participation in decision making processes. Although individuals are at the heart of empowerment, achieving a fairer distribution of power requires collective social action. (p. 1155)

Collective social action is at the core of social justice approaches to alleviate social, economic, and health inequalities among historically marginalized populations. Individuals benefit from increased self-esteem and personal empowerment. Latino communities benefit from advocating for social and economic

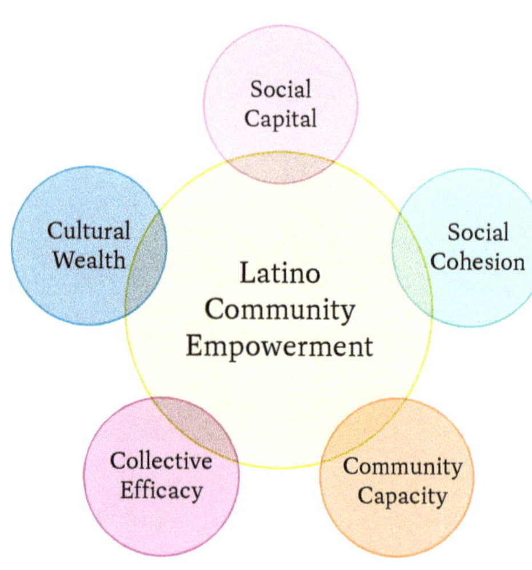

FIGURE 9.3 Latino Community Health and Empowerment

change collaboratively. Collective social action can lead to building Latino community capacity and empowerment but also depends on external investments from political and economic entities (Stokols, 1992). The empowerment of Latino communities is derived from social capital, social cohesion, community capacity, collective efficacy, and cultural wealth (Figure 9.3).

Latino community empowerment can lead to civic engagement wwith social, educational, and health institutions that facilitate building healthy and thriving communities. Access to social support networks, high levels of social cohesion, organizational flexibility and responsiveness, cooperation, and economic stability are the foundation for healthy communities (Stokols, 1992). Of course, one of the difficulties in establishing a sustainable, healthy Latino community is the lack of economic stability, one of the more important social determinants of health.

Advocating for a multilevel, social-ecological approach, Stokols (1992) states:

> The social-ecological perspective emphasizes the advantages of multilevel interventions that combine complementary or synergistic behavioral and environmental components. ... The ecological perspective suggests that multifaceted interventions that incorporate complementary environmental and behavioral components and span multiple settings and levels of analysis are more likely to be effective in promoting personal and public health than are those narrower in scope. (p. 18)

Thus, combining complementary interventions at the school, work, community, and individual levels may have more success in achieving the desired results of risk reduction, leading to lowering incidence and prevalence of disease and enhancing individual and community well-being. Nevertheless, acknowledging the lack of capital investment in Latino communities and other economic and financial challenges, the goal of building healthy Latino communities may be tenuous.

Social Justice in Public Health

Social epidemiology is an applied health science that seeks to eliminate social causes of preventable diseases in populations. Following from social epidemiological principles (Berkman et al., 2014), the social context in which the population resides is critical to the examination of the distribution of risk in populations. Additionally, risk exposure and risk behaviors are not randomly distributed in the population but rather are socially, culturally, and economically derived and tend to cluster with one another. For example, HIV risk behaviors are associated with many social (e.g., risk networks), cultural (e.g., homophobia), and economic (e.g., poverty) factors that create the social and biological context for HIV transmission to occur.

Applied social justice in public health is holistic in targeting institutions, policies, and personnel for changes in the status quo (Baum et al., 2009). Population approaches differ from individual approaches to risk reduction (Rose, 2001). *Population approaches* attempt to identify the causes of disease and reduce or eliminate them to reduce disease incidence, whereas *individual approaches* attempt to reduce risk behaviors among susceptible or high-risk individuals to avoid increasing prevalence (i.e., cases). Most public health research to date is focused on individual-level risk reduction because making significant changes at the macro level is more costly, time consuming, and difficult, and tangible results are more ephemeral to individual needs.

More research needs to be focused on reducing the incidence of health inequalities in vulnerable populations through the identification of social and behavioral factors that are linked to and within the social environment: the social determinants of health (Table 9.1).

TABLE 9.1 Social Determinants of Latino Health

Economic stability	Education	Community & social context	Neighborhood & built environment	Food	Health care system
Employment	Literacy	Ethnic enclaves	Affordable housing	Hunger	Health insurance coverage
Poverty/ net wealth	Language	Informal and formal social support networks	Transportation	Food swamps	Regular source of care
Living wage	Health literacy	Community cohesion	Safety	Food deserts	Cultural humility
Medical expenses	Early childhood education	Discrimination & racism	Green spaces	Access to healthy food options	Linguistic competency
	Vocational skills training	Generational status	Walkability		Quality of care

Health Outcomes

Mortality, Morbidity, Life Expectancy, Health Care Expenditures, Health Status, Functional Limitations

Multi-level analysis is fundamental to understanding both positive and negative macro- and micro-level influences on health outcomes (Stokols, 1992). For example, most research on substance abuse, mental illness, and HIV/AIDS examines fundamental macro and micro factors that contribute to disease incidence: socioeconomic status, poverty, lack of access to health care, racism, immigration status, gender orientation, and behaviors that confer increased risk. All these influences are part of the social and cultural environment in which the individual is embedded (Table 9.1).

Health promotion science is the application of evidence based, theory-driven interventions that focus on reducing multiple health risk behaviors and increasing the health and psychological well-being of the individual or community. Pennucci et al. (2022) provides a framework for identifying the interaction between personal values and community values in pursuit of behavior change (Figure 9.4).

Individual and community values (social values in Figure 9.4) are reciprocal and enhance health education, self and community activation, and engagement of individuals and communities in the health promotion process, leading to increased individual and community empowerment. According to Wallerstein (1993), *community empowerment* is "a social action process that promotes the participation of people toward goals of increased individual and community decision making and control, equitable resources and improved quality of life" (p. 219).

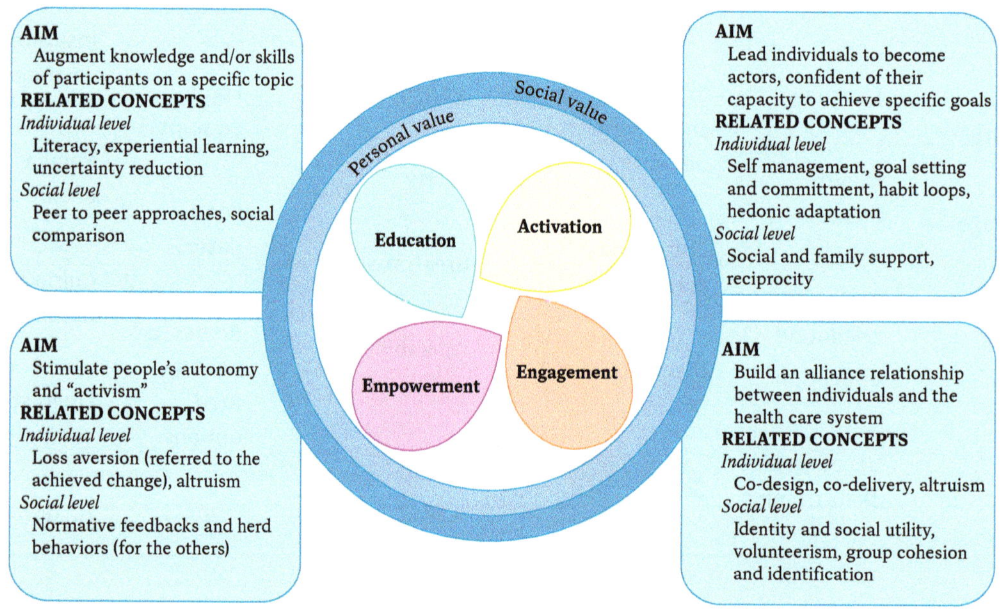

FIGURE 9.4 A Framework for Improving the Design and Implementation of Health Promotion Interventions

Social justice is an elusive concept, but within the field of public health it embraces equitable access to health care, nutrition, affordable housing, quality education, and physical environments free of toxic exposure (Beauchamp, 1976; Ruger, 2004). A sustained focus on eliminating negative influences of social determinants and enhancing positive influences can reduce health inequalities among historically marginalized populations in the United States. Buettner-Schmidt and Lobo (2012) defined five characteristics of social justice: (a) fairness; (b) equity in the distribution of power, resources, and processes that affect the sufficiency of the social determinants of health; (c) just institutions, systems, structures, policies, and processes; (d) equity in human development, rights, and sustainability; and (e) sufficiency of well-being. Together, these elements are hypothesized to increase the overall health of individuals and communities. The focus should also include individual and community capacity building to effectively garner resources for improved living spaces, or "health promotive environments," like green spaces, bicycle trails, and safer neighborhoods.

Health promotion in the community places greater emphasis on the role of individuals, groups, and organizations as active agents in shaping public health practices and policies to optimize both individual wellness and community well-being (Moore-Monroy et al., 2013; Stokols, 1992; Wilkinson-Lee et al., 2018). Stokols's (1992) conceptualization of "health promotive interventions" (Table 9.2) provides a framework for locating personal health behaviors within a social ecological context that "emphasizes the integration of person-focused and environment-focused strategies to enhance individual and collective wellbeing" (p. 15).

TABLE 9.2 Policy Options for Health Promotion and Disease Prevention

Health promotive interventions	Examples of health promotive policies and programs
Person-focused strategies (biogenetic)	Preventive public health programs for risk screening, genetic counseling, and inoculation; medical treatment regimens
Psychological and behavioral	Individual counseling and psychotherapeutic interventions; health behavior modification; lifestyle appraisal and modification pertaining to diet, exercise, smoking, safety practices, and so on; risk reduction
Environment-focused strategies (geographic)	Health and safety-oriented urban planning; land use policy and environmental law at municipal and regional levels; strategic siting of health care facilities in the community; focus on social determinants
Architectural and technological	Ergonomic and safety-oriented environmental design and facilities management; design of safe and health-promoting products; community sanitation systems; green spaces
Sociocultural	Organizational development and conflict resolution; multilevel health promotion programs; community health education and media programming; health promoting legislation and improved housing

Adapted from: Stokols (1992)

Stokols et al. (2013) cite several important forms of capital necessary for obtaining the goal of community well-being;

- *Social capital:* coordinated action for mutual benefits.
- *Human capital:* value acquired (e.g., through education) that enables people to develop skills and capabilities.
- *Moral capital:* the investment of personal or organizational resources to achieve social justice.

To this I would add *cultural capital* that includes cultural wealth and "funds of knowledge" derived from the Latino community.

Each of these examples situates the person within their social and cultural environments, acknowledging that individual behavior change does not occur in isolation to larger social environmental circumstances and that sustaining behavior change is a consequence of positive health promotive environments. Strategies that reduce the negative influences of social and cultural determinants on Latino health should be multilevel to effect sustained community and individual well-being.

Several socioenvironmental, psychosocial/behavioral, and genetic-environmental theories have been advanced to account for health inequalities among Latinos (LaVeist, 2011, Weber et al., 2018; see Chapter 5). Perhaps the most thoroughly researched are the Latino epidemiological paradox, immigration and acculturation hypotheses, and the biopsychosocial racism model. Length of residence in the United States and generational status are important health determinants for Latinos. Research by Alegría and colleagues (2007a, 2007b, 2017) has clearly demonstrated that mental illness is associated with these determinants. Additionally, Latinos of Mexican descent have lower mortality rates, with some exceptions, than non-Latino White Americans and non-Latino Black Americans. Nevertheless, discrimination and racism have been shown to increase psychological stress and depression among Latinos, which are known precursors to developing chronic diseases (Castañeda et al., 2016; Menselson et al., 2008; Molina et al., 2016; Pérez et al., 2008).

More recent studies have examined social epigenetic processes associated with Latino aging and intergenerational transmission of trauma among Latinos (see Chapter 8). The relationship between the transmission of intergeneration trauma, adverse childhood experiences (ACEs), maternal stress and intrauterine development of the fetus, and epigenetic modifications require multidisciplinary approaches that can identify linkages and points for prevention and intervention.

The need for developmental and longitudinal research on ACEs is critical based on the unequivocal evidence showing extremely high population attributable risk (PAR) for chronic diseases, including mental illness, in adulthood (Anda et al., 2006; Brown et al., 2009; Gilbert et al., 2015). Attention directed toward providing nurturing and caring social environments for children could potentially reduce PARs associated with adverse childhood experiences, especially among high-risk children (Asmussen et al., 2019). Especially effective are intervention programs that assist in strengthening family bonds early in the child's life and building resilience. For example, increases in positive parenting skills and stable and nurturing relationships through home visitation have been proven to be effective (CDC, n.d.; Garner, 2013). In other words, prevention and intervention efforts should focus on eliminating negative social and cultural influences on health.

Advancing health theory and practice that have the potential to decrease the burden of disease among Latinos can enhance their health status, increase access to needed medical care, and interrupt chronic disease progression that leads to serious complications like end-stage renal disease and lower limb amputations associated with type 2 diabetes. Other notable Latino health inequalities include lack of access to health care, certain types of cancers, obesity-related diseases (e.g., metabolic syndrome, cardiovascular disease, cerebrovascular disease, gallbladder disease) and communicable diseases, including HIV, sexually transmitted infections, and lack of vaccination coverage.

One of the better-known theories regarding the adoption of evidence-based interventions is derived from Rogers's (1983) diffusion of innovation theory. Rogers et al. (2014) proposed that the adoption of innovative interventions is based on several important factors: relative advantage, compatibility, complexity, trialability, and observability (Table 9.3). Together, these constructs provide a critical assessment of the costs versus benefits, cultural compatibility and acceptability, difficulty of performing risk reduction strategies, and immediacy of outcomes. The adoption or diffusion of the intervention is weighted against these considerations.

TABLE 9.3 Rogers's Diffusion of Innovation Theory

Construct	Definition
Relative advantage	Does the intervention proposed offer an advantage over existing interventions? What are the potential benefits and disadvantages?
Compatibility	Is the proposed intervention perceived as being compatible with existing values, lived experiences, and the needs of population?
Complexity	Is the proposed intervention perceived as too complex or difficult to understand or practice?
Trialability	Is the proposed intervention acceptable to the population? Can the intervention be modified? Is it scalable?
Observability	Are the outcomes of the proposed intervention tangible or immediate? Is the intervention adopted or advocated by role models the community deems credible?

Source: Rogers et al. (2014)

The importance of theoretically driven, evidence-based health promotion models is that they provide the basis for the empirical validation of the conceptual underpinnings of health promotion theory that ultimately allow for a more thorough understanding of factors that influence risk reduction and that provide for a more focused and individualized approach to reducing behavioral risks. According to Eccles and Mittman (2012), "Implementation research is the scientific study of methods to promote the systematic uptake of research findings and other evidence-based practices into routine practice, and, hence, to improve the quality and effectiveness of health services and care" (p. 1). Implementation science theories should be applicable to the scientific issues examined and congruent with the population to be served (Birken et al., 2017). They should also provide evidence for adoption in practice (i.e., be scalable) and culturally appropriate. This means that interventions must be adequately evaluated using culturally appropriate methods (Allison, 2021; CDC, 2014).

Health promotion interventions have been guided by several major theoretical models:

- Health belief model (HBM; Becker, 1974; Becker & Maiman, 1975; Janz & Becker, 1984)
- Social cognitive learning theory (SCLT; Bandura, 1985; Bandura & Walters, 1977; Rosenstock et al., 1988)
- Transtheoretical model of behavior change (TMC; Prochaska, 2008; Prochaska & DiClemente, 1982, 1983; Velicer et al., 1998)
- Theory of reasoned action (TRA) and the complementary theory of planned behavior (TPB; Azjen & Fishbein, 1988; Chang, 1998; Madden et al., 1992; Montano & Kasprzyk, 2015).

Each of these theories attempts to explain behavior change as a process involving cognitive and sociocultural expectations, as well as proposing potential points of intervention to reduce risk behaviors or maintain healthy behaviors.

Singer (1991, p. 258) rhetorically questioned the use of ethnic culture in many health promotion interventions: "Does ethnic culture matter in behavioral interventions?" Singer proposed several useful typologies to gauge the level of cultural approaches included in interventions:

- *Culturally sensitive approaches:* attempt to be "socioculturally empathetic." That is, these interventions use culture to enhance the physical climate of an organization, make a client feel at-ease and comfortable, and speak the same language.
- *Culturally appropriate approaches:* incorporate a specific awareness of the cultural and linguistic patterns of the community in which the intervention is based. This could mean displaying culturally inspired art, acknowledging the familial cultural hierarchy, or understanding and using specific Spanish dialects.
- *Culturally innovative approaches:* find ways to use culture therapeutically to both reach potential clients and to assist them in making behavioral changes to reduce their risks. Some researchers believe that Latinos are a "hard to reach" population, but if they incorporate Latino cultural concepts like confianza, respeto, and simpatia, they can effectively access this population. Moreover, "using culture" can include measuring levels of familism and self-efficacy to trigger behavior change.
- *Socioculturally congruent approaches:* are those community-based interventions that assist clients to view their culture as empowering. Latino cultural strengths can be enhanced and provide motivation to change an aspect of their environment to promote healthy living.

Each of these cultural approaches differ from one another by the inclusion of "ethnic culture" symbolically or as an empowerment tool to motivate people to change their risk behaviors.

Theory-Driven Interventions That Promote Latino Health

Theory-driven interventions have the advantage of being "tried and tested" with various populations, including Latinos (De Silva et al., 2014; Austin et al., 2023). They also provide a research and evaluation framework that examines adherence to intervention design and allows consistent verification of the driving and intervening concepts underlying important theory-driven interventions that promote the health of Latinos.

Social-Cognitive and Behavioral Interventions

Most of the intervention strategies that fall under this category use social cognitive theories to promote healthy behaviors and reduce risk behaviors on an individual or group basis, especially among social networks. Most of the theories do not explicitly include ethnic culture. Some of the theories have been used to improve access to health care, reduce obesity-related risk factors, and provide better educational outreach for Latinos.

The Health Belief Model (HBM)

The HBM is perhaps the most widely used behavioral change model in public health interventions. It has been effectively applied to marginalized populations, like African Americans and Latinos, and to an array of health inequalities, like type 2 diabetes and HIV/AIDS prevention and intervention programs (Anastasia & Bridges, 2015; Chen et al., 2007; Davis et al., 2013; Moore de Peralta et al., 2015; Rodríguez-Reimann et al., 2004; Scarinci et al., 2012; Wilson et al., 2017). The HBM and its major components are illustrated in Figure 9.5.

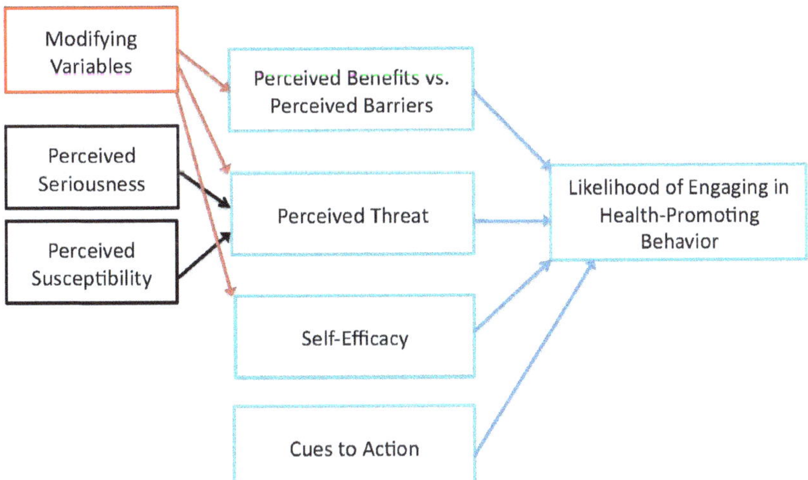

FIGURE 9.5 The Health Belief Model

Theoretically, the importance of one's health is informed by the perceived seriousness and perceived susceptibility to disease. If a disease is perceived as an existential threat to one's health, there should be strong motivation to prevent one from acquiring the disease. Modifying variables in Figure 9.5 include gender, age, race and ethnicity, socioeconomic status, and other social and personal characteristics of the individual. These antecedent perceptions and modifying variables influence perceived benefits and barriers to taking preventive action and perceived threat of the disease. Two important components of the theory are "self-efficacy" and "cues to action." *Self-efficacy* is defined as the ability to make personal behavioral changes. *Cues to action* are those internal and external triggers that motivate personal or group behavior change. Barriers to taking preventive action must also be acknowledged to overcome personal and interpersonal challenges to behavior change. Together, perceived benefits are weighted against perceived barriers to change. Each of the components in the HBM are used to predict the likelihood of engaging in health promoting behaviors (Table 9.4).

Chen et al. (2007) examined the HBM in relation to influenza vaccination coverage rates among Latino Americans, non-Latino Black Americans, and non-Latino White Americans and found that Latino Americans were significantly less concerned than non-Latino White Americans about the likelihood of getting influenza. Concern about getting influenza had the strongest and most significant association with getting an influenza vaccine among non-Latino White Americans and non-Latino Black Americans in comparison to Latino Americans.

In a study applying the HBM to cancer beliefs among non-Latino Black Americans, White Americans, and Latino Americans, Davis et al. (2013) did not find statistically significant differences between racial/ethnic groups for perceived severity, perceived barriers, and cues to action. The researchers did find that Latino Americans, compared to non-Latino White Americans, were 2.24 times more likely to believe that a perceived benefit was that cancer can typically be cured when detected early. However, Latino Americans were less likely to believe they had the ability to lower their risk of developing cancer than did both non-Latino Black Americans and White Americans. Latino Americans also believed they had a lower chance of acquiring cancer in the future compared to non-Latino White Americans. Latino Americanss cited structural barriers as the major factors preventing HPV vaccination, as well as cost, lack of health insurance, and transportation.

TABLE 9.4 Health Belief Constructs and Definitions

Construct	Definition
Perceived severity	The opinion of how *serious* the disease and its consequences are
Perceived barriers	The opinion that certain things will *interfere* with adopting the new behavior
Cues to action	Things that will *motivate* an individual to change behavior (i.e., events, people, or media)
Perceived susceptibility	The personal assessment of the *risk* of getting a certain disease
Perceived benefits	The belief that the new behavior is more *beneficial* to reduce risk for a disease
Self-efficacy	The confidence an individual has in their *ability* to do something

Source: Davis et al. (2013)

The applicability of the traditional HBM to tuberculosis and Latinos was found to be inadequate by Rodríguez-Reimann et al. (2004). They found that by adapting the HBM to include acculturation level among Latinos, the model became a "better fit." In this study the authors specifically included an Anglo

Orientation Scale and a Mexican Orientation Scale derived from Cuellar et al.'s (1995b) Acculturation Scale for Mexican Americans (ARSMA-II). The study found that Latinos of Mexican descent who were more Mexican-oriented reported higher perceived susceptibility and seriousness, more barriers, and greater attention to cues regarding tuberculosis prevention than "highly integrated bicultural" Latinos.

There are many more studies that have used the HBM with Latinos, with varying degrees of success, or model fit. Some research has demonstrated that the inclusion of Latino cultural concepts like acculturation and cognitive referents of acculturation (e.g., fatalism, familism) have more predictive ability in facilitating behavior change (Anastasia & Bridges, 2015; Wilson et al., 2017). Importantly, some studies demonstrate the efficacy of including cognitive referents of acculturation that provide more explanatory power to the HBM model and constructs (Moore de Peralta et al., 2015; Scarinci et al., 2012). For example, Moore de Peralta et al. (2015) examined three cultural concepts—acculturation, familism, and fatalism—in relation to cancer screening behaviors. They found that only familism was a significant predictor, together with other HBM constructs, of obtaining a PAP screening in the next 3 years.

Social Cognitive Learning Theory (SCLT)

Bandura's social cognitive learning theory (SCLT) is another widely used behavioral intervention that has been shown to be effective in reducing health promotion and risk reduction with Latinos (Cortés et al., 2013; Jimenez et al., 2023). The model and its major components are shown in Figure 9.6.

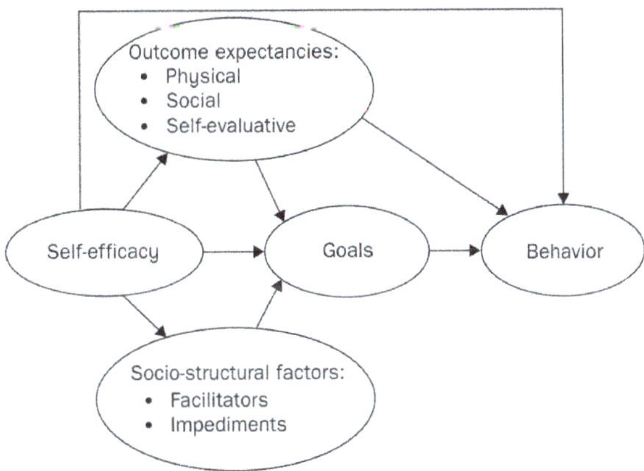

FIGURE 9.6 Social Cognitive Learning Theory

According to SCLT, self-efficacy is the primary driving force in behavior change. However, self-efficacy is influenced by social and normative characteristics that are valued or endorsed by society ("sociostructural factors" in Figure 9.6) and messaging by important and relevant role models. Moreover, outcome expectations (what one hopes to achieve) are associated with goal setting, which in turn influences behavior change (Table 9.5).

TABLE 9.5 SCLT Constructs and Definitions

Construct	Definition
Reciprocal determinism	The dynamic and reciprocal interaction of person (individual with a set of learned experiences), environment (external social context), and behavior (responses to stimuli to achieve goals).
Behavioral capability	A person's actual ability to perform a behavior through essential knowledge and skills.
Observational learning	People can witness and observe a behavior conducted by others and then reproduce those actions. This is often exhibited through "modeling" of behaviors.
Reinforcements	Internal or external responses to a person's behavior that affect the likelihood of continuing or discontinuing the behavior. This construct of SCLT is most closely associated with the reciprocal relationship between behavior and the social environment.
Outcome expectations	The anticipated consequences of a person's behavior. People anticipate the consequences of their actions before engaging in the behavior, and these anticipated consequences can influence successful completion of the behavior.
Self-efficacy	A person's belief in their ability to change their behavior. Self-efficacy is influenced by a person's specific capabilities and other individual factors, as well as by socioenvironmental factors (facilitators and impediments/barriers).
Facilitators	Personal, social, cultural assets than can facilitate behavior change.
Impediments	Personal, social, cultural barriers than can prevent behavior change.
Response efficacy	The person's assessment of the cost versus benefit of changing behavior.

Sources: Bandura and Walters (1977); LaMorte (2022)

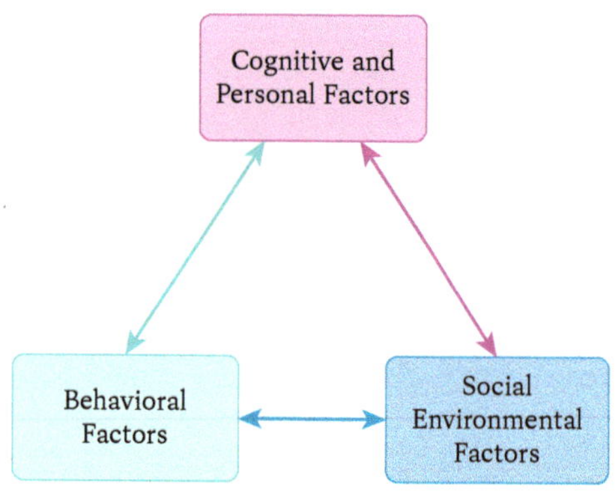

FIGURE 9.7 Reciprocal Determinism in SCLT

An important aspect of SCLT is the notion of *reciprocal determinism*, where cognitive and personal factors, behavior, and the social environment interact with one another (Figure 9.7). Bandura's notion of reciprocal determinism suggests that human action is influenced by three factors: the social environment, cognitive and personal characteristics, and behavior, all of which reinforce each other.

Social cognitive learning theory has been successfully used to reduce obesity among Latino youth and adults (Contento et al., 2010). Increases in self-efficacy and social support from friends and family facilitated risk reduction among Latino adolescents in the Contento et al. (2010) study. Similarly,

Cortés et al. (2013) delivered a nutrition education intervention to Latinos based on social learning/cognitive theory. After receiving between three and five home-based nutrition education sessions and a supermarket tour over a 6-month period, many Latino families adopted instructions on buying budget-friendly, healthier alternative foods. Findings indicated that participating families decreased the total number of calories and calories per dollar purchased from baseline to post education.

Hu et al. (2016) developed a family-focused intervention to reduced diabetes risks among Latino youth with type 2 diabetes, operationalizing familism by assessing the social-environmental support of family members and friends, neighborhood, and community to the individual. They found significant improvement in diabetes knowledge and diabetes self-efficacy among youth, and family members had improvements in diabetes knowledge and physical health-related quality of life.

Another study applying cognitive social learning theory to Latinos was conducted by Jimenez and colleagues (2023). They employed community health workers (CHWs) as lead informants to provide health education to older Latino individuals living with HIV/AIDS. The health promotion intervention included a social and physical activation session, a moderately intense group walk led by a CHW for 45 min, three times a week for 16 weeks, and scheduling pleasant events (e.g., going to brunch with friends). Group activities were also culturally adapted (e.g., foods, interactions). Learning within a social context and having a CHW lead discussions and provide positive reinforcements for behavior change were important aspects of applied SCLT (Van Servellen & Lombardi, 2005).

The Theory of Reasoned Action and Planned Behavior

The *theory of reasoned action and planned behavior,* also known as the *integrative behavioral model* (Montano & Kasprzyk, 2015), places importance on personal attitudes, subjective norms, motivations to comply to others' expectations, and perceived behavioral control are antecedent to behavioral intentions to change behaviors, which in turn leads to actual behavior change (Table 9.6). Behavioral intentions, then, are directly related to behavioral risk reduction. "Perceived behavioral control" is often used synonymously with "self-efficacy" in some health promotion research.

An integrative behavioral model comprising elements of both the theory of reasoned action (TRA) and the theory of planned behaviors (TPB) is shown in Figure 9.8. The TRA includes three constructs: attitudes toward the behavior, subjective norms regarding the behavior, and behavior intention to change behavior (Table 9.5). This model has also been used successfully in interventions with Latinos (Boyas et al., 2021; Diaz et al., 2009; Guinn et al., 2007; Kam et al., 2009; Martin et al., 2007; Villarruel et al., 2004; Vissman et al., 2013).

Villarruel et al. (2004) examined components of TPB in predicting condom use among Latino youth. They found that attitudes, subjective norms, self-efficacy, partner and parental approval, and impulse control beliefs were significant predictors of intentions to use condoms among their sample. Diaz et al. (2009) examined acculturation level and gender in association with TPB and dietary outcomes among Latino adolescents in California. They found support for the theoretical constructs, but with noted differences among women compared to men and lower compared to higher acculturated Latinos. Specifically, women had stronger intentions, more positive attitudes, and greater subjective normative influences than men, and higher acculturation had negative effects on intention for giving up liked food items and support and encouragement for eating a healthy diet in Latino adolescents, with less acculturated groups showing more favorable outcomes.

TABLE 9.6 Theory of Reasoned Action/Planned Behavior Constructs and Definitions

Construct	Definition
Attitudes toward behavior (behavioral beliefs and evaluations of behavioral outcomes)	The individual's positive or negative opinion of the behavior to change.
Subjective norms	The opinions of important others regarding the behavior.
Social norms	Societal, group, or cultural beliefs regarding the behavior.
Motivation to comply	The willingness of the person to comply to important others' beliefs regarding behavior change.
Perceived behavioral control (control beliefs and perceived power)	One's own belief that they can change their behavior. This would also include the ability and skills to change behavior.
Behavioral intentions to perform behavior	The likelihood that one will undertake behavioral changes.

Source: Ajzen and Fishbein (1988)

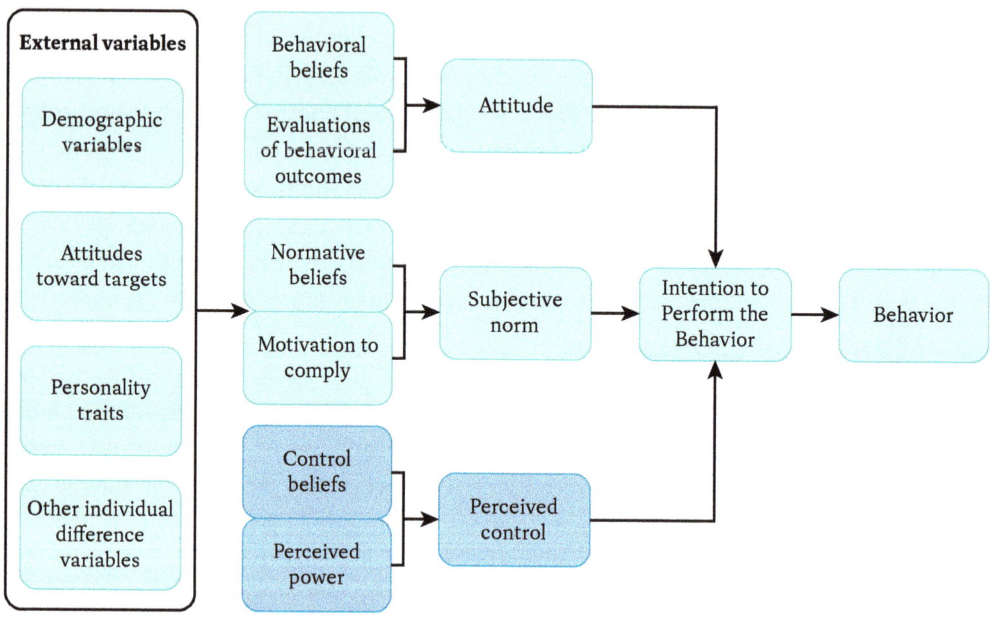

FIGURE 9.8 The Theory of Reasoned Action and Planned Behavior: The Integrative Behavioral Model

A study by Shi et al. (2023) examined the willingness to seek mental health care among Latinos, non-Latino White Americans, and non-Latino Black Americans. They found differences between the groups, with Latinos reporting lower levels of perceived norms and perceived behavioral control than non-Latino White Americans. Additionally, Latinos reported more favorable attitudes than non-Latino White Americans toward having a conversation with someone close about that person's mental health issues. Non-Latino Black Americans reported more favorable attitudes toward help-seeking from their social networks than non-Latino White Americans and had more favorable attitudes than non-Latino White Americans toward having a conversation.

The Transtheoretical Model—Stages of Change

A favorite of clinicians because of the staging process involved, the *transtheoretical model* of behavior change, also known as the *stages of change model*, has been widely used with various populations and risk reduction for disease, including smoking cessation and HIV/AIDS risk behaviors (Prochaska, 2008, Prochaska & DiClemente, 1982, 1983; Stevens & Estrada, 1996; Velicer et al., 1998). An individual can enter and exit stages at any point. An important aspect of the stages of change model is the acknowledgment of relapse back to negative health behaviors (Figure 9.9).

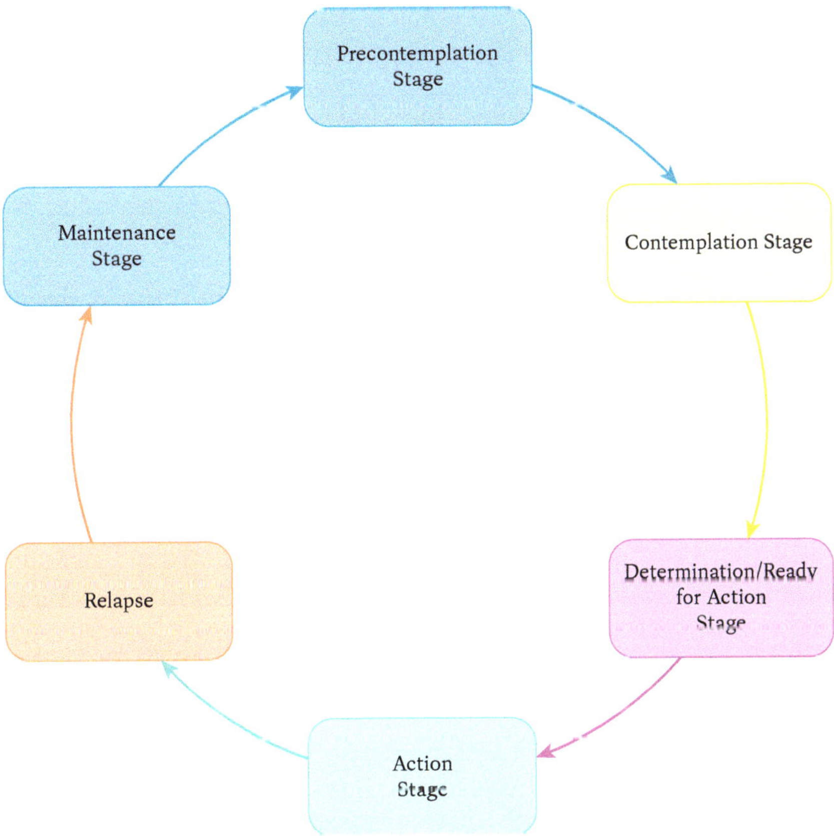

FIGURE 9.9 Stages of Change Model

In the *precontemplative stage*, the focus is on educating the person on the risks and benefits and positive outcomes associated with behavioral risk reduction behavior (see Table 9.7). In the *contemplative stage*, the focus is on identifying barriers and facilitators for behavior change, mustering social support, and addressing any concerns the person may have regarding the difficulty of changing risk behaviors (e.g., losing social networks). In the *determination/ready for action stage*, the person is cognitively ready to set realistic goals and provide an initial timeline for change. During this stage it is particularly important to provide social support and reinforcement for positive behavior change. In the *action stage*, the person is beginning to make positive changes in risk reduction behavior. Social support and reinforcement are critical to avoid relapse and continue to the maintenance stage. During the *maintenance stage*, positive reinforcement should continue, and goal attainment should be celebrated.

TABLE 9.7 Stages of Change Constructs and Definitions

Construct	Definition
Precontemplative stage	In this stage people are not intending to change their behavior in the foreseeable future. They may be in denial or unaware that their behavior is risk-inducing.
Contemplative stage	In this stage people are beginning to weigh the costs and benefits of changing behavior and thinking of ways to do it.
Determination/ready for action stage	In this stage people are intent on making behavioral change and are preparing for it.
Action stage	In this stage people are acting, putting a plan in place to make the desired behavior change.
Maintenance stage	In this stage people are sustaining their behavior change through positive reinforcements.
Relapse	In this stage people fall back into negative, risk-inducing behaviors. This stage can occur at any point in the process.

Source: Velicer et al. (1998)

The transtheoretical model or stages of change model has been used successfully with Latino populations with some cultural adaptation (Fernandez et al., 2007; Keller & McGowan, 2001; Kenya et al., 2015; Ruggiero et al., 2011; Smith & Ryan, 2006; Surís et al., 1998; Tung et al., 2016). Cultural adaptations included translation of research materials into the vernacular Spanish spoken in the study or by including an acculturation measure in the study.

For example, Surís et al. (1998) found that Latinas who were less educated, low income, and less acculturated clustered more in the precontemplative stage, and the most acculturated clustered in the contemplative and action stages. Tung et al. (2016) examined the relationship between cancer screening, self-efficacy, and stages of change among Latinas. They found that the highest self-efficacy scores were among Latinas in the action or maintenance stages, and the lowest self-efficacy scores were among Latinas in the precontemplative stage. The study also found that Latinas in the precontemplative or relapse stage perceived significantly higher barriers than those in contemplation, determination, action, and maintenance stages.

Kenya et al. (2015) were able to "stage" participants in their study using constructs from the transtheoretical model. An acculturation measure was also included in the study, finding that most Latinos were low to moderately acculturated. They classified 30% of their Latino sample in the precontemplative and contemplative stages, 31% in the determination stage, and 39% in the action or maintenance stages. However, acculturation level was not examined in relationship to stages.

Theory-Driven Community-Based Interventions

These types of interventions require time, external and internal financial investments, personnel, and community involvement advocating for policy change. Interventions for groups and communities are complex and require multilevel collaboration with both internal and external agencies. Community interventions are more inclusive of race, ethnicity, gender, and cultural factors and, as such, require an intersectionality perspective. Most of the approaches employ strategies to reduce the negative effects of the social determinants of health.

Social Ecological Approaches

Based on Bronfenbrenner's (1977) social ecological model, this approach considers macro-level influences on individual health behavior (Figure 9.10).

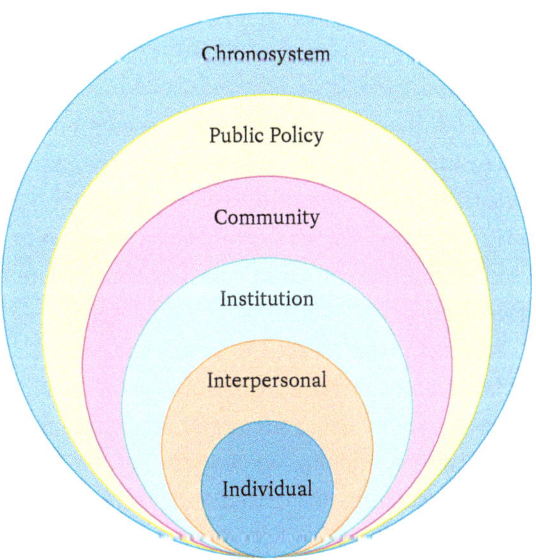

FIGURE 9.10 A Social Ecological Approach

Adapted from Bronfenbrenner (1977)

Individuals are "nested" within and are impacted by many external factors. Identifying important influences on the individual begins at the outer level. National, state, and local public policy significantly influences access to health care, the availability of specialty services, and the contribution of external resources. For example, undocumented individuals and families are not eligible for health care under the Affordable Care Act. Within the community level, organizational relationships and mutual collaboration can improve social conditions that contribute to increased risk for chronic and communicable diseases. Additionally, informal social networks contribute to increased community social cohesion. Institutional structures formulate rules and regulations that can have the effect of hindering or facilitating access to health care among Latinos. For example, hours of operation, bilingual staffing, and translators and interpreters are governed by medical institutions. Institutional cultural competence is an important aspect for providing adequate care to Latinos. At the interpersonal level, formal and informal social support networks provide a safety net for persons who may not have access to needed goods and services. Knowledge, attitudes, behaviors, and beliefs of the individual are at the inner level. One's cultural identity, self-concept, and self-efficacy have been shown to mitigate the effects of discrimination and racism among Latinos and enable the adoption of healthy lifestyles (Table 9.8).

TABLE 9.8 Bronfenbrenner's Social Ecological Model Constructs and Definitions

Construct	Definition
Microsystem (individual)	The layer closest to the person that includes the person's immediate setting (parents, family, home).
Mesosystem (interpersonal)	All the interactions within the microsystem.
Exosystem (institutional and community)	The extended family, friends, social welfare policies, community, and mass media.
Macrosystem (public policy)	The next layer after the exosystem includes cultural values, language, attitudes, economy, and policies.
"Chronosystem"	The outermost layer that examines transitions over the lifetime and shifting social and cultural expectations.

Source: Bronfenbrenner (1977)

In Williams et al.'s (2011) proposed model (Figure 9.11), acculturative stressors are explicitly included and influences and are influenced by broader social and physical environmental factors. These external factors influence the family domain, which includes family attributes, behaviors, functioning, and parenting factors. All these factors are antecedent to the child's physical activity and dietary behaviors, which influence the child's weight status. The model includes an explicit focus on social determinants of health.

A systematic literature review conducted by Kiraly et al. (2017) found empirical support for using the social ecological framework to focus on Latino youth and obesity. However, issues around sustainability of interventions using the social ecological model remains problematic given the number of resources in time, staffing, and money needed.

Latino community-based social ecological approaches have proven effective in establishing community social and health priorities; developing multilevel, reciprocal interactions to facilitate community well-being; and empowering communities to take political and social action to improve their lives (Blanco-Vega et al., 2007; Cacari Stone et al., 2022).

Within socioecological theory, the promotora de salud model is the most applied intervention with Latino communities. This model was developed to engage Latino participants where they live and attempt to facilitate social, and behavior change through peer-directed implementation. Derived from community health worker (CHW) models, promotoras de salud provide health education, knowledge, service awareness, and client-health navigation instruction to other peers in the community (Balcazar et al., 2006; Medina et al., 2007; Meister et al., 1992). Balcazar and colleagues (Balcázar et al., 2005; Medina et al., 2007)

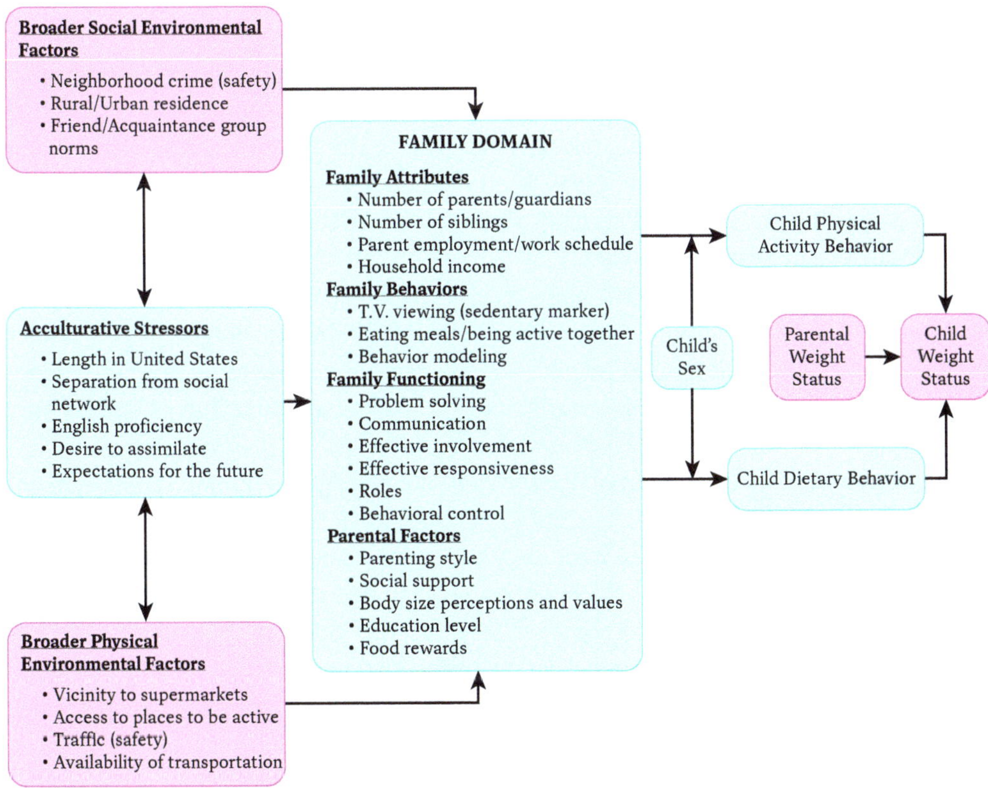

FIGURE 9.11 Social Ecological Model Examining the Social Environmental and Cultural Influences on Childhood Obesity

highlight the positive effects of promotora models in reaching Latino populations and fostering change in "heart-healthy living." Wilkinson-Lee et al. (2018) use a promotora model as part of their community-based participatory research design to increase awareness of sexually transmitted infections and depression among Latinas in the community. They found that promotoras can effectively engage and educate Latinas on these culturally sensitive topics.

However, a review of CHWs and promotoras conducted by Ahmed et al. (2022) found mixed results for the efficacy of CHW models. Though they were effective in building community capacity, many communities still experienced inequalities in access to health care. The authors concluded, "We need to move beyond seeing CHWs as a temporary sticking plaster, and instead build meaningful partnerships between CHWs, communities and policymakers to confront and address the underlying structures of inequity" (Ahmed et al., 2022, p. 1).

As the quote above makes clear, there continues to be a perception that CHWs and promotoras are "sticking plaster" or Band-Aid approaches to important Latino health inequalities. However, until there are more physicians in the Latino community and greater access to health care, there will always be a need for community approaches to promote health and navigate health systems.

Community-Engaged Research Approaches

The popularity of community-engaged research approaches was a result of involvement and active participation with community residents in identifying their social and health priorities. It represents a grassroots approach, with public health professionals taking a backseat to the "funds of knowledge" brought to the table by the community (González et al., 2006; Moll et al., 2006). The central concept of the funds of knowledge approach is that the Latino community possesses knowledge and practices they have produced and acquired through their lived experiences.

Community-engaged research is built upon trust between academia and the community. This is a hard sell to many Latino communities and other historically disadvantaged populations based on historical violations of trust and mutual respect (e.g., fumigation of Mexican migrants, the infamous Tuskegee Experiment with African Americans, and the forced sterilization of Latina and African American women).

Sanders Thompson and colleagues developed the community-engaged research continuum to facilitate working with communities (Goodman & Sanders Thompson, 2017; Sanders Thompson et al., 2021). The continuum shown in Figure 9.12 provides a strategy for empowering communities through continuous community engagement where all stakeholders have a voice in decision making (Table 9.9).

According to Goodman and Sanders Thompson (2017, p.490), "Successful partnerships are developed and sustained when the constituent members contribute their perspectives, resources, and skills creating an amalgam for research synergy allowing the partnership to obtain outcomes that no one constituent member could have produced on their own."

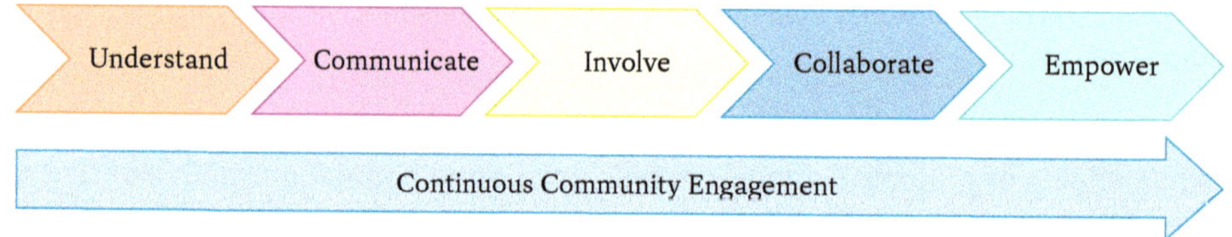

FIGURE 9.12 Community-Engaged Research Continuum

Adapted from: Sanders Thompson et al. (2021)

TABLE 9.9 Community Engagement Constructs and Definitions

Construct	Definition
Understand	To provide the community with balanced and objective information, to assist them in understanding the problem, alternatives, and solutions, and to understand the perspectives of the community.
Communicate	To obtain community feedback on analysis, alternatives, and decisions to build relationships and connect with community leaders.

Involve	To work with the community throughout the process to ensure that their concerns and aspirations are consistently understood and addressed.
Collaborate	To partner with the community in each aspect of the decision-making process from development to solution.
Empower	Shared leadership of community-led projects with final decision making at the community level. Acknowledge cultural strengths and build trust.

Adapted from: Sanders Thompson et al. (2021).

Several community engagement approaches have shown promising results in reducing health inequalities and empowering Latino communities to advocate for their health and social well-being (Alicea-Alvarez et al., 2016; Calva et al., 2020; Comfort et al., 2018; Fernandez, 2018; García et al., 2021; Kuo et al., 2017). The goal is to make "community engagement" synonymous with "community participation" (Lasker & Weiss, 2003). For example, Lasker and Weiss (2003) provide a process for community participation related to individual empowerment, bridging social ties among community members and partners, and creating synergy among community members to accomplish their goals.

Similarly, Fernandez (2018) identified several important processes and attitudes for cultivating community engagement among Latinos of Mexican descent residing in Chicago. She found that advocating for social justice, challenging racist perceptions of the Latino community, and including everyone's voice (democratic leadership) in the decision-making process elicited strong community support.

The identification of health priorities, from the community's perspective, is one example of community-engaged research. García et al. (2021) used focus groups comprised primarily of Latino and African American community members to identify needs. In their study, three themes emerged: the identification of social determinants that affected their health (i.e., lack of access to health care, costs associated with health care), the perceived power imbalances between researchers and community members, and the need for developing mutual trust and respect in collaborative research. Active listening, genuine caring, and nonjudgmental attitudes were cited as important ingredients to building trust with community members.

Community-Based Participatory Research (CBPR) Approaches

Israel et al. (2010) have demonstrated the utility of using CBPR approaches to develop and build academic–community partnerships to eliminate health disparities through multiple points of engagement, including policy change. According to Goodman and Sanders Thompson (2017), CBPR principles are centered on building trust among partners, mutual respect for each partner's expertise and contributions, with equitable and shared decision-making. CBPR principles are very similar to community-engaged research principles, and both have been used interchangeably in research literature (Minkler & Wallerstein, 2011; Shalowitz et al., 2009). Is the difference between them only semantic? Perhaps, but for the sake of simplicity let's say one is focused on *engagement* and the other on *participation*.

Wallerstein et al. (2008) developed a comprehensive CBPR model that is inclusive of all stakeholders and links inputs to outcomes (Figure 9.13). One of the more important outcomes of CBPR, especially with historically marginalized populations, is what Wallerstein et al. (2008) refer to as *emancipatory* in co-creating knowledge. They also recognized the importance of several other factors, including the role of context (historical, governance, and power differentials) and its influence on group dynamics, cultural issues (cultural humility, culturally centered interventions, cultural revitalization), and the role of CBPR in creating change and producing positive health outcomes for the community. This model best exemplifies Singer's (1991) definition of *socioculturally congruent approaches* with its focus on contexts, group dynamics/equitable partnerships, appropriate and culturally tailored interventions, and outcomes that include cultural renewal and social justice.

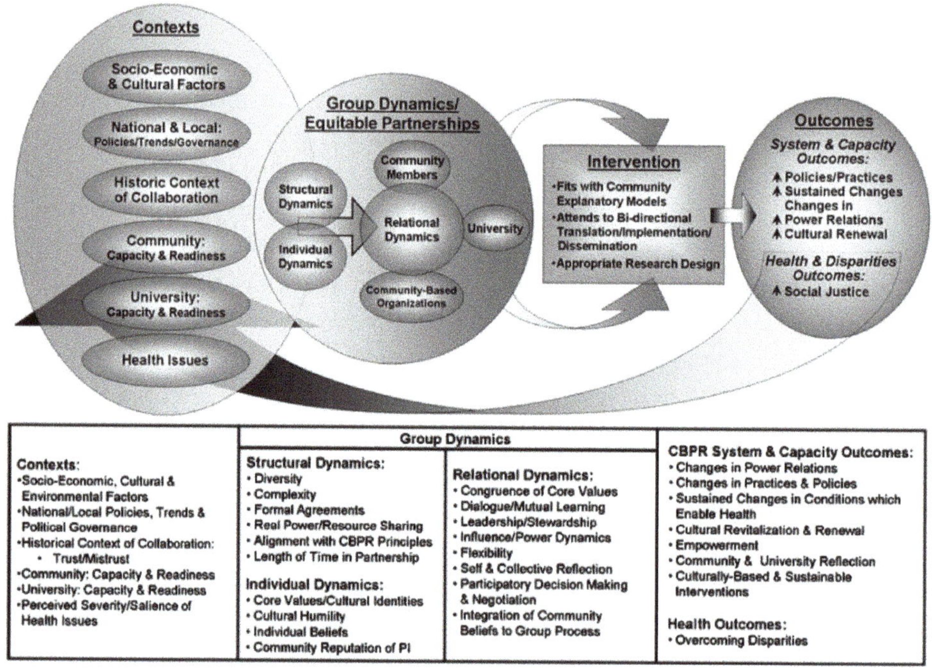

Contexts:	Group Dynamics		CBPR System & Capacity Outcomes:
•Socio-Economic, Cultural & Environmental Factors •National/Local Policies, Trends & Political Governance •Historical Context of Collaboration: • Trust/Mistrust •Community: Capacity & Readiness •University: Capacity & Readiness •Perceived Severity/Salience of Health Issues	**Structural Dynamics:** • Diversity • Complexity • Formal Agreements • Real Power/Resource Sharing • Alignment with CBPR Principles • Length of Time in Partnership **Individual Dynamics:** • Core Values/Cultural Identities • Cultural Humility • Individual Beliefs • Community Reputation of PI	**Relational Dynamics:** • Congruence of Core Values • Dialogue/Mutual Learning • Leadership/Stewardship • Influence/Power Dynamics • Flexibility • Self & Collective Reflection • Participatory Decision Making & Negotiation • Integration of Community Beliefs to Group Process	• Changes in Power Relations • Changes in Practices & Policies • Sustained Changes in Conditions which Enable Health • Cultural Revitalization & Renewal • Empowerment • Community & University Reflection • Culturally-Based & Sustainable Interventions **Health Outcomes:** • Overcoming Disparities

FIGURE 9.13 Community-Based Participatory Research

CBPR has been successfully applied to a broad range of social and health issues and with various populations, including Latinos (e.g., Hull et al., 2010; Kia-Keating et al., 2017; Kim et al., 2005; Loi et al., 2017; McQuiston et al., 2005; Rhodes et al., 2013; Shattell et al., 2008). The use of "lay health educators" or promotoras de salud has been observed in many CBPR approaches with Latino communities, as noted above. Kim et al. (2005) used this approach to outreach to and educate members of the Latino community. They used CBPR principles to achieve their goals, which included collaborative partnerships with researchers, community residents, community-based organizations, and health officials. This research collaborative recommended six strategies for creating a successful CBPR approach with Latino communities, which echoes suggestions of other studies (Loi et al., 2017):

- Involve members of the targeted group as partners.
- Include existing community agencies and social networks.
- Collaborate with other community programs.

- Foster Latino community pride and self-sufficiency.
- Provide resources.
- Be culturally responsive to the needs of the Latino community (e.g., acknowledge gender roles, family dynamics, cultural preferences, etc.).

A large body of evidence supports the application of CBPR approaches to identify social and health issues in the Latino community. There is little doubt that CBPR approaches facilitate community engagement, social cohesion, social capital, and empowerment (O'Mara-Eves et al., 2015; Popay et al., 2007). Nevertheless, findings are equivocal on whether CBPR approaches have a direct effect in reducing the incidence and prevalence of health inequalities in the communities targeted. In fact, Popay et al.'s (2007) review of the literature showed they did not have *any* positive impact on mortality, morbidity, health behaviors, or health inequalities.

Another systematic meta-analysis to examine whether community engagement had any impact on health and health inequalities among disadvantaged populations was conducted by Cyril et al. (2015). They found that of the 24 studies that met their inclusion criteria, 21 (87.5%) had positively impacted health behaviors, public health planning, health service access, health literacy, and a range of health outcomes. But overall, the review found little consistency in the effectiveness of CBPR in improving the health of historically marginalized populations. The studies reviewed by Cyril et al. (2015) that showed a positive impact on community health were characterized by their incorporation of cultural and ethnic perspectives, including community members in the development and implementation of research protocols (e.g. client recruitment), genuine power-sharing, bidirectional learning, and involvement in the community needs assessment (e.g. translation, feedback, and interpretation).

Negative, unanticipated outcomes have also been found. Attree et al. (2011), for example, found the process of engaging community members lead to "burnout" among the consortia. The researchers acknowledged that community participants perceived benefits for their physical and psychological health, increased self-confidence, increased self-esteem, and a sense of personal empowerment and improved social relationships. However, their review indicated that there were unintended negative consequences of community engagement for some members, which they conjecture may be detrimental to psychological well-being. In addition, inconsistent measures of health or mental health outcomes, lack of evaluation, and inadequate research designs contribute to a lack of intervention effectiveness (O'Mara-Eves et al., 2015).

Latino Culturally Responsive Interventions

Theory-driven interventions using these behavioral change models have demonstrated some utility in risk reduction among various racial/ethnic groups. However, none of these health promotion theories explicitly incorporates culture as an important component in behavior change. All have had to be adapted to address specific cultural factors and their influence on health behavior among Latinos.

Latino Cultural Adaptation of Theoretical Interventions

As noted in many meta-evaluations reviewed, cultural adaptation of theoretical interventions has been successfully applied to Latino populations. The extent of cultural adaptation varies considerably from the translation of materials into Spanish, hiring bilingual/bicultural personnel, involvement of community members in all aspects of the research endeavor, and using cultural concepts like acculturation level and cultural values like respeto and fatalism.

Latino cultural adaptations have flourished over the past several decades in a variety of disciplines, like social welfare, psychology, education, and public health (Benson-Floréz et al., 2017; Bernal & Domenech Rodríguez, 2009; Domenech Rodríguez et al., 2011; García et al., 2017; Gallardo & Curry, 2009; Hernandez et al., 2018; Jani et al., 2009; Leng et al., 2022; Leyva et al., 2022; Nelson et al., 2020; Rosas et al., 2020; Stein & Guzman, 2015).

Bernal et al. (1995) provide a very useful framework for adapting Latino culture to theoretical behavior change interventions. The framework includes eight components that are considered essential for successful Latino cultural adaptation (Table 9.10).

TABLE 9.10 Culturally Innovative Components and Dimensions for Cultural Inclusion

Intervention	Culturally innovative elements
Language	Culturally appropriate; culturally syntonic language
Persons	Role of ethnic/racial similarities and differences between client and therapist in shaping therapeutic relationship
Metaphors	Symbols and concepts shared with the population; sayings or "dichos" in treatment
Content	Cultural knowledge: values, customs, and traditions; uniqueness of groups (social, economic, historical, political)
Concepts	Treatment concepts consonant with culture and context: dependence vs. Interdependence vs. Independence; emic (within culture, particular) over etic (outside culture, universal)
Goals	Transmission of positive and adaptive cultural values; support adaptive values from the culture of origin
Methods	Development and/or cultural adaptation of treatment methods. Examples: "modeling" to include culturally consonant traditions (e.g., cuento therapy [therapy based on folk tales]); cultural reframing of drug abuse as intergenerational cultural conflicts; use of language (formal and informal); cultural hypothesis testing; use of genograms; "cultural migration dialogue"
Context	Consideration of changing contexts in assessment during treatment or intervention: acculturative stress; phase of migration; developmental stage; social supports and relationship to country of origin; economic and social context of intervention

Source: Bernal et al. (1995)

The application of these Latino cultural components to behavior change interventions requires specific attention to process and documentation of cultural adaptation and implementation strategies and Latino community feedback (Domenech Rodríguez et al., 2011). The absence of detailed documentation on how the intervention was culturally adapted and the processes involved severely limits the adoption and use of cultural interventions and the goal of using culture to assist in behavioral change. Still, cultural adaptation does not address the underlying social determinants of health unless there is a sustained focus on empowering the community to act in addressing and eliminating the underlying causes of health inequalities among Latinos.

Cultural adaptation should move beyond using constructs like acculturation level due to its conflation of socioeconomic status and language. When studies find that lower acculturated Latinos possess less knowledge about disease symptoms, or have less access to health care, or have better health outcomes than higher acculturated Latinos, what does that mean? Are they implying that Latinos should change their culture to become more Americanized? That Latinos should become bicultural? Are these studies continuing to perpetuate negative perceptions of Latino culture, like the cultural deficit theories discussed in a previous chapter? Acculturation level contributes little to the understanding of cultural influences associated with behavioral intentions, risk behaviors, or using culture to facilitate behavioral risk reduction among Latinos (Rudmin et al., 2017).

However, the examination of the ABCs (affective, behavioral, and cognitive) of acculturation (Cuellar et al., 1995a) and the sociocultural context in which interventions are performed provides a mechanism for applying them effectively for behavioral change and risk reduction among Latinos through cultural reframing.

Increased acculturation to mainstream U.S. societal customs and behaviors is a risk factor for Latinos. Several studies have demonstrated how risk behaviors increase with increasing levels of acculturation and length of residence in the United States. Likewise, the Latino cultural concepts of *machismo* and *marianismo* can be negative influences on help-seeking behaviors, health promotion, and risk reduction. Cultural reframing, as an example, is shown in Table 9.11.

TABLE 9.11 Examples of Cultural Reframing

Cultural influences on risk behaviors	Cultural reframing
Acculturation: increases the risk for substance abuse, psychiatric disorders, poorer eating habits.	Latino enculturation: strengthens Latino cultural values.
Machismo: negative influences on Latino health, help-seeking behaviors, engagement in behavioral risks.	Reorient toward *machismo* as a positive aspect for protecting family, self-esteem, and self-efficacy.
Marianismo: negative influences on Latina health, help-seeking behaviors.	Reorient toward *marianismo* as a positive aspect of caring for oneself to care for others (self-empowerment).
Fatalism: the belief that the disease was inevitable.	Reorient toward fatalism as embracing life and that there's still more to accomplish.

The Importance of Latino Cultural Context and Cognitive Referents of Acculturation

Cultural adaptation is a dynamic process that occurs within various social-ecological contexts (Lopez-Class et al., 2011). Lopez-Class et al. (2011) advocate for a social ecological perspective that includes the examination of attitudes, behaviors, and values that change because of acculturation processes, especially those changes associated with the health behaviors of Latinos.

Castro et al. (2007) included a measure of traditional family values and ethnic pride as predictors of alcohol and tobacco use among Latino adolescents. For Latino boys, they reported a positive correlation between traditional family values and ethnic pride, and positive correlations between traditional family values and self-efficacy to avoid tobacco. They also found positive correlations between ethnic pride and negative benefits of cigarette smoking. Acculturation level was not correlated with either of these intermediate outcomes. Similar findings were reported for Latino girls, with the exception that acculturation level was positively associated with alcohol use. As hypothesized in the literature, they found that acculturation level was negatively correlated in both boys and girls with traditional family values and ethnic pride, suggesting that as Latinos acculturate there is erosion of cultural strengths (Sabogal et al., 1987). These results provide a strategy for using Latino cultural strengths to reduce substance use risks: strengthening family values and increasing ethnic pride rather than becoming bicultural or changing something inherently negative about Mexican culture.

Cuellar et al.'s (1995a) seminal research on the association between acculturation and Mexican American cultural values ("cognitive referents of acculturation") led to a more nuanced consideration of cultural influences on behavior and intentions. Cuellar et al. developed five measures of cultural constructs: familism, fatalism, *machismo, personalismo,* and folk beliefs (a composite scale of use, belief in the supernatural, and folk practice beliefs). The authors found that four of these cognitive referents (fatalism, familism, *machismo,* and folk beliefs) were negatively associated with acculturation level, indicating that as acculturation level increases, cognitive referents decrease. The application of these findings can be used to identify cultural triggers that can motivate behavioral change and risk reduction among Latinos and identify cultural barriers to change. A more complete understanding of behavioral risk reduction among Latinos is to include specific cultural factors in health interventions. The inclusion of cultural factors in models of behavior change has been referred to by Castro and Alarcon (2002) as "culturally rich research" (p. 791).

There have been several studies that have included Latino cultural values to examine their influences on health behaviors (Germán et al., 2009; Gil et al., 2000; Romero & Ruiz, 2007; Santisteban et al., 2012). Most of these studies only included familism as an influence on risk behaviors. Santisteban et al. (2012) examined which family processes were involved as mediators in acculturation-based problem behaviors among Latino adolescents. Noting that Latino adolescent problem behavior increased with acculturation level and parenting, the study used a validated familism measure (Sabogal et al., 1987) to assess family processes. The findings showed that parents of Latino children who were less acculturated had parenting practices that were "characterized by higher levels of involvement, positive parenting, effective discipline, and lower levels of discipline avoidance" (Santisteban et al., 2012, p.8). They also found that higher levels of familism were associated with higher levels of positive parenting practices but did not find support for familism as a mediator of acculturation influences; rather, it was a distinct factor.

Context is especially critical in the examination of cultural and subcultural values among marginalized populations. Quintero and Estrada (1998a, 1998b) used qualitative, in-depth interviews to ascertain the perceptions of *machismo* among those who inject drugs. We identified several features of *machismo* within the context of Latino intravenous drug use subculture and created a scale consisting of 11 items based on the interviews (Table 9.12). Other cognitive referents of acculturation like familism, traditionalism, and religiosity were similarly constructed.

TABLE 9.12 *Machismo* Within Latino Intravenous Drug Use Subcultural Context

• For me, being macho means always having drugs.
• Being macho is an important part of who I am.
• A woman should give in to her husband in almost all matters.
• It is a man's right to drink and use drugs if he wants to.
• For me, being macho is controlling my drug use.
• It is macho to get high on any drug available.
• Drug use makes my friends think I am macho.
• It is macho to have lots of money and drugs.
• To be macho, you can never let your guard down.

Important questions to consider when including Latino cognitive referents of acculturation are derived from Singer (1991):

- How does Latino culture and subcultures of risk interact? Which may have precedence over behaviors and risks?
- What aspects of Latino culture can be used in behavioral interventions to trigger motivation to change risk behaviors?
- To what extent can behavior change models include Latino cognitive referents of acculturation to examine their influence on intentions to change behavior or lower risk?
- Does the addition of Latino cultural values provide more insight on how they are involved in behavior change and risk reduction?

Applied Cultural Humility in Latino-Focused Interventions to Promote Health

There is accumulating evidence, as noted above, that risk reduction for chronic and communicable diseases can be achieved through the development and implementation of culturally responsive interventions. Culturally responsive interventions for Latinos consider their cultural values, beliefs, practices, and familial hierarchies. Additionally, cultural strengths are identified and incorporated into risk reduction interventions. An assessment of risk exposure in the Latino community requires a multilevel analytic approach that interrogates how historical, political, and social factors have both undermined the health of Latinos and have provided the cultural, social, and biological resiliency to survive adversity.

Cultural competency and cultural humility have been discussed previously in Chapter 4. Understanding one's cultural knowledge limitations is the first step in applying cultural humility with interventions targeted at historically disadvantaged populations. Cultural humility is a lifelong learning process and moves away from cultural competency as a skill that can be mastered. Fisher-Borne et al. (2015) noted that the major criticisms of cultural competency include the focus on comfort with "others" framed as self-awareness (as opposed to "self"), the use of culture as a proxy for racial/ethnic identity, the emphasis on attempting to "know" and become competent in understanding another's culture or cultures, and the lack of a transformative social justice agenda that addresses and challenges social inequalities (Table 9.13).

TABLE 9.13 Differences Between Cultural Competency and Cultural Humility

	Cultural competency	Cultural humility
Perspective on culture	• Acknowledges the layers of cultural identity. • Challenges stereotypes. • Difference is seen in the context of systemic discrimination.	• Acknowledges the layers of cultural identity. • Recognizes that working with cultural differences is a lifelong and ongoing process. • Emphasizes not only understanding the "other" but understanding ourselves as well.
Assumptions	• Assumes the problem is a lack of knowledge, awareness, and skills to work across lines of difference. • Individuals and organizations develop the values, knowledge, and skills to work across lines of difference.	• Assumes that to understand clients, we must also understand our communities, colleagues, and ourselves. • Requires humility and recognition of power imbalances that exist in client–provider relationships and in society.
Components	• Knowledge • Skills • Behaviors	• Challenging power imbalances • Institutional accountability • Ongoing critical self-reflection
Stakeholders	• Practitioner (primarily) and students	• Practitioner • Client • Community • Institution/organization

	Cultural competency	Cultural humility
Critiques	• Focuses on knowledge acquisition • Issues of social justice not inherent • Regarded as a "cookbook" approach • Leads to stereotyping the other • Suggests an endpoint	• Lack of empirical data • Lack of conceptual framework

Source: Fisher-Borne et al. (2015)

Cultural humility must be incorporated as an ethos into all aspects of a behavioral change intervention with Latinos, not only to reduce behavioral risk factors but also to engage policymakers and other important stakeholders in making changes that reduce social, economic, and environmental causes.

The development of culturally responsive interventions for Latinos should also include rigorous research design methods—qualitative and quantitative—guided by grounded theory and/or efficacious theoretical models targeting individual and collective behavioral change with Latinos.

Reimagining Latino-Centered Health Promotion Interventions

Theories that are congruent with Latinos' lived experiences are needed to provide an intersectional perspective. Multiple layers of oppression exact a high cost in terms of increased allostatic load and toxic stress that can lead to physical and psychological diseases. Intersectionality is ever present and enacted in Latino communities through classism, racism, gendered violence, discrimination, labor exploitation, sexism, and nationality (Dinwiddie et al., 2014; Weber et al., 2018; Zambrana & Dill, 2006; Zambrana et al., 2021). According to Weber and Parra-Medina (2003), "Intersectional models assume a connection between oppression and resistance, between gaining knowledge of oppressive systems and engagement in social activism to challenge them" (p. 188).

Zambrana and colleagues' advocacy for using an intersectionality lens to expose multiple synergies of oppression provides a theoretical basis for examining social and cultural influences on Latino health inequalities. For instance, Dinwiddie et al. (2014) found that cardiovascular disease risk factors among Latinos differed by education, nativity, and gender, with higher education associated with increased risk for diabetes among Mexican women and men—an "intersectional paradox."

Gloria Anzaldúa, a prominent Chicana author and activist, argues that Latinos of Mexican descent require theories that explain "our realities, our existential existences and our transcendental experiences with conflicts" (Del Castillo et al., 2012, p. 17). They then provide the following quote by Anzaldúa: "*Necesitamos teorias* [We need theories] that will rewrite history using race, class, gender, and ethnicity as categories of analysis, theories that cross borders, that blur boundaries—new kinds of theories with new theorizing methods" (Del Castillo et al., 2012, p. 18).

In other words, we need theories that have an intersectionality perspective and that are based on the lived experiences of Latinos. For example, the concept of *mestizaje* means more than just racial blending.

Rather, it is a concept that conveys renewed cultural pride in our Indigenous roots and incorporates the voices of people from the margins of society (Koegeler-Abdi, 2013). It is representational, democratic, and self-empowering. The intersection of class, race, and gender forms a new type of liberating consciousness that can effectively resist oppressive structures and institutions (Del Castillo et al., 2012).

As an orienting philosophy in developing Latino-centered health promotion interventions, acknowledging cultural strengths, and including them in interventions is critical, from outreach to the community to dissemination of findings. Health promotion interventions that include a transformative process of cultural reawakening, ethnic self-identity, and Latino community and individual empowerment hold the promise of impacting macro-level influences on health behaviors. Derived from working in the Latino community, *razalogia* is a concept of Latino community inclusiveness and empowerment:

> a community learning for creating knowledge, nurturing personal and group power and advancing human/social transformation by sharing life experiences of family, culture and community; it represented the base of knowledge of the Raza experience; knowledge of India/o-Latina/o people derived from their realities and struggles for social justice and human actualization. (Vargas & Martinez, 1984, p. vii)

Raza refers to people who have their origins in Mexico and the American Southwest. It is not a term that signifies racial purity or race per se. Thus, the razalogia concept is built on Mexican cultural values, funds of knowledge, and the perceptions of racial social discourse that has led to discrimination, racism, and the need for social justice strategies to remedy health inequalities.

Many of the health promotion models discussed do not include this perspective, and only a few studies reviewed have included cultural values or acculturation level adaptations to these interventions. Only some community-based participatory research interventions have included aspects of Latino culture and social justice (Wallerstein et al., 2008).

Perhaps applying what has been learned from Indigenous, Native American models may shed light on developing and implementing a *raza*-based intervention. According to Chino and DeBruyn (2006), "An indigenous model must reflect indigenous reality. It must integrate the past, the present, and the people's vision for the future. It must acknowledge resources and challenges and allow communities to build a commitment to identifying and resolving health concerns and issues" (p. 599).

Several decolonial paradigms have been advanced that may be appropriate for use with Latinos of Mexican descent based on their historical, geopolitical, and social experiences. For example, Walters and Simoni (2002) proposed a stress-coping paradigm that situates Native women's health within the larger context of their status as a colonized people (Figure 9.14). The model directly links trauma to health outcomes, including HIV risk, morbidity, alcohol/drug use and abuse, and PTSD and depression.

Cultural buffers are hypothesized to moderate the direct effect on these health outcomes. Therefore, a model that strengthens cultural buffers and reduces the impact of historical trauma on health outcomes is one that can be applied to Latinos of Mexican descent. Identity attitudes could be replaced by ethnic pride; spiritual coping with resiliency and religiosity; traditional health practices with Mexican folk healing practices, including the use of sweat lodges. There are many parallels but also stark historical and social differences between American Indigenous populations and Latinos of Mexican descent. Again, the historical, social, and geopolitical context must be taken into consideration in the development of a *raza*-centered approach to behavioral risk reduction.

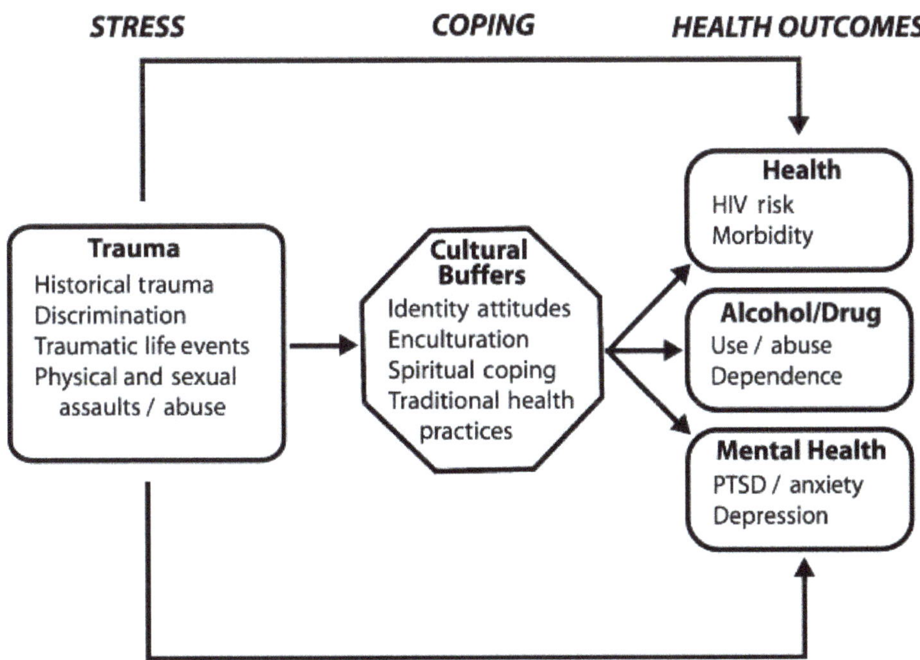

FIGURE 9.14 "Indigenist" Coping Model

Similarly, Mohatt et al. (2014) provides a model that focuses on historical trauma and present-day health outcomes among Indigenous peoples (Figure 9.15).

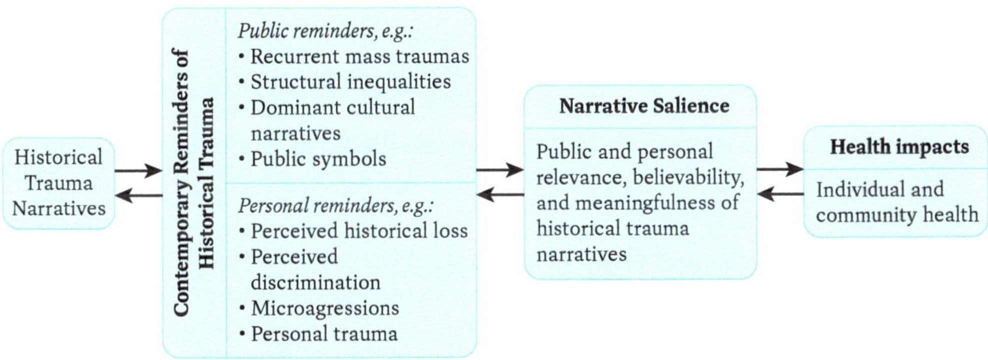

FIGURE 9.15 Historical and Intergenerational Trauma and Health Outcomes

The Mohatt et al. (2014) model examines social, cultural, and historical narratives in perpetuating historical trauma and the influence of historical trauma narratives on health. Relative to Latinos of Mexican descent, loss of two thirds of their landmass, policies instituted against speaking Spanish, and discrimination and other microaggressions could constitute a historical trauma narrative (*testimonios*), with contemporary reminders through structural inequalities, dominant cultural narratives, and anti-Latino sentiment. The impact of these narratives depends on their salience to the lived experience of Latinos.

Testimonios are Latino narratives that explicitly draw attention to social, cultural, and gender inequalities and bear witness to structural and symbolic trauma.

A health promotion model that embodies an Indigenous perspective, incorporating aspects of cultural humility and examining the role of historical trauma and intergenerational transmission of trauma, may illuminate an effective and acceptable approach for Latinos of Mexican descent. Matching important cultural elements within Indigenous paradigms to Latino paradigms may prove useful since there are many similarities: the use of community and cultural strengths, interdependence, the value of elders, social networks, and building trust with academic researchers and health officials.

Sustained individual and community behavior change and risk reduction depends in large part on policies that create healthy living environments. Focusing on macro-level organizations and systems that can provide an equitable distribution of resources requires multiple strategic initiatives that can eliminate health and social inequalities among historically marginalized populations.

Developing a Culturally Innovative Intervention for Latinos

The research literature has a substantial amount of information regarding acculturation, acculturative stress, cultural humility, and the importance of Latino cultural values in developing health promotion and risk reduction interventions. However, few prevention practitioners have ready access to this information or have the time to digest the hundreds of academic articles on the topic. Using information contained in the book, consider the following set of questions in developing a culturally responsive intervention for Latinos of Mexican descent.

At the core of cultural innovative interventions is possessing cultural humility. Acknowledging the funds of knowledge that the Latino community possesses initiates the engagement process with an overarching respect for Latino cultural strengths. Building on this foundation allows for strategic priority setting with Latino community leaders and residents. The identification of community health priorities becomes a shared process with community buy-in. A researcher who believes they know what is best for the Latino community based on their reading of the studies (e.g., diabetes mellitus) will not gain the full cooperation of the Latino community unless the community prioritizes it as such. Once the mutual identification of a health issue is accomplished, one can then begin to go through the checklist in Table 9.14. The predominant goal is to eliminate health inequalities *together*, using both sets of expertise: the community's and the public health professionals.

A community may wish to focus on decreasing obesity rates to reduce incidence and prevalence of type 2 diabetes. The short-term goal would be to identify some modifiable behaviors that would lead to a reduction in obesity with the long-term goal of achieving reduced incidence and prevalence of type 2 diabetes.

Equally important is identifying the "dynamics of difference" in the Latino community—that is, the historical, geopolitical, social, and cultural characteristics of the community and how they synergize to create health inequalities. Moreover, the identification of Latino cultural strengths is key in moving away from cultural deficit models that blame Latinos for their social and health inequalities. Using Latino culture to motivate behavior change is an important contribution to health promotion interventions. Also, acknowledging and identifying cultural values that hinder help-seeking or increase risk behaviors can prove useful in reframing negative to positive aspects of culture (e.g., *machismo*).

Theoretical behavior change models can and should be applied to Latinos with significant inclusion of Latino culture. Rethinking the use of acculturation measures is warranted given their limitations behavioral research, especially in the U.S.-Mexico border region. Cognitive referents of acculturation may prove more useful in identifying cultural influences on behavior. The following questions provide guidance in developing culturally innovative public health interventions with and for Latinos (Table 9.14).

TABLE 9.14 Guiding Questions in the Development of Latino Culturally Innovative Interventions

Questions to consider	Goal
Who are the key stakeholders in the community? How do they prioritize community health concerns? What are some formal and informal social networks in the community?	• Ensuring community support and buy-in. • Identifying community health priorities and goals. • Identifying individuals who can assist in the development of an intervention.
What are the modifiable risk behaviors you would like to reduce? What is their prevalence in the Latino population? How do they contribute to disease causation? What are some of the factors that may also contribute to these risky behaviors (social, demographic, psychological, and/or cultural)?	• Understanding the incidence and prevalence of disease in the community. • Examination of factors related to disease causation. • Understanding of social, psychological, and cultural factors involved.
What are some of the important sociocultural characteristics of the Latino population? • Poverty rates • Literacy rates • Residency/immigration status • Access to health care	• Understanding some of the important sociocultural characteristics of the population—the "dynamics of difference."
How are these characteristics related to the risk behaviors you want to reduce? For example, do they act as barriers to care? Do they contribute to risk behaviors?	• Understanding how social, economic, and cultural characteristics are associated with risky behaviors and impede access to care.
What are some Latino cultural strengths that you think could be used to facilitate risk reduction? • How can they be integrated with existing evidence-based practices? • How can they improve the feasibility and efficacy of the risk reduction program? • Are they salient to the local Latino population? • How can Latino cultural strengths be used to trigger behavior change?	• Using a cultural strengths approach to empower Latino individuals and communities. • Integrating Latino cultural strengths into risk reduction interventions.

(continued)

TABLE 9.14 (*continued*)

Questions to consider	Goal
What are some important Latino cultural or linguistic barriers that you think could interfere with risk reduction? How can they be modified or reduced? How can we work with these identified cultural barriers?	• Understanding Latino cultural values that might interfere with risk reduction interventions, like *machismo, marianismo*, and fatalism. • Reframing cultural barriers as facilitators to action.
Which theory-based behavior change models come to mind when you think about interventions to reduce these risk behaviors among Latinos? • What are some of their key components? • How could they be adapted to the Latino population? • How could you infuse these models with Latino cultural factors?	• Utilizing theory-based approaches to change risk behaviors. • Infusing Latino culture values and acknowledging funds of knowledge with interventions.
How would you develop a culturally innovative intervention based on how you answered the above questions?	• A holistic understanding of the strengths and limitations of culturally innovative approaches and their success in changing risk behaviors.

CHAPTER SUMMARY

Long-standing social inequalities have significantly contributed to health inequalities experienced by Latinos of Mexican descent. Additionally, tension and mistrust between public health agencies and the Latino community has led to fragmented health care delivery systems and a lack of preventive health care among Latinos of Mexican descent.

Latinos of Mexican descent have been portrayed as disease carriers, from typhus to COVID-19. They have been characterized as "filthy," "dirty," and having "poor personal hygiene," in part based on their supposed "inferior" culture and Indigenous roots. Latinos crossing the U.S.-Mexico border were forced to be fumigated and take kerosene baths to rid themselves of body lice so they would not pose a threat to Americans. A legacy of disempowerment, disenfranchisement, and racism has paradoxically implanted a sense of Latino cultural resilience. In the face of adversity, Latinos have utilized their cultural capital to sustain and build collective efficacy.

The multilevel social ecological approach as advocated by many scholars provides a systematic approach to disentangling the effects of macro and micro influences on Latino health inequalities. This approach highlights the need to examine both life-enhancing and life-threatening aspects characterizing the social determinants of health. Applied social justice in public health targets those social determinants that limit the equitable distribution of health care, quality education, and other aspects of the social and built environment.

Health promotion to reduce health inequalities among Latinos is guided by a multilevel framework that links personal and social values to education, activation, engagement, and empowerment. Likewise, health promotive interventions focus on person-focused strategies, psychological and behavioral strategies, environmental strategies, and sociocultural strategies to improve population health.

Several health inequality theories are relevant to health risks experienced by Latinos. The biopsychosocial racism model and the Latino epidemiologic paradox have been most often applied to investigations of Latino health inequalities. Health risks are not randomly distributed in the U.S. population but rather tend to cluster in low-income communities primarily comprised of Latinos and other ethnic groups. Research on "upstream" causes of Latino health inequalities have included maternal and child stress, fetal origins of adult disease, adverse childhood experiences, and social epigenetics associated with the intergenerational transmission of stress and increased risk for certain diseases.

Adopting evidence-based practices that reduce or eliminate Latino health inequalities depends on their relative advantage, compatibility with Latino cultural values, complexity in performing behavior change, acceptability to the Latino community, and tangible outcomes. Moreover, Latino interventions should include cultural approaches that are congruent with expected outcomes. Culturally sensitive, culturally appropriate, culturally innovative, and socioculturally congruent approaches differ with respect to cultural inclusiveness and community involvement.

Overall, two types of interventions have been used to promote Latino health: (a) theory-driven social-cognitive behavioral interventions (e.g., the health belief model, social cognitive learning theory, theory of reasoned action and planned behavior, stages of change) and (b) theory-driven community-based interventions (social ecological, community-engaged, community-based participatory research). Each has their strengths and weaknesses, processes of Latino cultural inclusion, and differential impacts. Almost all have had to be culturally adapted for Latinos to either increase explanatory power of the models or to engage the Latino community in culturally responsive interventions targeting the social determinants of health. The inclusion of the Latino community as important stakeholders and partners is critical for effective capacity building and for evaluation of an intervention's success in promoting Latino health.

Frameworks for Latino cultural inclusion argues for processes that have meaningful involvement of the Latino community in all phases of intervention development. Additionally, cultural adaptation should move beyond measures of acculturation to fully embrace Latino cultural values, or cognitive referents of acculturation, as influences on intentions and behavior. Regarding potential negative Latino cultural influences (e.g., acculturation, *machismo, marianismo*), reframing them in the positive may facilitate health promotion. Moreover, consideration of the sociocultural context and real-life experiences is important in developing Latino culturally informed risk reduction interventions.

Cultural humility, rather than cultural competency, must be embodied by the personnel working with Latinos to promote healthy behaviors and reduce risk behaviors. Conceptual frameworks integrate social, cultural, and personal characteristics to promote healthy behaviors. Sustained efforts focused on eliminating negative social determinants, however, require macro-level change.

The reimagining of Latino-centered health promotion interventions capitalizes on intersectionality theory to examine multiple layers of oppression that prevent Latinos from fully actualizing their health potential. Health promotion interventions that include a transformative process of cultural reawakening, ethnic self-identity, and Latino community and individual empowerment hold the promise of impacting macro-level influences on health behaviors. Examining decolonial theories, spiritual healing, and narratives that promote health and reduce risks may be applicable to the intergenerational trauma experienced by Latinos of Mexican descent.

QUESTIONS TO CONSIDER

1. Do health promotion interventions need to be theoretically driven? Why, or why not?
2. Does Latino culture matter in the development of health promotion interventions?
3. Describe the usefulness of acculturation measures versus cultural values (cognitive referents of acculturation) in identifying risk behaviors among Latinos.
4. Are there other, more practical ways of achieving health equity among historically marginalized and disadvantaged populations in the United States?

SUGGESTED READINGS

Allison, K. G. (2021). Planning, implementing, and evaluating culturally appropriate health programs. In M. Perez & R. Luquis (Eds.), *Cultural competence in health education and health promotion*. John Wiley & Sons.

Banyard, V., Hamby, S., & Grych, J. (2017). Health effects of adverse childhood events: Identifying promising protective factors at the intersection of mental and physical well-being. *Child Abuse & Neglect, 65*, 88–98.

Bauer, G. R. (2014). Incorporating intersectionality theory into population health research methodology: Challenges and the potential to advance health equity. *Social Science & Medicine, 110*, 10–17.

Baum, F. E., Bégin, M., Houweling, T. A., & Taylor, S. (2009). Changes not for the fainthearted: Reorienting health care systems toward health equity through action on the social determinants of health. *American Journal of Public Health, 99*(11), 1967–1974.

Bernal, G., Bonilla, J., & Bellido, C. (1995). Ecological validity and cultural sensitivity for outcome research: Issues for the cultural adaptation and development of psychosocial treatments with Hispanics. *Journal of Abnormal Child Psychology, 23*, 67–82.

Buettner-Schmidt, K., & Lobo, M. L. (2012). Social justice: A concept analysis. *Journal of Advanced Nursing, 68*(4), 948–958.

Calva, A., Matthew, R. A., & Orpinas, P. (2020). Overcoming barriers: Practical strategies to assess Latinos living in low-income communities. *Health Promotion Practice, 21*(3), 355–362.

Davis, J. L., Buchanan, K. L., & Green, B. L. (2013). Racial/ethnic differences in cancer prevention beliefs: Applying the health belief model framework. *American Journal of Health Promotion, 27*(6), 384–389.

Domenech Rodríguez, M. M., Baumann, A. A., & Schwartz, A. L. (2011). Cultural adaptation of an evidence based intervention: From theory to practice in a Latino/a community context. *American Journal of Community Psychology, 47*, 170–186.

Fernandez, M. (2018). Increasing community engagement in Latino residents to improve health outcomes. *Local Environment, 23*(9), 920–933.

Israel, B. A., Coombe, C. M., Cheezum, R. R., Schulz, A. J., McGranaghan, R. J., Lichtenstein, R., Reyes, A. G., Clement, J., & Burris, A. (2010). Community-based participatory research: A capacity-building approach for policy advocacy aimed at eliminating health disparities. *American Journal of Public Health, 100*(11), 2094–2102.

Rosenstock, I. M., Strecher, V. J., & Becker, M. H. (1988). Social learning theory and the health belief model. *Health Education Quarterly, 15*(2), 175–183.

Sanders Thompson, V. L., Ackermann, N., Bauer, K. L., Bowen, D. J., & Goodman, M. S. (2021). Strategies of community engagement in research: Definitions and classifications. *Translational Behavioral Medicine, 11*(2), 441–451.

Shi, W., Donovan, E. E., Quaack, K. R., Mackert, M., Shaffer, A. L., De Luca, D. M., Nolan-Cody, H., & Yang, J. (2023). A reasoned action approach to social connection and mental health: Racial group differences and similarities in attitudes, norms, and intentions. *Health Communication, 21*, 1–14.

Singer, M. (1991). Confronting the AIDS epidemic among IV drug users: Does ethnic culture matter? *AIDS Education and Prevention: Official Publication of the International Society for AIDS Education, 3*(3), 258–283.

Stokols, D. (1992). Establishing and maintaining healthy environments: Toward a social ecology of health promotion. *American Psychologist, 47*(1), 6–22.

Wallerstein, N. (1993). Empowerment and health: The theory and practice of community change. *Community Development Journal, 28*(3), 218–227.

Williams, J. E., Kabukuru, A., Mayo, R., & Griffin, S. F. (2011). Commentary: A social-ecological perspective on obesity among Latinos. *Ethnicity and Disease, 21*(4), 467.

Zambrana, R. E., Parra-Medina, D., & Butler, C. (2021). Social determinants of health: Intersectional impacts of race, class, ethnicity and place. In S. C. Scrimshaw, S. D. Lane, et al. (Eds.), *The SAGE handbook of social studies in health and medicine*. SAGE.

REFERENCES

Ahmed, S., Chase, L. E., Wagnild, J., Akhter, N., Sturridge, S., Clarke, A., Chowdhary, P., Mukami, P., Kasim, A., & Hampshire, K. (2022). Community health workers and health equity in low-and middle-income countries: Systematic review and recommendations for policy and practice. *International Journal for Equity in Health, 21*(1), Article 49.

Ajzen, I., & Fishbein, M. (1975). A Bayesian analysis of attribution processes. *Psychological Bulletin, 82*(2), 261.

Ajzen, I., & Fishbein, M. (1988). *Theory of reasoned action: Theory of planned behavior.* University of South Florida.

Alegría, M., Álvarez, K., & DiMarzio, K. (2017). Immigration and mental health. *Current Epidemiology Reports, 4*, 145–155.

Alegría, M., Mulvaney-Day, N., Torres, M., Polo, A., Cao, Z., & Canino, G. (2007a). Prevalence of psychiatric disorders across Latino subgroups in the United States. *American Journal of Public Health, 97*(1), 68–75.

Alegria, M., Sribney, W., Woo, M., Torres, M., & Guarnaccia, P. (2007b). Looking beyond nativity: The relation of age of immigration, length of residence, and birth cohorts to the risk of onset of psychiatric disorders for Latinos. *Research in Human Development, 4*(1–2), 19–47.

Alicea-Alvarez, N., Reeves, K., Lucas, M. S., Huang, D., Ortiz, M., Burroughs, T., & Jones, N. (2016). Impacting health disparities in urban communities: Preparing future healthcare providers for "neighborhood-engaged care" through a community engagement course intervention. *Journal of Urban Health, 93*, 732–743.

Allison, K. G. (2021). Planning, implementing, and evaluating culturally appropriate health programs. In M. Perez & R. Luquis (Eds.), *Cultural competence in health education and health promotion.* John Wiley & Sons.

Amado, M. L. (2012). The "new mestiza," the old mestizos: Contrasting discourses on mestizaje. *Sociological Inquiry, 82*(3), 446–459.

Anastasia, E. A., & Bridges, A. J. (2015). Understanding service utilization disparities and depression in Latinos: The role of fatalismo. *Journal of Immigrant and Minority Health, 17*, 1758–1764.

Anda, R. F., Felitti, V. J., Bremner, J. D., Walker, J. D., Whitfield, C. H., Perry, B. D., Dube, S. R., & Giles, W. H. (2006). The enduring effects of abuse and related adverse experiences in childhood: A convergence of evidence from neurobiology and epidemiology. *European Archives of Psychiatry and Clinical Neuroscience, 256*, 174–186.

Artiga, S., & Hinton, E. (2018, May 10). *Beyond health care: The role of social determinants in promoting health equity.* Kaiser Family Foundation. https://www.kff.org/racial-equity-and-health-policy/issue-brief/beyond-health-care-the-role-of-social-determinants-in-promoting-health-and-health-equity/

Asmussen, K., McBride, T., & Waddell, S. (2019). The potential of early intervention for preventing and reducing ACE-related trauma. *Social Policy and Society, 18*(3), 425–434.

Attree, P., French, B., Milton, B., Povall, S., Whitehead, M., & Popay, J. (2011). The experience of community engagement for individuals: A rapid review of evidence. *Health & Social Care in the Community, 19*(3), 250–260.

Austin, R. R., McLane, T. M., Pieczkiewicz, D. S., Adam, T., & Monsen, K. A. (2023). Advantages and disadvantages of using theory-based versus data-driven models with social and behavioral determinants of health data. *Journal of the American Medical Informatics Association, 30*(11), 1818–1825.

Balcazar, H., Alvarado, M., Hollen, M. L., Gonzalez-Cruz, Y., Hughes, O., Vazquez, E., & Lykens, K. (2006). Salud Para Su Corazon-NCLR: A comprehensive promotora outreach program to promote heart-healthy behaviors among Hispanics. *Health Promotion Practice, 7*(1), 68–77.

Balcázar, H., Alvarado, M., Luna Hollen, M., Gonzalez-Cruz, Y., & Pedregon, V. (2005). Evaluation of Salud para Su Corazón (Health for Your Heart)—NCLR national dissemination promotora outreach projects. *Preventing Chronic Disease, 2*(3), 1–9.

Bandura, A. (1985). Model of causality in social learning theory. In M. J. Mahoney & A. Freeman (Eds.), *Cognition and psychotherapy* (pp. 81–99). Springer.

Bandura, A. (1991). Social cognitive theory of self-regulation. *Organizational Behavior and Human Decision Processes, 50*(2), 248–287.

Bandura, A., & Walters, R. H. (1977). *Social learning theory* (Vol. 1). Englewood cliffs.

Banyard, V., Hamby, S., & Grych, J. (2017). Health effects of adverse childhood events: Identifying promising protective factors at the intersection of mental and physical well-being. *Child Abuse & Neglect, 65*, 88–98.

Bauer, G. R. (2014). Incorporating intersectionality theory into population health research methodology: Challenges and the potential to advance health equity. *Social Science & Medicine, 110*, 10–17.

Baum, F. E., Bégin, M., Houweling, T. A., & Taylor, S. (2009). Changes not for the fainthearted: Reorienting health care systems toward health equity through action on the social determinants of health. *American Journal of Public Health, 99*(11), 1967–1974.

Beauchamp, D. E. (1976). Public health as social justice. *Inquiry, 13*(1), 3–14.

Becker, M. H. (1974). The health belief model and sick role behavior. *Health Education Monographs, 2*(4), 409–419.

Becker, M. H., & Maiman, L. A. (1975). Sociobehavioral determinants of compliance with health and medical care recommendations. *Medical Care, 13*, 10–24.

Benson-Flórez, G., Santiago-Rivera, A., & Nagy, G. (2017). Culturally adapted behavioral activation: A treatment approach for a Latino family. *Clinical Case Studies, 16*(1), 9–24.

Berkman, L. F., Kawachi, I., & Glymour, M. M. (2014). *Social epidemiology* (2nd ed.). Oxford University Press.

Bernal, G., Bonilla, J., & Bellido, C. (1995). Ecological validity and cultural sensitivity for outcome research: Issues for the cultural adaptation and development of psychosocial treatments with Hispanics. *Journal of Abnormal Child Psychology, 23*, 67–82.

Bernal, G., & Domenech Rodríguez, M. M. (2009). Advances in Latino family research: Cultural adaptations of evidence-based interventions. *Family Process, 48*(2), 169–178.

Birken, S. A., Powell, B. J., Shea, C. M., Haines, E. R., Alexis Kirk, M., Leeman, J., Rohweder, C., Damschroder, L., & Presseau, J. (2017). Criteria for selecting implementation science theories and frameworks: Results from an international survey. *Implementation Science, 12*(1), 1–9.

Blanco-Vega, C. O., Castro-Olivo, S. M., & Merrell, K. W. (2007). Social-emotional needs of Latino immigrant adolescents: A sociocultural model for development and implementation of culturally specific interventions. *Journal of Latinos and Education, 7*(1), 43–61.

Boyas, J. F., Woodiwiss, J. L., & Nahar, V. K. (2021). Examining intentions to engage in sun protective behaviors among Latino day laborers: An application of the theory of planned behavior. *Health Promotion Perspectives, 11*(3), 351.

Bronfenbrenner, U. (1977). Toward an experimental ecology of human development. *American Psychologist, 32*(7), 513.

Brown, D. W., Anda, R. F., Tiemeier, H., Felitti, V. J., Edwards, V. J., Croft, J. B., & Giles, W. H. (2009). Adverse childhood experiences and the risk of premature mortality. *American Journal of Preventive Medicine, 37*(5), 389–396.

Buettner-Schmidt, K., & Lobo, M. L. (2012). Social justice: A concept analysis. *Journal of Advanced Nursing, 68*(4), 948–958.

Cacari Stone, L., Sanchez, V., Bruna, S. P., Muhammad, M., & Zamora, C. (2022). Social ecology of hypertension management among Latinos living in the U.S.-Mexico border region. *Health Promotion Practice, 23*(4), 650–661.

Calva, A., Matthew, R. A., & Orpinas, P. (2020). Overcoming barriers: Practical strategies to assess Latinos living in low-income communities. *Health Promotion Practice, 21*(3), 355–362.

Castañeda, S. F., Buelna, C., Giacinto, R. E., Gallo, L. C., Sotres-Alvarez, D., Gonzalez, P., Fortmann, A. L., Wassertheil-Smoller, S., Gellman, M. D., Giachello, A. L., & Talavera, G. A. (2016). Cardiovascular disease risk factors and psychological distress among Hispanics/Latinos: The Hispanic Community Health Study/Study of Latinos (HCHS/SOL). *Preventive Medicine, 87*, 144–150.

Castro, F. G., & Alarcon, E. H. (2002). Integrating cultural variables into drug abuse prevention and treatment with racial/ethnic minorities. *Journal of Drug Issues, 32*(3), 783–810.

Castro, F. G., Garfinkle, J., Naranjo, D., Rollins, M., Brook, J. S., & Brook, D. W. (2007). Cultural traditions as "protective factors" among Latino children of illicit drug users. *Substance Use & Misuse, 42*(4), 621–642.

Centers for Disease Control and Prevention. (n.d.). Adverse childhood experiences (ACEs). Retrieved October 1, 2023, from https://www.cdc.gov/violenceprevention/aces/index.html

Centers for Disease Control and Prevention. (2014). *Practical strategies for culturally competent evaluation*. U.S. Dept of Health and Human Services. https://www.cdc.gov/asthma/program_eval/cultural_competence_guide.pdf

Centers for Disease Control and Prevention. (2022). *Suicide Prevention Resource for Action: A compilation of the best available evidence*. National Center for Injury Preventions and Control. https://www.cdc.gov/suicide/pdf/preventionresource.pdf

Chang, M. K. (1998). Predicting unethical behavior: A comparison of the theory of reasoned action and the theory of planned behavior. *Journal of Business Ethics, 17*, 1825–1834.

Chen, J. Y., Fox, S. A., Cantrell, C. H., Stockdale, S. E., & Kagawa-Singer, M. (2007). Health disparities and prevention: Racial/ ethnic barriers to flu vaccinations. *Journal of Community Health, 32*, 5–20.

Chino, M., & DeBruyn, L. (2006). Building true capacity: Indigenous models for Indigenous communities. *American Journal of Public Health, 96*(4), 596–599.

Comfort, M., Raymond-Flesch, M., Auerswald, C., McGlone, L., Chavez, M., & Minnis, A. (2018). Community-engaged research with rural Latino adolescents: Design and implementation strategies to study the social determinants of health. *Gateways: International Journal of Community Research & Engagement, 11*(1), 90.

Constantine, M. G., Myers, L. J., Kindaichi, M., & Moore, J. L., III. (2004). Exploring Indigenous mental health practices: The roles of healers and helpers in promoting well-being in people of color. *Counseling and Values, 48*(2), 110–125.

Contento, I. R., Koch, P. A., Lee, H., & Calabrese-Barton, A. (2010). Adolescents demonstrate improvement in obesity risk behaviors after completion of choice, control & change, a curriculum addressing personal agency and autonomous motivation. *Journal of the American Dietetic Association, 110*(12), 1830–1839.

Cortés, D. E., Millán-Ferro, A., Schneider, K., Vega, R. R., & Caballero, A. E. (2013). Food purchasing selection among low-income, Spanish-speaking Latinos. *American Journal of Preventive Medicine, 44*(3), S267–S273.

Cuellar, I., Arnold, B., & Gonzalez, G. (1995a). Cognitive referents of acculturation: Assessment of cultural constructs in Mexican Americans. *Journal of Community Psychology, 23*(4), 339–356.

Cuellar, I., Arnold, B., & Maldonado, R. (1995b). Acculturation Rating Scale for Mexican Americans-II: A revision of the original ARSMA scale. *Hispanic Journal of Behavioral Science, 17*, 275–304.

Cyril, S., Smith, B. J., Possamai-Inesedy, A., & Renzaho, A. M. (2015). Exploring the role of community engagement in improving the health of disadvantaged populations: A systematic review. *Global Health Action, 8*(1), 29842.

Davis, J. L., Buchanan, K. L., & Green, B. L. (2013). Racial/ethnic differences in cancer prevention beliefs: Applying the health belief model framework. *American Journal of Health Promotion, 27*(6), 384–389.

Del Castillo, R., Wycoff, A., & Cantu, S. (2012). Curanderismo as decolonization therapy: The acceptance of mestizaje as a remedio. *NACCS Annual Conference Proceedings*. https://scholarworks.sjsu.edu/naccs/2012/Proceedings/7

Delgado, A. (2022). From bath riots to blocking asylum. Public Health and Race at the us-mexico border. *Perspectives on History, Summer 2022*. Available from https://www.historians.org/research-and-publications/perspectives-on-history/summer-2022/from-bath-riots-to-blocking-asylum-public-health-and-race-at-the-us-mexico-border

De Silva, M. J., Breuer, E., Lee, L., Asher, L., Chowdhary, N., Lund, C., & Patel, V. (2014). Theory of change: a theory-driven approach to enhance the Medical Research Council's framework for complex interventions. *Trials, 15*, 1–13.

Diaz, H., Marshak, H. H., Montgomery, S., Rea, B., & Backman, D. (2009). Acculturation and gender: Influence on healthy dietary outcomes for Latino adolescents in California. *Journal of Nutrition Education and Behavior, 41*(5), 319–326.

Dinwiddie, G. Y., Zambrana, R. E., & Garza, M. A. (2014). Exploring risk factors in Latino cardiovascular disease: The role of education, nativity, and gender. *American Journal of Public Health, 104*(9), 1742–1750

Domenech Rodríguez, M. M., Baumann, A. A., & Schwartz, A. L. (2011). Cultural adaptation of an evidence based intervention: From theory to practice in a Latino/a community context. *American Journal of Community Psychology, 47*, 170–186.

Eakin, B. L., Villarruel, A. M., Jemmott III, J. B., & Jemmott, L. S. (2005). Physical activity in Latino adolescents: Understanding influences on activity intentions. *Hispanic Health Care International, 3*(3), 125.

Eccles, M., & Mittman, B. (2012). Welcome to implementation science. 2006. *Implementation Science, 1*(1).

Fernandez, M. (2018). Increasing community engagement in Latino residents to improve health outcomes. *Local Environment, 23*(9), 920–933.

Fernandez, M., Wippold, R., Williams, J., Longoria, J., Byrd, T., Coughlin, S., & Vernon, S. (2007). Development of a tailored interactive colorectal cancer screening intervention for Latinos. *Cancer Epidemiology Biomarkers & Prevention, 16*(Suppl. 11), B33–B33.

Fisher-Borne, M., Cain, J. M., & Martin, S. L. (2015). From mastery to accountability: Cultural humility as an alternative to cultural competence. *Social Work Education, 34*(2), 165–181.

Gallardo, M. E., & Curry, S. J. (2009). Shifting perspectives: Culturally responsive interventions with Latino substance abusers. *Journal of Ethnicity in Substance Abuse, 8*(3), 314–329.

Gallois, C., McCamish, M., & Terry, D. J. (2015). *The theory of reasoned action: Its application to AIDS-preventive behaviour.* Garland Science.

García, A. A., West Ohueri, C., Garay, R., Guzman, M., Hanson, K., Vasquez, M., Zuñiga, J., & Tierney, W. (2021). Community engagement as a foundation for improving neighborhood health. *Public Health Nursing, 38*(2), 223–231.

Garcia, E., Wijesekera, K., & Lester, P. (2017). A family-centered preventive intervention within pediatric oncology: Adapting the FOCUS intervention for Latino youth and their families. *Journal of Educational and Psychological Consultation, 27*(3), 393–410.

Garner, A. S. (2013). Home visiting and the biology of toxic stress: Opportunities to address early childhood adversity. *Pediatrics, 132*(Suppl. 2), S65–S73.

Germán, M., Gonzales, N. A., & Dumka, L. (2009). Familism values as a protective factor for Mexican-origin adolescents exposed to deviant peers. *The Journal of Early Adolescence, 29*(1), 16–42.

Gil, A. G., Wagner, E. F., & Vega, W. A. (2000). Acculturation, familism, and alcohol use among Latino adolescent males: Longitudinal relations. *Journal of Community Psychology, 28*(4), 443–458.

Gilbert, L. K., Breiding, M. J., Merrick, M. T., Thompson, W. W., Ford, D. C., Dhingra, S. S., & Parks, S. E. (2015). Childhood adversity and adult chronic disease: An update from ten states and the District of Columbia, 2010. *American Journal of Preventive Medicine, 48*(3), 345–349.

Gillmore, M. R., Archibald, M. E., Morrison, D. M., Wilsdon, A., Wells, E. A., Hoppe, M. J., Nahom, D., & Murowchick, E. (2002). Teen sexual behavior: Applicability of the theory of reasoned action. *Journal of Marriage and Family, 64*(4), 885–897.

González, N., Moll, L. C., & Amanti, C. (Eds.). (2006). *Funds of knowledge: Theorizing practices in households, communities, and classrooms*. Routledge.

Goodman, M. S., & Sanders Thompson, V. L. (2017). The science of stakeholder engagement in research: Classification, implementation, and evaluation. *Translational Behavioral Medicine, 7*(3), 486–491.

Guinn, B., Vincent, V., Jorgensen, L., Dugas, D., & Semper, T. (2007). Predicting physical activity among low-income Mexican American women: Application of the theory of planned behavior. *American Journal of Health Behavior, 31*(2), 115–122.

Harvey, V. M., Oldfield, C. W., Chen, J. T., & Eschbach, K. (2016). Melanoma disparities among U.S. Hispanics: Use of the social ecological model to contextualize reasons for inequitable outcomes and frame a research agenda. *Journal of Skin Cancer*, Article 4635740.

Hernandez, R., Cheung, E., Carnethon, M., Penedo, F. J., Moskowitz, J. T., Martinez, L., & Schueller, S. M. (2018). Feasibility of a culturally adapted positive psychological intervention for Hispanics/Latinos with elevated risk for cardiovascular disease. *Translational Behavioral Medicine, 8*(6), 887–897.

Hu, J., Amirehsani, K. A., Wallace, D. C., McCoy, T. P., & Silva, Z. (2016). A family-based, culturally tailored diabetes intervention for Hispanics and their family members. *The Diabetes Educator, 42*(3), 299–314.

Hull, P. C., Canedo, J. R., Reece, M. C., Lira, I., Reyes, F., Garcia, E., Juarez, P.,Williams, E., & Husaini, B. A. (2010). Using a participatory research process to address disproportionate Hispanic cancer burden. *Journal of Health Care for the Poor and Underserved, 21*(10).

Israel, B. A., Coombe, C. M., Cheezum, R. R., Schulz, A. J., McGranaghan, R. J., Lichtenstein, R., Reyes, A. G., Clement, J., & Burris, A. (2010). Community-based participatory research: A capacity-building approach for policy advocacy aimed at eliminating health disparities. *American Journal of Public Health, 100*(11), 2094–2102.

Jani, J. S., Ortiz, L., & Aranda, M. P. (2009). Latino outcome studies in social work: A review of the literature. *Research on Social Work Practice, 19*(2), 179–194.

Janz, N. K., & Becker, M. H. (1984). The health belief model: A decade later. *Health Education Quarterly, 11*(1), 1–47.

Jimenez, D. E., Weinstein, E. R., & Batsis, J. (2023). You gotta walk the walk to talk the talk: Protocol for a feasibility study of the Happy Older Latino Adults (HOLA) health promotion intervention for older HIV-positive Latino men. *Pilot and Feasibility Studies, 9*(1), 1–12.

Kam, J. A., Matsunaga, M., Hecht, M. L., & Ndiaye, K. (2009). Extending the theory of planned behavior to predict alcohol, tobacco, and marijuana use among youth of Mexican heritage. *Prevention Science, 10*(1), 41–53.

Keller, C. S., & McGowan, N. (2001). Examination of the processes of change, decisional balance, self-efficacy for smoking and the stages of change in Mexican American women. *Southern Online Journal of Nursing Research, 4*(2).

Kenya, S., Lebron, C. N., Chang, A. Y. H., Li, H., Alonzo, Y. A., & Carrasquillo, O. (2015). A profile of Latinos with poorly controlled diabetes in South Florida. *Journal of Community Hospital Internal Medicine Perspectives, 5*(2), Article 26586.

Kia-Keating, M., Santacrose, D. E., Liu, S. R., & Adams, J. (2017). Using community-based participatory research and human-centered design to address violence-related health disparities among Latino/a youth. *Family & Community Health, 40*(2), 160–169.

Kim, S., Flaskerud, J. H., Koniak-Griffin, D., & Dixon, E. L. (2005). Using community-partnered participatory research to address health disparities in a Latino community. *Journal of Professional Nursing, 21*(4), 199–209.

Kiraly, C., Turk, M. T., Kalarchian, M. A., & Shaffer, C. (2017). Applying ecological frameworks in obesity intervention studies in Hispanic/Latino youth: A systematic review. *Hispanic Health Care International, 15*(3), 130–142.

Koegeler-Abdi, M. (2013). Shifting subjectivities: Mestizas, nepantleras, and Gloria Anzaldúa's legacy. *Multi-Ethnic Literature of the United States, 38*(2), 71–88.

Kuo, A. A., Sharif, M. Z., Prelip, M. L., Glik, D. C., Albert, S. L., Belin, T., McCarthy, W. J., Roberts, C. K., Garcia, R. E., & Ortega, A. N. (2017). Training the next generation of Latino health researchers: A multilevel, transdisciplinary, community-engaged approach. *Health Promotion Practice, 18*(4), 497–504.

LaMorte, W. W. (2022). *The social cognitive theory.* Boston University School of Public Health. https://sphweb.bumc.bu.edu/otlt/MPH-Modules/SB/BehavioralChangeTheories/BehavioralChangeTheories5.html.

Lasker, R. D., & Weiss, E. S. (2003). Broadening participation in community problem solving: A multidisciplinary model to support collaborative practice and research. *Journal of Urban Health, 80*, 14–47.

LaVeist, T. A. (2011). *Minority populations and health: An introduction to health disparities in the United States.* Jossey-Bass.

Leng, J., Lui, F., Narang, B., Puebla, L., González, J., Lynch, K., & Gany, F. (2022). Developing a culturally responsive lifestyle intervention for overweight/obese U.S. Mexicans. *Journal of Community Health, 47*(1), 28–38.

Leyva, D., Weiland, C., Shapiro, A., Yeomans-Maldonado, G., & Febles, A. (2022). A strengths-based, culturally responsive family intervention improves Latino kindergarteners' vocabulary and approaches to learning. *Child Development, 93*(2), 451–467.

Loi, C. X. A., Alfonso, M. L., Chan, I., Anderson, K., Tyson, D. D. M., Gonzales, J., & Corvin, J. (2017). Application of mixed-methods design in community-engaged research: Lessons learned from an evidence-based intervention for Latinos with chronic illness and minor depression. *Evaluation and Program Planning, 63*, 29–38.

Lopez-Class, M., Castro, F. G., & Ramirez, A. G. (2011). Conceptions of acculturation: A review and statement of critical issues. *Social Science & Medicine, 72*(9), 1555–1562.

Luszcynska, A., & Schwarzer, R. (2015). Social cognitive theory. In M. Conner & P. Norman (Eds.), *Predicting health behaviour* (3rd ed., pp. 127–169). Oxford Universtiy Press.

Madden, T. J., Ellen, P. S., & Ajzen, I. (1992). A comparison of the theory of planned behavior and the theory of reasoned action. *Personality and Social Psychology Bulletin, 18*(1), 3–9.

Marmot, M. (2007). Achieving health equity: From root causes to fair outcomes. *The Lancet, 370*(9593), 1153–1163.

Martin, J. J., Oliver, K., & McCaughtry, N. (2007). The theory of planned behavior: Predicting physical activity in Mexican American children. *Journal of Sport and Exercise Psychology, 29*(2), 225–238.

McQuiston, C., Parrado, E. A., Martínez, A. P., & Uribe, L. (2005). Community-based participatory research with Latino community members: Horizonte Latino. *Journal of Professional Nursing, 21*(4), 210–215.

Medina, A., Balcázar, H., Hollen, M. L., Nkhoma, E., & Mas, F. S. (2007). Promotores de salud: Educating Hispanic communities on heart-healthy living. *American Journal of Health Education, 38*(4), 194–202.

Meister, J. S., Warrick, L. H., De Zapien, J. G., & Wood, A. H. (1992). Using lay health workers: Case study of a community-based prenatal intervention. *Journal of Community Health, 17*(1), 37–51.

Menselson, T., Rehkopf, D. H., & Kubzansky, L. D. (2008). Depression among Latinos in the United States: A meta-analytic review. *Journal of Consulting and Clinical Psychology, 76*(3), 355.

Minkler, M., & Wallerstein, N. (Eds.). (2011). *Community-based participatory research for health: From process to outcomes.* John Wiley & Sons.

Mohatt, N. V., Thompson, A. B., Thai, N. D., & Tebes, J. K. (2014). Historical trauma as public narrative: A conceptual review of how history impacts present-day health. *Social Science & Medicine, 106*, 128–136.

Molina, K. M., Little, T. V., & Rosal, M. C. (2016). Everyday discrimination, family context, and psychological distress among Latino adults in the United States. *Journal of Community Psychology, 44*(2), 145–165.

Molina, N. (2006). *Fit to be citizens? Public health and race in Los Angeles, 1879–1939.* University of California Press.

Moll, L., Amanti, C., Neff, D., & Gonzalez, N. (2006). Funds of knowledge for teaching: Using a qualitative approach to connect homes and classrooms. In N. Gonzales, L. C. Moll, & C. Amanti (Eds.), *Funds of knowledge* (pp. 71–87). Routledge.

Montano, D. E., & Kasprzyk, D. (2015). Theory of reasoned action, theory of planned behavior, and the integrated behavioral model. *Health Behavior: Theory, Research and Practice, 70*(4), 231.

Moore de Peralta, A., Holaday, B., & McDonell, J. R. (2015). Factors affecting Hispanic women's participation in screening for cervical cancer. *Journal of Immigrant and Minority Health, 17*, 684–695.

Moore-Monroy, M., Wilkinson-Lee, A. M., Verdugo, L., Lopez, E., Paez, L., Rodriguez, D., Wilhelm, M., & Garcia, F. (2013). Addressing the information gap: Developing and implementing a cervical cancer prevention education campaign grounded in principles of community-based participatory action. *Health Promotion Practice, 14*(2), 274–283.

Nelson, A., Ayers, E., Sun, F., & Zhang, A. (2020). Culturally adapted psychotherapeutic interventions for Latino depression and anxiety: A meta-analysis. *Research on Social Work Practice, 30*(4), 368–381.

Nisson, C., & Earl, A. (2020). The theories of reasoned action and planned behavior. In *The Wiley encyclopedia of health psychology* (pp. 755–761). Wiley.

O'Mara-Eves, A., Brunton, G., Oliver, S., Kavanagh, J., Jamal, F., & Thomas, J. (2015). The effectiveness of community engagement in public health interventions for disadvantaged groups: A meta-analysis. *BMC Public Health, 15*, 1–23.

Pennucci, F., De Rosis, S., Murante, A. M., & Nuti, S. (2022). Behavioural and social sciences to enhance the efficacy of health promotion interventions: Redesigning the role of professionals and people. *Behavioural Public Policy, 6*(1), 13–33.

Pérez, D. J., Fortuna, L., & Alegria, M. (2008). Prevalence and correlates of everyday discrimination among U.S. Latinos. *Journal of Community Psychology, 36*(4), 421–433.

Popay, J., Attree, P., Hornby, D., Milton, B., Whitehead, M., French, B., Kowarzik, U., Simpson, N., & Povall, S. (2007). *Community engagement in initiatives addressing the wider social determinants of health: A rapid review of evidence on impact, experience and process.* University of Lancaster.

Prochaska, J. O. (2008). Decision making in the transtheoretical model of behavior change. *Medical Decision Making, 28*(6), 845–849.

Prochaska, J. O., & DiClemente, C. C. (1982). Transtheoretical therapy: Toward a more integrative model of change. *Psychotherapy: Theory, Research & Practice, 19*(3), 276.

Prochaska, J. O., & DiClemente, C. C. (1983). Stages and processes of self-change of smoking: Toward an integrative model of change. *Journal of Consulting and Clinical Psychology, 51*(3), 390.

Qunitero, G. A., & Estrada, A. L. (1998a). Cultural models of masculinity and drug use: Machismo, heroin, and street survival on the U.S.–Mexico border. *Contemporary Drug Problems, 25*, 147–168.

Quintero, G. A., & Estrada, A. L. (1998b). Machismo, drugs and street survival in a U.S.–Mexico border community. *Free Inquiry in Creative Sociology, 26*, 3–10.

Rhodes, S. D., Duck, S., Alonzo, J., Daniel-Ulloa, J., & Aronson, R. E. (2013). Using community-based participatory research to prevent HIV disparities: Assumptions and opportunities identified by the Latino partnership. *Journal of Acquired Immune Deficiency Syndromes, 63*(0 1), S32–S35.

Rodríguez-Reimann, D. I., Nicassio, P., Reimann, J. O., Gallegos, P. I., & Olmedo, E. L. (2004). Acculturation and health beliefs of Mexican Americans regarding tuberculosis prevention. *Journal of Immigrant Health, 6*, 51–62.

Rogers, E. (1983). *Diffusion of innovations.* Free Press.

Rogers, E. M., Singhal, A., & Quinlan, M. M. (2014). Diffusion of innovations. In D. W. Stacks, M. B. Salwen, & K. C. Eichhorn (Eds.), *An integrated approach to communication theory and research* (pp. 432–448). Routledge.

Romero, A. J., & Ruiz, M. (2007). Does familism lead to increased parental monitoring?: Protective factors for coping with risky behaviors. *Journal of Child and Family Studies, 16*, 143–154.

Romo, D. D. (2014). *Ringside seat to a revolution: An underground cultural history of El Paso and Juarez, 1893–1923.* Cinco Puntos Press.

Rosas, L. G., Lv, N., Xiao, L., Lewis, M. A., Venditti, E. M., Zavella, P., Azar, K., & Ma, J. (2020). Effect of a culturally adapted behavioral intervention for Latino adults on weight loss over 2 years: A randomized clinical trial. *JAMA Network Open, 3*(12), e2027744–e2027744.

Rose, G. (2001). Reiteration. Sick individuals and sick populations. *International Journal of Epidemiology, 30*(3), 427–432.

Rosenstock, I. M., Strecher, V. J., & Becker, M. H. (1988). Social learning theory and the health belief model. *Health Education Quarterly, 15*(2), 175–183.

Rudmin, F., Wang, B., & de Castro, J. (2017). Acculturation research critiques and alternative research designs. In. S. J. Schwartz & J. B. Unger (Eds.), *The Oxford handbook of acculturation and health* (pp.75–96). Oxford Universtiy Press.

Ruger, J. P. (2004). Health and social justice. *The Lancet, 364*(9439), 1075–1080.

Ruggiero, L., Oros, S., & Choi, Y. K. (2011). Community-based translation of the diabetes prevention program's lifestyle intervention in an underserved Latino population. *The Diabetes Educator, 37*(4), 564–572.

Sabogal, F., Marín, G., Otero-Sabogal, R., Marín, B. V., & Perez-Stable, E. J. (1987). Hispanic familism and acculturation: What changes and what doesn't? *Hispanic Journal of Behavioral Sciences, 9*(4), 397–412.

Sanders Thompson, V. L., Ackermann, N., Bauer, K. L., Bowen, D. J., & Goodman, M. S. (2021). Strategies of community engagement in research: Definitions and classifications. *Translational Behavioral Medicine, 11*(2), 441–451.

Santisteban, D. A., Coatsworth, J. D., Briones, E., Kurtines, W., & Szapocznik, J. (2012). Beyond acculturation: An investigation of the relationship of familism and parenting to behavior problems in Hispanic youth. *Family Process, 51*(4), 470–482.

Scarinci, I. C., Bandura, L., Hidalgo, B., & Cherrington, A. (2012). Development of a theory-based (PEN-3 and health belief model), culturally relevant intervention on cervical cancer prevention among Latina immigrants using intervention mapping. *Health Promotion Practice, 13*(1), 29–40.

Shalowitz, M. U., Isacco, A., Barquin, N., Clark-Kauffman, E., Delger, P., Nelson, D., Quinn, A., & Wagenaar, K. A. (2009). Community-based participatory research: A review of the literature with strategies for community engagement. *Journal of Developmental & Behavioral Pediatrics, 30*(4), 350–361.

Shattell, M. M., Hamilton, D., Starr, S. S., Jenkins, C. J., & Hinderliter, N. A. (2008). Mental health service needs of a Latino population: A community-based participatory research project. *Issues in Mental Health Nursing, 29*(4), 351-370.

Shi, W., Donovan, E. E., Quaack, K. R., Mackert, M., Shaffer, A. L., De Luca, D. M., Nolan-Cody, H., & Yang, J. (2023). A reasoned action approach to social connection and mental health: Racial group differences and similarities in attitudes, norms, and intentions. *Health Communication, 21*, 1-14.

Singer, M. (1991). Confronting the AIDS epidemic among IV drug users: Does ethnic culture matter? *AIDS Education and Prevention, 3*(3), 258–283.

Smith, C., & Ryan, A. (2006). Change for Life/Cambia tu vida: A health promotion program based on the stages of change model for African descendent and Latino adults in New Hampshire. *Preventing Chronic Disease, 3*(3).

Soderlund, P. D. (2017). The social ecological model and physical activity interventions for Hispanic women with type 2 diabetes: A review. *Journal of Transcultural Nursing, 28*(3), 306–314.

Stein, G. L., & Guzman, L. E. (2015). Prevention and intervention research with Latino families: A translational approach. *Family Process, 54*(2), 280–292.

Stern, A. M. (1999). Buildings, boundaries, and blood: Medicalization and nation-building on the U.S.-Mexico border, 1910–1939. *Hispanic American Historical Review, 71*(1), 41–81. https://doi.org/10.1215/00182168-79.1.41

Stevens, S. J., & Estrada, A. L. (1996). Reducing HIV risk behaviors: Perceptions of HIV risk and stage of change. *Journal of Drug Issues, 26*(3), 607–618.

Stokols, D. (1992). Establishing and maintaining healthy environments: Toward a social ecology of health promotion. *American Psychologist, 47*(1), 6–22.

Stokols, D., Lejano, R. P., & Hipp, J. (2013). Enhancing the resilience of human-environment systems: A social ecological perspective. *Ecology and Society, 18*(1).

Surís, A. M., del Carmen Trapp, M., Diclemente, C. C., & Cousins, J. (1998). Application of the transtheoretical model of behavior change for obesity in Mexican American women. *Addictive Behaviors, 23*(5), 655–668.

Tung, W. C., Smith-Gagen, J., Lu, M., & Warfield, M. (2016). Application of the transtheoretical model to Cervical cancer screening in Latina women. *Journal of Immigrant and Minority Health, 18*, 1168–1174.

Turin, T. C., Chowdhury, N., Haque, S., Rumana, N., Rahman, N., & Lasker, M. A. A. (2021). Meaningful and deep community engagement efforts for pragmatic research and beyond: Engaging with an immigrant/racialised community on equitable access to care. *BMJ Global Health, 6*, Article e006370.

Van Servellen, G., & Lombardi, E. (2005). Supportive relationships and medication adherence in HIV-infected, low-income Latinos. *Western Journal of Nursing Research, 27*(8), 1023–1039.

Vargas, R., & Martinez, S. C. (1984). *Razalogia: Community learning for a new society.* Razagente Associates.

Velicer, W. F., Prochaska, J. O., Fava, J. L., Norman, G. J., & Redding, C. A. (1998). Detailed overview of the transtheoretical model. *Homeostasis, 38*, 216–233.

Villarruel, A. M., Jemmott, J. B., III, Jemmott, L. S., & Ronis, D. L. (2004). Predictors of sexual intercourse and condom use intentions among Spanish-dominant Latino youth: A test of the planned behavior theory. *Nursing Research, 53*(3), 172–181.

Vissman, A. T., Young, A. M., Wilkin, A. M., & Rhodes, S. D. (2013). Correlates of HAART adherence among immigrant Latinos in the southeastern United States. *Aids Care, 25*(3), 356–363.

Walker, D. (2023). In 1916, the U.S. began forcing Mexicans crossing the southern border to take kerosene baths. That tactic was later studied by the Nazis. *Business Insider.* https://www.msn.com/en-us/news/world/in-1916-the-us-began-forcing-mexicans-crossing-the-southern-border-to-take-kerosene-baths-that-tactic-was-later-studied-by-the-nazis/ar-AA1jETQT

Wallerstein, N. (1993). Empowerment and health: The theory and practice of community change. *Community Development Journal, 28*(3), 218–227.

Wallerstein, N., Oetzel, J., Duran, B., Tafoya, C., Belone, L., & Rae, R. (2008). What predicts outcomes in CBPR. *Community Based Participatory Research for Health: From Process to Outcomes, 2*, 371–392.

Walters, K. L., & Simoni, J. M. (2002). Reconceptualizing Native women's health: An "indigenist" stress-coping model. *American Journal of Public Health, 92*(4), 520–524.

Weber, L., & Parra-Medina, D. (2003). Intersectionality and women's health: Charting a path to eliminating health disparities. In M. T. Segal & V. Demos (Eds.), *Gender perspectives on health and medicine* (Vol. 7, pp. 181–230). Emerald Group Publishing.

Weber, L., Zambrana, R. E., Fore, M. E., & Parra-Medina, D. (2018). Racial and ethnic health inequities: An intersectional approach. In P. Batur & J. R. Feagin (Eds.), *Handbook of the sociology of racial and ethnic relations* (pp. 133–160). Springer.

Wilkinson-Lee, A. M., Armenta, A. M., Leybas Nuño, V., Moore-Monroy, M., Hopkins, A., & Garcia, F. A. (2018). Engaging promotora-led community-based participatory research: An introduction to a crossover design focusing on reproductive and mental health needs of a Latina community. *Journal of Latina/o Psychology, 6*(4), 291.

Williams, J. E., Kabukuru, A., Mayo, R., & Griffin, S. F. (2011). Commentary: A social-ecological perspective on obesity among Latinos. *Ethnicity and Disease, 21*(4), 467.

Wilson, A. R., Mulvahill, M. J., & Tiwari, T. (2017). The impact of maternal self-efficacy and oral health beliefs on early childhood caries in Latino children. *Frontiers in Public Health, 5*, 228.

Zambrana, R. E., & Dill, B. T. (2006). Disparities in Latina health: An intersectional analysis. In A. Schultz & L. Mullings (Eds.), *Race, class, gender and health* (pp. 192–227). Jossey-Bass.

Zambrana, R. E., Parra-Medina, D., & Butler, C. (2021). Social determinants of health: Intersectional impacts of race, class, ethnicity and place. In S. C. Scrimshaw, S. D. Lane, et al. (Eds.), *The SAGE handbook of social studies in health and medicine* (p. 38). SAGE.

Figure Credits

Fig. 9.1: Alexandra Minna Stern, "Border Quarantine Certification Card," *The Hispanic American Historical Review*, vol. 79, no. 1, p. 47. Copyright © 1999 by Duke University Press.

Fig. 9.2: Leonard Nadel, "Contract Mexican Laborers Being Fumigated with the Pesticide DDT in Hidalgo, Texas, in 1956," https://commons.wikimedia.org/wiki/File:Contract_Mexican_laborers_being_fumigated_with_the_pesticide_DDT_in_Hidalgo,_Texas,_in_1956.jpg, 1956.

Fig. 9.4: Francesca Pennucci, "A Framework for Improving the Design and Implementation of Health Promotion Interventions," https://www.researchgate.net/figure/Framework-for-improving-the-design-and-implementation-of-health-promotion-and_fig1_334492990. Copyright © 2019 by Cambridge University Press.

Fig. 9.5: Copyright © by Laurenhan (CC by 3.0) at https://commons.wikimedia.org/wiki/File:The_Health_Belief_Model.pdf.

Fig. 9.6: Aleksandra Luszczynska and Ralf Schwarzer, "Social Cognitive Learning Theory," https://www.researchgate.net/publication/284667057_Social_Cognitive_Theory, p. 226. Copyright © 2015 by McGraw-Hill Education.

Fig. 9.8: Icek Ajzen and Martin Fishbein, "The Theory of Reasoned Action and Planned Behavior - The Integrative Behavioral Model," https://www.simplypsychology.org/theory-of-reasoned-action.html. Copyright © 1975 by Simply Psychology.

Fig. 9.11: Joel Williams, Rachel Mayo, Annah Kabukuru, and Sarah Griffin, "Social Ecological Model Examining the Social Environmental and Cultural Influences on Childhood Obesity," https://www.researchgate.net/publication/221721064_Commentary_A_social-ecological_perspective_on_obesity_among_Latinos, p. 469. Copyright © 2011 by Taylor & Francis Group.

Fig. 9.13: Nina Wallerstein, John Oetzel, Bonnie Duran, and Gregory B. Tafoya, "Community-Based Participatory Research," https://www.researchgate.net/publication/285496812_What_predicts_outcomes_in_CBPR, pp. 381. Copyright © 2008 by American Public Health Association.

Fig. 9.14: Karina L. Walters and Jane M. Simoni, "Indigenist Coping Model," https://www.ncbi.nlm.nih.gov/pmc/articles/PMC1447108/. Copyright © 2002 by American Public Health Association.

Fig. 9.15: Nathaniel Vincent Mohatt, Azure B. Thompson, Nghi D. Thai and Jacob Kraemer Tebes, "Historical and Intergenerational Trauma and Health Outcomes," https://www.ncbi.nlm.nih.gov/pmc/articles/PMC4001826/. Copyright © 2014 by Elsevier B.V.

Index

D

M

www.ingramcontent.com/pod-product-compliance
Ingram Content Group UK Ltd.
Pitfield, Milton Keynes, MK11 3LW, UK
UKHW050141280726
14058UKWH00006B/775